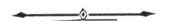

ISBN 978-0-484-37327-2
PIBN 10042029

62

OXFORD

LOOSE-LEAF

SURGERY

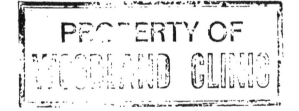

OXFORD

LOOSE-LEAF

SURGERY

BY VARIOUS AUTHORS

EDITED BY

F. F. BURGHARD, AND ALLEN B. KANAVEL

M S. (LOND), F R.C.S (ENG).
COLONEL, A.M S

LECTURER ON SURGERY AND SURGEON TO
KING'S COLLEGE HOSPITAL CONSULTING SUR-
GEON TO THE CHILDREN'S HOSPITAL PADDING-
TON GREEN. LONDON. ENG.

A.B., M D., F.A.C.S., LIEUT.
COL. U.S.A.

ASSOCIATE PROFESSOR OF SURGERY NORTHWEST-
ERN UNIVERSITY MEDICAL SCHOOL ATTENDING
SURGEON WESLEY AND COOK COUNTY HOSPI-
TALS CHICAGO ILL

IN FIVE VOLUMES

OVER 1800 ILLUSTRATIONS

VOL. II

NEW YORK

OXFORD UNIVERSITY PRESS

AMERICAN BRANCH . 35 WEST 32ND STREET
LONDON, TORONTO, MELBOURNE, AND BOMBAY

1919

PREFACE

SURGERY is no longer "a mere mechanic art." Out of the old surgery which placed so great a stress upon technique a new surgery is being evolved, a new conception is being formed, the application of which belongs to no passing event, the future of which no one can prophesy.

Functional surgery, if one may use the term, belongs to all the future. Take, for example, abdominal diagnosis, where the mechanism of pain is a question of vast complexity, and the evaluation so essential to diagnosis. Again, the latter-day investigation of anæsthesia opens a new field and warns the surgeon that every function of the nervous system must be given detailed consideration. The study of antiseptics has linked Ehrlich's conception of chemical action with the daily technique of the operating room and extended the domain of bacteriology in the scientific treatment of wounds. It is such advances as these that we have attempted to incorporate with the portrayal of the technique of various surgical clinics. The foundation was found in Burghard's Surgery, whose various contributors in collaboration with the editors have added proved procedures from American clinics and revised the various chapters in the light of the developments in surgical practice produced by experience in war.

The loose-leaf form of the Oxford Surgery will permit the editors to present the future changes in British surgery and incorporate the best thought of the leading American clinics.

The originality and individuality obtained in these volumes will be sought rather than a colourless enumeration of operative procedures. Categorical enumeration of operations of historical interest only and procedures not demonstrated by actual experience to be of value will be avoided.

The editors wish to express to the various contributors and to those whose contributions are being prepared for future insertions the appreciation of the surgeons of America and Great Britain for their unstinted and unselfish labour during a time when they are so occupied by duties necessitated by the exigencies of war.

F. F. BURGHARD.
ALLEN B. KANAVEL.

CONTRIBUTORS TO THIS VOLUME

F. F. BURGHARD, M.S. (Lond.), F.R.C.S. (Eng.), Colonel A.M.S.

Lecturer on Surgery and Surgeon to King's College Hospital.

Operations for Non-tuberculous Affections of Joints

SIR HAROLD J. STILES, M.B., F.R.C.S. (Edin.), Lieutenant-Colonel R.A.M.C.(T.)

Surgeon to Chalmers Hospital, Edinburgh, and to the Royal Hospital for Sick Children, Edinburgh.

Operations for Tuberculous Affections of the Bones and Joints

EDMUND OWEN, F.R.C.S. (Eng.), D.Sc. (Hon.)

Late Consulting Surgeon to St. Mary's Hospital and to the Hospital for Sick Children, London.

Operations for Hare-lip and Cleft-palate

G. LENTHAL CHEATLE, C.V.O., C.B., F.R.C.S. (Eng.), Surgeon General R.N.

Surgeon to King's College Hospital and to the Italian Hospital.

Operations for Cancer of the Lips and Face

C. H. FAGGE, M.S. (Lond.), F.R.C.S. (Eng.), Major R.A.M.C.(T.)

Assistant Surgeon to Guy's Hospital.

Operations upon the Jaws

VILRAY P. BLAIR, A.M., M.D., F.A.C.S., Major M.R.C.

Professor of Oral Surgery, Washington University Dental School, St. Louis, Mo.

Deformities of the Lower Jaw

T. P. LEGG, M.S. (Lond.), F.R.C.S. (Eng.), Lieutenant-Colonel R.A.M.C.(T.)

Surgeon to the Royal Free Hospital; Assistant Surgeon to King's College Hospital.

Plastic Surgery

J. M. H. MacLEOD, M.A., M.D., F.R.C.P. (Lond.)
Physician for Diseases of the Skin, Victoria Hospital for Children.

Burns and Scalds

H. D. GILLIES, F.R.C.S., L.R.C.P., Major R.A.M.C.(T.)
Surgeon to the Queen's Hospital for Sailors and Soldiers suffering from Facial Injuries. Surgeon to Throat and Ear Department, Prince of Wales Hospital, W.

Principles of Plastic Surgery

H. J. WARING, M.S. (Lond.), F.R.C.S. (Eng.), Brev. Col. R.A.M.C.
Surgeon to and Joint-Lecturer on Surgery, St. Bartholomew's Hospital.

Operations upon the Tongue

GEORGE E. WAUGH, F.R.C.S. (Eng.)
Surgeon to the Hospital for Sick Children, Great Ormond St.

Operations upon the Tonsils

WILFRED TROTTER, M.S. (Lond.), F.R.C.S. (Eng.), Captain R.A.M.C.(T.)
Assistant Surgeon to University College Hospital.

Operations upon the Pharynx

SIR BERKELEY MOYNIHAN, M.S. (Lond.), F.R.C.S. (Eng.), Lieutenant-Colonel R.A.M.C.(T.)
Surgeon to the Leeds General Infirmary.

Operations upon the Stomach

PROFESSOR RUTHERFORD MORISON, F.R.C.S., Staff Surgeon R.N.V.R.
Consulting Senior Surgeon, Northumberland War Hospital.

Surgery of the Stomach

DAVID LIGAT, M.D., F.R.C.S. (Eng.)
Late House Surgeon, Middlesex Hospital.

Hyperalgesia as an aid to Diagnosis in Abdominal Disease

SIR G. H. MAKINS, K.C.G.M., C.B., F.R.C.S. (Eng.)
Surgeon to St. Thomas's Hospital and President of the Board of Examiners for the Naval Medical Service.

Operations upon the Intestines

CONTENTS

SECTION I

OPERATIONS FOR NON-TUBERCULOUS AFFECTIONS OF JOINTS

By FRED^C. F. BURGHARD, M.S. (Lond.), F.R.C.S. (Eng.), Colonel A.M.S.

Lecturer on Surgery and Surgeon to King's College Hospital; Consulting Surgeon to the Children's Hospital, Paddington Green

CHAPTER I

GENERAL CONSIDERATIONS

CHAPTER II

OPERATIONS UPON THE WRIST-JOINT

CHAPTER III

OPERATIONS UPON THE ELBOW-JOINT

CHAPTER IV

OPERATIONS UPON THE SHOULDER-JOINT

SECTION II

OPERATIONS FOR TUBERCULOUS AFFECTIONS OF THE BONES AND JOINTS

PART I

OPERATIONS FOR TUBERCULOUS AFFECTIONS OF THE BONES

By SIR HAROLD J. STILES, M.B., F.R.C.S. (Edin.), Lieutenant-Colonel
R.A.M.C.(T.)

Surgeon to Chalmers Hospital, Edinburgh, and to the Royal Hospital for Sick Children, Edinburgh

CHAPTER I

OPERATIONS FOR TUBERCULOUS OSTEOMYELITIS
OF THE DIAPHYSES OF THE LONG BONES

CHAPTER II

OPERATIONS FOR TUBERCULOUS OSTEOMYELITIS
OF THE SHORT LONG-BONES

CHAPTER III

OPERATIONS FOR TUBERCULOUS OSTEOMYELITIS
OF THE BONES OF THE VAULT OF THE SKULL

CONTENTS

PART II

OPERATIONS FOR TUBERCULOUS AFFECTIONS OF THE JOINTS

By SIR HAROLD J. STILES, M.B., F.R.C.S. (Edin.), Lieutenant-Colonel R.A.M.C.(T.)

Surgeon to Chalmers Hospital, Edinburgh, and to the Royal Hospital for Sick Children, Edinburgh

SECTION III

OPERATIONS UPON THE LIPS, FACE, AND JAWS

PART I

OPERATIONS FOR HARE-LIP AND CLEFT-PALATE

By EDMUND OWEN, F.R.C.S. (Eng.), D.Sc. (Hon.)

Late Cons. Surgeon to St. Mary's Hospital and to the Hospital for Sick Children, London

CHAPTER I

OPERATIONS FOR HARE-LIP

CHAPTER II

OPERATIONS FOR CLEFT-PALATE

PART II

OPERATIONS FOR CANCER OF THE LIPS AND FACE

By G. LENTHAL CHEATLE, C.V.O., C.B., F.R.C.S. (Eng.), Surgeon-General R.N.

Surgeon to King's College Hospital and to the Italian Hospital

CHAPTER III

OPERATIONS FOR CANCER OF THE LIPS AND FACE

PART III

OPERATIONS UPON THE JAWS

By C. H. FAGGE, M.S. (Lond.), F.R.C.S. (Eng.), Major R.A.M.C.(T.) Assistant Surgeon to Guy's Hospital

CHAPTER IV

OPERATIONS UPON THE UPPER JAW

CHAPTER V

OPERATIONS UPON THE LOWER JAW AND THE TEMPORO-MAXILLARY JOINT

CHAPTER VI

CORRECTION OF DEVELOPMENTAL OR ACQUIRED DEFORMITIES OF THE LOWER JAW

By VILRAY P. BLAIR, A.M., M.D., F.A.C.S., Major M.R.C.

Professor of Oral Surgery, Washington University Dental School, St. Louis, Mo.

SECTION IV

PLASTIC SURGERY

By T. P. LEGG, M.S. (Lond.), F.R.C.S. (Eng.), Lieutenant-Colonel R.A.M.C.(T.)

Surgeon to the Royal Free Hospital; Assistant Surgeon, King's College Hospital

CHAPTER I

GENERAL PRINCIPLES: SKIN-GRAFTING

CHAPTER VI

PRINCIPLES OF PLASTIC SURGERY

By H. D. GILLIES, F.R.C.S., L.R.C.P., Major R.A.M.C.(T.)

Surgeon to the Queen's Hospital for Sailors and Soldiers suffering from Facial Injuries; Surgeon to Throat and Ear Department, Prince of Wales Hospital, N.

SECTION V

OPERATIONS UPON THE TONGUE, TONSILS, PHARYNX, AND ŒSOPHAGUS

PART I

OPERATIONS UPON THE TONGUE

By H. J. WARING, M.S. (Lond.), F.R.C.S. (Eng.), Brev. Colonel R.A.M.C.

Surgeon to and Joint-Lecturer in Surgery, St. Bartholomew's Hospital

CHAPTER I

OPERATIONS FOR NON-MALIGNANT AFFECTIONS OF THE TONGUE

CHAPTER II

OPERATIONS FOR MALIGNANT DISEASE OF THE TONGUE AND FLOOR OF THE MOUTH

CHAPTER III

OPERATIONS UPON THE TONSIL

By GEORGE E. WAUGH, M.D., F.R.C.S. (Eng.)

Surgeon to the Hospital for Sick Children, Great Ormond Street

CHAPTER IV

OPERATIONS FOR PHARYNGEAL ABSCESS

CHAPTER V

OPERATIONS FOR MALIGNANT DISEASE OF THE ORAL AND LARYNGEAL PARTS OF THE PHARYNX

By WILFRED TROTTER, M.S. (Lond.), F.R.C.S. (Eng.), Captain
R.A.M.C.(T.)

Assistant Surgeon, University College Hospital

PART II

OPERATIONS UPON THE ŒSOPHAGUS

By C. H. FAGGE, M.S. (Lond.), F.R.C.S. (Eng.), Major R.A.M.C.(T.)

Assistant Surgeon to Guy's Hospital

CHAPTER VI

OPERATIONS UPON THE ŒSOPHAGUS

SECTION VI

OPERATIONS UPON THE STOMACH AND INTESTINES

PART I

OPERATIONS UPON THE STOMACH

By SIR BERKELEY MOYNIHAN, M.S. (Lond.), F.R.C.S. (Eng.), Lieutenant-Colonel R.A.M.C.(T.)

Surgeon to the Leeds General Infirmary

CHAPTER I

PREPARATION AND AFTER TREATMENT OF PATIENTS OPERATED UPON FOR DISEASES OF THE STOMACH

CHAPTER II

GASTROTOMY: GASTROSTOMY: PARTIAL GASTRECTOMY

CONTENTS

PART II

OPERATIONS UPON THE INTESTINES

By SIR G. H. MAKINS, K.C.G.M., C.B., F.R.C.S. (Eng.)

Surgeon to St. Thomas's Hospital, and President of the Board of Examiners for the Naval Medical Service

LIST OF ILLUSTRATIONS

SECTION I

OPERATIONS FOR NON-TUBERCULOUS AFFECTIONS OF JOINTS

BY

FRED^C. F. BURGHARD, M.S. (Lond.), F.R.C.S. (Eng.),
Colonel A.M.C.

Lecturer on Surgery and Surgeon to King's College Hospital ; Consulting
Surgeon to the Children's Hospital, Paddington Green

CHAPTER I

GENERAL CONSIDERATIONS

IT will be best to discuss briefly the general considerations applying to each type of operation practised upon joints, reserving for special description in subsequent pages special points in these operations upon individual joints.

ARTHROTOMY

Arthrotomy, or simple incision of a joint, is useful in many affections and is much more frequently resorted to at the present day than at any previous period in the history of surgery. Formerly, to incise a joint of any size was to imperil its movements and possibly to entail amputation of the limb or loss of life. Owing to the complexity of most of the joint surfaces and the number of recesses in connexion with them they are difficult to drain and, should sepsis occur, the results are likely to be more serious than they would be in a wound that can be drained freely.

Indications. (i) Arthrotomy is often required for simple *exploration* of the joint in order to determine the nature of the lesion and to settle the appropriate treatment.

(ii) In *suppurative arthritis* a free incision must be made into the joint in order to establish effective drainage.

(iii) Arthrotomy is called for in cases of *acute non-purulent effusion* of rheumatic, gonorrhœal, or traumatic origin in which the effusion refuses to respond to other measures and threatens to weaken the joint permanently by overstretching its ligaments. It is especially indicated in those cases in which there is any doubt as to the exact nature of the case, as the possibility of some internal derangement must always be borne in mind.

(iv) For the extraction of a *movable body* in the joint, or in the rarer cases of a foreign body.

(v) At the present day arthrotomy is probably most frequently practised as a preliminary to the removal of a *displaced semilunar cartilage*. It is also a preliminary to the operations for various other internal derangements of the joint.

Operation. In all cases the most scrupulous care must be taken

3

to disinfect not only everything that comes into contact with the wound but also a wide area of the patient's skin. In nearly all these cases the surgeon desires to have the joint moved in some particular direction during the course of the operation so that he may obtain better inspection of or better access to certain parts of the joint. For this purpose the assistant has to bend the joint, and it is quite common to see him grasp the limb by some portion that has escaped purification prior to the operation; this mistake, of course, may lead to very serious consequences. The limb on both sides of the joint should be securely wrapped up in sterilized cloths bandaged firmly on so that they cannot get displaced.

The position of the limb and the surgeon and the site and length of the incision will be determined partly by the individual joint and partly by the particular object of the operation; this is dealt with more fully in connexion with the individual joints. In all cases it is important to arrest all hæmorrhage before the joint is opened, and it is well to distinguish between the capsule of the joint and the synovial membrane and open each by a separate incision. In the earlier stages of the operation, before the joint has been incised, the use of chemical antiseptics is admissible, if the surgeon be in the habit of employing them. When, however, the synovial cavity has been opened, all chemical antiseptics should be abandoned, as their use is likely to irritate the synovial membrane; sterilized salt solution at a temperature of 100° F. should be substituted.

All manipulations of the joint cavity should be of the gentlest description consistent with the object in view. The edges of the synovial membrane may be caught in fine-toothed catch forceps and held apart by an assistant. If retractors be used they should be blunt hooks, and no force should be employed. All manipulations inside the joint should be done with forceps if possible, and the finger should only be introduced if it be absolutely necessary; in this way unnecessary bruising is avoided. All traction should be as light as possible and any incisions should be cleanly made with instruments as fine as is consistent with the effective performance of their duties.

When the object of the operation has been attained, great care must be taken to see that bleeding from the joint cavity has ceased entirely before the synovial membrane is sutured. Hæmorrhage generally ceases readily, except when an artery has been wounded, and this should be picked up and tied. Exposure to the air or douching with saline solution at a temperature of 115° F. usually suffices to stop oozing quickly; it is inadvisable to employ drainage if it can be avoided. The articular cavity should be closed in two separate layers if possible, one suture of the finest catgut taking up the cut edges of the synovial membrane, the other, rather stouter, approximating the incision in the capsule; the skin wound is sewn up separately. When possible a flap should be raised over the proposed incision in the capsule, so that when the wound is sutured the cicatrices in the various structures do not correspond.

ARTHROPLASTY

From the early days of surgery it has always been an important object to obtain mobility in ankylosed limbs. Many plans have been adopted and much time and trouble have been expended, but it must be confessed that the results have hitherto been disappointing. Within recent years, however, the work of Murphy has opened up wider possi-bilities in this direction. Briefly stated, his method may be said to imitate by art what occurs in nature when an ununited fracture results from the interposition of soft structures between the fractured ends.

The operative technic for arthroplasty on the knee, hip, elbow, and shoulder joints as originated by John B. Murphy and modified in some of the details by Kreuscher, deals entirely with attached pedicled flaps of fat and fascia. In every instance the part to be operated upon is most carefully prepared by shaving and cleansing the skin thoroughly the day preceding the operation. Immediately before the operation is begun and after the patient has been placed in the proper position on the operating table, the skin is again cleansed with alcohol and ether, fol-lowed by a coating of gutta-percha solution, which is a 1% solution of gutta-percha in acetone. Throughout the entire operation the strictest asepsis and the non-hand-contacting technic is used. No portion of the instrument which has touched the gloved hand is introduced into the wound. The ligatures and sutures are all tied with forceps.

Operation. The actual details of the operation will vary with the individual joint for which the operation is done, but generally speaking the steps of the operation are as follows:—The joint is fully exposed by whatever incision may be most suitable. The union between the bones is divided by knife, saw, or chisel according to the nature of the uniting medium. The articular surfaces are then shaped in any way that the surgeon may think will best facilitate movement, the most essential point being that the surfaces are chiselled or scraped until they are perfectly smooth. The next step is to see that there are no contracted structures that will interfere with the desired movements of the joint, and with this object attempts are made to carry the limb through the full range of the movements desired. This is done by the assistant whilst the surgeon examines for the presence of tight bands or ligamentous structures and divides them freely. If the obstacles to move-ment be contracted muscles, their tendons should be lengthened instead of being divided.

The contraction preceding the ankylosis may have been so great that vessels or nerves may be endangered by the straightening process. Here it will be a consideration whether the limb should be gradually stretched by extension and the arthroplasty finished at a subsequent date when the limb is straight, or whether sufficient bone should be cut away to enable the limb to be brought into the desired position without endangering these important structures. This question will be largely determined by the joint in question. For instance, the sacrifice of bone in the upper extremity is a matter of small importance as compared with the lower extremity, in which it affects locomotion considerably.

The most important part of the operation is the means adopted for maintaining the movement thus obtained, and the work of Murphy holds out considerable promise in this direction. A thick layer of the neighbouring soft structures is detached in the form of a flap correspond-ing in its dimensions to the cross-section of the joint, and is laid in between the bone ends and fastened in position by sutures. The origin of this flap is not a matter of great importance, but it should contain plenty of fat and areolar tissue. This substance seems to be most suited for promoting movement, as it develops bursæ readily, and in practice it has been found to answer the purpose better than anything else. The incision in the capsule is closed without a drainage tube.

After-treatment. Passive movement is begun as soon as possible. When the ligamentous connexions between the articular ends have not been divided too freely it may be practised from the third or fourth day; when the contrary is the case a week or ten days should be allowed to elaspse. At first passive movement will have to be done under gas, but it must be persisted in regularly and the range of movement should be steadily increased; this should be accompanied by massage. The object is to develop a fairly thick layer of connective tissue between the two joint ends, and the formation of a bursa in this to act as a synovial cavity. Very promising results have been obtained by persever-ing attempts in this direction.

ARTHRODESIS

This operation is the converse of the one just described and has for its object the replacement of an unduly movable joint by a stiff one.

Indications. The aim of this operation is to produce ankylosis in a paralysed and flail-like joint, and so to allow movements to be carried out in a limb which were previously impossible. The operation is applicable in both extremities, and is called for in bad cases of infantile paralysis in which it is impossible to restore movement by tendon-grafting or muscle-transplantation. Thus it may be very useful to stiffen a flail knee-joint, as the patient will then be able to walk, provided that there be enough power left in the muscles moving the ankle to allow the weight to be borne upon that joint without its giving way. Similarly, by fixing a flail shoulder-joint the upper extremity may be moved by the scapular muscles, or by fixing a flail elbow the hand may be rendered much more useful.

Operation. The operation has for its object removal of the articular cartilage so as to leave large areas of raw bone, which are then brought into apposition and kept immovable until bony union has taken place between them. Removal of the cartilage is best effected with a chisel, and the operation should be done with the least possible damage to the soft parts, so as not to weaken the limb more than is necessary. The steps of the operation for the exposure of the articular surfaces must of course vary with the joint operated upon.

Results. The limb is kept rigid until firm bony union has occurred. Unfortunately, however, although this would probably follow in healthy subjects, it may not occur in these cases, possibly owing to defective nutrition of the parts. However, union may occur later on if the limb be kept in some light casing. Even when the operation fails to secure firm bony union the patient's condition is often considerably improved. Fibrous union takes the place of the useless flail-like limb, and at the worst some light splint has to be employed in the place of the cumbersome and heavy metal apparatus that would otherwise have to be worn.

ARTHRECTOMY

The term arthrectomy strictly implies the removal of the joint surfaces. As the term is generally applied at the present day to removal of tuberculous disease from a joint it is therefore somewhat of a misnomer. Strictly speaking, operations such as excision and arthrodesis are also arthrectomies. The term is a bad one and should be banished from surgical terminology; its true significance being the extirpation of tuberculous disease from a joint it does not fall into the scope of this article and will be dealt with by Mr. Stiles.

EXCISION

By excision of a joint is understood the removal of the articular surfaces.

Indications. In non-tuberculous cases this operation is done chiefly for extensive injury to the bones entering into the formation of a joint. It may also be required for a dislocation which is not reducible by other methods, or to rectify ankylosis by producing a movable joint or by removing the deformity. The primary object of the operation in non-tuberculous cases is to remove the articular ends of the bone in order to produce either mobility or stability, or, in cases of extensive injury, to preserve a limb which would otherwise have to be amputated. The synovial membrane is only excised in so far as it is removed along with portions of the bone. Operations of this type are done in adults for tuberculous disease of the joints; they will be dealt with by Mr. Stiles.

As these operations vary entirely according to the joint affected, no general rules apply to them, and each individual joint will be treated separately in the following chapters.

CHAPTER II

OPERATIONS UPON THE WRIST-JOINT

THE only operation of importance in connexion with the wrist-joint is excision. The joint may be opened in an operation for a badly united Colles's fracture, but in that case the operation is not primarily one upon the joint itself.

EXCISION OF THE WRIST

Indications. Complete excision of the wrist will scarcely ever be required for any condition save tuberculous disease—a condition that does not come into the scope of this article. Partial excisions are, however, not infrequently practised for fractures of various carpal bones, the knowledge of which is becoming increased by the use of radiography. When these fractures are compound, the bones, or portions of them, may be extracted by enlarging the existing wound; otherwise one or both of the incisions recommended by Lord Lister (*vide infra*) may be used.

Operation. Several methods of excising the wrist have been introduced; of these only ·Lord Lister's will be described here, as it is an excellent dissecting-room exercise, and may also be used for a partial excision in cases of injury. It is described as follows by the late Mr. Timothy Holmes (see Holmes's *System of Surgery,* vol. iii, p. 748) :—

' An incision is made commencing in front over the second metacarpal bone internal to the tendon of the extensor secundi internodii pollicis, and running ₌long the back of the carpus, internal to the same tendon, as high as to the base of the styloid process of the radius. The soft parts, including the extensor secundi internodii and the radial artery, being cautiously detached from the bones external to this incision, and the tendons of the radial extensors of the wrist being also severed from their attachments, the external bones of the carpus will be exposed. When this has been done sufficiently, the next step is to sever the trapezium from the other bones with cutting-pliers, in order to facilitate the removal of the latter, which should be done as freely as is found convenient. The operator now turns to the ulnar side of the incision and cleans the carpal and metacarpal bones as much as can be done easily. The ulnar incision is now made (see Fig. 1). It should be very free, extending from about 2 inches above the styloid process down to the middle of the fifth metacarpal bone, and lying near the anterior edge of the ulna. The dorsal line of this incision is then raised along with the tendon of the extensor carpi ulnaris, which should not be isolated from the skin, and should be cut as near its insertion as possible. Then the common

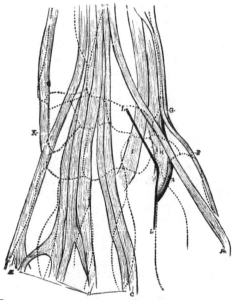

FIG. 1. STRUCTURES CONCERNED IN LISTER'S EXCISION OF THE WRIST (Holmes's *System of Surgery*). A, The radial artery; B, Tendon of the extensor secundi internodii pollicis; C, Metacarpal of index finger; Tendons of—D, Extensor communis digitorum; E, Extensor minimi digiti; F, Extensor primi internodii pollicis; G, Extensor ossis metacarpi pollicis; H, I, Extensor carpi radialis longior and brevior; K, Extensor carpi ulnaris; L L, Line of radial incision.

extensor tendons should be raised, and the whole of the posterior aspect of the carpus denuded, until the two wounds communicate quite freely together; but the radius is not as yet cleaned. The next step is to clean the anterior aspect of the ulna and carpus, in doing which the pisiform bone and the hooked process of the unciform are severed from the rest of the carpus, the former with the knife, the latter with the cutting-pliers. In cleaning the anterior aspect of the carpus, care must be taken not to go so far forward as to endanger the deep palmar arch.

Now, the ligaments of the internal carpal bones being sufficiently divided, those bones are to be removed with blunt bone-forceps. Next the end of the ulna is made to protrude from the incision, and is sawn off, as low down as is consistent with its condition, but in any case above its radial articulation. The end of the radius is then cleaned sufficiently to allow of its being protruded and removed. If this can be done without disturbing the tendons from their grooves, it is far better. If the level of the section is below the upper part of the cartilaginous facet for the ulna, the remainder of the cartilage must be cut away with the pliers. The operator next attends to the metacarpal bones, which are pushed out from one or the other incision and cut off with the pliers so as to

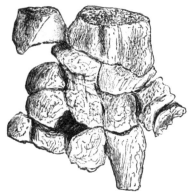

FIG. 2. THE PARTS REMOVED IN EXCISION OF THE WRIST BY LORD LISTER'S METHOD (Holmes's *System of Surgery*).

remove the whole of their cartilage-covered portions. The trapezium bone, which was left in the early stage of the operation, is now carefully dissected out, so as to avoid any injury to the tendon of the flexor carpi radialis or to the radial artery, and the articular surface of the first metacarpal bone is then exposed and removed. Lastly, the cartilaginous portion of the pisiform bone is taken away; but the non-articular part is left behind, unless it is diseased, in which case it should be removed entire. The same remark applies to the hooked process of the unciform.

' The operation is one of the most tedious and difficult in surgery, but it appears to me to give very satisfactory results, and therefore should, I think, always be adopted in such cases as are favourable for any operation at all. It is advisable, if not necessary, to put on Esmarch's bandage; so that the view of the parts should not be obstructed by blood. It is also very desirable to break down any adhesions which the tendons may have formed while the patient is under anæsthesia previous to the operation.

'No tendons are necessarily divided in this operation except the extensors of the wrist, for the flexor carpi radialis is inserted lower down than the point at which the metacarpal bone is usually divided.

'In order to ensure motion, particularly in the fingers, passive movements should be performed from a very early period after the operation. For this purpose, Mr. Lister places the limb on a splint with the palm of the hand raised by a large wedge of cork, fixed below it; so that the joints of the fingers can be moved without taking the limb off the apparatus. Special arrangements are made for keeping the splint steady, and for preventing displacement of the hand to either side. Careful and methodical passive motion should be used to each several joint—to those of the finger and thumb almost from the day of the operation, and to the wrist as soon as the parts have acquired some firmness, each movement, pronation and supination, flexion and extension, abduction and adduction, being separately exercised; and the patient should be encouraged to make attempts at voluntary motion as early as possible. In order to exercise the fingers, the portion of the splint which supports them may be removed, while that on which the wrist is received is still left. Finally, when the rigid splint is left off, some flexible support is still to be worn for a long time.'

Lord Lister was always careful to provide against stiffness of the thumb in the adducted position by having a notch or deep groove cut in the lateral aspect of the splint, so that the thumb could hang down well away from the other fingers. The functional results after the operation are very fair, but a moulded wristlet must be worn for several months in order to counteract the tendency to displacement of the hand to the radial side.

CHAPTER III

OPERATIONS UPON THE ELBOW-JOINT

ARTHROTOMY AND DRAINAGE

Indications. (i) The elbow-joint is not infrequently the seat of *acute suppurative arthritis,* which is often of traumatic origin and follows septic wounds about the point of the elbow, leading to suppuration in the olecranon bursa and subsequent infection of the joint. It is also occasionally attacked in the course of pyæmia, but is rarely affected in acute infective osteomyelitis.

(ii) In *compound fractures of the olecranon* acute suppuration often occurs, owing to the direct nature of the injury and the certainty of infection of the joint, and will necessitate arthrotomy and drainage.

Operation. As a rule the joint can be drained effectually through vertical incisions in the posterior part of the capsule on either side of the olecranon. That on the inner side must carefully avoid the ulnar nerve; that on the outer side should be just behind the external intermuscular septum and extend downwards far enough to open the radiohumeral joint. As a rule this will give sufficient drainage, but if necessary the soft parts may be raised from the front of the internal condyle and the capsule exposed and the joint opened from the front also.

The limb should be put up on a light sterilizable metal splint with the elbow at right angles, and it will be well to practise continuous irrigation of the joint with normal saline solution circulating through the drainage tubes. Should this be impracticable the joint should be immersed in a large arm-bath containing normal saline solution or boric lotion frequently renewed.

If this fail to drain the joint satisfactorily, a vertical incision should be made down to the bone as for excision (see p. 17). The triceps tendon is split centrally as in that operation, and the olecranon process is chiselled across at its base and removed, the wound being left open widely, so as to secure efficient drainage. The limb is placed in an elbow-bath.

OPERATIONS FOR INTRA-ARTICULAR FRACTURES

Operations for fractures involving the articular surfaces of the lower end of the humerus almost invariably require operative interference if the functional result is to be satisfactory. Owing to the complicated nature of the articular surfaces the least irregularity will give rise to limitation of movement.

Operation. The exact incision will be determined mainly by the nature and extent of the fracture, which in its turn can only be satisfactorily ascertained beforehand by means of stereoscopic radiograms. The best method of access will generally be by vertical incisions along the supra-condylar ridges reaching well down the condyles, so as to expose the lateral aspects of the lower end of the humerus. In the majority of cases it will probably be necessary to make an incision on each side. The soft parts are carefully peeled off the capsule front and back, so that the joint can be opened, the fracture examined, and the fractured surfaces got accurately into apposition and held there whilst the lower end of the bone is drilled from side to side by a long fine electrically-driven drill; fixation pins are then made to transfix the fragments from side to side. The exposure of the lower end of the humerus may have to be very free, especially in the case of a T-shaped fracture into the joint. In all these cases the soft parts should be peeled off the capsule first and the latter then incised freely; at the end of the operation the incisions in the capsule are sutured. In fractures involving the articular ends of the bone it is almost always necessary to pass the fixation pins from side to side, as nothing can be applied to the articular surfaces for fear of causing a projection upon them that would interfere with movement. When there is a T-shaped fracture, however, it will be necessary to fix the reconstructed articular end to the shaft after pinning the condyles together in this fashion, and this may be done by the application of plates, wires, tacks, or any other fixation method that the surgeon may deem most advisable. After fixation has been accomplished, the joint is kept steady in the position in which it is to be put up, which will generally be at right angles, and the wound is then sutured and a splint applied that takes a firm grip of the limb, but is hinged at the elbow to allow of flexion and extension. A metal excision splint is a useful form, as it allows flexion and extension of the elbow and pronation and supination of the forearm to be practised.

After-treatment. The chief difficulty in the after-treatment is to promote union between the fragments whilst avoiding stiffness in the joint; with this end in view the most careful attention must be paid to the after-treatment. Pronation and supination should be practised from the first, but the limb should remain undisturbed on the splint for about ten days, when the sutures may be taken out. From this time onwards careful passive movements of the elbow-joint must be practised. This should be done at first while the limb is on the splint, the region of the fracture being steadied with one hand whilst the other grasps the forearm and flexes and extends the elbow gently.   In about three weeks' time the range of movement may be increased considerably, and in a month the patient should be practising movements for himself.

OPERATIONS FOR FRACTURE OF THE OLECRANON

Indications.   Operative interference is not so essential for fractures of the olecranon as it is for those of the patella, because the results of non-operative treatment in the former cases are not entirely unsatisfactory.   All healthy persons under forty years of age who are the subject of the fracture of the olecranon accompanied by marked separation of the fragments, however, should have the fragments fixed by operation.   For those to whom the strength of the limb is important, operation is necessary.   In many cases, however, admirable mobility and even a fair amount of power follow non-operative treatment.

Operation.   In all its essential details this resembles that for fracture of the patella (see p. 66).   There are a few points, however, in which the two operations differ.

The incision should be crescentic or horseshoe-shaped, with its convexity upwards and its upper limit just above the point of the olecranon. Its lower extremities should be about half an inch below the line of fracture.   The flap thus marked out is turned down and the olecranon bursa and the fracture are exposed.   All clot is turned out and the joint is cleared of blood by irrigation with saline solution.   Apposition is quite easy and it is unnecessary to pass the wire, or whatever uniting medium is employed, through the articular surfaces.   The bone is drilled from its posterior subcutaneous surface to the middle of the fractured surface, care being taken to see that the point at which the drill emerges on the fractured surface corresponds on the two sides.   This can be ensured by bringing the fractured surfaces into apposition when the drill is protruding through the first hole and making its point mark a depression in the opposite fractured surface.   A silver wire (No. 4 French catheter gauge) is introduced through the drill holes and twisted as for fractured patella. It brings the fragments together accurately without any part of it being within the joint cavity.

Wire is probably much the best material for fastening these fractures. It should be of the gauge recommended above, and it is well to cut a shallow groove or recess in the subcutaneous surface of the olecranon, in which the twist can be embedded so as to be quite out of the way of pressure of any kind.   If this simple precaution be taken there will be no necessity to remove it on account of irritation.   Screws and nails introduced through the upper surface of the olecranon parallel with its long axis and driven into the shaft of the ulna have been much advocated and employed. I have used them more than once and have been disappointed with them, although the result on the operating table was excellent. The softening of the bone that a foreign body like a screw sets up almost immediately weakens it as a uniting medium, and it is not uncommon to find a certain amount of separation occur in a few days' time and to see the screw pushed out from the bone.

After-treatment. The limb should be put up almost fully extended on an internal splint with a hinge at the elbow. Flexion should be increased gradually during the first fortnight, when the stitches may be taken out, and gentle massage and passive movements employed. At the end of three weeks the patient should be encouraged to move the limb freely for himself, and in a month from the operation the functions of the limb should be completely restored.

Operations for fractures of long standing. These operations are very rare indeed nowadays and do not call for any extended notice, as they follow exactly the lines for similar operations upon fractures of the patella (see p. 74). If necessary for coaptation the triceps tendon, which is fairly thick, can be lengthened (see Vol. I, p. 626).

OPERATIONS FOR DISLOCATIONS

Indications. Operation may be required for a dislocation of the elbow-joint which has passed unrecognized owing to excessive effusion in the neighbourhood of the injury, which has been deemed to be due to a fracture. Unless a radiogram be obtainable the existence of a dislocation may not be ascertained for a long time, when it may be impossible to reduce the dislocation after a careful trial under full anæsthesia. As a rule reduction may be effected safely within six weeks from the date of the injury, and it should always be attempted up to that time. After that, however, the adhesions may become so dense that the force required to break them down may fracture the humerus or stretch the ulnar nerve unduly, giving rise to paralysis; for dislocations that have lasted longer than this operation is advisable without attempting reduction first.

Occasionally it may be necessary to operate upon dislocations of recent origin. This will probably be due to the fact that the coronoid process or some other portion of the articular surface has been fractured and either causes recurrence of the dislocation or mechanically prevents reduction. These cases strictly come under the heading of operations for fractures involving articular surfaces and are dealt with in exactly the same way, the dislocation being easily reduced before the fractured surfaces are fastened together.

In cases of unreduced dislocations of long standing, the operation will often take the form of an excision, as it may be impossible to get the dislocated surfaces into proper position. Reduction of the dislocation, however, should be possible, provided that sufficient exposure of the parts is obtained and that there is no fracture of the articular surfaces complicating reduction by altering the joint surfaces.

Operation.   The best exposure of the joint is obtained by two vertical incisions, one over each condyle.   The inner one should be about five inches long, the outer slightly less, as it must not extend lower down than the head of the radius for fear of damaging the radial nerve.   By careful dissection the soft parts are raised from the front of the capsule, which is left intact, and a thin flexible spatula is passed beneath them from the inner to the outer incision so as to lift them out of the way. This gives perfect access to the front of the joint, and it may then be possible to effect reduction by traction, checking its effects by the fingers in the wound placed over the front of the joint.   If this fail, the soft parts are peeled from the capsule behind as far as the margin of the olecranon, and the joint is opened on the inner side by dividing the remains of the internal lateral ligament.   The finger can be then passed into the joint and the condition of affairs ascertained.   Any tight structures should be divided, and traction should then bring the bones into position without any risk of doing damage either to the vessels or the ulnar nerve.

After reduction the joint is closed as accurately as possible and the elbow and forearm are supported in a large sling.   Movement is practised early and vigorously.   It will probably be necessary to move the limb frequently under anæsthesia.

EXCISION OF THE ELBOW

Indications.   (i) The affection for which excision of the elbow is most frequently done is *tuberculous disease;* this is dealt with by Mr. Stiles, and the operation for it will not be described here.

(ii) *Injuries to the elbow* frequently require partial or complete excision of the joint.   These are generally fractures involving the condyles, which have united with the fragments in a faulty position or with superabundant callus.

(iii) *Unreduced dislocations* may require excision of the joint, but as a rule this will not be called for unless they are complicated by a fracture of the articular surfaces, which prevents proper reduction of the dislocation (*vide supra*).

(iv) The most common non-tuberculous affection for which excision of the elbow is required is *ankylosis*. The results of excision of the elbow, both with regard to the range of movement obtained and the power that can be exerted, are so satisfactory that a patient may always be safely advised to undergo excision with the object of substituting a movable elbow for a stiff one, provided that he has reached the age when growth in the bones has ceased. Excisions prior to this age are apt to be disappointing, owing to the large amount of bone thrown out sub-

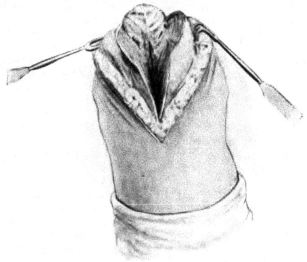

FIG. 3. REFLECTION OF THE SOFT PARTS IN EXCISION OF THE ELBOW. The triceps aponeurosis is being turned off the condyles.

sequently; this limits movement considerably, and may even reproduce the ankylosis.

(v) In *acute suppurative arthritis* the joint may have to be drained by a modified excision of the joint, namely, removal of the olecranon (see p. 13).

(vi) *A fracture of the head of the radius* may necessitate a partial excision of the joint; this will be limited to removal of the fractured portion of the bone.

(vii) *Unreduced dislocation of the radius* will necessitate a similar procedure.

Operation. Only one form of operation, that by the classical vertical incision of Langenbeck, will be described here. This is, on the whole, the most suitable method for most of the conditions enumerated above; other methods, which are more suited for tuberculous disease, will be described by Mr. Stiles.

The assistant holds the limb so that the upper arm is vertical and the elbow is flexed at an angle of 135°, while the surgeon, standing on the affected side, makes an incision four inches long with its centre over the

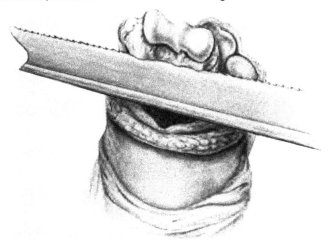

Fig. 4. Sawing the Humerus in Excision of the Elbow. The saw is applied above the level of the condyles.

tip of the olecranon in the middle line of the limb. This incision should go down to bone throughout, the lower half reaching the subcutaneous surfaces of the ulna and the olecranon, whilst the upper half opens the joint and enters the olecranon fossa of the humerus (see Fig. 3). The tendinous expansion of the triceps and anconeus is now turned off each side of the olecranon, partly with the point of a stout short-bladed knife kept closely in contact with the bone, and partly with a Farabeuf's rugine (see Fig. 271, Vol. I), which is excellent for this purpose. The beginner is apt to damage the soft parts unduly by scraping at them with the rugine to the entire exclusion of the use of the knife. The latter is a most useful instrument provided that the surgeon knows how and where to use it, and that he keeps command over it lest its point slip and cut across the expansion of the triceps, which would seriously interfere with the functional results of the operation. As the soft parts are turned off the sides of the olecranon the posterior ligament of the joint is reached and opened, and while this is being done the assistant extends the limb somewhat, so as to relieve the tension on the soft parts. Each condyle is cleared in turn, and, when the soft parts have been turned sufficiently far forward to clear the front of the condyle, the joint is fully flexed, so that the bones project through the incision. The lateral ligaments

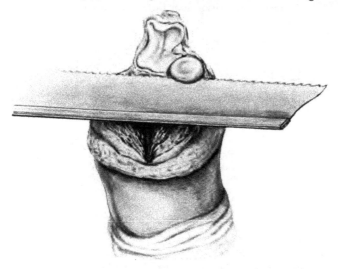

FIG. 5. SAWING THE RADIUS AND ULNA IN EXCISION OF THE ELBOW. The saw is applied above the level of the orbicular ligament.

are now divided and this allows the bones to come apart. By flexing the elbow acutely the lower end of the humerus is made to project freely from the wound, and, after clearing its lower end from the soft parts by a few touches of the knife, the saw is applied just above the level of the condyles (see Fig. 4) and the whole of the articular surface is removed.

The articular ends of the bones of the forearm are next removed. They are cleared by a few touches with the point of the knife and are made to protrude prominently from the soft parts by the assistant, who thrusts them up by grasping the wrist. The saw is applied just at the commencement of the head of the radius, so as to preserve the slightly expanded portion of the neck which retains the bone in the orbicular ligament (see Fig. 5). This structure should be carefully preserved from injury during the operation; should it have been divided, it should be sutured before the wound is closed. Retention of the movements of pronation and supination largely depends upon the integrity of the orbicular ligament and the retention of the neck of the radius in its grasp. All bleeding points are secured, and, if any sharp projecting points have been left on the humerus, these are removed with a gouge or · cutting-pliers.

The result of the removal of bone is the production of a gap of two inches or more between the ends of the bones. This may appear a formidable amount to the inexperienced operator, but, as a matter of fact, the mistake made is nearly always that too little is removed, and the result is more likely to be a stiff elbow afterwards than a flail one. The vertical incision through the triceps is brought together by a few fine catgut sutures and a drainage tube is inserted into the joint. The limb is put up in the almost fully extended position, with the forearm midway between pronation and supination, upon an internal splint furnished with an adjustable hinge at the joint. It is also well to provide a hand-piece, which is capable of rotation.

After-treatment. The arm is raised upon a pillow, slightly away from the side. The drainage tube should be removed in forty-eight hours, and after that the dressing need not be disturbed until the stitches have to be removed, which will be in about fourteen days. The movements of pronation and supination should be practised passively from the day after the operation, and flexion and extension may be begun after the first dressing, viz. about the third day. The range of the movements must be increased regularly, and after the removal of the stitches the patient should be encouraged to move the arm as fully and as frequently as possible.

Results. The results of this operation are in all respects excellent, provided it be done after the age at which growth ceases. Before that time the vigour of the reparative process is very great, and large amounts of bone are thrown out both in the region of the triceps tendon and the lower end of the humerus, and defective movement is frequently the result. In a typically good case there is perfectly good movement, and the only drawback is some loss of power when forcible movements, especially extension of the forearm, are attempted.

ARTHRODESIS

The earlier steps of the method of excision described above are eminently suited for the operation of arthrodesis. The access to the joint is excellent and the triceps, being paralysed, offers no difficulty in peeling the soft structures off the condyles. When the lateral ligaments have been divided and the end of the humerus protruded through the wound

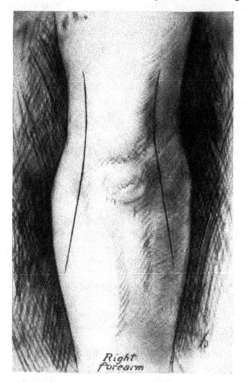

Fig. 6. Arthroplasty of Elbow for Complete Bony Ankylosis between the Humerus and Ulna in a Position of Complete Extension. Posterior view of the right elbow showing the location and direction of the two longitudinal incisions, one on the radial and one on the ulnar side of the olecranon. (*Murphy.*)

(see p. 20) the cartilage should be removed from the ulna, except that of the radio-ulnar joint and the corresponding amount from the lower end of the humerus; this is best done with a gouge. The cartilage in contact with the head of the radius should be left intact and none should be removed from the head of the radius. The limb is then fixed at right angles in a plaster of Paris casing.

ARTHROPLASTY (MURPHY)

Two lateral incisions are made, one on either side of the olecranon (see Fig. 6); although only one such incision may be necessary, depending on whether or not it is possible to work freely through an external incision without injuring the ulnar nerve.

If there is any danger of inflicting injury on this nerve, the second or inner lateral incision should be made. We must always insist on

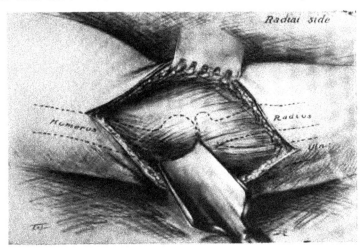

FIG. 7. EXPOSURE OF THE CAPSULE OF THE JOINT FROM THE RADIAL SIDE. The positions of the humerus, radius, and ulna are indicated by dotted lines. Note the direction in which the curved chisel is applied to separate the bones on the radial side of the joint. Note also that the curve of the chisel selected for the division corresponds exactly to the normal curve of the articular surface of the elbow joint, thus reproducing in the artificial joint the exact contour of the original. (*Murphy.*)

finding the nerve, freeing it from adhesions, and retracting it out of the field of operation (see Fig. 8).

The length of this lateral incision will depend on how much of an area one wishes to expose. As a rule, an incision about 5 inches in length is sufficient, although there is no reason why it should not be made longer if necessary. The incisions are made about one-half inch to either side of the olecranon and extend through the skin and superficial fascia. The edges of the wound are then retracted widely so as to give easy access to the joint (see Fig. 7).

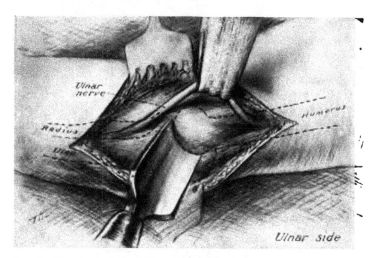

FIG. 8. EXPOSURE OF THE ULNAR NERVE AND CAPSULE OF THE JOINT FROM THE ULNAR SIDE. (*Murphy.*)

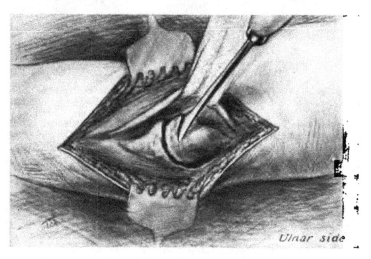

FIG. 9. REMOVAL OF ULNAR SIDE OF HUMERUS. (*Murphy.*)

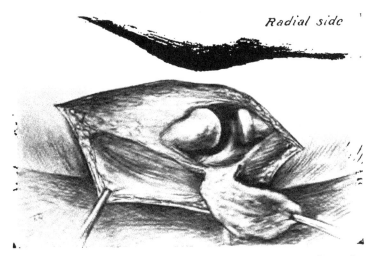

FIG. 10. PEDICLED FAT AND FASCIA FLAP PREPARED FROM THE OUTER SIDE OF THE ARM FOR INSERTION INTO THE JOINT FROM THE RADIAL SIDE. (*Murphy.*)

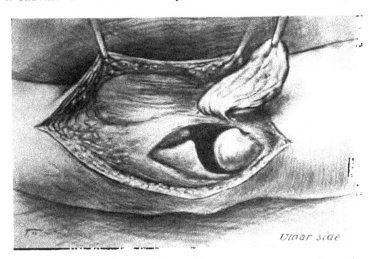

FIG. 11. PEDICLED FAT AND FASCIA FLAP PREPARED FROM THE INNER SURFACE OF THE FOREARM FOR INSERTION INTO THE JOINT FROM THE ULNAR SIDE. (*Murphy.*)

The interposing flap in these cases is taken from the aponeurosis of the supinator longus and from the fascia and fat on the inner side of the joint. The bases of these flaps are directed upward. The flaps are made sufficiently wide so as to cover the freshened surfaces of the bone and long enough so as to reach across from one side of the joint to the other (see Figs. 10 and 11).

The ankylosis in the case of the elbow usually exists between the olecranon process of the ulna and the humerus. This is carefully di-

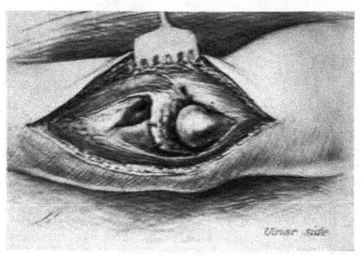

FIG. 12. ULNAR FLAP INTERPOSED AND SUTURED INTO POSITION BETWEEN THE ULNA AND HUMERUS. (Murphy.)

vided by means of a curved chisel, twisted laterally, until free mobility of the joint is secured (see Fig. 9).

Sometimes there is a bony ankylosis between the head of the radius and the lesser sigmoid cavity. When this exists it is also chiselled free. The bony deposit is removed, all exostoses are cut away, and absolute freedom of motion is secured. If necessary, the olecranon fossa may be deepened, so that the extension of the arm may be complete. Ample bone should be removed from the humerus and radius to permit of free flexion and extension without force and the anterior capsule of the joint fully and completely divided.

Having secured the desired mobility of the joint and having freshened all bony surfaces, the next step in the operation is to place and secure the interposing flaps (see Figs. 12 and 13). As stated before, these flaps are drawn into the joint and secured on all sides with chromicized catgut sutures. The ulnar nerve which was exposed at the commencement of the operation, so as to protect it from injury, is now replaced in its groove and surrounded by fat. The remainder of the opera-

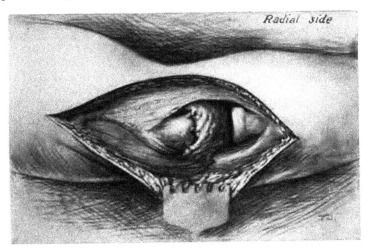

FIG. 13. RADIAL FLAP INTERPOSED AND SUTURED INTO POSITION BETWEEN THE HUMERUS AND THE RADIUS AND ULNA. The deep stitches which fasten together the radial and ulnar flaps in the depths of the wound have not been shown in these illustrations. (*Murphy.*)

tion consists of the steps already described, such as closing the wound and applying the powder and dressings.

The elbow is immobilized at an angle of about 30 to 40 degrees. The patient is encouraged to make active and passive motion and, if necessary, is ordered to carry sand-bags or other weights for the purpose of securing as much extension of the arm as is possible. Massage may now be of service in increasing the function of the joint. It should never be severely painful or prolonged.

CHAPTER IV

OPERATIONS UPON THE SHOULDER-JOINT

ARTHROTOMY AND DRAINAGE

Indications. The shoulder is not a frequent seat of suppurative arthritis, either pyæmic or secondary to acute infective osteomyelitis of the humerus or scapula; it may, however, have to be drained for either of these conditions.

Operation. The joint is difficult to drain from the front, owing to the obliquity of the insertion of the capsule, which extends much further down on the inner than on the outer side. It will be necessary, therefore, to make a counter-opening at the most dependent spot in all cases. This will be on the axillary aspect of the joint, and care will be needed to avoid damage to the important structures in that region.

The first step is to open the front of the joint, and here there will be some difficulty, owing to the necessity of avoiding injury to the tendon of the biceps, which would cause serious disability subsequently. The only safe plan is to dissect down upon the front of the joint with care and deliberation, exposing the parts fully and ascertaining the whereabouts of the structures to be avoided. An almost vertical incision downwards for about two inches from just in front of the acromion process will give good access. The deltoid fibres are separated and the muscles inserted into the outer tuberosity are exposed. By incising them vertically downwards in the line of the skin incision the joint will be opened well outside the biceps tendon, which will lie in its groove undisturbed. Its position can be felt by the finger in the wound, and if necessary it can be drawn out of harm's way by rotating the limb firmly inwards. A drainage tube is inserted into the joint beneath the acromion.

A second incision for through-and-through drainage will be required, and this must be made at the most dependent spot in the axilla. It is not easy to hit off this spot exactly as the conformation of the joint makes it difficult to pass forceps across from the previous incision. Perhaps the best plan is to raise the arm above the head so as to render the head of the humerus as prominent in the axilla as possible, and then to cut down upon this by an incision about two inches long just below the axillary vessels. These are identified and pulled upwards so as to expose the capsule below and behind. The head of the bone can be made out by the finger in the axilla. The capsule may be opened by cutting down directly upon the head of the bone; this may be facilitated by bringing the arm down, and passing a long pair of dressing forceps across the joint from the upper incision and making their points protrude beneath the capsule so that they can be cut down upon and made to seize the drainage tube and pull it into position.

OPERATIONS FOR FRACTURES INVOLVING THE SHOULDER-JOINT

Indications. Owing to the small portion of the bone contained within the capsule of the joint and the fact that the commonest form of fracture, viz. that through the surgical neck, is outside the joint, arthrotomy is not often called for in connexion with fractures of the upper end of the humerus. Moreover the articular surfaces are in such loose apposition that slight irregularities do not materially impair the movements of the joints. However, fractures such as those of the anatomical neck, as well as those of the great trochanter, will generally require operative treatment in order to secure the best possible result. These cases are now recognized more quickly and more certainly than they were formerly, owing to the great assistance afforded by stereoscopic radiograms. By means of them it will generally be possible to tell not only the cases that should be operated upon, but also the most suitable position for the arthrotomy incision.

Operation. Into the steps of the operation it is unnecessary to go in detail. It will consist of two parts—arthrotomy, followed by removal of the detached portion of the bone or fixation of it in place by some of the mechanical methods already described (see Vol. I, p. 705). The incision for exposure of the joint will vary according to the precise affection for which the operation is done. For a fracture of the anatomical neck the incision advised for use in the reduction of dislocations (see p. 31) is perhaps the most useful, while for fractures involving the greater tuberosity the one beneath the acromion (see p. 21) will lead down to the seat of injury more directly. The treatment of the fracture after the joint has been opened will be determined by the conditions present. If the head of the bone be separated it is as well to remove it entirely, gouging and smoothing off the fractured surface left, so that movement may be unimpeded afterwards. The question of some form of arthroplasty (see p. 5) will have to be considered in this connexion. For any other form of fracture mechanical fixation will probably be required and the most appropriate method should be adopted (see Vol. I, p. 705). The joint should be closed without a drainage tube.

After-treatment. The chief point is to promote early movement. The arm should be carried in a sling only, and passive movement should be practised from the first few days and pushed vigorously.

OPERATIONS FOR DISLOCATIONS OF THE SHOULDER

It may become necessary to have recourse to operative measures for the reduction of a dislocation at various periods after the receipt of the injury. It is usual to divide the operations into two classes, viz. those done while the dislocation is recent, and those for dislocations of long standing. This is, however, not a good plan, as the distinction between recent dislocations and those of long standing is rapidly disappearing with the advance of aseptic surgery, and the conviction is growing that no dislocation should be allowed to reach the stage in which it may be said to be an unreduced dislocation of long standing. Radiograms will clear up doubts as to the nature of the condition and the remedy for it is becoming more widely agreed upon; it is, that the joint should be opened and an attempt made to replace the head of the bone as soon as a fair trial of reduction by manipulation under an anæsthetic has been made and has failed. Operation will be required for:

Indications. (i) All cases of dislocation complicated by fracture of the upper end of the humerus. These cases should be operated upon directly they come under notice. The prospects of obtaining a good result are directly proportionate to the celerity and thoroughness with which operative restoration is performed. The procedure will be reposition of the head, suture of the capsule, and mechanical fixation of the fragments.

(ii) All cases of dislocation complicated by fracture of the glenoid cavity. This accident has only received just recognition since radiographic examination has become the rule. It is likely to lead to a crippled joint unless early operation be practised for the removal of detached bone and suture of the torn structures.

(iii) Any dislocation that cannot be reduced after two or three careful attempts at reduction under full anæsthesia. These, of course, will be recent cases. Operation should be practised within the first week, preferably within the first three days.

(iv) Any unreduced dislocation that has lasted for less than six weeks after a careful attempt at reduction under anæsthesia has failed. The attempt should be by manipulation only, and operation should be carried out forthwith if it fails; this avoids further adhesions which would make an operation carried out at a later period more difficult.

(v) All cases of dislocation that have lasted longer than six weeks without any previous attempt at reduction, provided that the patient's age, health, and degree of disability render an operation advisable. In this connexion it is well to remember that some patients have excellent, though limited, use of the arm in spite of the unreduced dislocation, and that operation will not always improve upon this. In old and fat people the restoration of function is often very defective, especially when the head of the bone cannot be replaced and the joint has to be excised.

Operation in recent cases. In recent cases very little difficulty may be met with, except when there is an extensive fracture complicating the dislocation. A very good incision is that suggested by Mr. Keetley (*Lancet,* 1904, vol. i, p. 211), following Tiling and Paulet, along the anterior margin of the deltoid, just external to the cephalic vein, from the clavicle nearly to its insertion. The anterior fibres of the deltoid are separated along the line of the incision, and a transverse cut is made from its inner edge for about two or three inches through the deltoid half an inch below the clavicle and acromion. This latter part of the incision is not always necessary in recent cases, but it is very useful, as by employing it the whole area concerned in the dislocation can be exposed quite satisfactorily and without causing any risk to the nerve-supply of the deltoid, which it is very important to preserve intact.

When this incision has been well retracted, the dislocated head of the bone will be seen, and, if the case be one of simple dislocation unaccompanied by fracture (as a radiogram will demonstrate), the arm should be manipulated for reduction by an assistant while the surgeon ascertains and overcomes any obstacle to reduction, such as the tendon of the subscapularis, by pulling it aside. When reduction has been accomplished, the rent in the capsule is sewn up if it can be reached, the deltoid, if cut, is sutured (see Vol. I, p. 623), and the wound is closed without a drainage tube. The arm is bound lightly to the side and the elbow supported in a large sling. Passive movements, while the arm is supported by the sling, are practised from the first. After the sutures have been removed, the elbow is supported in a sling for another week, but overhead movements should not be allowed for a month after operation for fear of recurrence of the dislocation. Abduction can be restricted by fixing a strap round the thorax and another round the arm, and connecting them with a light chain of suitable length.

When a fracture complicates dislocation it will be necessary to remove any loose fragments of bone from the joint cavity if the fracture involve the glenoid cavity, after which the treatment is as above, care being taken to smooth down any rough surface of bone left. When the fracture is in the upper end of the humerus, the dislocation is first reduced and the rent in the capsule sutured, after which the fragments are fixed by mechanical means (see Vol. I, p. 705). Some difficulty may be experienced in handling the upper fragment when reducing the dislocation if the fracture be high up, since it is difficult to get a hold upon it. This may necessitate the use of special forceps (see Fig. 273, Vol. I); in one case I was successful after transfixing the head of the bone with a drill which served as a handle to manipulate the bone with. After successful reduction and fixation, the limb is put up as for fracture of the neck of the humerus, the wrist being supported by a sling and the shoulder-joint fixed by a moulded cap of poroplastic material or gutta-percha, the elbow being allowed to hang unsupported.

In the *after-treatment* the condition of the shoulder-joint must not be overlooked, and it will be necessary to guard against stiffness by practising free passive movement from an early date, steadying the seat of fracture carefully meanwhile. It is very difficult to obtain a perfectly satisfactory result in these cases; much depends upon the thoroughness with which the passive movements are carried out.

Operations for unreduced dislocation. When the dislocation has remained unreduced for a long time the operations for its cure are really two in number, viz. re-position of the head of the humerus in the glenoid cavity or excision of the joint. As it is impossible to tell beforehand which of these methods is likely to be successful, and as in practice the surgeon always attempts to replace the head of the bone before he convinces himself that it will be necessary to excise it, these two operations will be described as portions of one procedure.

The purification of the soft parts in these operations, as in the corresponding ones upon the hip, must be both thorough and extensive. The entire pectoral, scapular, and axillary region must be shaved and cleansed and the upper limb must be secured in sterilized towels, for the manipulations are likely to be severe and prolonged, and the hands have to be carried well under the back in order to fix the scapula.

For exposure of the operation area no incision is better than that advised by Keetley (*loc. supra cit.*). The anterior fibres of the deltoid are split and the posterior fibres are divided by a horizontal incision outwards below the clavicle, enabling the muscle to be pulled backwards from the upper end of the bone, thus exposing the displaced head lying beneath the coracoid process, where it will have contracted dense adhesions and have formed a false joint. Before there will be any chance of getting the head into the glenoid cavity, the muscles passing from the scapula to the humerus, which are all shortened, must be separated. The best way to do this is, as Keetley advises, to chisel off the greater tuberosity with the muscles attached to it and to divide the coracoid process with the coraco-brachialis arising from it. The tendon of the biceps may be divided by a very oblique section if necessary, and the lesser tuberosity with the insertion of the subscapularis may also be detached if its tendon cannot be hooked out of the way. The soft structures forming the new false capsule must be opened up freely and the head and neck of the bone separated from the adjacent soft parts. This is the most difficult stage of the operation, since the axillary vessels and nerves may be closely adherent to the inner surface of the neck. By keeping very close to the bone and using Farabeuf's sharp rugines (see Fig. 271, Vol. I), this danger will be got over. Finally the glenoid cavity is examined, and if it be filled up by the remains of the capsule, which has fallen over and become adherent to its anterior surface, as will probably be the case, it must be removed with knife and scissors before the head is put in place.

Nothing now remains to be done but to attempt to replace the head of the bone in the glenoid cavity. How this is to be done each operator must determine for himself. It should be by manipulation methods if possible, after dividing any structures that oppose reduction and can be divided with impunity. Pulleys were frequently used and are still advocated, but it seems more reasonable to submit cases obstinate enough to demand such extreme force, to some form of excision. Powerful bone forceps, retractors, and levers may be required to lift the head of the bone on to the glenoid surface. When it is there, manipulations will complete the reduction. If the head of the bone should have undergone distortion from traumatic arthritis, as it may have done in cases of very long standing, it will be necessary to pare it away and leave it very smooth and of proper shape. Redundant capsule must be cut away, but any that is likely to come in useful in the formation of a new capsule should be retained.

If the attempts at reduction are successful, the next step is to restore the various muscular insertions that have been divided. The tuberosities are fastened in place with tacks, the coracoid process is wired on, and the biceps tendon sutured if it has been divided. The deltoid fibres are sutured (see Vol. I, p. 623) and any remnants of capsule are brought together to form a new capsule for the joint. The wound is closed without a drainage tube, and the *after-treatment* is similar to that for recent cases (see p. 32), except that the convalescence will be longer.

If these attempts at reduction fail, however, there is no alternative but to excise the joint (*vide infra*). In several reported cases the wound has been closed after it was found that reduction could not be effected, but this only serves to make the patient's condition worse than it was before, and excision is probably preferable.

After the head of the bone has been sawn (see p. 38) the raw surface

is rounded off and made as smooth as possible, and it will be well to
' practise arthroplasty (see p. 5) by bringing in a flap of soft parts over
the cut surface so as to encourage movement subsequently.　The detached
muscular attachments are fastened in place once more (*vide supra*) and
divided tendons and muscles sutured.　The *after-treatment* is similar to
that of excision generally (see p. 38), except that passive movement
must be begun earlier and persevered in more energetically, under full

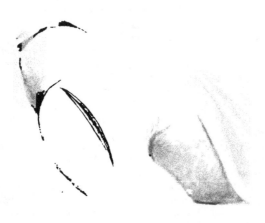

FIG. 14. INCISION FOR EXCISION OF THE SHOULDER-JOINT.　This is the anterior
incision described in the text.　The limb is in the position in which it should be
held when the incision is made.

anæsthesia, if necessary, on account of the readiness with which adhesions form in the disorganized joint.

EXCISION OF THE SHOULDER

Indications.　(i) *Tuberculous disease* of the joint is the affection
for which this operation is most frequently performed.　This does not
come within the scope of the present article, however.

(ii) *Compound fractures* of the upper end of the humerus may occasionally be best treated by excision in order to preserve the movements of the joint.

(iii) *Unreduced dislocations* of long standing that resist all attempts to get the head of the bone into the glenoid cavity may be treated by excision and a wider range of movement thereby assured.

(iv) *Ankylosis* of the shoulder in a young subject is often a fit subject for excision with the object of obtaining a range of movement

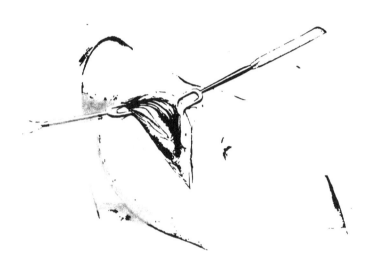

Fig. 15. Preservation of the Biceps Tendon in Excision of the Shoulder-joint. The tendon has been lifted out of its groove.

that is unobtainable without it. The operation should not be undertaken for this purpose, however, without a careful selection of cases, as the functional results are not nearly so good in elderly subjects as in younger people.

Operation. (*a*) **For injury.** An incision five inches long (see Fig. 14) is begun upon the clavicle above the coracoid process, and carried downwards and outwards along the anterior border of the deltoid, which is separated from the clavicular portion of the pectoralis major by the cephalic vein. The latter is drawn to the inner side along with the pectoralis major, while the deltoid is drawn outwards. The front portion of the deltoid will probably have to be detached from the clavicle, and some of the branches of the acromio-thoracic artery ligatured.

When these muscles have been retracted, the outer surface of the capsule of the joint is exposed; in the lower part of the wound the tendon

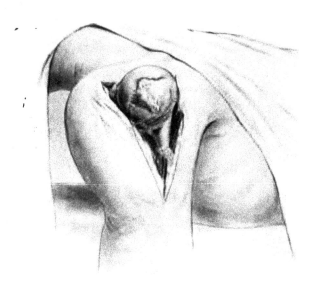

FIG. 16. DISARTICULATION OF THE HEAD OF THE HUMERUS IN EXCISION OF THE SHOULDER-JOINT. The arm is vertical and the head of the bone can be pushed well up out of the wound.

of insertion of the pectoralis major is seen. The arm is rotated inwards and the sheath of the biceps tendon is opened along the outer lip of the bicipital groove. The sheath is slit up to the edge of the glenoid cavity, and the biceps tendon is freed and drawn inwards (see Fig. 15). The tendon must be carefully preserved throughout the operation. The incision into the sheath of the biceps tendon opens the capsule of the joint, and the next step is to separate the attachment of the tendons inserted into the upper end of the humerus, viz. the subscapularis into the lesser tuberosity, the supraspinatus, infraspinatus, and the teres minor into the greater tuberosity. This is done by means of vertical cuts close to the bone made parallel to the bicipital groove, the humerus

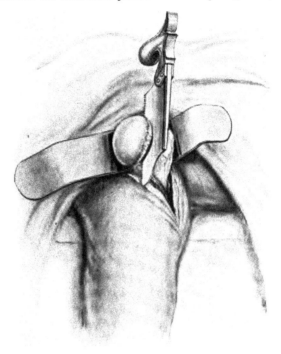

FIG. 17. SAWING THE HEAD OF THE HUMERUS IN EXCISION OF THE SHOULDER-JOINT. The soft parts are protected by a spatula.

being meanwhile rotated first outwards and then inwards; no transverse cuts should be made in the capsule, as it is essential for a good result that it should be detached undamaged. While this is being done, the assistant holds the arm nearly horizontal, and at right angles to the trunk. When the humerus must be exposed farther downwards, the anterior and posterior circumflex arteries and the circumflex nerve, which surround the surgical neck, must be borne in mind, and the former if necessary ligatured. The nerve must on no account be injured.

The head of the bone can now be made to project from the capsule and should be pushed up out of the wound by the assistant (see Fig. 16). In determining how much bone to remove in these cases the surgeon is guided by the desire to get free movement, since there is no disease requiring to be removed. A free removal of bone may be practised if care be taken to preserve those portions of the tuberosities into which the rotators of the bone are inserted. The saw is applied parallel to and just outside the line of the anatomical neck (see Fig. 17). Whatever the amount of bone removed, the line of section should be obliquely from without downwards and inwards, so as to avoid any projecting edge against the axillary vessels or nerves. When the section is complete it is well to go over the whole of the inner aspect of the cut surface and pare this down with a gouge or a burr, so that it is as smooth as possible and presents no prominences that will interfere with movement. It is also an excellent plan to fashion a flap from the soft structures around and fasten it over the raw bone surface in order to promote movement subsequently (see p. 5). Foreign substances, such as thin sheet rubber or gold foil, have been used with a similar object.

The remaining steps of the operation are concerned with the closure of the wound. Before this is done the insertions of the supraspinatus, infraspinatus, and teres minor are sutured to the greater tuberosity and the tendon of the subscapularis to the lesser with stout catgut. The biceps tendon is replaced in its groove and its sheath is sutured over it. A drainage tube should be inserted into the joint cavity, as a large ' dead ' space is left in which blood would otherwise collect. A small pad is placed in the axilla to prevent the head of the humerus being drawn inwards, and the elbow and forearm are supported in a sling. The arm is fastened lightly to the side.

Passive movements are begun from the first and the patient is encouraged to swing his arm about in the sling as much as he can. The support should be removed from the elbow about the third or fourth day, the sling only taking in the wrist.

(b) **For unreduced dislocation.** This has been already referred to separately in connexion with the operations for unreduced dislocations (see p. 33).

(c) **For ankylosis.** There is often considerable difficulty in these cases owing to the want of proper exposure of the parts. The anterior oblique incision described above does not give enough room for the very important soft structures on the inner aspect of the joint to be properly protected while the head of the bone is being sawn or chiselled through *in situ,* as it has to be in cases of ankylosis. When the head of the bone can be protruded from the wound, as it can be in ordinary cases, there is no risk to the axillary structures, but when division has to be effected in-ankylosed cases the saw or chisel may easily do very serious damage. Even when a Gigli's saw is employed and is introduced by pulling it round the bone with the aid of a suitably curved director insinuated between the soft parts and the inner aspect of the joint the procedure is difficult, as it may be hard to protrude the humerus from the wound after simple division of the ankylosis. Therefore an operation that will give the fullest exposure of the joint with the least damage to the functional powers of the muscles subsequently is greatly to be desired.

Kocher's posterior resection. On the whole these conditions are better fulfilled by the posterior method introduced by Kocher. The following is his description of the operation (*Textbook of Operative Surgery,* translated by Stiles, 1903, p. 376) :—

' The skin incision is carried from the acromio-clavicular joint over the top of the shoulder and along the upper border of the acromion to the outer part of the spine of the scapula (root of the acromion), and from thence downwards in a curved direction towards the posterior fold of the axilla, ending two fingers' breadth above it. The upper limb of the incision passes through the superior ligament right into the acromio-clavicular joint (the strong fibres of which are divided), and the rest of its course divides the insertion of the trapezius along the upper border of the spine of the scapula. The descending limb of the incision divides the dense fascia at the posterior border of the deltoid, and exposes the fibres of the latter. The thumb is now introduced beneath the smooth under surface of the deltoid so as to separate it from the deeper muscles (with which it is connected merely by loose cellular tissue) up to its origin from the acromion, and its posterior fibres are divided. The finger is now carried along the upper border of the infraspinatus muscle so as to free it opposite the outer border of the spine and the root of the acromion.

' In a similar manner the supraspinatus is detached with a blunt dissector from the upper border of the spine of the scapula, in order that the finger may be passed from above underneath the root of the acromion. The root of the acromion, which is now freed, is chiselled through obliquely, and, along with the deltoid, is forcibly pushed forwards with the thumbs over the head of the humerus.

' In chiselling through the bone care must be taken not to injure the suprascapular nerve which passes under the muscles from the supraspinous into the infraspinous fossa; the nerve is also protected by the transverse ligament of the scapula. It is desirable before chiselling the bone to bore the holes required for the subsequent suture.

' Instead of dividing the root of the acromion, the formation of the posterior flap may be simplified by merely detaching the scapular origin of the deltoid subcortically: this allows of very firm union subsequently.

' After reflecting the acromio-deltoid flap, the head of the bone is readily accessible in its upper, outer, and posterior aspects, covered by the tendons of the external rotators, viz. the supraspinatus, infraspinatus, and teres minor muscles. The posterior surfaces of these muscles are also exposed. An incision is now made over the head of the bone, and in order to avoid unnecessary injury this must be done accurately. The arm being rotated outwards, a longitudinal incision is carried down to the bone in the coronal plane. Commencing at the upper part of the posterior lip of the bicipital groove, it extends upwards through the capsule along the anterior edge of the insertions of the external rotator muscles and over the highest part of the head of the humerus, so as to expose the tendon of the biceps as far as its attachment to the upper edge of the glenoid cavity. The insertions of the external rotators are now separated from the greater tuberosity and drawn backwards. The biceps tendon is freed from its groove and drawn forwards, so that its sheath may be inspected.

' In this way the entire head of the humerus and the glenoid fossa can be freely exposed, and if it is not necessary to do a complete excision, the anterior wall of the capsule and the insertions of the anterior muscles can be preserved. In other cases the insertion of the subscapularis into the lesser tuberosity is detached upwards and inwards.

' The circumflex vessels and nerve which come out from under the teres minor can be preserved: indeed, if the operation be properly performed there need be no fear of injuring them.'

When the upper and back part of the joint has been freely exposed in this manner it becomes a much easier task to protect the soft parts on the anterior and inner aspects of the joint and to divide the bone. On the whole it is perhaps best to perform the section with a broad chisel which is sunk into the line of ankylosis, which can always be identified. A few gentle strokes with the hammer and a little manipulation of the arm by one assistant while another fixes the scapula will generally suffice to mobilize the head of the humerus. Fine spatulæ can then be slipped down behind the neck of the bone and the rest of the operation carried out as for an ordinary excision (see p. 38).

ARTHRODESIS

Indications. In the rare cases in which the muscles passing from the scapula to the humerus are paralysed, it will be considerable help to the patient if his shoulder-joint can be fixed firmly enough to enable the scapulo-thoracic movements to be substituted for those of the shoulder. This can be done to some extent by arthrodesis, but it must be confessed that the results may be disappointing since the bone surfaces cannot always be kept closely enough in contact for firm bony union to occur, and this is required if the arm is to be useful. The leverage is so great that fibrous union soon stretches. Close approximation of the denuded articular surfaces is difficult to maintain, owing to the dependent position of the limb and the fact that the muscles maintaining apposition in the normal joint are paralysed here. Mechanical fixation (see Vol. I, p. 705) may be employed with advantage.

Operation. The first stages of the operation will be the same as for an excision (see p. 35). It is immaterial what incision is used for the purpose. The oblique anterior one recommended above is as good as any, but in this case a large deltoid flap may be raised, if desired, as this muscle will be paralysed by the affection for which the operation is done, and there is therefore no objection to injuring it, as there is in the ordinary excision operation.

When the head of the bone has been protruded from the wound (see Fig. 16), the cartilage is carefully removed from the whole of it with a chisel. Besides this it will be advisable to flatten the rounded surface of the head somewhat so as to ensure a broad surface of contact when it rests against the glenoid cavity; otherwise, it will only touch at one point. As these operations are generally done in growing children, it will be unsafe to use the saw for this purpose, as the epiphyseal line might be injured; more delicate and certain work can be done with the chisel.

The next point is to remove the cartilage from the glenoid cavity. This is rather difficult to get at, but removal must be thorough and methodical, and is best done with a gouge. An electrically-driven burr is an excellent instrument, and it has the further great advantage that a flat surface can be made of the glenoid cavity to fit accurately against the flattened head of the bone.

The two raw surfaces of bone are now placed in apposition, and I have found it best to fasten them together in order to prevent them falling asunder and to promote bony union, which is very essential. A simple and satisfactory plan is to transfix the head of the bone with a steel pin driven in through the greater tuberosity and passing through the head of the humerus and the glenoid cavity well into the neck of the scapula. The end of the pin protrudes through the wound and can be enveloped in the dressings and removed when union has occurred. The humerus is held in apposition to the glenoid cavity by the assistant while the peg is being driven in, and care must be taken to see that it is somewhat inwardly rotated while this is being done, otherwise it will be difficult to bring the forearm to the chest afterwards.

ARTHROPLASTY (MURPHY)

The skin and deltoid are split and the fascia is separated along its anterior margin for a distance of four inches and elevated so as to expose the bony union between the glenoid and the head of the humerus. A curved chisel is then used to separate these and an additional excavation on the surface of the glenoid is made. An incision is then made at right angles to the original incision across the chest, over the middle of the pectoralis major muscle; a flap of fat, aponeurosis of the pectoralis major muscle is then made, 4½ inches long and 3½ wide, with its pedicle left attached to the humerus. It is swung upward and interposed between the head of the humerus and glenoid, completely covering the bony surfaces. In lieu of this simple procedure, the following may be adopted, as described by Coville: He made a 4-inch incision, starting below the clavicle and passing external to the coracoid process, down along the arm, following the fibres of the deltoid muscle. This muscle is incised just outside of the delto-pectoral groove, when the shoulder-joint will be found to be exposed freely. Coville then extracted the head of the humerus and divided it from the remainder of the bone, at the level of the anatomic neck. The long strip of deltoid muscle was cut transversely, the superior portion being left adherent. A piece 4 inches wide was taken from the transverse section and interposed between the head of the bone and the glenoid cavity.

Coville perforated the capsule with a probe so as to prevent wounding the musculo-spiral nerve, and made a counter-incision at the same level, passing a thread through its opening. This thread surrounded the extremity of the muscular strip in the form of a loop, and by tightening this loop the strip of muscle is applied to the articular cavity.

Besides using a muscle flap in the manner described above, one may substitute and use as an interposing flap the anterior portion of the deltoid, inserting it anterior to the coraco-brachialis and short head of the biceps.

EXCISION OF THE SCAPULA

Indications. (i) *For sarcoma of the bone.* This is practically the only condition that is likely to require complete excision of the scapula, although parts of the bone may be removed for other conditions.

(ii) *For necrosis of the scapula.* This results from acute infective osteomyelitis in young subjects and may require a partial excision of the bone; it is, however, hardly ever likely to demand complete removal.

(iii) The scapula is removed together with the entire upper extremity in the *interscapulo-thoracic amputation* of Berger. This, however, is a special operation which is not really excision of the scapula.

Operation. Various incisions may be employed; the one in most common use is a vertical incision along the vertebral border of the bone, from the superior to the inferior angle, joined by another along the whole length of the spine of the scapula as far as the tip of the acromion. This gives two triangular flaps which are dissected up and down. I personally prefer a somewhat I-shaped incision, the upper horizontal limb of which is longer than the lower and extends from the tip of the acromion to the superior angle of the scapula. The lower crosses the lower angle and is about four inches long. The mid-points of these two incisions are joined by an incision, which marks out two rectangular flaps which are dissected up inwards and outwards, and which expose the entire scapular area to view.

It is a great advantage to retain a portion of the acromion if this can be done with safety, but it is rarely advisable to do so since the bone is usually removed for a periosteal sarcoma. If a part of the acromion is to be left behind, it is divided at the desired spot with a saw or chisel, otherwise the incision extends right into the acromio-clavicular joint. When the operation is done for growth, the various muscles attached to the scapula must be removed as completely as possible; when this is not the case, however, they may be cut long. This is only really important as far as the deltoid and the trapezius are concerned; if they can be cut long they may be sutured together at the end of the operation with great advantage to the patient. The scapular muscles are of course not needed after the scapula has been removed.

After the flaps have been well reflected, the first muscle to be divided is the deltoid, beneath the fibres of which the fingers can be thrust so that the muscle may be hooked up and divided at its origin from the acromial spine, or its scapular fibres can be separated from the clavicular ones, and removed entirely down to their insertion. The tendons inserted into the upper end of the humerus are now cut through in order, beginning with the subscapularis and going on to divide the tendon of the biceps, the supraspinatus, the infraspinatus, and the teres minor. The insertion of the teres major will also have to be severed. The circumflex nerve must be preserved, if possible, but the dorsalis scapulæ artery and perhaps the posterior circumflex will be exposed and should be ligatured at this stage.

The fingers are now passed beneath the fibres of the trapezius, which is lifted from the acromion, and its insertion into the spine of the scapula divided throughout. Beneath the anterior fibres of the muscle the acromial branches of the acromio-thoracic artery must be secured. This renders the borders of the scapula freely visible and the muscles which attach the bone to the trunk are then divided in regular order. Beginning along the upper border from the neck of the bone, the omohyoid will be detached and the suprascapular artery ligatured at the same time; then the levator anguli scapulæ will be cut away from the upper angle of the bone and the posterior scapular artery will be ligatured. This only leaves the rhomboids and the serratus magnus connecting the bone with the trunk, and these are divided in turn, the posterior scapular giving no trouble as it has been already divided. This separates the bone entirely, with the exception of the structures attached to the coracoid process and the front portions of the capsule of the shoulder-joint; the latter is easily divided, the finger being hooked round the neck of the scapula, which is pulled up so that the capsule is rendered prominent and can be divided. The soft parts are then pushed carefully away from the front of the neck and the under aspect of the coracoid process. This is the really difficult part of the operation, as the first part of the axillary artery and vein lie in close connexion with this structure. If the surgeon be doubtful of his ability to clear it without damaging these vessels, the coracoid process may be cut across at its base with a pair of cutting-pliers, and then dissected out. With care it is, however, easy to push the structures away sufficiently to render evident the tendons of the coraco-brachialis and the pectoralis minor, which are detached from the bone, and the latter is then removed.

The flaps are brought together, a large drainage tube is placed at the most dependent spot, and the dressings are firmly bandaged round the thorax so as to obliterate any space in which blood might collect.

Difficulties and dangers. If done as above described there will be little risk of bleeding, which is the chief danger in these operations. The great point is to secure perfect exposure of the parts, to divide the muscles *seriatim*, and to know where to look for the principal vessels.

Results. The results are excellent; the patient retains all movements of the limb, with the exception that he is unable to abduct the arm above a right angle from the trunk.

CHAPTER V

OPERATIONS UPON THE ANKLE-JOINT: OPERATIONS UPON THE TARSAL BONES AND JOINTS

ARTHROTOMY AND DRAINAGE OF THE ANKLE-JOINT

THE ankle is a difficult joint to drain effectively, since it is divided into two parts by the astragalus, which projects up into the tibio-fibular arch and separates the posterior sac between the tendo Achillis and the astragalus (talus) almost completely from the anterior one between that bone and the extensor tendons.

Indications. Fortunately suppuration in the ankle-joint is rare and drainage is not often required.

(i) *Acute suppurative arthritis,* either of pyæmic origin or due to acute infective osteomyelitis of the os calcis or the bones of the leg, will require the freest possible drainage.

(ii) *Compound fractures into the ankle-joint,* particularly the variety known as Pott's, are not infrequently followed by acute suppuration, since from the nature of the injury the wound may be contaminated with dirt which escapes the cleansing processes.

Operation. There are two chief methods for arthrotomy and drainage. Of these the simpler plan is to make free incisions on each side of the joint front and back, and to pass tubes through from side to side; this should succeed unless the infection be very virulent or the case be seen too late.

Simple arthrotomy. An incision is made behind the external malleolus, avoiding the sheaths of the peronei tendons, and the posterior ligament, which will be distended with the pus in the joint, is exposed and opened. Through this opening dressing forceps are passed across the back of the joint and made to project behind the inner malleolus; here the points are cut down upon and a drainage tube is pulled through from side to side across the back of the joint. In making this incision the tendon sheaths behind the inner ankle and the posterior tibial vessels and nerve must be avoided. The best way to do this is to dissect down with a blunt instrument after the skin has been divided until the points of the dressing forceps are reached. Similar incisions are next made in

45

the front of the joint and a drainage tube is drawn across from side to side in that situation. The tendon sheaths should not be opened and the dorsalis pedis must be avoided. The drainage through these tubes can be supplemented by continuous irrigation if desired.

Excision of the astragalus. In bad cases, however, it will be necessary to lay all the recesses of the joint into one large cavity if drainage is to be effectual, and this can only be done by excising the astragalus (talus). This method of treatment has been strongly advocated by Bolton (*Ann. of Surg.*, 1906, vol. xliv, p. 959); it is of course of drastic once since the utility of the foot must be permanently impaired by it, but it must not be forgotten that this will also probably be the case whenever there is suppuration in the ankle, and it is an open question whether the functions of the joint after excision of the astragalus are not better performed than after drainage followed by ankylosis with the foot in the right-angled position. In any case operation is imperative unless the temperature drops and the general conditions undergo amelioration after simple drainage practised as recommended above; no time must be lost, and the astragalus should be removed (see p. 51) as an alternative to amputation of the leg.

The wound must be left widely open, and it will be well to make a counter-opening on the inner side and insert a large tube. The large cavity left by the removal of the astragalus may be mopped out with a saturated solution of chloride of zinc, so as to hinder septic absorption from the freshly cut surfaces, and then lightly packed with strips of gauze for the first three days, after which the large drainage tubes alone will suffice. The chief care must be to keep the foot from becoming displaced on the leg.

ARTHROTOMY FOR THE TREATMENT OF FRACTURES INTO THE ANKLE-JOINT

Indications. (i) *Recent Pott's fracture.* In certain cases operative interference is required for recent Pott's fractures. These will comprise all compound fractures, and those simple forms in which reduction under an anæsthetic cannot be effected satisfactorily.

(ii) *Dupuytren's fracture or fractures of the astragalus* are frequently followed by such severe disability as to render operative interference imperative. Now that stereoscopic radiograms can show the exact displacement of fractures in this situation, immediate operation will probably be resorted to in future for all these cases, while it is comparatively easy to rectify displacements or to remove detached portions of bone which might otherwise give rise to much trouble and possibly interfere with a satisfactory result from operation subsequently. Hitherto operation has been largely confined to cases of long standing, accompanied by great disability.

Operations for compound Pott's fracture. The seat of fracture and the ankle-joint should be fully exposed after the parts have been purified. The method of purification resembles that for compound fractures, being essentially thorough purification of the skin, after shutting off the joint cavity from the surface by means of a gauze plug, with subsequent removal or disinfection of soiled surfaces in the deeper structures. The wound, which is practically always on the inner side of the ankle, should be enlarged for the purpose of disinfection and exploration, and this gives the opportunity of discovering and removing soiled tissues both in the soft parts and the bone, and also enables the dislocation accompanying the fracture to be properly reduced and the fractured internal malleolus fastened in its normal position by means of tacks or a metal plate (see Vol. I, p. 707). Should the bone not be fractured, but only the internal lateral ligament torn, this structure should be sutured accurately. Provision must be made for drainage in case the purification of the soft parts does not suffice to prevent infection, but no opening should be left over the region of the fracture in the tibia if this can be avoided; the skin wound should be sewn up completely and a counter-opening for drainage made at a more dependent spot. If skin has been cut away in this region the raw surface that would otherwise be left may be covered by sliding a flap from the skin of the leg above. Healing will probably be more rapid if the seat of fracture about the malleolus and the mechanical fixation apparatus are covered with healthy skin.

Operations for simple recent Pott's fracture. Operative interference will be required when the surgeon cannot effect complete reduction of the dislocation under an anæsthetic. These cases are comparatively rare; they are generally due to the interposition of some structure between the bone surfaces, such, for instance, as the tendon of the tibialis posticus (posterior) or a portion of bone, generally a fragment of the internal malleolus or of the astragalus. This not only prevents reduction but interferes materially with the subsequent usefulness of the foot.

The objects of the operation will not be limited to getting the astragalus into position; the fractured surfaces of the tibia should also be fastened together. A good incision is a curved one with its concavity forward, commencing just in front of the inner border of the tibia, about two inches above the joint level, curving around the tip of the internal malleolus, and extending as far forward as the tubercle of the scaphoid (navicular). The incision is deepened down to the bone, taking care to avoid damage to the tendon of the tibialis posticus (posterior), and the joint is opened through the fracture at the base of the internal malleolus, or, if that does not exist, through the ruptured internal lateral ligament. The parts are fully retracted and the cause of the difficulty in reduction is ascertained. Should this be the tendon of the tibialis posticus (posterior), this is hooked out of the way with a retractor, and the astragalus pushed into place. If it be a loose piece of bone, this is removed, if small, and the surface from which it has been detached is smoothed off with a gouge or burr; if large, it is re-attached to the surface from which it was broken.

The final stage of the operation consists in fastening the internal malleolus back into place or suturing the rent in the internal lateral ligament, according to which lesion is present. The wound is closed without a drainage tube, and the foot is put up at right angles to the leg in plaster of Paris, in a slightly inverted position, so as to relax all the structures on the inner side of the foot. The sutures are removed at the end of ten days, and passive movement and massage are begun, if necessary, under an anæsthetic within the first few days.

Operations for simple Pott's fracture of long standing are required when there is considerable deformity and disability, as the patient is frequently crippled and unable to follow his employment. The outward dislocation associated with this deformity throws the weight of the body upon the inner border of the foot and flattens its arch; this, combined with partial ankylosis of the joint, gives rise to much pain and disability.

The ankle-joint must be opened and an attempt made to restore the bones to their normal positions. A stereoscopic radiogram helps greatly to determine what the condition of affairs is, and therefore what procedure is most likely to be effectual. Not infrequently the inability to reduce the deformity is due to the internal malleolus having become deflected outwards and united to its base in that position. This will necessitate exposure of the joint from the inner side, through the incision recommended above, and detachment of the malleolus, after which attempts must be made to rectify the outward displacement of the astragalus. This may require re-fracture of the fibula in order to allow its lower end to be rotated upon the inferior tibio-fibular ligaments, so that the astragalus may carry with it the external lateral ligament and the tip of the malleolus as it is pushed inwards. If this can be done, the result will probably be satisfactory; it will be necessary to smooth down with a gouge any callus about the base of the malleolus and then to fasten the tip of that process in position with tacks or bone plates.

In many cases, however, this theoretically ideal operation cannot be performed, as the two articular surfaces will not work accurately together, in spite of all attempts to make them do so. Under these circumstances there is the choice of two methods:—

(a) To pare down the articular surfaces until the astragalus rests in the tibio-fibular arch with the foot in its normal position, so that the patient can bear his weight upon the normal points of support. In order to do this, the fracture in the fibula will certainly have to be reproduced so as to allow the external malleolus to be pushed inwards into proper position. The bone surfaces that have been pared away to make the astragalus (talus) fit must be rendered as smooth as possible, and it is a good plan to fasten over the raw surfaces thus left a flap of the fatty structures from the immediate neighbourhood; this facilitates movement in the joint subsequently (see p. 5). The foot is put up strictly at right angles to the leg, and should be kept rigid for the first ten days, after which time careful movement may be begun; the greatest care must be taken to see that there is no lateral deflexion of the foot.

(b) The other alternative is to excise the astragalus (see p. 51). This operation gives a movable ankle but rather a weak joint in an adult; in children, in whom the functional results are excellent, these fractures rarely, if ever, occur.

Operations for fractures of the astragalus. The steps of the operation cannot be given in detail, as they depend so largely upon the condition of affairs present. The joint may be exposed through an internal or an external incision (see p. 51), or by both combined, and the subsequent steps are similar to those described for Pott's fracture. Detached portions of bone should be removed, if small, or fastened back into place, if large, and the most careful attempt should be made to restore the condition of the joint as accurately as possible. It may be necessary to excise the astragalus entirely (see p. 51).

ARTHRODESIS

Indications. Arthrodesis of the ankle-joint may be usefully employed in cases of advanced infantile paralysis in which all the muscles around the joint are paralysed, giving rise to a flail-limb that is unable to bear the patient's weight. By means of apparatus it will of course be possible to prevent the joint from collapsing when weight is put upon it, but this is cumbrous and expensive, and may prove too much for the patient's strength, especially when there is also paralysis of some of the muscles moving the knee. Under these circumstances a more useful limb can be obtained if the ankle-joint be steadied by producing ankylosis.

Operation. The joint may be opened by the lateral incisions described below (see p. 51), but in these cases it is quicker to open the joint by a transverse incision across the front, dividing some, or if necessary all, of the extensor tendons. The muscles moving these are paralysed, and they are therefore useless, but if desired, it is easy to identify and suture them at the end of the operation. The anterior route gives better access, and it is important in these cases to remove the cartilage as completely as possible; this is done with a chisel or gouge, which clears the articular surfaces of the tibio-fibular arch, the malleoli, and the astragalus as completely as possible. The bony surfaces are then put back into apposition, the wound and the divided tendons are sutured, and the limb is put up in plaster of Paris with the foot strictly at right angles to the leg. The stitches are removed in ten days' time and an immovable plaster casing is then put on; it should be worn for nearly six months after the operation.

Results. The chief difficulty is to obtain firm bony union. Fibrous union is obtained in many cases, and when bony union does occur it may be extremely slow.

EXCISION OF THE ANKLE-JOINT

True excision of the ankle as distinct from excision of the astragalus on the one hand and arthrotomy for fractures on the other is never performed save for tuberculous disease. By the term is meant complete removal of the articular surfaces, both bony and synovial; this will be dealt with by Mr. Stiles.

OPERATIONS UPON THE TARSAL BONES AND JOINTS

EXCISION OF THE ASTRAGALUS

Indications. Excision of the astragalus (talus) alone is fairly often done, although it is most frequently practised as a part of the modern form of excision of the ankle. Apart from excision it may be done :—

(i) *In cases of injury.* These may be either severe comminution of the bone or such extensive contamination of it with dirt that there is no hope of avoiding sepsis otherwise.

(ii) *In extreme talipes equinus following infantile paralysis.* Here the pointing of the foot gradually protrudes the astragalus from the tibio-fibular arch, with the result that the bone becomes too broad in front to enable it to be returned beneath it when the tendo Achillis is divided; in order to get the foot at right angles to the leg the astragalus must either be removed or so cut down as to allow it to pass into position. As these cases are usually met with in children in whom the functional results of removal of the astragalus are extremely good, it is better to remove the bone than to pare it down.

(iii) *In cases of extreme congenital talipes varus.* In order to overcome the extreme deformity it may be necessary to remove the astragalus (talus), after which the foot can be got into good position.

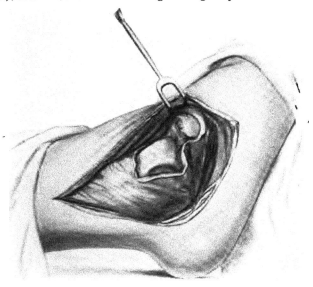

Fig. 18. Incision for Excision of the Astragalus. The peronei tendons have been divided by an oblique section. The ankle-joint has been opened as well as the astragalo-scaphoid joint.

Operation. The incision that I have used most frequently for the above conditions is a crescentic one over the outer ankle, commencing immediately behind the fibula two and a half inches above the tip of the external malleolus, extending down to the tip of that structure and forwards along the outer aspect of the foot as far as the prominence on the base of the fifth metatarsal (see Fig. 18). This incision is deepened, and the structures in front of it are dissected up for a short distance in the form of a flap. The foot is now plantar-flexed and everted in order to relax the peronei tendons, which are then separated from the back of the fibula, turned out of their groove beneath the external malleolus, and entrusted to an assistant, who keeps them out of danger beneath a hook. This may be very difficult, and a much easier plan is to divide the tendons by an oblique section and suture them at the end of the operation. The external lateral ligament is divided and the incision carried forwards so

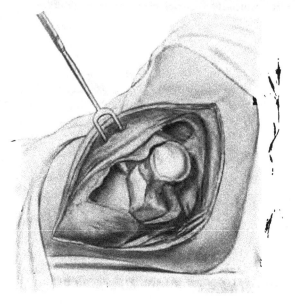

Fig. 19. Exposure of the Astragalus. The head of the bone has been separated from the scaphoid and the interosseus ligament has been divided.

as to expose the head of the astragalus (talus) and open the joint between it and the scaphoid (navicular). In order to do this the foot is forcibly inverted and the toes bent inwards. When the astragalo-scaphoid (talo-navicular) joint has been opened, the point of the knife can be passed along the under surface of the former bone and made to divide the inter-osseous ligament between the astragalus (talus) and the os calcis (cal-caneus), when the former bone can be made to start up prominently in the wound by further inverting the foot, which is dislocated inwards almost completely (see Fig. 19). The head of the astragalus (talus) is seized in lion forceps, and a few touches of the knife will remove it altogether (see Fig. 20).

The os calcis (calcaneus) is then brought up against the malleoli, and in young children will fit fairly well without much risk of dislocation. In adults, however, the projection of the sustentaculum tali makes the bone too broad to fit beneath the malleoli, and it is well, therefore, to pare down the articular surfaces so as to make them fit. A portion may be

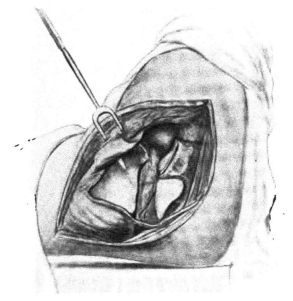

FIG. 20. REMOVAL OF THE ASTRAGALUS. The articular surfaces of the tibia and the os calcis are seen, as well as the divided interosseous membrane.

taken off each side of the os calcis (calcaneus), and the articular surfaces of the malleoli may also be cut away, but the whole of the sustentaculum tali should not be removed, as it is required for the support of the tibialis posticus (posterior) tendon passing beneath it.

The wound is closed without a drainage tube, and the limb should be put up in a plaster of Paris casing; there must be no lateral deflexion of the foot, which should be at right angles to the limb. Throughout the after-treatment the most important point is to see that no lateral displacement of the foot occurs, and for this purpose a plaster of Paris casing strengthened with metal at the sides should be used for the first three months, followed later on by an apparatus with lateral irons and a hinge at the ankle-joint. This will have to be worn for nearly two years in the case of a child; an adult will probably have to wear it for a much longer period.

Excellent results follow the simpler method of excising the bone after dividing the extensor tendons, and the operation is preferred by some to the one described above. A large flap is made upon the front of the ankle with its convexity downwards towards the toes. The incision reaches from one malleolus to the other, and its lowest point is on a level with the tubercle of the scaphoid. All the tendons are divided over the front of the joint, and the dorsalis pedis artery and the anterior tibial nerve are cut across and the ankle-joint opened from the front. This gives very free access to the astragalus, which is first freed from its attachments to the lateral ligaments of the ankle-joint and then from the scaphoid (navicular) in front. In order to remove the bone it is then only necessary to divide its connexions with the os calcis (calcaneus). The ends of the extensor tendons are identified and united at the end of the operation; speedy union occurs in aseptic cases and there is no loss of power on this account.

EXCISION OF THE OS CALCIS

Indications. (i) *For tuberculous disease.* The operations for this condition will be described by Mr. Stiles.

(ii) *For injury.* Severe comminuted fractures of the os calcis (calcaneus), especially when they are compound, will require an operation in order to secure the best results. This, however, will usually be only a partial excision.

(iii) *For new growths of the bone.* In the majority of cases an amputation of the foot will be the safer procedure, but in innocent tumours and in myelomata the bone may be excised and the progress of affairs watched.

Operation. The operation is difficult, owing partly to the want of elasticity in the cutaneous structures, but chiefly to the difficulty of dissecting out the sustentaculum tali. A good method of gaining free access to the bone is by making a vertical incision along the outer edge of the tendo Achillis, beginning an inch and a half above the upper edge of the os calcis (calcaneus) and reaching down to just above the outer margin of the sole. A second incision is carried at right angles to the first, horizontally round the back of the heel and along the outer border of the foot, from a point a finger's breadth behind the internal malleolus to the tuberosity of the fifth metatarsal bone.

This incision gives two large flaps, of which the upper is dissected off the posterior and outer aspects of the os calcis first. In doing this the tendo Achillis is divided above, the external lateral ligament on the outer aspect of the bone, and the ligaments of the calcaneo-cuboid joint in front. The lower or plantar flap is now raised as far as the flexibility of the skin permits, and then the foot is firmly inverted, the peronei tendons are hooked out of the way, and the calcaneo-astragaloid (talo-calcaneal) joint is opened and the firm interosseous ligament divided. The remaining ligaments of the calcaneo-cuboid joint are cut through, and all that remains to be done is to sever the attachments of the bone on the inner side. In order to do this in the easiest way the foot must be very forcibly inverted and the tendon of the tibialis posticus (posterior) looked for as it passes under the sustentaculum tali in its special groove. It is raised from this and held out of the way with a hook. When this has been done, the knife is passed along the inner side of the bone from end to end, dividing the internal lateral ligament of the ankle and the ligaments connecting the os calcis (calcaneus) and astragalus (talus) on the inner side. A few touches of the knife then complete the removal of the bone.

A drainage tube should be inserted in the large and irregular cavity thus made. The cavity soon shrinks up, and the patient can walk well upon the heel provided that a small pad be placed beneath it. The stump is quite sound in about six weeks.

CHAPTER VI

OPERATIONS UPON THE KNEE-JOINT

REMOVAL OF DISPLACED SEMILUNAR CARTILAGES

Indications. In cases of recurrent displacement of the semilunar cartilage operation is now a safe and easy way of putting an end to a troublesome and often crippling affection. For a first or even a second attack it is not necessary to operate, since careful massage and suitable movements will often bring about a permanent cure; should the displacement recur in spite of this, however, early operation is indicated, since by it the displaced cartilage (which is practically always the internal one) can be removed and subsequent attacks prevented. The functions of the joint are unimpaired after removal of the cartilage, provided that this be done before the affection has lasted long enough for the recurrent inflammatory attacks to set up chronic changes in the joint resembling those of osteo-arthritis; in such cases removal of the cartilage will not necessarily be followed by complete restoration of the functions of the joint.

Operation. Various incisions may be used to expose the inner tuberosity of the tibia, along the upper border of which lies the cartilage. This should be felt for carefully before the skin incision is made, and the examination should be repeated before the capsule is opened by putting the finger on the joint and flexing and extending it. It is easy to mistake the level of the knee-joint, and, although this is not of much importance in other operations on the knee, in this particular one the difference of a quarter of an inch in the level of the incision in the capsule changes the operation from a simple to a difficult one.

In this operation, as in all of those upon the knee-joint, the limb should be purified from mid-thigh to mid-calf and wrapped up securely in sterilized cloths so that the assistant's hands cannot come into contact with unsterilized parts during the manipulations of the leg that may be necessary during the operation.

The surgeon faces the inner side of the knee, which should be semi-flexed and outwardly rotated. He makes an incision exposing the upper border of the inner tuberosity of the tibia from the inner margin of the ligamentum patellæ backwards to the junction of the inner with the posterior surface of the tibia. A very useful incision for this purpose is a crescentic one with its convexity forwards. This gives a flap which can be extended backwards by prolonging the horns of the incision if necessary; the advantage of this is that the skin incision does not lie over that in the capsule. Before raising the flap small cuts or scratches may be made across the incision so as to identify the corresponding points when the flap has to be sutured at the end of the operation, by which time its outline will have become somewhat altered. If preferred, however, a transverse or a vertical incision may be made. The vertical incision is parallel to the vessels and nerves of the limb and so saves them from injury, but it is rather difficult to get proper exposure through it unless it be very long, and a second incision posterior to the first may be required in order to get at the cartilage satisfactorily.

The flap is dissected back and the capsule of the joint over the inner condyle exposed. After all bleeding points have been ligatured, the capsule is opened by a horizontal incision parallel to and about a quarter of an inch above the upper margin of the inner tuberosity of the tibia, which should be carefully defined by the finger; the capsule only should be divided and not the synovial membrane. There is often free bleeding from the articular arteries in doing this, and this should be checked before proceeding further. The synovial membrane which is thus exposed is caught up with fine-toothed forceps and snipped through with scissors in order to open the articular cavity, and the incision is enlarged sufficiently to give a good view into the joint.

The condition of the internal semilunar cartilage can now be made out by retracting the edges of the wound in the capsule; the limb will have to be flexed rather acutely to display the front of the joint well. Various lesions of the cartilage, such as detachment from its insertion or transverse or longitudinal ruptures, partial or entire, may be met with; but these are of little importance, since the only effective method of treatment is to remove as much of the cartilage as can be got at through the incision in the capsule.

In order to remove the cartilage, its convex edge, which will have been torn away from the head of the tibia by the accident, is seized in catch forceps, and the cartilage is raised and, if necessary, separated from its lateral attachments so that a pair of fine curved scissors can be slipped round its anterior extremity and made to divide its attachment in front, if that has not already been separated by the original injury. This is seized in forceps and the back part of the cartilage is put upon the stretch, freed by scissors, and divided as far back in the joint as the scissors can reach. The whole operation can be done without any further interference with the joint than the introduction of the scissors into it. Very little bleeding accompanies the intra-articular part of the operation; it is easily stopped by douching the joint with hot saline solution. Some surgeons make a point of removing the entire cartilage, but this is a much more difficult matter, and, as far as my experience goes, is not necessary. The simplest way of doing it is to make a second small incision in the capsule just behind the condyle and to divide the posterior end of the cartilage through that, as it would weaken the joint unduly to divide the capsule and the internal lateral ligament over the whole of the cartilage.

When all bleeding has been arrested, a fine catgut suture unites the cut edges of the synovial membrane. A somewhat stouter one sutures the capsule, after which the skin wound is brought together with a separate suture. Outside the dressing the joint is enveloped in a thick mass of wool, bandaged on firmly so as to exert an elastic compression which will prevent effusion and restrict movement. No splint is needed; the knee is slightly flexed and the limb is elevated upon a comfortable pillow.

After-treatment. The patient may move his limb inside the dressing if he desires to do so. After a week a lighter dressing may be substituted and the patient encouraged to move the limb more freely. The sutures are removed on the tenth or twelfth day, and vigorous active and passive movements should then be employed. Perfect use of the limb should be regained within three weeks from the operation.

Difficulties and dangers. The chief danger is *sepsis*, the risk of which cannot be over-estimated. No one should perform this operation who is not confident of commanding complete asepsis throughout. Should sepsis occur, the joint must be opened immediately and drained freely (see p. 60). Another danger is *hæmorrhage* into the joint at the close of the operation, which may easily happen unless the surgeon be careful to secure every bleeding point as he goes on. It is always best to apply a ligature to all of these, as very slight bleeding in the joint may give rise to anxiety as to the progress of the case and a definite retardation in convalescence; the patient may be left with a distended capsule, for which prolonged treatment may be required. It is sometimes difficult to find the displaced cartilage; this generally results from incising the capsule too high above the cartilage. In order to get properly at the cartilage the joint has then to be opened unduly freely, and some weakness of the capsule may result. The best way to avoid this is to palpate the parts well while the joint is being moved after the skin incision has been made. The sharp edge of the tibia is unmistakable and will guide the surgeon to the right spot.

It occasionally happens that the joint remains weak for some little time after the operation. This is only likely to occur when the patient has had recurrent attacks for a long time before seeking surgical aid. The interior of the joint at this stage will show a widely thickened and inflamed synovial membrane, and this condition may persist for a considerable time after removal of the exciting cause. In these cases massage and exercises designed to strengthen the thigh muscles and thereby tighten up the capsule are most beneficial.

ARTHROTOMY AND DRAINAGE

Indications. The knee-joint rarely requires to be drained for any affection other than suppurative arthritis. It has been proposed to incise and drain the knee-joint as treatment for gonorrhœal or simple acute rheumatism, with the view of relieving tension, alleviating pain, and promoting restoration of function more rapidly than can be done by non-operative measures. The only experience that I have in this direction is in connexion with gonorrhœal rheumatism. On five occasions I have incised freely a knee-joint which was acutely distended as the result of gonorrhœal arthritis, and in all the cases the relief of pain was very striking. In four out of the five the swelling had subsided completely within six weeks, and the functions of the joint were left unimpaired. In the remaining case the synovial membrane remained thickened for three months after the wound had healed.

Operation. The knee is a difficult joint to drain, and drastic measures have been proposed in order to effect this. In early days a large drainage tube was passed through the joint from side to side beneath the patella. A useful improvement upon this was the plan of effecting drainage by continuous irrigation, while more recently the late Mr. Harold Barnard (*Clin. Soc. Trans.*, vol. xxxvi, p. 150) proposed a very thorough drainage scheme for this complex joint. The most radical method is excision of the articular surfaces so as to open up the joint cavity and to obliterate most of its recesses. This method can hardly be recommended at the present day, however. Its chief result will be to open up large areas of cancellous bone to septic infection. A better plan would be to adopt the line of treatment suggested and practised by Mr. Eve (*loc. sup. cit.*), who cut across the front of the joint, divided the patella, and flexed the knee fully so as to expose the recesses of the joint. Such a method must of course result in a stiff limb, and nothing but the desperate state of the patient would justify recourse to it. It is hardly likely that such extreme measures would be called for when infection has followed a surgical operation, such as removal of a semilunar cartilage, or wiring of the patella. Here the surgeon would be alive to the nature of the case very early, and less radical measures should suffice to secure recovery with a more or less movable limb. It may therefore be advisable to divide the operations for drainage of the joint into two groups: those in which the infection is slight, *e.g.* those in which the infection follows a surgical operation, and those in which the infection is severe, as in neglected cases of injury to the joint, or those accompanying infection from acute infective osteomyelitis.

In cases of mild infection. These probably form the majority of cases met with in practice at the present day, and good results may be looked for if the treatment be undertaken early enough and be sufficiently thorough. Effective drainage may be obtained by opening the joint by two free vertical incisions, each about a finger's breadth from the edge of the patella and reaching from the level of its lower margin to a full inch above its upper border. This exposes the front and lateral aspects of the joint fully, and enables the surgeon to inspect the interior and to ascertain the extent of the subcrural pouch above the patella, whereby he can judge whether it is necessary to employ direct drainage of this space. If so, a pair of dressing forceps is thrust from one of the lateral wounds to the upper limit of the pouch and its points are cut down upon through the skin in the middle line; a large drainage tube is drawn through from this opening in the skin and made to project through one of the lateral incisions, generally the inner one. In the majority of cases it is well to drain the outer side of the joint also, and this can be done by passing down a pair of sinus forceps over the outer condyle to the lowest limit of the joint and thrusting them through the capsule in that situation. An incision is made through the skin over the points of the forceps and a drainage tube introduced from behind into the outer recess of the joint. In doing this care must be taken to divide only the skin with the knife, otherwise the external popliteal nerve may be endangered. A large tube is passed across the front of the joint from the inner to the outer incision beneath the patella, and the joint cavity can be drained freely in this manner in the majority of cases. The tubes can be arranged so as to permit of continuous irrigation of the joint, the fluid being run into the joint through the tube above the patella or through one end of the tube passing across the front of the joint. Before the first dressings are applied the whole of the interior of the joint should be flushed out freely with sterilized salt solution.

In cases of acute infection. In the cases suited for the preceding operation the infection is mainly in the front and lateral aspects of the joint, but in the more severe ones there is a tendency for the posterior sacs to be acutely infected, and it is difficult to drain these from the front. The late Mr. Barnard (*loc. sup. cit.*) drew attention to the importance of these synovial sacs which contain the corresponding condyle. They lie between the head of the gastrocnemius and the bone, and the outer pouch sends a prolongation along the popliteus. He strongly advocated separate incisions for the drainage of each of these sacs. On the inner side the prominent inner condyle can be cut down upon when the limb is extended and forceps, carrying a drainage tube, can be introduced into the joint. On the outer side a vertical incision should be made between the biceps tendon and the outer head of the gastrocnemius just behind the external popliteal nerve, going through skin only. The capsule of the joint over the condyle is exposed with a blunt dissector, incised, and a drainage tube inserted. In addition to these incisions, drainage of the front of the joint should be effected by vertical incisions on either side of the patella and a median one above it for draining the subcrural pouch. Mr. Barnard noted the frequency with which pus under pressure spurted out from the outer posterior pouch when it was incised.

After-treatment. The dressings require to be changed frequently, and it is a good plan to employ peroxide of hydrogen (10 vols. per cent.) at each dressing. As the discharge diminishes, the drainage tubes are gradually shortened and finally withdrawn. Passive movement is begun as early as possible, the limb meanwhile being kept upon a splint in order to prevent the contraction which the powerful hamstring muscles would otherwise produce. The most important point in the after-treatment is to keep the patella from becoming adherent to the front of the condyles, and this must therefore be moved freely at each dressing. It is remarkable that excellent functional results have been obtained in this manner even after the most severe infection.

REPAIR OF THE CRUCIAL LIGAMENTS

This operation is a very rare one, and has, as far as my knowledge goes, only been performed once (Mayo Robson, *Clin. Soc. Trans.,* vol. xxxvi, p. 92). The joint was opened by a curved incision across the front, dividing the ligamentum patellæ about its middle. Both the crucial ligaments had been torn from their upper attachments and had to be stitched in position with catgut sutures. The anterior ligament was fastened to the synovial membrane and adjacent tissues on the inner side of the external condyle; the posterior had to be split in order to lengthen it, and was fastened by sutures to the synovial membrane and cartilage on the outer side of the inner condyle. The patient made an uneventful recovery with perfect use of his limb. He was seen six years after the operation, when the abnormal mobility present before the operation had been entirely lost, and there was no interference with movement except some limitation of flexion, the knee becoming fixed when it was flexed just beyond a right angle. There was fine creaking felt in the joint on movement, and the patient said it was more liable to pain in damp and cold weather.

This operation seems worthy of being added to the list of recognized surgical operations, since the injury is by no means as uncommon as might be thought. I have recently seen two cases resulting from severe hunting accidents in which, however, the degree of disability was not extreme enough to demand operative interference in a well-to-do patient. The description of the above case, however, shows that in those who follow laborious occupations the operation has a definite field of usefulness. The patient operated upon by Mr. Mayo Robson was a miner and followed his occupation from the time of his discharge from the Leeds Infirmary without any trouble.

REMOVAL OF THE SYNOVIAL MEMBRANE OF THE KNEE

Indications. The joint is frequently opened for the removal of diseased synovial membrane. As a rule, however, this affection is tuberculous, and the operation for this condition does not fall within the scope of the present article and is dealt with by Mr. Stiles.

The synovial membrane, however, or a considerable part of it, may not infrequently have to be removed for other reasons. Thus it may become hypertrophied and covered with papillary outgrowths, which give rise to so much inconvenience in locomotion as to call for active surgical interference. This affection may be diffused over almost the whole of the synovial membrane, or it may be limited to a few spots, generally in the neighbourhood of the inner condyle and the margin of the patella. This condition is apparently distinct from the ordinary osteo-arthritis. Occasionally the joint is opened for the removal of osteophytic outgrowths or polypoid masses of synovial membrane occurring in osteo-arthritis and acting as a mechanical obstruction to movement.

Operation. As a rule it is well to open the joint by a free incision, and for this purpose none is better than a long vertical incision about a finger's breadth to the inner side of the patella. This gives admirable access to the whole of the inner side and most of the anterior part of the joint, and the synovial membrane can be dissected out with ease and accuracy. Should it be deemed necessary, a similar incision can be added on the outer side of the patella, and any portion of the affected synovial membrane on the front of the joint that cannot be reached from the inner wound may be removed from that.

It is needless to say that the most scrupulous attention must be paid to disinfection of the skin. The whole of the joint must be purified carefully front and back, and the limb above and below securely wrapped up in sterilized towels, as it will be necessary to move the joint frequently during the course of the operation. It is well to raise the skin as a flap, so that the incision in it does not lie directly over the incision in the capsule. The steps of this part of the operation are similar to those for removal of a displaced semilunar cartilage (see p. 56).

When the joint has been incised, its interior is inspected and the particular portion of the synovial membrane that has to be removed is identified. This patch should then be marked out by carrying an incision around it with the knife or scissors, and the whole thickness of that part of the synovial membrane should be dissected off. This is generally effected best with blunt-pointed scissors, which serve both as cutting and dissecting instruments. An attempt should be made to remove the affected area in one mass, however large may be the extent of synovial membrane that has to be removed. After removal, all bleeding points are ligatured with fine catgut, and any oozing is stopped by douching the joint freely with sterilized salt solution at a temperature of 115° F. When all the bleeding has ceased, the incision in the joint is closed accurately, the capsule being united by a separate fine continuous catgut suture; no drainage tube is employed. The dressing should consist of a roll of gauze, which is wound round the limb so as to prevent swelling from extravasation of blood. No splint is required.

After-treatment. The patient is encouraged to bend his knee from the first, and massage and passive movements should be employed, beginning at the end of the first week. When the stitches are removed, the massage should be vigorous and the patient should be encouraged to walk at as early a date as possible.

Results. The results of some of these cases are really remarkable. I have on several occasions removed almost the whole of the excisable portion of the synovial membrane for a papillary non-tuberculous synovitis which had resisted all previous treatment for many months, and was the source of complete incapacity to the patient. The pain and swelling were not only cured, but perfect movement in the limb resulted without any difficulty whatever and without any necessity for the use of passive movements under an anæsthetic. With complete asepsis and the use of non-irritating lotions the most extensive raw surfaces may be left in contact within the joint without impairing movement.

OPERATIONS FOR INTRA-ARTICULAR FRACTURES

Although strictly speaking operation for the fixation of a fracture about the lower extremity of the femur is practically always in the nature of an arthrotomy in that the joint is always incised, yet as a rule the operation itself is performed mainly outside the joint, and the chief interest in the case centres in the approximation of the fragments rather than the technique of the joint surgery. Occasionally it may be necessary to open the joint freely for the treatment of a fracture of the spine of the tibia, in which case the operation will be very similar to that for suture of the crucial ligaments (see p. 61). A very important fracture involving the knee-joint is that of the patella, the operations for which it will be well to consider here.

OPERATIONS FOR FRACTURE OF THE PATELLA

There are several operations for fracture of the patella, all of which have for their object the close approximation and fixation of the fragments so that true bony union shall result.

Indications. Much difference of opinion has occurred during the last twenty years as to the indications for operative interference in fractures of the patella. Even at the present day there are still surgeons who consider that the age of the patient and his occupation should influence the question whether an operation should be done or not. Neither the age of the patient nor his occupation should determine the question. The only points of real importance are the nature of the fracture and the patient's ability to undergo any ordinary operation.

In a fit subject for operation, any fracture of the patella, either recent or of long standing, which is of the transverse variety and is accompanied by separation of the fragments should be operated upon, as this condition of affairs inevitably ends in fibrous union and probably in considerable disability of the joint. The stellate or longitudinal fractures which are readily differentiated by the X-rays, and which are not accompanied by any marked separation of the fragments, are excluded from this category; in them excellent bony union usually results without operation.

As the steps of the operation, and to some extent its results, differ somewhat according to whether the operation is done for recent cases or those of long standing, these two groups will be described separately.

OPERATIONS FOR RECENT FRACTURES

Before discussing the methods by which a fractured patella may be united, it is important to consider the question of *when to operate*. Some difference of opinion still exists upon this point, but the tendency is in favour of early, if not immediate, operation. It would appear reasonable that the sooner the joint is opened, the blood cleared out of it, and all bleeding points secured the better; moreover, the sooner the broken ends are brought into apposition the more accurately they fit, and this to some extent makes the operation easier, as the surgeon sees exactly what he has to do, and his view is not obscured by the blood-clot which clings very tenaciously to the fractured surfaces when the injury is a few days old. It was formerly thought that sepsis was more likely to occur if operations were carried out immediately after receipt of the injury; this was attributed partly to the inflammatory reaction following the injury, and partly to the difficulty of securing perfect asepsis of the skin. While it is now recognized that the first objection has no foundation in fact, the second one, namely, the difficulty of securing asepsis, may be of importance in certain cases. The skin over the front of the knee is rough, thick, and, in labouring men, often deeply ingrained with dirt, so that it may be a matter of extreme difficulty to get it into a condition approaching that of sterility, except after prolonged saturation of the superficial layers of the epidermis with antiseptics so that they can be actually scraped off and the surface beneath purified. Personally, it is my invariable custom to operate upon all these cases as soon after they are seen as is convenient, but in the case of a labouring man whose skin is thick and dirty there is no objection to postponing the operation for two or three days, so that in the meantime cleansing methods may have a fair chance. The old rule, however, of leaving the case for ten days or a fortnight until most of the effusion has become absorbed should not be followed. This is a bad rule, as it allows coagulation of the effused blood to take place and the clot to become so closely adherent to the broken bone and the torn synovial membrane that it is difficult to remove it without doing more damage to the delicate articular structures than the joint should be exposed to.

In preparing the limb for operation it should be shaved from mid-leg to mid-thigh and thoroughly scrubbed with ether soap, followed by 1 in 20 carbolic lotion, which has a considerable power of penetrating epidermis. A compress of sterilized gauze, wet with 1–2,000 sublimate solution, should then be bandaged over the knee and kept from evaporating by gutta-percha tissue placed outside. This forms a wet dressing, which is removed in six hours, and the skin again scrubbed with ether soap and hot water, followed by another application of the wet 1–2,000 sublimate dressing, and a final purification with ether soap and 1–500 sublimate solution is carried out just before the operation. This method of purification applies to ordinary cases; in labouring men with dirty horny skin it should be repeated every eight hours until the operation takes place, and it should be done at least three times.

Operation. The only operation of which I have personal experience is that rendered classical by Lord Lister. I have always found it give such excellent results that I have never been tempted to practise any other.

Lord Lister's method. The surgeon and his assistants should wear gloves, and all instruments, sponges, &c., should be wrung out of sterilized salt solution. As little interference with the structures of the joint as possible should be permitted, and everything should be done with the greatest gentleness.

The best *incision* is a semilunar one, with its convexity upwards and its extremities on a somewhat lower level than the fracture. The left thumb and forefinger are placed on either side of the patella at a distance of about three-quarters of an inch from its margin and about half an inch below the level of the fracture, and between these two points the convex incision is marked out, its upper limit reaching just to the upper border of the patella. This gives a flap the cicatrix of which is nowhere exposed to pressure. In order to facilitate accurate suture of the flap at the end of the operation I always make two or three small cross cuts when marking out the incision at the commencement of the operation, so that the corresponding points on the two sides of the incision can be easily recognized when the flap has to be sewn up. The flap is turned down by a few touches of the knife; it rarely requires much dissection, as the first incision usually opens into the distended prepatellar bursa, which communicates with the fracture; a few small vessels will require clamping. The turned-down flap is covered with gauze while the fracture is inspected; this usually occurs about the junction of the lower with the middle third of the bone, and is prolonged on either side as a considerable rupture of the capsular ligament. As it is important to get a good view of the interior of the joint in order to wash out clot and effect accurate coaptation, the capsule should be incised on either side if the fracture of the patella has not already ruptured it.

The next step is to wash away all blood and clot from the fractured surfaces and the surrounding tissues, and to see how many pieces the patella is split into; it not infrequently happens that the lower fragment is split up into two or more portions. All bleeding points should be secured, and before drilling the bone the surgeon determines whether he will put in one or two wires, and how thick the wire shall be. When the fracture is a simple transverse one, consisting merely of an upper and lower fragment, the latter being of reasonable size, I have always found

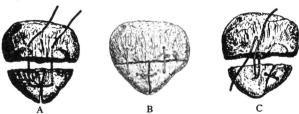

A   B   C

FIG. 21.   METHODS OF INSERTING SUTURES IN COMMINUTED FRACTURES OF THE PATELLA. A shows a mattress suture applied so as to approximate three fragments. B shows the same fragments secured by three separate sutures, while c shows a good method when only a small portion is chipped off the lower fragment. Here the larger one is approximated by the usual stout median wire and the small portion is united to it by a fine lateral one.

it sufficient to use a single median wire of gauge No. 5 (French catheter scale).

When, however, the patella is split into three fragments, it may be necessary to use more than one wire. A simple method of fastening three fragments together by one wire is by means of a mattress suture

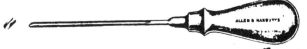

FIG. 22.   BONE DRILL FOR WIRING. There is a large groove in the end of the drill which serves as a guide for the passage of the wire (see Fig. 23).

(see Fig. 21), which takes a secure hold on all three. Occasionally it may be necessary to use three sutures (see Fig. 21), a fine wire to join the lower fragments together and two stouter ones to join the united lower ones to the upper. In either of these cases the wire used need only be of gauge 4, as the strain upon it will not be so great as when a single median wire is employed.

Drilling the bone is best done by means of an electrically driven drill, as the high speed at which the drill runs enables it to penetrate the fragments with the least amount of damage to the joint structures and the least application of force; the surgeon is, therefore, able to direct the shaft of his drill more accurately and with less chance of deflexion.

The most difficult part of the operation lies in drilling the fragments
so as to make the drill-holes correspond exactly to one another on the
fractured surface. If a hand-drill be used Fig. 22 shows the usual pattern. The bone is drilled from its anterior surface to the fracture.
Before doing this, it is advisable to make a small incision through the
soft parts covering the bone, and to push them away from the spot at
which the drill will enter and from which the end of the wire will have to
emerge; it is convenient to keep the edges of this little cut apart by catch-

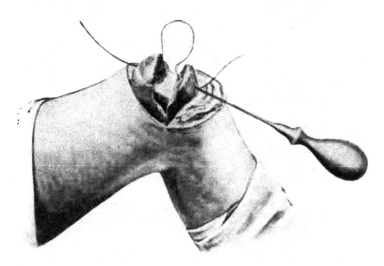

FIG. 23. PASSING THE WIRE IN FRACTURE OF THE PATELLA. The loop into
which the wire is bent is shown. The wire is being guided through the lower
fragment along the groove of the drill.

ing them in forceps. Unless this be done, the end of the wire as it
emerges from the hole in the bone may be caught in the soft tissues and
burrow its way through them for some distance without emerging
directly.

The drill is made to penetrate the upper fragment first and passes
from its anterior aspect to the fractured surface. It is entered nearly
half an inch above the line of fracture and emerges from the fractured
surface just in front of the articular cartilage (see Fig. 23). The lower
fragment is drilled in a similar manner, the drill being entered on the
anterior surface of the bone as near its apex as possible and made to

appear on the fractured surface exactly opposite the hole in the upper fragment and just in front of the articular cartilage. The wire passing through the fragments, therefore, will be outside the articular cavity.

After a little practice it is easy to make the two holes on the fractured surfaces correspond, but for a beginner a simple way of ensuring regularity is to drill the lower fragment first in the manner described above and then to bring the lower fragment into careful apposition while the drill remains *in situ;* if the drill be pushed on slightly, a depression is marked on the fractured surface of the upper fragment. The drill is then withdrawn from the lower fragment and entered at the puncture thus made on the fractured surface of the upper fragment and made to penetrate the fragment from below upwards instead of from above downwards as just described.

When introducing the wire certain precautions are necessary to ensure a good result. A portion of the wire about one foot long is carefully unrolled and straightened, and one end cut somewhat obliquely with cutting-pliers. Great care must be taken to avoid kinking, as a kink in stout wire of this sort is almost impossible to obliterate without removing the wire entirely. In order to introduce the wire, therefore, the portion to be used is made quite straight and one end is introduced through the upper fragment from its anterior aspect and made to emerge through the opening on the fractured surface. The fragment is rotated so that this surface looks well upwards, and the wire is pulled through until only about four inches remains projecting from the anterior surface of the patella. The remainder of the wire is then bent into an easy curve so that it can be carried through the lower fragment from the fractured surface to the anterior aspect (see Fig: 23). If the grooved hand-drill (see Fig. 22) be employed this may be used to guide the wire as it emerges from the front of the lower fragment.

When wire has been passed, its ends are grasped in suitable forceps and firm traction is made upon them in opposite directions. This straightens out the wire and allows an assistant to push the two fragments threaded upon it closely together; when they have been made to meet, the ends of the wire are brought together, twisted round in two complete twists over the upper fragment (see Fig. 24), and the ends cut short with cutting-pliers. The section of the wire should be very oblique, and the ends are hammered down with a fine punch so that they are buried beneath the soft tissues over the front of the patella; a small slit should be made for their reception. If this be done carefully the ends will be buried effectually, and it is unlikely that the wire will require removal subsequently.

All that now remains to be done is to bring together with catgut sutures the rent in the capsule on either side of the fracture and the torn fibrous tissues over the front of the bone. The knee is dressed with gauze loosely rolled around the limb from below upwards so as to exercise a certain amount of compression, but not too much, and outside this is applied a large amount of wool bound on fairly tightly so as to exert good elastic compression and to act to some extent as a splint. No splint is required; it is sufficient to restrain any involuntary movement of the limb

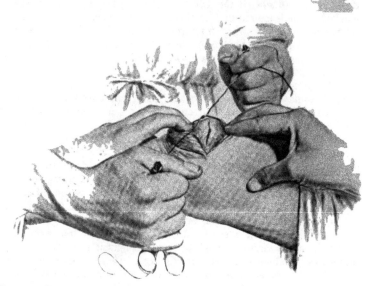

Fig. 24.   Twisting the Wire in Fracture of the Patella.   The fragments
have been pushed together along the wire.

by the use of sand-bags for the first few hours. Two or three pillows should be placed beneath the limb so that the hip is flexed at an angle of about twenty degrees.

After-treatment.   The patient is not discouraged from moving th leg in bed if he desires to do so; he will probably keep it rigidly stiff fo the first week, after which he will gradually attempt some movements; he should be encouraged to do this more and more, so that after the first ten days he will be able to effect a fair amount of flexion. The wound need not be inspected until the end of the first week, when a collodion dressing may be applied and the wool around the limb diminished, in order to allow the patient to move the limb more freely. The stitches may be removed on the tenth day, and the patient may get up between the tenth and fourteenth day. From the fourteenth day onwards I have always been in the habit of allowing my patients to get about with the aid of a stick, trusting entirely to the wire to retain the fragments in position. The patients readily regain the use of the limb, and usually

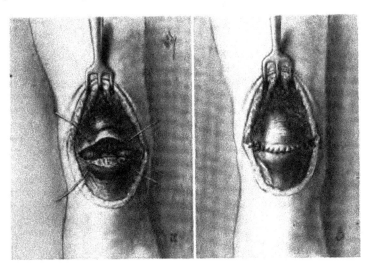

Fig. 25. Suturing the Lateral Capsule for Fracture of the Patella. A represents the lateral tension sutures being placed through the capsule at the side of the patella. The second row of sutures shown in B represents bilateral sutures and running suture suturing the periosteum and fibrous tissue over the patella.

are walking about quite well without any artificial aid at the end of a month from the operation. It is a good plan, however, to have them fitted for the first six weeks or so after the operation with an apparatus that does not allow more than twenty degrees of flexion, so as to prevent any sudden strain from stumbling, &c.

Suture of the Lateral Capsule for Fracture of the Patella. When a simple transverse fracture of the patella exists there is always a tear in the lateral ligaments on either side of the knee-joint. The length of the tear depends upon the amount of separation of the two fragments of the patella. When the edges of the torn ligament are approximated, the fragments of the patella will of necessity be brought into position, thus making it unnecessary to use any suture in the substance of the patella. This method of treatment is common among American surgeons.

Technic. A curved incision is made with the convexity downward. The incision is carried from a point lying just below the condyles of the femur, the lower portion of the convexity being well below the lower border of the patella when in position. A flap is dissected upward, care being taken to avoid injury to the blood-supply. As this flap is dissected upward, the tear in the soft tissues and the fracture line of the patella will come into view. The blood clots in the joint are carefully removed, preferably with tissue forceps or wiped out with soft wet sponges to avoid trauma to the articular surfaces of the joint. The edges of the torn lateral capsule are brought into view, and if ragged the contused parts should be trimmed away with a pair of scissors.

A strong suture either of kangaroo tendon or heavy chromicized catgut is passed through the lateral capsule on either side of the patella. Each suture closely hugs the lateral surface of the patella and includes both the upper and lower margins of the torn lateral capsule (see Fig. 25). When these two sutures are tied, thus closing the patellar end of the tear in the lateral capsule on either side, the fragments of the patella will be brought into close approximation. The remaining portion of the torn lateral capsule on either side is sutured with strong catgut (see Fig. 25). Under certain conditions it is possible to dissect back some of the aponeurosis lying on the dorsum of the patella and this may now be sutured, thus aiding in the fixation and approximation of the patella. The skin wound is now closed with running locked silk stitch and a dressing applied. A posterior moulded splint immobilizes the part until the patient has fully recovered from his anæsthetic.

Passive motion of the joint may be instituted within three or four days, care being taken to avoid overaction with a possible tearing of the sutured capsule.

OPERATIONS FOR FRACTURES OF LONG STANDING

Indications. Surgical interference in fractures of the patella of long standing is only practised to overcome disability of the limb. There are three principal classes of cases in which operation may be called for:

(i) Cases of *re-fracture of the patella after previous wiring*. These may be looked upon as practically recent fractures.

(ii) Cases marked by *a wide gap between the fragments* filled in with fibrous tissue. This condition is not uncommon after non-operative treatment, and in such cases the gap may either be very wide from the first, or the union, which at first was close and satisfactory, may gradually stretch owing to the inability of the fibrous union to bear the strain put upon it. The mere size of the gap between the fragments is not necessarily any criterion as to the necessity for operation or not; the important point is the functional value of the limb. In considering the question of whether to operate on cases of long-standing fracture of the patella, it is important to remember that, quite apart from the question of sepsis, the operation is by no means as easy as it is in the recent cases, and that therefore, in a patient of fairly advanced years with a wide gap between the fragments but a fairly useful limb, it may be a rash procedure to interfere, since the amount of permanent shortening of the muscles present renders the after-treatment necessarily long and the prognosis somewhat uncertain.

(iii) Cases in which the gap between the fragments, although slight, shows distinct evidence of *widening*. Unless the patient be too advanced in years, it is best to interfere at once in these cases and unite the fractured surfaces in the hope of getting firm bony union. The results of operation at this period are more satisfactory than when further stretching has taken place.

Operation. The steps of the operation are exactly similar to those for recent fractures up to the exposure of the fragments. In cases of long standing, changes will have occurred in the fractured surfaces which will interfere with the process of union if they are simply placed in apposition; the bone surfaces require to be refreshed by cutting a thin slice from each fragment with a chisel or saw. If the conditions allow of it these surfaces should be cut at right angles to the long axis of the bone; in any case the two surfaces should be parallel to one another. The fragments are then drilled as described above (see p. 67). It is here that the greatest care is required, as the bone is soft and fatty owing to non-use, and too much traction upon the wires will make them cut their way out of the bone. One way of avoiding this very unpleasant accident is to make use of a mattress suture, as originally suggested by Sir Hector Cameron, and this is an excellent method when the size of the fragments allows (see Fig. 21). The contraction of the quadriceps must also be overcome and reduced to a minimum, and this may offer so great a resistance that it may even be necessary to divide its tendon partially. Before any attempt is made to draw the fragments together it is important to see that the upper fragment is freely mobile. The finger is passed between it and the condyles of the femur, and any adhesions are broken down so that the bone moves freely and can be pulled down. The assistant then extends the knee fully and flexes the extended limb upon the pelvis so as to relax the quadriceps to the utmost. The surgeon takes one fragment in each hand and pushes them together forcibly until they come into contact. If this can be done it will be safe to pass a wire in the ordinary manner; the steps of this are identical with those for recent fractures (see p. 67). If, however, the fragments will not come together satisfactorily in spite of manœuvres of this sort, the surgeon has to make his choice of measures designed for still further relaxation. Three methods are open to him :—

(*a*) Division of the quadriceps extensor tendon.

(*b*) Division and lengthening of the quadriceps muscle.

(*c*) Approximation of the fragments in two stages.

Of these, division of the quadriceps extensor tendon is of very slight value as, in order for it to be effective, the patella must be cut away from its attachments very freely, and its blood-supply and consequently the union of the fragments are thereby seriously endangered. Lengthening the quadriceps muscle gives a more satisfactory result, and may perhaps be the method of choice when the patient is young and the muscular development is good. In elderly subjects, however, it is somewhat difficult to get proper restoration of muscular power after the somewhat weak muscles have been divided.

Another suggested method is to chip off the tubercle and the attachment of the ligamentum patellæ to the tibia, and thus displace the lower fragments upwards and lessen the gap. This operation is more fascinating in theory than useful in practice, and gives very little gain.

For the majority of cases the approximation of the fragments in two stages, as proposed and practised by Lord Lister, is on the whole the soundest in principle and in practice. His description of it, quoted from the *British Medical Journal*, 1908, vol. i, p. 849, is as follows :—

Realizing that a method practised by M. Lucas-Championnière, who, finding himself unable to approximate the fragments, contented himself with connecting them with a long wire and left the wire in position, was open to objections as a permanent arrangement, Lord Lister determined to adopt it as a temporary expedient in order to stretch the quadriceps, and, when the stretching had been brought about, he operated a second time and brought the fragments together. The case he describes is that of a woman who had sustained a fracture of both patellæ four years previously. There were five inches of separation on the left side and the upper fragment was very small. On the right side, however, the upper fragment was of good size and the separation less, and the following operation was performed on it :—

' I made two short longitudinal incisions (A B and C D) over the two fragments (shown in dotted line) (see Fig. 26), and having exposed them by a little dissection, drilled two holes in the upper one, and passed through them, from without inwards, the ends of a piece of the usual stout silver wire, so that, when the ends were pulled upon, the middle of the loop of wire would press upon the surface of the fragment (see Fig. 26 A).

'Next, passing into the lower incision a blunt instrument (a broad raspatory), I detached from the front of the femur the soft parts lying between the incisions, consisting, of course, only of skin and fat, as the muscle was absent at that part. Then passing a strong pair of forceps from the lower incision under the skin till their blades appeared in the upper incision, I seized the ends of the wire and drew them down into the lower incision. I then drilled two holes in the lower fragment and

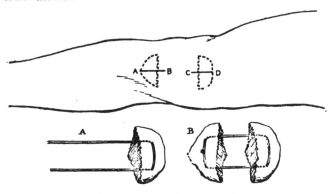

FIG. 26.   LORD LISTER'S OPERATION FOR UNION OF A FRACTURE OF THE PATELLA
OF LONG STANDING WITH WIDE SEPARATION OF THE FRAGMENTS.

passed the ends of the wire through them from within outwards, and, after drawing the upper fragment well down, secured them in the usual way and cut the ends short. The immediate result, so far as the fragments were concerned, is indicated in this diagram (see Fig. 26 B). The incisions in the skin were then brought together by sutures and a dressing (the double cyanide gauze) applied.

'In drawing down the upper fragment I found a great advantage from the use of a very strong sharp hook, the point of which was inserted in the tendon of the quadriceps at its attachment. By this means I was able to exert much greater traction upon the bone than can be done by simply pulling upon the wire; and, in order to relax the quadriceps as much as possible, the limb was placed in the vertical position before the fragment was pulled down. The dressing having been put on, a trough of Gooch's splint was applied to the limb still in the elevated position, and the same attitude was maintained as the patient was removed to the ward, and continued by attaching the end of the splint to a rope connected with the tripod and pulley used in applying Sayre's plaster of Paris jacket. This position of the limb did not cause the patient material inconvenience, and after two or three days the rope was slackened a little so as to allow the end of the splint to come down every two days or so, till the limb could be placed quite horizontal.

' This preliminary operation is of the simplest character, no paring of the broken surfaces being done at this stage, and there being almost no bleeding and no shock. The wound having healed (I need hardly say without suppuration), the patient was allowed to leave her bed, and left the hospital soon after to practise using the limb.

' Before long she was readmitted, and the second operation was performed. The lower cicatrix was opened and the wire removed, and two interrupted wire sutures placed in the tracks of the previous continued one: the fragments, of course, being this time pared to clear them of fibrous tissue of new formation and produce smooth surfaces for coaptation. This was all satisfactorily effected, though not without the use of the powerful hook and the vertical position of the limb. The result was restoration of the use of the joint in a manner so satisfactory that I determined to try the same procedure in the other limb. The only difference which I made in this case was that, as the upper fragment was too small to bear drilling, I passed the ends of the wire, in dealing with that fragment, through the tendon of the quadriceps just above the upper border of the bone: the lower fragment, which was, of course, very substantial, being drilled as in the other limb. By this means, aided by the vertical position of the limb and the hook, I was able to bring down the upper fragment very satisfactorily, so much so that I did not feel it needful to have the patient use the limb in walking before proceeding to the second operation, but did this before she left her bed, soon after the wounds had healed. In the second operation I applied two interrupted sutures, passing them, as in the first operation, through the track in tendon and bone which the first wire had occupied.'

After-treatment. The after-treatment of all these cases, whatever be the operation, is similar; it consists in securing at first the maximum relaxation of the quadriceps extensor by fully extending the knee-joint and flexing the extended limb upon the pelvis at an angle of 45° or less. The flexed position is maintained for a fortnight or longer, but it is relieved by gradually lowering the limb every two days by a few degrees until, at the end of the fortnight, it lies flat on the bed. Massage should then be begun and carefully practised for another ten days, at the end of which time cautious passive movements may be performed, but flexion must be very carefully carried out, as otherwise the tension upon the wires may be too great. The patella should, however, be kept from adhering to the condyles of the femur by moving this bone from side to side repeatedly, and these movements may be practised from the time that the wound has healed.

EXCISION OF THE KNEE

Indications. By excision of the knee is meant removal of the articular ends of the bone with or without the entire synovial membrane. The operation may be required for several conditions:

(i) *For tuberculous disease.* This is by far the most important condition for which excision of the knee is done. Operations for tuberculous disease of the joints, however, do not fall into the scope of this article and are dealt with by Mr. Stiles.

(ii) *For injury.* A true set excision of the knee is very rarely indeed performed for injury at the present day. Operative interference in cases of compound fracture involving the knee now takes a much more conservative form. If mechanical fixation of the fragments is deemed impossible or inadvisable the operative measures will probably be limited to removal of small portions of bone, followed by strenuous attempts to preserve the movements of the joint, which of course would be entirely lost after a set excision of the knee on account of the firm bony ankylosis that follows it.

(iii) *For ankylosis in a faulty position.* When the knee has become firmly ankylosed, either in the flexed or the hyper-extended position, the deformity will call for rectification, and this will generally take the form of an excision. The milder forms of these deformities may be remedied by a linear osteotomy, but as a rule the deformity is so great that an excision of the joint, which in reality, however, is a cuneiform osteotomy, will be required before the deformity can be satisfactorily remedied. It must be noted that excision necessarily involves the epiphyseal line in these cases, and therefore the operation should not be undertaken in those who are much under the age of twenty-one.

(iv) *For arthrodesis.* This operation (see p. 6) is very useful in many situations. In the knee, however, it is open to the serious objection that, although it gives a firm basis of support, a stiff leg is very objectionable to many and, except when a patient's means or vocation render the operation essential, some form of apparatus will probably be preferred.

(v) *For intractable suppurative arthritis.* This has been given as an indication for excision of the knee for many years. It seems, however, one of the worst possible methods of treatment for such a serious affection. Although excision may open up the joint cavity effectually and render its recesses accessible, yet it exposes a patient already gravely ill to the serious risk of infection of the large cancellous bone surfaces by virulent organisms, and it is hardly surprising that a high mortality has attended these cases in the past. Unless arthrotomy and drainage (see p. 59) are successful in bringing down the temperature and relieving the symptoms amputation should be preferred.

Operation. The chief question in excision of the knee for affections other than tuberculous disease is the best method of obtaining

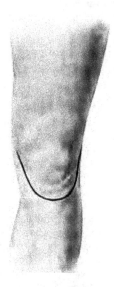

FIG. 27. INCISION FOR EXCISION OF THE KNEE.

access to the articular ends of the bones. Clearly this is by a transverse incision across the joint over the middle of the patella, followed by division of that bone, and this is the best plan if there be no objection to division of the patella. When the operation is done in order to secure ankylosis it is immaterial whether the patella be divided or not, and therefore in the operation for arthrodesis it will be best to open the joint by this transverse incision, sawing across the patella. When operating for ankylosis in a faulty position, also, this incision will be the best. In cases of injury, however, the patella should not be divided unless this step will greatly facilitate the work, since the necessary wiring of the patella afterwards may add in some degree to the tendency to ankylosis when a movable joint is desired. In these cases of excision or partial excision for injury arthroplasty (see p. 5) may be usefully employed.

When the patella is to be preserved intact, a curved incision (see Fig. 27) extending from the back of one condyle to the corresponding point on the back of the other is made across the front of the knee. The surgeon stands somewhat to the right of and facing the knee, which is flexed at an angle of 135°. He places his left thumb and middle finger upon the two points mentioned above, and carries his knife over the front of the joint in a bold sweep with its convexity downwards, crossing the ligamentum patellæ close to its insertion into the tubercle of the tibia. This incision is carried down to the deep fascia all round and the patella is raised in the large U-shaped flap thus marked out. This may be done either by cutting across the ligamentum patellæ about its centre and dissecting it and the patella up after opening the knee-joint, or by chiselling off the insertion of the ligament into the tuberosity of the tibia. On the whole the latter method is probably preferable, as it ensures firmer union subsequently, since the bony surfaces unite readily when replaced in contact, whereas the tendinous structures are more difficult to unite satisfactorily. The patella and the flap are raised together, the capsule of the point being opened freely right back to the posterior limits of the incision. As this is done the assistant bends the knee and renders the articular surfaces visible. There is often free bleeding from the articular arteries, which, however, is easily controlled either by pressure forceps or by under-running and tying the bleeding points with fine catgut. The subsequent steps of the operation will vary with the condition for which the operation is being performed.

(i) **In cases of excision for injury** two courses are open. The first is to excise the articular surfaces in the orthodox manner so as to leave large surfaces which subsequently become firmly united by bone, giving the patient a stiff but strong leg.

Extensive removal of the articular surfaces. In order to do this the crucial ligaments are divided, which allows the tibia to be separated from the femur and the lower end of the latter bone to be projected from the wound. A few touches of the knife divide the remnants of the lateral ligaments and clear the end of the femur for the application of the saw. The posterior ligament, with the popliteal vessels behind it, is pushed back out of the way and is protected by a spatula which is passed in behind the bones.

The saw is applied parallel to the transverse plane of the condyles, and, in order to make the section through the shaft from front to back in the right direction, it is held so that the plane of its blade corresponds with the transverse plane of the long axis of the leg when the joint is at an angle of 135° (see Fig. 28). The amount of bone removed will vary according to the affection for which the excision is done. The less taken away the better, since the shortening is thereby minimized. It is never necessary to apply the saw high enough to remove the entire cartilaginous surface on the front of the femur.

The head of the tibia is now cleared, the leg being held vertical with the sole of the foot planted firmly upon the table. It is only necessary to clear the extreme top of the tibia so as to cut a level surface; this will remove most of the cartilage together with the semilunar cartilages and the projecting spine of the tibia. The structures behind the knee-joint are not endangered in this part of the operation, as they are at some distance from the posterior margin of the articular surface. The

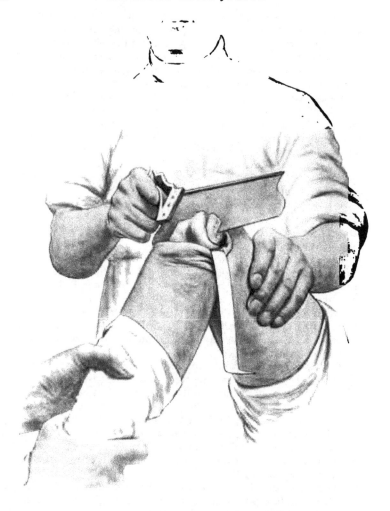

FIG. 28. SAWING THE CONDYLES OF THE FEMUR IN EXCISION OF THE KNEE. The
retractor guards the soft parts at the back of the joint from injury.

saw is applied from before backwards, and its blade is held strictly
horizontal (see Fig. 29). If the bone section has been made accurately

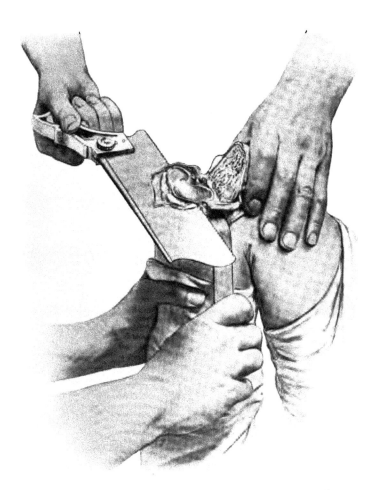

Fig. 29. Sawing the Tibia in Excision of the Knee. The sole of the foot rests flat upon the operating table.

the cut surfaces should fit exactly when applied together, giving the knee a slight inclination inwards.

The wound is now closed, but previous to doing this many surgeons are accustomed to fasten the bone ends together by some mechanical means, such as wires, pegs, pins, or screws. There is no objection to using any of these means should it be thought desirable. The only reason that can be urged against them is that they are not necessary and there is a possibility of their having to be removed at some later date. I never use them and have never experienced any need for them. If the limb be put up accurately and immovably on a splint there is no risk of displacement, and bony union takes place rapidly and satisfactorily.

Various splints are employed; I prefer a roll of Gooch's splinting in which the limb is wedged with suitable pads. An excellent method is

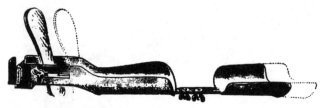

Fig. 30. Howse's Excision Splint. The splint is of metal and can be sterilized. The narrow posterior bar lies behind the popliteal space, so that the region of the operation can be inspected without removing the splint. The latter may be fixed on by means of plaster of Paris or waxed bandages.

to employ Howse's excision splint (see Fig. 30), in which the limb can be fixed firmly and need not be disturbed for dressings. A similar splint can be made by placing a malleable iron bar along the middle line of the popliteal surface and incorporating its ends in plaster of Paris bandages which surround the ankle and leg up to the middle of the calf below and the upper two-thirds of the thigh above. This leaves the whole area of the operation exposed for the change of dressings. At the present day, however, this is of slight importance, as the dressings can be left undisturbed for three weeks, when the sutures may be removed without any risk of displacing the bone surfaces.

Union follows the usual course and the patient should be able to walk on the limb comfortably in six weeks.

The use of the Esmarch bandage is frequently advocated for this operation. I have no hesitation, however, in strongly condemning its use. It is essential for success that all bleeding shall have ceased when the limb is put up, so that there may be no collection of blood beneath the skin, no drainage tube employed, and no chance of sepsis. If the Esmarch bandage be employed, the oozing after its removal is persistent and difficult to stop. It has been advised that firm pressure by means of a bandage drawn as tightly as possible over a large mass of wool and dressing should be applied before the Esmarch is removed, so as to check the bleeding by pressure. This plan is not advisable; however efficient it may be in checking serious bleeding a certain amount of blood must necessarily be extravasated into the soft parts, and all recent experience shows the risk of sepsis from such a procedure. When no tourniquet is used the bleeding vessels can be caught up and tied as they are met with, and a dry wound at the end of the operation is thereby assured.

When only a portion of the articular surface is to be removed the chief aim will be to retain the movements of the knee. As little of the bone as possible is removed, the gouge and chisel being used in such a way as to leave the raw surfaces of bone quite smooth and of such shape as to interfere least with movement. In order to prevent union between the raw bone surfaces some method of arthroplasty (see p. 5) may well be adopted. A flap of sufficient size, with a wide base so as to secure proper nourishment and containing as large a proportion of fat as possible, is fashioned if possible from the extra-articular structures, turned in over the raw surfaces, and fastened by fine sutures to any suitable adjacent structures. Throughout the operation the object should be to damage the joint structures as little as possible. The joint is closed as after simple arthrotomy (see p. 4), and the limb should not be put up on a splint; a firm mass of dressing should be applied to check synovial effusion, and the patient should be encouraged to move the limb.

Gentle attempts at passive movement may be made from the first, but after the fourth or fifth day it will be well to commence regular movement under anæsthesia. This will probably have to be repeated about twice a week for some time, but great pains should be taken to promote movement. Massage and passive and active movements should be practised freely and frequently.

(ii) **Excision for arthrodesis** does not require so extensive a removal of bone, as the object of the operation is to secure a stiff joint with the least amount of shortening. This can be done by merely removing the cartilage from the articular surfaces with a broad chisel or gouge. The joint is opened by a trans-patellar incision and the latter bone is sawn across. This gives good exposure of the joint, so that it may be possible to remove the cartilage without dividing the crucial ligaments, which is an advantage, as it prevents dislocation backwards of the tibia upon the femur; this, however, is not of great importance, since most of the muscles are paralysed in the cases for which arthrodesis is done and will therefore have little influence.

The cartilage should be removed from the under surfaces of each condyle with a broad chisel; some amount of bone must be taken away also in order to get a sufficiently large bony area to unite with that of the tibia. It is also well to remove all the cartilage from the patella and from its articular facet on the front of the femur. The posterior ligament is not interfered with, nor are the posterior fibres of the lateral ligaments. The two halves of the patella are united by two moderately stout catgut sutures at the end of the operation; these are sufficiently strong for the purpose, as there is no tendency to separation of the fragments owing to the paralysis for which the operation is done. The limb should be put up in the extended position in a plaster of Paris splint, which may be applied either immediately after the operation or as soon as the sutures have been removed. The tendency in these cases is for non-union to occur, and the limb may have to be kept in a rigid casing for many weeks.

(iii) **Excision for ankylosis in a faulty position.** A transverse incision should be made across the prominent angle of the deformity, and the patella divided if it be adherent to the bone. If, however, the patella be even partially movable, the incision should run below the bone and the ligamentum patellæ should be detached from its insertion into the tibia, the patella being turned upwards in the flap.

When the operation is done in young children the union between the bones will rarely be entirely bony, and it will often be possible to divide it with a chisel or knife, aided by forcible flexion of the limb. This greatly facilitates the operation, as the operator can clear the articular ends and can see exactly how much bone should be removed; the operation is also simplified, because the structures in the popliteal space can be then effectually protected from injury. No attempt should be made to straighten the limb forcibly after the ankylosis has been broken down; such a procedure is likely to end disastrously to the structures in the popliteal space, which are often shortened and adherent in their new position. Enough bone must therefore be removed in order to allow the limb to be straightened without stretching them unduly. To do this it will probably be necessary to encroach upon the epiphyseal line of the femur, and therefore, as has already been pointed out, this operation should not be undertaken in young children or in any one under the age of eighteen. The subsequent steps of this form of the operation are exactly similar to those just described. Occasionally it may be possible to straighten the limb after removing so little bone that it will be worth while to attempt to obtain a movable joint by means of arthroplasty (see p. 5).

When the ankylosis is completely bony it will be necessary to do a cuneiform osteotomy and remove a wedge from the knee with its base forwards. The difficulty in this part of the operation is to avoid damaging the structures in the popliteal space, either when dividing the bone or when straightening the limb subsequently. The bone should be exposed by a transverse incision across the most convex part of the limb. The patella should be sawn across if it lies beneath the incision, and in any case should be removed entirely. The seat of ankylosis should be bared completely so as to allow the surgeon to estimate the amount of bone that must be removed. In case of any doubt on this point it is well to remove less than is actually necessary, as it is easy to remove more towards the end of the operation with perfect safety. In order to guard the structures in the popliteal space the soft parts are separated from the bone just around the lateral margins of the tibia opposite the point at which the apex of the wedge is to be situated, and a narrow spatula is inserted along the posterior surface of the bone on each side between it and the soft parts. The bone can now be sawn without risk of damaging the popliteal structures, since the spatula protects the soft parts laterally and the bone will fracture before the section is complete. When this has happened there is no further risk to the structures in the popliteal space, as the soft parts can be pushed back from the bone with rapidity and safety. The opposite side of the wedge is then sawn through and the desired portion of bone is removed. The limb is cautiously straightened, and if the surfaces then fit without any projection backwards in the popliteal space or tension on the posterior ligament the wound is closed and the case is treated as an ordinary excision (see p. 82). If, however, there be a projection of osteophytic outgrowths backward into the popliteal space these must be carefully trimmed away. If there be any undue tension on the structures behind, more bones must be removed until a perfect fit is obtained.

ARTHROPLASTY (MURPHY)

The usual preparations are made. An Esmarch constrictor is placed around the thigh high up. Two incisions are made, one on the inner, the other on the outer surface of the knee, parallel to the long axis of the limb (see Fig. 31). Each of these incisions is about 5 inches in length and extends 3½ inches above and 1½ inches below the point where the new joint is to be made. These incisions pass through the skin and fat down to the fascia. The wound margins are retracted and the skin freed sufficiently to expose the field of operation.

Next the interposing flaps are prepared, the outer one including a portion of the vastus externus and such portion of the capsule and ligaments as may be present on the outer side of the knee. The inner one is made up of a portion of the vastus internus and the capsule and

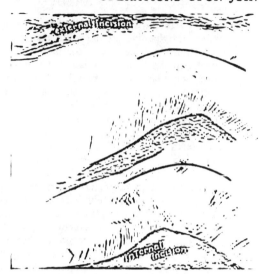

FIG. 31.   INCISION IN ARTHROPLASTY OF KNEI

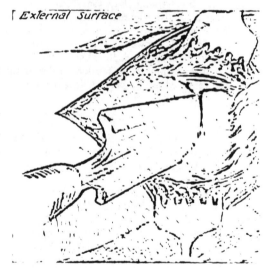

FIG. 32.   FREEING TIBIA FROM FEMUR WITH CURVED C
prepared.   (*Murphy.*)

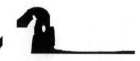

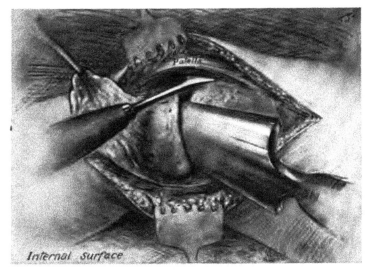

FIG. 33. FREEING ANKYLOSED PATELLA FROM FEMUR WITH 'ARTIST' CHISEL.
Interposing flap prepared.   Freeing tibia from femur with curved chisel.
'Murphy.)

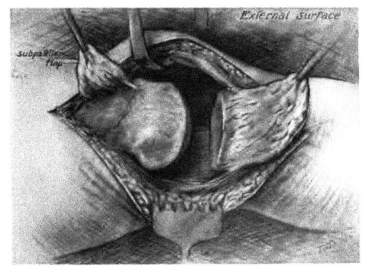

FIG. 34.   ARTICULAR SURFACES OF FEMUR AND TIBIA READY FOR INSERTION OF
INTERPOSING FLAP.   Subpatellar flap prepared.   (Murphy.)

ligaments on the inner side of the knee-joint. These flaps should be 3½ inches long and 2½ inches wide, with the base left attached on the tuberosities of the tibia just below the line of bone division for the new joint. After these flaps are prepared they are placed into towels or sterile gauze and held downward out of the field of operation. If the patella is ankylosed to the femur, it is freed by the use of a flat chisel, preferably the thin-bladed artist's chisel, maintaining of course the normal groove in the femur (see Fig. 33). When the skin is fully re-

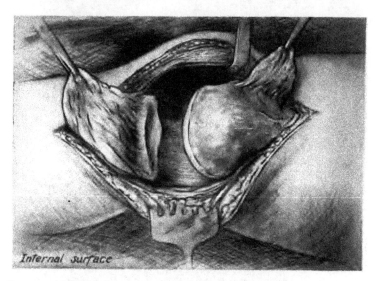

Internal surface

Fig. 35. Articular Surfaces of Femur and Tibia ready for Insertion of Interposing Flaps. Subpatellar flap prepared. (*Murphy.*)

tracted the operator chooses the line in which he wishes to make the new joint, remembering that the normal joint is just under the lower tip of the patella when the leg is fully extended. The curved chisel then separates the tibia from the femur on each side, maintaining the normal anatomic conformation of the joint surface (see Fig. 32). Five-eighths of an inch distal to this incision the chisels are again driven from either side, this time cutting through the upper end of the tibia and thus taking out a wedge of bone ⅝ of an inch wide. By artistic shaping with chisel and bone rasp one makes depressions to resemble the normal articular concavities of the external and internal tuberosities of

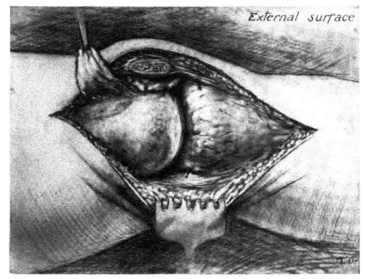

FIG. 36. SHOWS EXTERNAL TIBIO-FEMORAL FLAP INSERTED AND OUTER END OF
INTERNAL PATELLAR FLAP. (*Murphy.*)

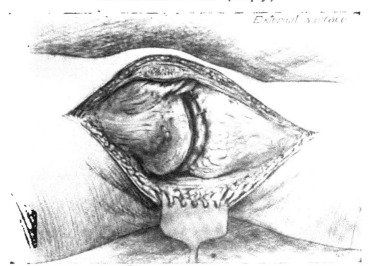

FIG. 37. SHOWS THE OVERLAPPING OF INTERNAL AND EXTERNAL INTERPOSING
FLAPS. (*Murphy.*)

the tibia. The intercondyloid ridge must be preserved. The intercondyloid groove of the femur must be excavated deep enough to accommodate itself to the ridge of the tibia (see Fig. 34).

If the ankylosis is in a flexed position, then a sufficient wedge must be removed to permit the leg to be fully extended without putting undue tension on the vessels and nerves in the popliteal space. It is to be re-

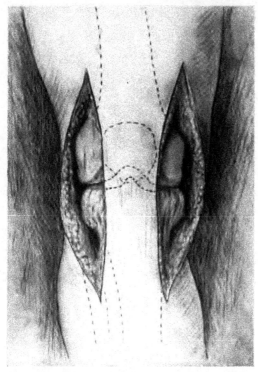

Fig. 38. Schematic. Showing the Bone and Anterior Flap Relations at Completion of Operation. (*Murphy.*)

membered that most of the bone is removed from the upper end of the tibia, as in this way one has the least amount of denuded bone surface to cover. The interposing flaps which were previously prepared are now drawn over the upper end of the tibia and sutured firmly in position, so that no raw surface remains exposed (see Fig. 37). It is not necessary to cover the femur. The newly made joint is now closed, usually without drainage (see Fig. 38), and the limb is placed into a moulded wire or plaster of Paris trough. A Buck's extension of from 8 to 12 pounds is applied. Passive motion is begun about the twelfth day. If the patella is ankylosed, a small piece of fascia is passed between it and the femur and sutured in position so that it may not again adhere to the femur (see Figs. 35 and 36).

CHAPTER VII

OPERATIONS UPON THE HIP-JOINT

ARTHROTOMY OF THE HIP

Indications. The hip-joint may be exposed and opened for a large number of conditions, of which the following are the most important:—

(i) *As a preliminary to excision of the joint.* Excision of the hip is rarely performed for any other than a tuberculous affection of the joint; this is part of the subject dealt with by Mr. Stiles. Excision of the joint for injury is very rare indeed; if it be required, as possibly it may be in military surgery, it will probably take the form of an arthrotomy, followed by piecemeal removal of fragments of bone and smoothing off of the portion remaining. Excision may be necessary in septic suppurative arthritis due to acute epiphysitis or pyæmia; the head of the bone may have to be removed in order to allow satisfactory drainage to be established.

(ii) It forms the first stage of the operation for re-position of a *congenital dislocation of the hip* by the open method (see p. 113).

(iii) When it is desired to rectify *ankylosis of the hip* in a faulty position it is often employed as a preliminary to division of the neck of the femur or a trans-trochanteric division of the bone.

(iv) It must be done in all those cases of *intra-capsular fracture* of the neck of the femur in which it is desired to fasten the fragments together (see p. 95).

(v) It is a preliminary stage of a cuneiform osteotomy of the neck of the femur for *coxa vara* (see p. 94).

The steps of the operations appropriate to each of the above conditions are described separately, but to avoid unnecessary repetition the operation for exposure of the neck of the bone, which is common to them all, will be described first.

Operation. The patient lies flat on his back and the surgeon stands on the outer side of the limb. It is most important that the entire thigh and buttock should be thoroughly purified and the thigh securely fastened in a sterilized towel, as free manipulation of the limb will probably be required during the course of the operation.

The incision begins at the anterior superior iliac spine and runs downwards and inwards for four or five inches parallel with the outer edge of the sartorius, in the interval between it and the tensor fasciæ femoris. This intermuscular space leads at once down to the neck of the bone without division of any important structure. There may be fairly smart bleeding from the anastomosis of the external circumflex when the neck of the bone is reached, but this is easily stopped. The finger defines the anterior surface of the neck of the femur, when the muscles are well retracted and the capsule of the joint is opened by an incision parallel to the long axis of the neck; whatever further steps are necessary can then be undertaken. As these vary considerably they will be described separately.

DRAINAGE OF THE HIP-JOINT

The first step towards securing efficient drainage of this joint is to remove the head of the bone. In acute suppurative affections this may be quite easy, owing to dislocation having taken place. In that case, after the joint has been opened as described above, the neck is sawn *in situ* and the head removed. The sawing is accomplished with an Adams's osteotomy saw or a Gigli's wire saw passed round the neck of the bone, and should be done without disturbing the parts until the section of the neck is complete. The head can then be turned out with a large raspatory, and this gives free access to the front of the joint. In order to provide satisfactory drainage, however, it will be necessary to perforate the posterior part of the capsule and to insert a large drainage tube, which will project posteriorly through the skin in the post-trochanteric region. For this purpose an incision is made in the posterior part of the capsule large enough to allow the passage of a pair of long dressing forceps, which are thrust through it and made to perforate the soft parts over the back of the joint until they can be clearly felt beneath the skin of the buttock about midway between the tuber ischii and the great trochanter. They are then cut down upon through an incision about two inches long and made to protrude through the skin. Their blades are cautiously dilated and the orifice in the posterior aspect of the capsule is increased until a drainage tube as large as the thumb can be grasped by the forceps and pulled into the joint from the gluteal wound. The chief danger in doing this is in damaging the sciatic nerve, which lies in close relation to the back of the hip-joint. The only safe method is to employ large dressing forceps and to insinuate them carefully through the tissues; they then pass to one side of the sciatic nerve, which escapes damage. The drainage tube should be long enough to pass through the joint from front to back, and the openings in it should be so arranged that one of them is at the most dependent part of the joint cavity.

The articulation is washed out thoroughly and may be douched with peroxide of hydrogen solution (10 vols. per cent.) with advantage. Antiseptic dressings are applied front and back, and a weight extension of four or five pounds should be put on so as to keep the joint cavity as widely open as possible for the purpose of drainage and also to prevent the tube being compressed by the pull of the muscles forcing the neck of the bone into the acetabulum.

As soon as drainage is satisfactorily established, which will be in about three or four days, portions may be gradually cut off the tube by pulling it out of the posterior wound and removing a quarter of an inch at each dressing, until the anterior end of the tube lies flush with the opening in the posterior part of the capsule. The anterior wound can safely be allowed to close, but drainage from the posterior wound should be kept up until all discharge has ceased, when the tube may be gradually shortened and the extension of the limb dispensed with.

OSTEOTOMY OF THE NECK OF THE FEMUR

The neck of the bone is exposed in the usual manner (see p. 92) ; the neck of the femur may be divided with the saw or a wedge of the bone may be removed.

Simple osteotomy. This is done with Adams's subcutaneous osteotomy saw with the minimum disturbance of the soft parts, which are protected above and below the neck by the interposition of a thin metal spatula. The section of the bone should be made as near the trochanter as possible, in order to leave a wide surface for subsequent union if this should be desired; if the section be made in the immediate neighbourhood of the head of the bone, union may not be obtained subsequently, owing to separation of the fragments. In this connexion it may be remarked that Mr. Robert Jones of Liverpool is in favour of what he terms a trans-trochanteric incision, extending obliquely from the top of the greater to the lesser trochanter; this gives a broad surface for bony union after rectification of the malposition for which the operation has been done.

Cuneiform osteotomy. This may be required for *coxa vara*. At the present day, however, this affection will rarely require operation, as extended experience tends to show that all cases in young children are amenable to treatment by appropriate splints. In them, moreover, this particular operation could have no sphere of usefulness, as the neck of the femur is too small a structure to be satisfactorily treated in this way. Should it be necessary, however, to operate upon these cases in adults, which is doubtful, cuneiform osteotomy of the neck of the femur would be the operation of choice. The neck of the bone is exposed as described above, and more particularly that part of it from which the wedge is to be removed; this is best determined by previous stereoscopic radiography. As a rule the base of the wedge will be at the junction of the upper with the anterior aspect of the neck. With an Adams's osteotomy saw the surgeon marks out a wedge of a suitable size and performs the section either partially or entirely with this instrument; if there be any difficulty it may be finished with a few strokes of a broad chisel. The assistant then rotates the limb into the position in which the two cut surfaces fit one another accurately, and it is then seen whether this position returns the limb to its normal position; if not, more bone is removed to make the surfaces fit accurately when the limb is lying flat on the table with the anterior surface of the patella looking vertically upwards.

It is well not to remove any large portion of the posterior aspect of the neck, which may be retained as a sort of hinge to prevent displacement of the divided surfaces, and it is generally advisable to make use of some method of mechanical fixation to the same end; long pins or nails driven in through a separate incision over the outer surface of the great trochanter, when the limb is held in position by the assistant, answer admirably (see Fig. 39). The after-treatment will be similar to that of fractures of the neck of the femur (see p. 99).

OPERATIONS FOR FRACTURES OF THE NECK OF THE FEMUR

Indications. In theory, operative measures designed to secure accurate approximation and fixation of the fractured surfaces are called for in all cases of intra-capsular fracture, owing to the very unsatisfactory results obtained by any other method. Occasionally, it is true, actual bony union may occur, but even this is likely to be followed by much impaired mobility of the limb, either from mal-union or from the presence of osteophytic outgrowths in the region of the head of the bone. Any operation, therefore, that can bring the fractured surfaces into accurate apposition and keep them there should be welcomed as an improvement. The truth is, however, that operative interference in fractures of the neck of the femur is often very difficult to carry out and disappointing in its results. There are many reasons for this.

In the first place the hip-joint and the neck of the femur in the adult are deeply placed, covered by structures of importance, and therefore difficult of access in a wound which does not lend itself to manipulation. It is only in spare subjects that the joint is near enough to the surface to be at all amenable to surgical procedures with ease.

A second point is that the nature of the fracture renders accurate apposition of the fragments difficult to obtain and even more difficult to maintain. When the line of fracture is near the head of the bone there is no leverage by which this can be got into good position, and even if this can be done, the subjects in which this fracture occurs have such rarefied and brittle bony tissue that a fixation apparatus has not a really fair chance of keeping the fragments together. The leverage exerted by the weight of the limb is so great that displacement is very likely to occur.

Thirdly, even if union does occur, it is apt to be accompanied by the formation of so large a callus about the seat of the fracture that the movements of the limb may be seriously hampered by the mechanical contact of the callus with the acetabulum.

Finally, it must never be forgotten that the subjects of these fractures are always elderly and frequently in bad health and subject to chronic bronchitis. To them operative interference that entails the administration of an anæsthetic for a long period, and the necessarily prolonged convalescence and confinement to bed, means a risk that is not justified if good results can be obtained with early massage and the employment of a suitable splint. My own experience leads me to limit operative interference to patients who are comparatively young, spare, healthy, and active, and in whom the desire to be restored to the full vigour of life makes them willing to run some slight degree of risk.

Operation. Before operating, it is important to obtain a knowledge of the exact condition of the fracture, and for this purpose stereoscopic radiograms are essential.

The parts are thoroughly and widely purified in the usual manner, the trochanteric region and the buttock having special care devoted to them. The joint is opened and the fracture exposed in the manner already described for exposure of the neck of the bone (see p. 92). The incision should be free, and wide retraction will be required to expose the seat of fracture. A radiogram is most useful in indicating the direction in which exposure is most needed. It will probably be impossible to see the whole extent of the fracture, and it may be difficult to get the limb into proper position for fixation unless the surgeon has a clear notion of it.

In effecting apposition the greatest difficulty may be experienced in dealing with the proximal fragment, viz. the head of the bone and the adjacent portion of the neck. The distal fragment should be got out of the way by rotating the limb so as to make it clear the inner end of the fractured neck, and thus enable the surgeon to get at the head of the bone.

This must now be rotated so that, when the fractured surfaces of the neck are in apposition, the lower extremity will lie flat upon the bed with the foot pointing upwards. As there are no muscles attached to the head and neck of the femur it will remain in any position it is put, but it is often difficult to get a sufficiently firm hold of it to rotate it into the desired position.

The next step is to manipulate the lower limb so as to get the fractured surfaces into good apposition before fixing them. This is done by an assistant under the direction of the surgeon, who places the forefinger of one hand in the wound so as to ascertain the position of the fractured surfaces and the other hand upon the trochanter. When the fracture is in good position the limb is steadied and the fragments are fixed. This is the most important and the most difficult part of the operation, as the least movement may cause considerable displacement, which can neither be discovered nor rectified subsequently. Any means that may suggest themselves to the surgeon for fixing the fragments temporarily in position pending their permanent fixation should be adopted. On one occasion I have been lucky enough to be able to grasp the fragments in powerful bone forceps, such as Peters's, which have steadied them sufficiently to enable the neck to be drilled and pegged satisfactorily. On another occasion, when the fracture was somewhat oblique from before backwards, a bradawl run between the two fragments from front to back steadied the fracture until the long pins were inserted for permanent fixation.

Permanent fixation is best secured by pegs, pins, screws, or nails driven through from the outer surface of the great trochanter along the long axis of the neck well into the head of the bone. The application of wires, pins, screws, or nails to the neck itself is hardly to be recommended, since the leverage of the lower limb is likely to tear them from their place, while any foreign body projecting from the neck of the bone may mechanically interfere with the movements of the joint. On the whole I have found the best fixation apparatus to be stout steel knitting-needles or screws. I prefer knitting-needles, one end of which is sharpened and the other somewhat expanded so that it may be driven in with a hammer if necessary. This end projects through the skin, is enveloped in the dressings, and can therefore be removed when the surgeon deems it necessary. In order to introduce pins or screws, a vertical incision should be made over the outer surface of the great trochanter near its base, and the whole thickness of this structure is bored with a drill of suitable size from its outer surface right along the neck of the bone and into the head almost up to the cartilaginous surface. It is a good plan to make this incision in the skin and to drill the trochanter and the outer part of the neck before apposition has been effected. The drill is made to penetrate the neck of the bone until its end just projects on the fractured surface, and as soon as the two fragments have been got into apposition it is driven on into the head of the bone and the fractured surfaces are thereby fixed. By adopting this plan it is easy to tell how far into the neck and head of the bone the drill may go with safety. The screw or pin is introduced for the requisite distance, and the fracture should then be firm (see Fig. 39). When a screw is used it is important that it should be exactly the right length, and therefore a number of different lengths should be at hand.

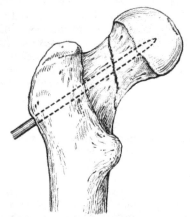

Fig. 39. Diagram illustrating the Method of pinning Fractures of the Neck of the Femur.

Steel pins should be about eight inches in total length. If they are used, it may be possible to run in two pins parallel to each other so as to give an extra firm hold. An electrically-driven drill is of the greatest service in drilling the bone; it requires no force, and the whole attention of the assistant can be directed to keeping the limb in position without having to resist the force which the surgeon must exert in using the hand-drill. ("The use of autogenous bone splints" is discussed in the chapter on Bone Transplantation in Fractures. See that section in this volume.)

From this time onwards the limb must be kept absolutely immovable in the corrected position, and this is one of the chief difficulties of the operation. The operation is greatly facilitated if some measures are adopted similar to those recommended for the application of a plaster of Paris splint after the operation for the re-position of congenital dislocations of the hip (see p. 117). This consists essentially in propping the patient's pelvis on a suitable support, like a bootmaker's last, so that plaster of Paris bandages can be applied immediately the wound is closed, which should be done by an assistant, the surgeon making himself responsible for the position of the limb from the time that the pegs are inserted to the time the patient is put back to bed. If the pelvis is raised in this manner and the thorax is elevated to a corresponding height upon pillows, the application of an immovable apparatus is quite simple; if necessary, the foot can be supported on a suitable telescopic rest standing on the floor. The plaster of Paris bandage should take in the knee and should be the usual figure-of-eight spica around the pelvis. It is put on exactly as for the congenital hip operation (see p. 117), and the limb is enveloped in a bandage of boric lint under the plaster casing.

The patient is kept under the anæsthetic until the plaster has set and is left upon the table until it is moderately dry. He is then put to bed with the utmost care. No care and attention bestowed upon the later stages of these operations, including the transference to bed, can be too minute, and personal experience convinces me that it is upon the proper observance of them that the success or failure of many of these cases depends.

After-treatment. The patient should be propped up in bed as soon as possible. The hip-joint is of course fixed, but a good range of movement is allowed in the lumbar region, and this should be utilized to the full. The wound need not be looked at until about the eighteenth day, when an anæsthetic should be given, the plaster casing removed, the stitches taken out, and a fresh plaster applied; this should again take in the knee for about a week or more, after which the portion embracing the joint can be cut away so that the knee can be bent. The patient should be got up on crutches with a patten on the sound foot as soon as possible after this plaster has been applied. It will probably be possible to dispense with the plaster casing at the end of four or five weeks, but the patient should still go about on crutches with a patten on the sound foot for another three or four weeks, during which time massage and passive movements of the affected limb are employed; after this, weight may be gradually borne upon the limb.

EXCISION OF THE HIP-JOINT

There are three principal routes by which this operation can be performed, viz. by an anterior incision, which has already been dealt with fully in connexion with arthrotomy (see p. 92), and will be considered again by Mr. Stiles in connexion with tuberculous disease of the hip; by a posterior incision, in which the structures behind the joint are divided and the back of the articulation exposed; or by the external route, by which both surfaces of the joint can be investigated.

Of these methods the anterior route has already been described in so far as it falls within the scope of the present subject. The posterior route sacrifices muscles whose functions the surgeon is anxious to preserve if possible; as a compensation for this it offers a very direct approach to the joint and good drainage. It might be called for in very bad tuberculous cases, but it will rarely be necessary for a non-tuberculous affection. The excision by the external incision is therefore the only one that will be described here.

EXCISION OF THE HIP-JOINT BY AN EXTERNAL INCISION

This is the method perfected by Kocher (*Operative Surgery*, trans. by Stiles, 2nd Ed., p. 360), from whom the description of the operation is taken.

Indications. There will be few non-tuberculous affections of the hip that will call for excision.

(i) In cases of bad *injury* to the joint in military surgery accompanied by extensive comminution of the upper end of the bone, it may be advisable to expose the entire neighbourhood of the joint and deal freely with it by excision.

(ii) In chronic cases of *suppurative arthritis* accompanied by sinuses and much caries the anterior incision will not suffice for proper access and safe drainage, and the external route will be preferable.

Operation. The following description follows that of Kocher very closely :—The surgeon stands on the outer side of the limb and the patient is rolled over well on to the sound side. The incision (see Fig. 40) is a somewhat curved one, running over the outer surface of the great trochanter from its base to its anterior superior angle; thence it passes obliquely upwards and backwards, following the direction of the fibres of the gluteus maximus. Over the outer surface of the trochanter the knife divides branches of the external circumflex artery and the dense aponeurotic insertion of the gluteus maximus, while it divides the fibres of the gluteus maximus in the upper part of the incision. At this stage some vessels of considerable size will be divided and must be ligatured. The insertion of the gluteus medius is seen at the outer side of the great trochanter and that of the gluteus minimus at its anterior border; these are detached from the bone and turned forwards. The anterior surface of the neck is now exposed, the limb being flexed and rotated outwards, and the ilio-femoral ligament is separated from the anterior inter-trochanteric line. The dissection is next carried out on the posterior surface; the capsule is incised along the lower border of the tendon of the pyriformis, the latter structure being detached from its insertion into the inner surface of the trochanter and turned backwards along with the external rotators; the periosteum covering the

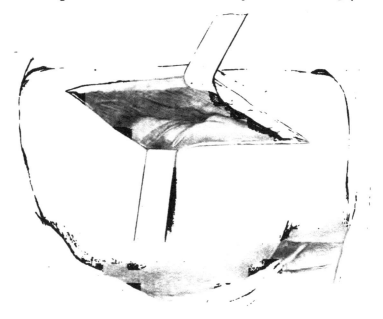

Fig. 40. Excision of Hip by Kocher's External Incision. The muscles are separated from their attachments, exposing the neck of the bone and the capsule of the joint.

inner surface of the trochanter is reflected along with the muscles enumerated above.

Kocher recommends this particular method of approach because the gluteus medius and minimus muscles supplied by the superior gluteal nerve are drawn forwards and upwards towards the tensor fasciæ femoris, which has the same nerve-supply. All these muscles play an important part in the future abduction of the thigh. The gluteus maximus, the pyriformis, and the obturators, which are supplied by the inferior gluteal nerve, are drawn downwards. When the joint is approached by this incision, admirable exposure of the entire posterior, external, and anterior surfaces of the head and neck of the femur is afforded, as well as of the trochanter itself. There is very little bleeding. Branches of the internal circumflex artery will be divided in front of the neck of the femur, while the transverse branch of the external circumflex artery may also need to be ligatured as it winds round the base of the trochanter

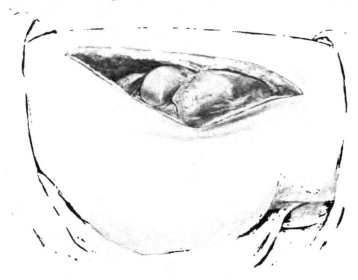

FIG. 41. EXPOSURE OF THE HEAD OF THE FEMUR IN KOCHER'S EXCISION OF THE HIP. The capsule has been opened and both sides of the neck are rendered easily accessible.

under the vastus externus. The ligamentum teres is reached and divided by cutting on to the head of the bone through the cotyloid ligament from behind and below, while an assistant fully adducts, flexes, and rotates the limb inwards. The head is thereby dislocated backwards and the acetabulum rendered visible.

This free exposure enables the necessary manipulations to be carried out with ease. In cases of injury these will be removal of the shattered portions of bone and resection of the neck to the extent required to make the surfaces smooth. No more bone should be removed than is actually necessary, and the trochanteric part of the neck should be rounded off as accurately and as smoothly as possible with chisels or gouges, in order that it may, if possible, take the place of the head of the bone which has been removed. In suppurative arthritis the neck should be sawn through quite close to the head and well rounded off after the latter has been removed. After all bleeding has been stopped, the displaced muscles are secured in position by sutures. In cases of injury the wound should be closed, without a drainage tube if possible; a tube will only be needed in compound fractures. In cases of suppurative arthritis the wound should be flushed out with 1 in 2,000 biniodide lotion, followed by a solution of 10 vols. per cent. of peroxide of hydrogen, and it is a good plan to swab the entire raw surface over with a saturated solution of chloride of zinc in order to retard the spread of the infection to the freshly cut surfaces. A large drainage tube is then inserted into the most dependent part of the joint.

After-treatment. Extension by means of weight and pulley, beginning with 4 to 5 lb., should be employed for the first fortnight; care must be taken to prevent eversion of the foot. In aseptic cases the sutures are then removed and the patient may get about on crutches, for the first fortnight in a Thomas's hip-splint and afterwards without it. In six weeks or two months after operation weight may be borne gradually upon the stump. In septic cases the drainage tube is gradually shortened until healing occurs. Much the same line of treatment is adopted as in aseptic cases, but the convalescence will be longer.

ARTHROPLASTY (MURPHY)

After having made the usual aseptic preparations, a U-shaped incision is made (see Fig. 42), the flap measuring about 3 inches in width with the base directed upward. Incision is begun 3 inches above the trochanter and extends downward 2 inches below the trochanter, so that it is placed exactly in the center of the U. The knife passes through the skin, superficial fat, and fascia lata, so that all these tissues are dissected and displaced upwards in the flap.

The next step in the operation is to free the trochanter, leaving its muscles attached to it from the shaft.

A large, curved, flat, blunt-pointed needle, chain-saw carrier, threaded with heavy silk, is passed around the base of the trochanter from before backward under the muscles attached to it. This serves as a carrier for the chain-saw, which is next brought into position. The trochanter is carefully sawed off downward and outward and is retracted upward out of the field of operation, carrying with it the attached muscles. The obturators and pyriformis are then divided and both ends transfixed with sutures for subsequent approximation (see Fig. 44). The joint is now freely exposed and the next step in the operation consists in incising the capsule of the joint without, however, separating it from its attachment to the acetabulum. It is loosened from the neck of the femur and stripped upward toward the head of

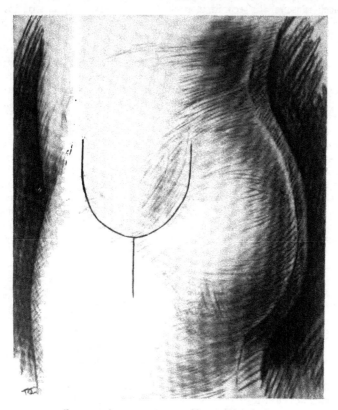

FIG. 42. ARTHROPLASTY OF HIP. (*Murphy.*)

the bone, so that it can be interposed later between the head of the bone and the acetabulum, if needed, so as to assist in the formation of a new lining for the acetabular cavity.

This is only one of the interposing tissues which may be used in the operation. It serves, in the main, to provide a perfectly smooth acetabular margin, so that it will at no time subsequently permit of the reformation of a bony ankylosis or bone collar formation.   This procedure thus far does not disturb the attachment of the gluteus maximus.

The next step is the formation of a new acetabular cavity and a new femoral head.   The first thing to be done is to separate the ankylosed

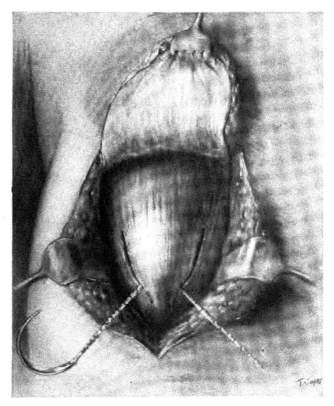

Fig. 43.   Arthroplasty of Hip.   (*Murphy.*)

head from the ilium as near the normal anatomic line as possible.   This is done by chiselling out the bony tissue, filling the acetabular cavity by means of a curved chisel about 1½ inches in width (see Fig. 45). With properly directed blows and sufficient force, the chisel is driven obliquely toward the acetabular cavity for the depth of 1 inch all the way around the head, as near the normal conformation as possible. When the chiselling process is complete, with the chisel as a lever and the thigh as an assistant, the head is fractured out of the acetabulum. The acetabular cavity is then fashioned with a special globular drill or

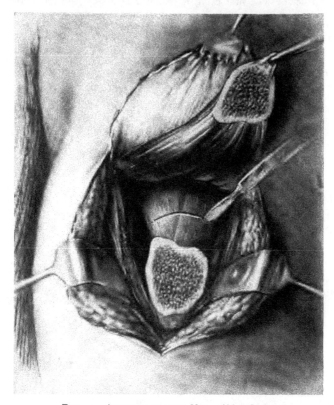

Fig. 44. Arthroplasty of Hip. (*Murphy.*)

reamer, so as to receive the new femoral head, which will be similarly fashioned from the bony mass chiselled out of the acetabulum. For this purpose use is made of a specially constructed cup-shaped end-mill, making it possible to provide a new femoral head of normal conformation and smoothness (see Fig. 46).

These two instruments used in fashioning the acetabulum and the femoral head constitute, in reality, parts of the same appliance; the globular portion fits into the cup-shaped portion in such a manner that unless the interposing tissues are in position the fit is perfect.

The main reliance for obviating the recurrence of the ankylosis is

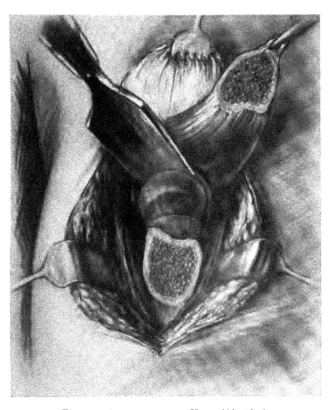

FIG. 45. ARTHROPLASTY OF HIP. (*Murphy.*)

placed on the flap of the deflected fascia lata, which is made by splitting the original U-shaped flap. This flap is dissected from the subcutaneous fatty tissue which formed a part of the original skin and fascia flap, the base of the U being directed upward so that the nutrition of the flap is preserved as much as possible to ensure its continued vitality (see

Fig. 47). Grasping the edge of the flap with tissue forceps, it is drawn into the joint and the edge sutured to the acetabular margin or to the remnant of the capsular ligament still attached to the neck of the bone with chromic catgut, thus forming a complete covering for the acetabular

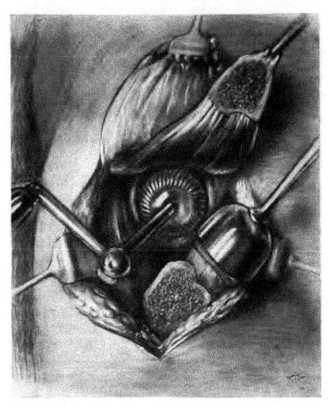

FIG. 46. ARTHROPLASTY OF HIP. (*Murphy.*)

cavity (see Fig. 48). When the head is placed into the acetabular cavity, this flap also serves as a lining for this cavity, reinforcing the capsular ligament, although the latter is used mainly for the purpose of preventing a ' locking ' of the joint by the formation of exostosis from the acetabular rim.

The next step is to replace the trochanter, which, it will be remembered, was sawed off from the bone without disturbing the muscular attachment. Then the ends of the obturator and pyriformis muscles are reunited. The trochanter is brought down, fitted on to its original position, and secured with chromic catgut. Occasionally a small nail

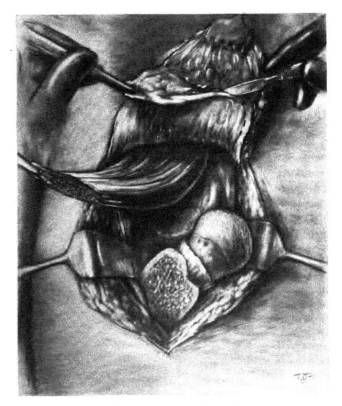

FIG. 47. ARTHROPLASTY OF HIP. (*Murphy.*)

may be used in addition to the sutures (see Fig. 49). The deep fascia is sutured and the skin closed with horsehair without drainage. The patient is placed into bed in a Travois splint and a Buck's extension with 12 to 15 pounds' weight applied to the leg. This weight prevents the pressure necrosis of the flap and overcomes the involuntary muscle contractions which so frequently cause pain. Passive motion is begun at the end of twelve to fourteen days.

OPERATIONS FOR TRAUMATIC DISLOCATIONS

In recent cases, Strictly speaking, these operations may be divided up into those performed for recent dislocations and those for similar

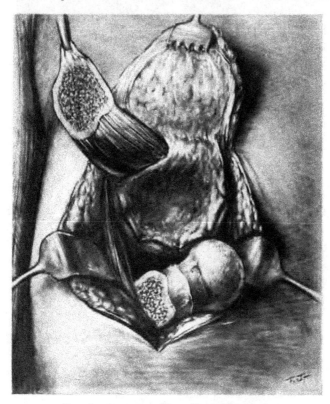

FIG. 48. ARTHROPLASTY OF HIP. (*Murphy.*)

injuries of long standing. It is, however, rare for a recent dislocation to require operative treatment for its reduction, as manipulation under an anæsthetic almost invariably succeeds. Occasionally, however, this is not so, especially when the dislocation is complicated with a fracture either of the acetabulum or of some portion of the head or neck of the bone. Under these circumstances, which should be diagnosed with certainty by means of a stereoscopic radiogram, it will be necessary to expose the joint and effect reduction without delay.

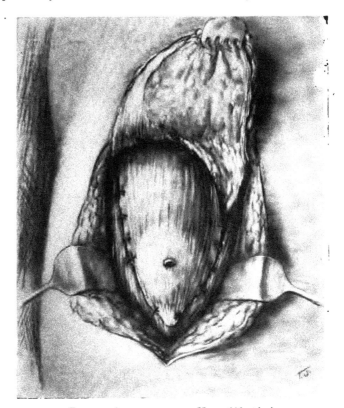

FIG. 49. ARTHROPLASTY OF HIP. (*Murphy*.)

Exposure of the joint for this purpose should be by the anterior route, since that gives the best access; the dislocation, if not primarily a posterior one, will certainly have become converted into one by the manipulations undertaken for its reduction, and the posterior route is unsuitable when the head of the bone lies behind the acetabulum. The operation need not be described in detail, since it follows the lines

already laid down for exposure of the neck of the femur (see p. 92).
When the head of the bone has been exposed, the finger is introduced
into the wound and the necessary manipulations for the reduction of the
dislocation according to Bigelow's instructions should be carried out;
any source of obstruction can be detected and removed or pulled aside.
It ought not to be necessary to divide the Y-ligament or any important
structures in these recent cases.

After reduction has been effected, the wound is sewn up and the
limb is steadied by a long Liston's splint for about a week after the
operation, when the patient may be fitted with a Thomas's hip-splint
and allowed to get about on crutches.   Passive movements should be
begun from the second or third day and gradually increased in range
and vigour.   The patient should be able to walk upon the limb within a
month of the operation.

In cases of long standing.   It is difficult to fix the exact time at
which operative interference should be preferred to attempts to reduce
the dislocation by manipulations, but it is best to give the benefit in any
case of doubt to operative interference, as the risk of damage to the
head of the bone or to important parts in the neighbourhood during
manipulation is very considerable owing to the powerful leverage that
can be brought to bear by means of the lower extremity.   It is probably
advisable to operate upon any case of unreduced dislocation that has
lasted for more than two or three weeks.   The exposure of the joint adds
little to the severity of the operation, while it undoubtedly simplifies
re-position, since this can be performed under the direct guidance of
the finger in the wound.

The operation should be done through an anterior incision.   The
posterior route is unsuitable because the head of the bone is always
dislocated behind the acetabulum and will interfere with access to that
cavity if the posterior route be chosen.   The acetabulum is easily inspected
through an anterior incision, on the other hand, especially if the incision
be prolonged upwards so as to detach the muscles from the outer side
of the ilium, and it can be prepared for the reception of the head of the
bone if necessary.

There are two principal difficulties in the operation which are directly
proportionate to the severity of the injury and the length of time that
the dislocation has remained unreduced; they are—partial obliteration
of the acetabulum and adhesions around the joint.   Most writers on the
subject mention the fact that the acetabulum is occupied by fibrous tissue
which must be removed before the head of the bone can be got into place.
The amount and consistency of this soft tissue will depend largely upon
the length of time that has elapsed since the dislocation, and therefore

this serious difficulty in the operation is likely to disappear as earlier operation becomes the practice.

The presence of dense adhesions around the joint may give rise to great difficulty in replacing the head of the bone. Here again the difficulty will be proportionate to the length of time that the dislocation has remained unreduced. The adhesions may have to be divided widely, and in doing this the position of the various important structures in the neighbourhood of the head of the neck of the bone must be remembered. If the adhesions be only trivial they may be broken down by rotating the limb freely in all directions. It is better to do this after the joint has been exposed, as any bleeding it causes can be checked at once. The capsule may have to be incised freely before the head of the bone can be got into position, since it will be much contracted and distorted. The principal structure that interferes with reduction is the Y-ligament, which may have to be partially or entirely detached from the neck of the femur before the head of the bone can be got back into place. In some of the published cases the rim of the acetabulum has been found to be fractured and portions have been removed. The head of the bone should be got into place if possible by manipulation methods rather than by traction, but it may be necessary to employ firm traction of this kind by means of pulleys; this, however, will only be called for in cases of long standing with extensive adhesions and considerable shrinkage of the ligamentous structures. In cases like this the whole upper extremity of the femur may need to be separated from its muscular attachments. The ligamentum teres is torn and as a rule cannot be traced.

After the head of the bone has been got into place the remains of the capsule are sutured over it and the soft parts are brought together as accurately as possible with buried catgut sutures. The wound is sutured without a drainage tube and the limb is steadied by a long Liston's splint. The after-treatment is similar to that for recent cases (*vide supra*).

OPERATIONS FOR CONGENITAL DISLOCATIONS

There are two principal methods for replacing a congenital dislocation of the hip, viz. Lorenz's so-called ' bloodless ' method, and the open operation. The former appears to be the more popular procedure at present, but in so far as it must necessarily be uncertain, since the surgeon can only guess and not see what he is doing, it is probable that, as surgeons gain more confidence in their power to treat large wounds in this region with safety, open operation will take its place, since it does with certainty what the misnamed ' bloodless operation ' can only do by guess. With regard to bleeding, there is no doubt that less blood is shed in the open operation than in the so-called 'bloodless method'; in the latter case free bleeding takes place into the tissues. Lorenz's method will not be described here, since it is not, strictly speaking, a surgical operation any more than is the setting of a fracture or the reduction of an ordinary dislocation.

Indications. (i) Operative measures are called for in congenital dislocations in children under four in which a careful attempt at re-position by Lorenz's method, checked by stereoscopic radiograms, has failed.

(ii) Operation is also required for all cases in children over the age of four as a primary measure. In these cases the alterations in the joint are so marked that experience upon the operating table shows it to be practically impossible to get the head of the bone properly into the acetabulum without a definite surgical operation. If Lorenz's manipulation be practised unsuccessfully the disturbance of the soft parts produced by it is so great as to interfere materially with the prospects of an open operation.

Operation. The writer is in the habit of dividing the operation into two stages. The first stage is the subcutaneous division of the shortened adductor muscles, which invariably offer considerable resistance to reduction and to the maintenance of the limb in position when the dislocation has been reduced. In order to avoid the severe bruising and extravasation of blood following Lorenz's manipulations the adductors are divided near their origin from the pelvis by a few sweeps of a tenotomy knife, which is inserted over the muscles as they are put on the stretch by abducting the limb. This is done a week before the main operation is undertaken, and the small wound will then have healed.

The most scrupulous care must be bestowed on the purification of the skin in these cases, and the only safe way is to purify the whole extremity as well as the groin and the buttock, as the manipulations during the operation are numerous and prolonged. The limb is enveloped in sterilized towels bandaged firmly on with a sterilized bandage wet with 1 in 2,000 biniodide solution. The child must lie upon sterilized cloths, and a sterilized towel should be pinned firmly round the waist so that there shall be no risk of the hands of the surgeon or his assistant coming into contact with unsterilized parts.

The incision, which is seen in Fig. 50, commences just below the anterior superior iliac spine, and is carried downwards and inwards between the outer margin of the sartorius and the adjacent edge of the extensor fasciæ femoris for about three inches. This incision is generally prolonged upwards parallel to and just over the outer edge of the iliac crest for about three inches. The incision below opens up the intermuscular interval which leads at once down to the neck and head of the bone.   As a rule the finger feels the rounded head projecting forwards, as the dislocation in these young children is practically always of the anterior variety.   The incision is deepened above so as to divide the extensor fasciæ femoris from its origin from the outer aspect of the ilium.   This gives excellent exposure of the whole hip area, and the

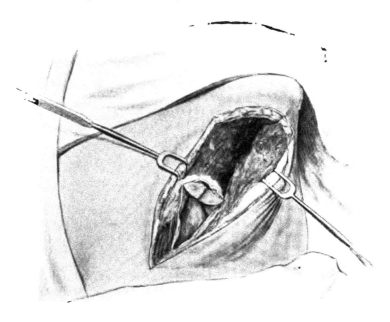

FIG. 50.   ANTERIOR INCISION FOR EXPOSURE OF THE HIP-JOINT.   The neck of the bone is seen exposed and the cotyloid ligament divided.   The incision has been prolonged above so as to detach the tensor fasciæ femoris from its origin.

capsule is then incised over the head of the bone, which is made to protrude forwards through it.

On introducing the finger through the capsule it will be found that the head of the bone has been lying in a diverticulum above and in front of the acetabulum.   The latter can always be identified by the finger and there is invariably a strong band derived from the Y-ligament stretched over its anterior aspect.   Between this band and the subjacent edge of the acetabulum the head of the bone has to pass before the dislocation can be reduced.   The surgeon now takes the limb in one hand

and attempts to reduce the dislocation, keeping the index finger of the other hand in the acetabulum as a guide. The best way to attempt reduction is to flex the limb fully and then to abduct it to its fullest limit, circumducting the whole limb outwards whilst doing so. This manœuvre is very like that practised for the reduction of an ordinary dislocation. No set instructions can be given for these manipulations, however, as they will vary with the alterations that have taken place in the neck of the femur. As a rule this is inclined unduly forward, so that when the head of the bone is in the acetabulum the limb is in a position of marked inward rotation. It will often be necessary to detach part of the capsule from the front of the acetabulum before the aperture becomes sufficiently large for the head of the bone to pass into it. There is never any doubt as to when reduction has been effected; the head of the bone slips in with a loud click and the joint at once becomes stable and remains so as long as that position is maintained. When the head is allowed to slip out of the acetabulum there is the characteristic sucking noise, and the finger is always able to examine the joint and see if the bone is in position or not.

When reduction has thus been attained, the position of maximum stability is determined; this is the position in which the head of the bone remains in the acetabulum with the least risk of displacement, and the limb must be kept in this position throughout the rest of the operation and must be immobilized in it subsequently. This position is often similar to that in which the limb is put up after Lorenz's manipulations, but it is not by any means always so; it is chiefly dependent upon the direction of the neck of the femur. In the last case in which I operated the limb was in a position of extreme inward rotation after reduction of the dislocation. It is nearly always necessary to keep the knee flexed in order to relax the tension of the hamstrings, which are otherwise apt to shoot the head of the bone out of the acetabulum.

The limb is entrusted to the assistant, who keeps it rigidly in the correct position. As long as this position is maintained there is no fear of dislocation recurring, and the child can be moved about with ease. The least alteration of the position, however, is apt to result in a sudden reproduction of the dislocation. The wound is now closed; before doing this I usually excise as much as possible of the redundant capsule, which is now unnecessary as the head of the bone is in the acetabulum. The edges of this are brought together with stout catgut and this forms a further barrier against reproduction of the dislocation. The soft tissues are brought together over the front of the joint with a few buried catgut sutures, and the wound is sutured completely without a drainage tube after every bleeding point has been tied.

Before sewing up the wound, the child is lifted on to the special support fixed to the table that Lorenz employs for the application of his plaster casings, and is held steady on this by an assistant, folded blankets or pillows being placed under the thorax to render the trunk horizontal. It is important to do it at this stage of the proceedings, since recurrence of the dislocation might occur from a clumsy movement on the part of the assistant, and if this occur before the wound is sewn up it is quite simple to reduce the dislocation under the guidance of the finger in the wound.

The dressings are applied and fastened in position by a few turns of a sterilized spica bandage. A pair of woollen combinations is then drawn on, and outside this a plaster of Paris spica is applied, taking in the knee in the flexed position. Before applying the bandage stout whip-cord, which has been steeped in melted beeswax, is laid over the combinations in the positions in which the casing is to be sawn for subsequent removal. These serve as guides for pulling through a Gigli's wire saw, which is the speediest and best method of removing the casing. The ends of the cord should project for several inches above and below the spica so that they may be tied together after the plaster has set, and then there will be no risk of their being pulled out. The spica is strengthened over the flexure of the knee and the front of the groin by applying strands of tow, which are teased out in plaster cream; this gives the bandages a toughness that prevents them from cracking. The child is kept under the anæsthetic during the application of the plaster and is not allowed to come round until it has set, when the edges are trimmed off and he is put back to bed.

After-treatment. The stitches are removed at the end of a fortnight. In order to do this the plaster of Paris casing must be removed. Another casing is applied immediately, and the utmost care must be taken to keep the limb in its original position throughout the removal of the plaster and the stitches and the application of the fresh casing. The child should always be under anæsthesia, from which it is not allowed to recover until the bandage has set. Fresh casings will have to be applied at intervals of two or three months, the limb meanwhile being brought down into its normal position by degrees, as each fresh plaster is applied. The knee is not included in the bandage after the first four months, and at the end of the first six months the child may be allowed to get about, the limb being still somewhat abducted. If the heel of the boot on the sound side be a little thickened it will tend to diminish the chance of the head of the bone slipping out of place. For further information upon this subject the reader may consult a paper by the author in the *Brit. Med. Journ.*, 1903, vol. ii.

SECTION II

OPERATIONS FOR TUBERCULOUS AFFECTIONS OF THE BONES AND JOINTS

PART I

OPERATIONS FOR TUBERCULOUS AFFECTIONS OF THE BONES

BY

HAROLD J. STILES, M.B., F.R.C.S. (Edin.), Lieutenant-Colonel, R.A.M.C.(T.).

Surgeon to Chalmers Hospital, Edinburgh, and to the Royal Hospital for Sick Children, Edinburgh

CHAPTER I

OPERATIONS FOR TUBERCULOUS OSTEOMYELITIS OF THE DIAPHYSES OF THE LONG BONES

THE operations upon the disease as it occurs in the long bones proper, that is to say, in those possessing an epiphysis at each end of the diaphysis, will be considered first. The seat of election for the disease to attack these bones is, in the writer's experience, undoubtedly the growing extremities of the diaphyses.

As the tuberculous focus in the end of the diaphysis develops, it sooner or later comes to invade the neighbouring structures. The nature of the operative treatment will not only be influenced by the particular bone involved, but will depend also on the extent and route of spread of the lesion, namely, whether it has made its way into the joint, into the soft parts outside the joint, or up the shaft of the bone. When the epiphysis is small, as is the case, for example, with the upper epiphysis of the femur and the lower epiphysis of the humerus, the adjacent diaphyseal extremities are very closely related to the cavity of the joint, as they are separated from it merely by the periosteum and the synovial membrane, with more or less intervening synovial fatty tissue. These anatomical relationships explain why the hip and elbow become so early involved secondary to a primary bone focus. In such cases the primary osseous lesion is dealt with at the same time that the joint is operated upon. When, however, the epiphysis adjacent to the juxta-epiphyseal focus is a large one, as is the case, for example, with the upper epiphysis of the humerus and the lower epiphysis of the femur, the neighbouring joint generally escapes. The disease meanwhile tends to advance either up the diaphysis or to the surface of the bone outside the joint.

In addition to the primary localized juxta-epiphyseal focus so commonly met with, we occasionally have to deal with tuberculosis of the diaphysis in a more diffuse form. It is this form of the disease which will be specially referred to under the heading of tuberculous osteomyelitis of the diaphysis. Although apparently of rare occurrence in other European countries, as well as in the American and Australian continents, it is by no means rare, at any rate in this country, as the writer has operated on upwards of fifty cases of the affection in the Royal Hospital for Sick Children, Edinburgh, during the last ten years.

OPERATIONS FOR PRIMARY TUBERCULOUS OSTEO-MYELITIS OF THE DIAPHYSIS

Primary tuberculous osteomyelitis of the diaphysis may start either in the spongy tissue at some distance from the epiphyseal cartilage or in the medullary canal, and in each situation the disease may present itself as a more or less circumscribed focus, or it may take the progressive infiltrating form, originally described by König. Occasionally the infiltration may involve the entire length of the medullary canal. It not infrequently happens, however, that a primary focus, beginning in the juxta-epiphyseal region (the metaphysis), spreads as a tuberculous infiltration into the medullary cavity, so that it is not always possible to draw a sharp distinction between metaphyseal and diaphyseal (medullary) tuberculosis.

The circumscribed form of the disease generally occurs as a soft, caseous, avascular focus, surrounded by an advancing zone of active tuberculous tissue, which is of a greyish colour, semi-translucent, and slightly vascular. The surrounding bone, apart from its increased vascularity, may appear almost normal; in some cases it is rarefied, while in others again, especially if the disease be very chronic and tending to heal spontaneously, it is more or less sclerosed. Sometimes the focus contains one or more small sequestra, but even when the sequestrum is single, it is seldom of large size. Only rarely is the focus represented by a chronic abscess, and when this is the case the wall of the abscess very seldom presents the smooth sclerosed surface met with in the chronic staphylococcal abscess, known as Brodie's abscess.

The congestion set up in the surrounding bone by the presence of the tuberculous focus spreads through the Haversian systems to the periosteum, with the result that a formative osteoplastic periostitis is set up, and this gives rise to the deposit of a layer of new vascular and porous bone between the periosteum and the cortex. It is this sheath of subperiosteal new bone which gives to the disease its most important and characteristic diagnostic sign, namely, thickening of the diaphysis; indeed, in the early stage of the disease this is the only physical sign present. Its importance, therefore, cannot be overestimated.

As the disease almost invariably occurs during childhood, congenital syphilis is the only affection with which it is likely to be confounded. There is seldom any difficulty in excluding the latter condition.

A good radiogram will not only confirm the diagnosis, but in many instances demonstrates quite distinctly the position, size, and shape of the focus, the presence or absence of a sequestrum, and the thickness and extent of the subperiosteal sheath of new bone. It follows, therefore, that a skiagram should always be taken before proceeding to operation, as it shows exactly how much bone requires to be removed.

As the tuberculous focus enlarges, first the cancellous, then the cortical, and ultimately the new subperiosteal bone becomes invaded at

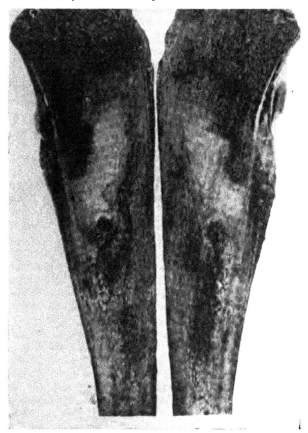

Fig. 51. Upper Two-thirds of the Diaphysis of a Tibia resected for Tuberculous Osteomyelitis. From a child aged 10 years. The upper end of the diaphysis was wrenched away from the epiphysis. The specimen is bisected, exposing two sawn surfaces. The light shadow represents an elongated and somewhat irregular caseous focus. Note the thick layer of new subperiosteal bone, especially posteriorly where the disease has reached the cortex. (*Photograph by Mr. Richard Muir.*)

one or other part of its circumference. Finally, the periosteum gives way, and a deep-seated abscess is produced; this sooner or later becomes super-ficial, and if left to itself ruptures externally, leaving a chronic sinus.

Operation. The operative treatment of primary tuberculous osteo-myelitis of the diaphysis consists in the first place of freely exposing the bone for a little distance beyond the extent of the disease. The incision is so planned that the dissection occasions the minimum of injury to the soft parts. An intermuscular plane is chosen which avoids injuring more especially the nerve-supply to the muscles.

The method usually adopted is, after freely opening up the bone with a chisel, to thoroughly gouge and scrape away the diseased focus. This having been done, either some preparation of iodoform or pure carbolic acid is applied to the wall of the cavity; the latter is then stuffed with iodoform gauze or filled with Mosetig-Moorhof's iodoform-wax filling.

While the above method is that which has been invariably employed by those surgeons who have recorded cases of this disease, the writer is strongly of opinion that such a procedure should be the exception rather than the rule. The early results of such a method of treatment are satisfactory enough, but unfortunately it too often happens that the patient sooner or later returns with the scar tuberculous and the seat of a sinus leading down to further disease in the bone. Such a result is not to be wondered at when we consider that it is almost impossible to remove all the affected area by the gouging process.

After a few such disappointments the writer has, for a number of years past, treated the affection by subperiosteal resection of the diseased part of the diaphysis. Care is taken to divide the bone well above and below the focus; in short, the disease is dealt with radically, as if it were a malignant tumour.

By the aid of skiagraphy the disease can be diagnosed in its early stage, before the focus has perforated the bone. Then is the most favour-able stage for operation, as the knife can be kept outside the infected area. No iodoform or other antiseptic need be applied to the wound, no stuffing is introduced, and the wound can almost invariably be closed without drainage.

The best instrument for dividing the shaft of the bone is Gigli's wire saw. This is passed round the shaft inside the periosteum, which has been previously thoroughly separated all round with a suitable elevator. For introducing the saw behind the bone the writer uses an instrument (Fig. 52) which resembles somewhat a broad flattened aneurysm needle with an oblique slit leading into a large eye placed as close as possible to its extremity. After the instrument has been passed behind the bone and the eye made to project on the opposite side between the bone and the periosteum, the loop at the end of the wire saw is hooked into the eye by means of the slit above mentioned. By withdrawing the instrument, the saw is carried behind the bone; the handles are then hooked on, and the bone is sawn across. In young children the bones of the forearm may be snipped across with ordinary bone-forceps, but this instrument leaves a bruised and less even section, with the result that there is often some irregularity subsequently where the new bone joins the old. By using Gigli's wire saw, on the other hand, it is often almost impossible, even with a skiagram, to tell, after the new bone has completely developed, where the bone had been divided.

After the diaphysis has been divided beyond one extremity of the lesion, a strong hook is introduced into the medullary canal, and while the divided end is forcibly dragged upwards the periosteum is separated from the deep surfaces of the bone until it is freed to a little beyond the opposite limit of the diseased focus. When this level has been reached, Gigli's saw is again applied and the bone divided. The sawn surfaces of the segment of bone removed are carefully examined to make sure that they are free from disease; if not, more bone must be removed.

If the disease has approached close to one end of the diaphysis, or if it has spread along it from a juxta-epiphyseal lesion, the diseased segment must be removed right up to the epiphysis. After sawing across the diaphysis, the separation of the diseased portion from the epiphysis is effected by seizing its divided end and wrenching it away from the epiphysis. When this has been done it will be found that the epiphyseal cartilage, instead of coming away with the diaphysis, is left firmly attached to the epiphysis. This is what one would expect on anatomical grounds; were it otherwise, the radical operation would be contra-indicated on account of the shortening which would result. As long as the disease has not actually involved the epiphyseal cartilage itself, the writer has found that the above operation does not give rise to any subsequent shortening.

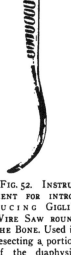

FIG. 52. INSTRU-
MENT FOR INTRO-
DUCING GIGLI'S
WIRE SAW ROUND
THE BONE. Used in
resecting a portion
of the diaphysis.
See also Fig. 72.

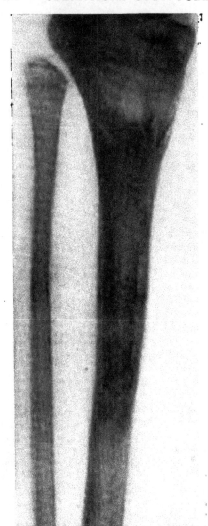

The bleeding from the periosteal tube seldom amounts to more than a general oozing which soon ceases. Occasionally, the main nutrient artery needs ligaturing. After the bleeding has practically ceased, the periosteal tube is closed with a buried catgut suture; care is taken to suture carefully the two extremities of the incision in the periosteum in such a way as to completely re-cover the sawn stumps of the bone. It is this precaution, combined with the use of Gigli's saw, which enables Nature to effect such a remarkably accurate fusion of the new bone with the old stump (Fig. 53). In suturing the periosteum, the writer prefers to use an interrupted rather than a continuous suture, for, should the periosteal tube become over-distended with blood, the tension is removed by some of the blood escaping between the sutures.

A few cutaneous catgut sutures are also employed to stitch the deep fascia, and, in the case of a deep bone such as the radius or fibula, the muscles are also stitched, either along with or separ-

FIG. 53. SKIAGRAM OF THE LIMB FROM WHICH THE SPECIMEN SEEN IN FIG. 51 WAS REMOVED. Shows new formation of bone one year after the operation. Note the delicate transverse line of sclerosis at the junction of the new and old bone. Ossification is still somewhat incomplete towards the upper part of the new diaphysis. (*By Dr. E. Price.*)

ately from the periosteal tube. The operation is completed by closing the skin wound with interrupted sutures of silkworm-gut.

If a sinus already exists at the time of operation it should first of all be well scraped and disinfected with pure carbolic acid. The orifice should be excised by including it in an elliptical incision, which may either form part of the main incision or be independent of it; in the latter case it may be taken advantage of for drainage.

It not infrequently happens that, by the time the patient reaches the surgeon, the focus has given rise to a chronic abscess in the soft parts. As regards situation, it may be either subperiosteal, intermuscular, or more superficial, depending on its duration. In such a case an endeavour is made to plan the incision so that it will give free access to the abscess cavity as well as to the diseased bone. If this be not possible a separate incision must be made. The whole abscess cavity should be freely laid open and any outlying pockets of pus must be followed out. After the cavity and its ramifications have been thoroughly curetted, some sublimated iodoform-bismuth paste is rubbed into the wall. This preparation, which the writer uses in all tuberculous cases, consists of a mixture of one part of iodoform and two parts of subnitrate of bismuth stored in a 1–1,000 solution of perchloride of mercury. Enough for the operation is removed from the stock jar with a spoon and transferred to a small sterilized vessel. This mixture is preferable to dry iodoform, to the glycerine emulsion, or to the ethereal solution. Its advantages are that it is less toxic, so that more can be used, and that it forms rather more of a paste than sublimated iodoform alone.

After-treatment. The after-treatment consists in keeping the limb quiet in good position for a few weeks, after which it is put up in a suitable splint or in plaster of Paris until the new bone is sufficiently well developed to allow the patient to begin to use the limb. If the disease has not involved the periosteum, the new bone, as already stated, is perfectly re-formed in from three to six months (Fig. 74). If, on the other hand, the periosteum has been invaded by the disease, the reproduction is less perfect.

The steps of the more typical operations for the localized as well as the more diffuse varieties of tuberculous osteomyelitis of the diaphyses of the various long bones will now be described.

OPERATIONS FOR TUBERCULOUS OSTEOMYELITIS OF THE DIAPHYSIS OF THE HUMERUS

If the skiagram shows a limited focus of tubercle at the *upper end of the diaphysis*, thorough scraping will usually suffice to bring about a cure. A dissection is made so as to expose the surgical neck of the humerus, where it is free from muscular attachments, namely, beneath the posterior part of the deltoid, immediately in front of the insertion of the teres minor and the upper fibres of origin of the outer head of the triceps. As the bone is deeply placed, the incision must be a comparatively long one; it is made along the middle three-fifths of the posterior border of the deltoid. After dividing the integuments and deep fascia, the posterior border of the muscle is freed and retracted

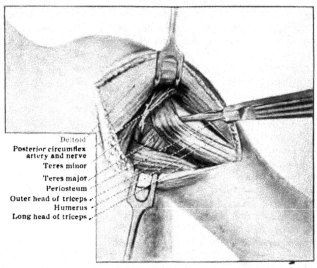

Deltoid
Posterior circumflex
artery and nerve
Teres minor
Teres major
Periosteum
Outer head of triceps
Humerus
Long head of triceps

FIG. 54.   EXPOSURE OF THE UPPER END OF THE DIAPHYSIS OF THE HUMERUS. The deltoid is retracted forwards, and the posterior circumflex vessels and nerve are seen coming through the quadrilateral space; the periosteum is divided longitudinally exactly in front of the upper part of the origin of the outer head of the triceps; a rugine is seen separating the periosteum from the bone.

well forwards. To reach the surgical neck of the humerus it will, as a rule, be found necessary to divide transversely the upper part of the posterior fibres of the deltoid. Some of the cutaneous branches of the circumflex nerve are divided, and forceps are applied to the accompanying superficial branches of the posterior circumflex artery. The lower border of the teres minor is now identified, and by following it to its insertion the humerus will be reached immediately above the surgical neck. The circumflex nerve and the posterior circumflex artery are then defined as they come through the quadrilateral space in the posterior wall of the axilla. The boundaries of this space as seen from behind are:

above, the lower border of the teres minor; below, the teres major; externally, the surgical neck of the humerus; internally, the long head of the triceps.

After carefully isolating and freeing the above vessels and nerves they may be retracted downwards so as to give sufficient room for applying the gouge. The bone is opened up in the first instance immediately below the capsule, and in gouging away the focus care is taken not to

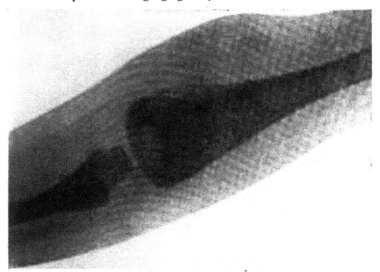

FIG. 55. SKIAGRAM SHOWING DIFFUSE TUBERCULOUS OSTEOMYELITIS OF THE LOWER THIRD OF THE DIAPHYSIS OF THE HUMERUS. From a child aged 1 year and 4 months. The disease has perforated the bone and given rise to a secondary abscess above the internal condyle. (*By Dr. H. Rainy.*)

open unnecessarily into the joint or to injure the epiphyseal cartilage. Should the focus extend for some little distance down the shaft, the circumflex vessels and nerves are retracted upwards, and the opening in the bone is enlarged downwards immediately in front of the origin of the outer head of the triceps, the periosteum being previously incised and stripped backwards and forwards. After thoroughly scraping away all the disease, sublimated iodoform-bismuth paste is rubbed into the cavity, or the latter is filled with Mosetig-Moorhof's iodoform-wax filling. The wound is closed without drainage.

Resection of the upper third of the diaphysis of the humerus is merely an extension of the operation above described. Instead of goug-

.ing into the bone, the periosteum is incised longitudinally from immediately below the capsular ligament downwards parallel to, and immediately in front of, the origin of the outer head of the triceps. The
circumflex vessels and nerves are retracted upwards. The periosteum
is divided in front of the outer head of the triceps, thereby avoiding
the musculo-spiral nerve and the superior profunda vessels. After sawing across the humerus with Gigli's saw, and hooking up its divided end

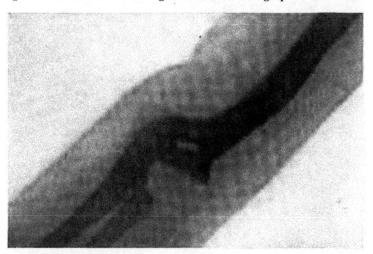

FIG. 56. SKIAGRAM OF THE ARM SHOWN IN THE PREVIOUS FIGURE. Taken
four months after subperiosteal resection of the lower third of the diaphysis of
the humerus. The elbow-joint has not been opened into. Note how well the
lower end of the bone has modelled itself. There is slight angular deformity at
the junction of the old and the new bone. (*By Dr. H. Rainy.*)

in the manner already described, the periosteum and the three muscles
inserted into the region of the bicipital groove are carefully separated
from the bone, which is then wrenched away from its upper epiphysis.
This can be done without opening into the joint. The periosteal tube
is carefully sutured with catgut and the wound closed.

After-treatment. The after-treatment must be directed towards
keeping the periosteal tube on the stretch so as to prevent shortening
as well as angular deformity at the junction of the new with the old
bone. For the first few weeks the patient is kept on his back with
extension applied to the arm in the abducted position. After this the
patient is allowed to get about with the limb in a rectangular splint

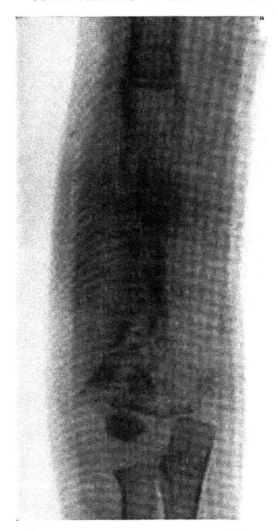

FIG. 57. SKIAGRAM SHOWING RE-FORMATION OF THE HUMERUS. Taken six weeks after subperiosteal resection of the lower two-thirds of the diaphysis for extensive tuberculous osteomyelitis in a child aged 6 years. The elbow-joint has not been opened into. Note the 'patchy' manner in which new bone is forming, and the ferrule of new subperiosteal bone surrounding the stump of the old bone. (*By Dr. E. Price.*)

and light weight extension applied to the lower fragment. In three months the bone is sufficiently re-formed to allow the patient to begin to use the arm.

In resection of the lower half of the diaphysis of the humerus the incision is begun on the back of the external condyle and carried vertically upwards immediately behind the external intermuscular septum as far as the musculo-spiral groove. The bone is reached by deepening the incision through the fleshy fibres of the inner head of the triceps. The musculo-spiral (radial) nerve and superior profunda vessels are carefully freed and retracted forwards and upwards. If the disease extends higher up than the middle of the shaft, some of the fibres of the outer head of the triceps must be divided in an upward and backward direction parallel to and behind the musculo-spiral nerve, the external cutaneous branches of which are divided. The periosteum is divided along the whole length of the wound, and the bone, after having been divided at the requisite level, is completely freed from the periosteum, and then wrenched away from the lower epiphysis. In spite of the fact that the capsule of the elbow-joint is attached to the diaphysis considerably above the level of the epiphyseal cartilage, it is interesting to note that on both occasions on which the writer has done this operation he was able to wrench the lower end of the diaphysis away from the epiphyseal cartilage subperiosteally without opening into the joint.

After-treatment. The after-treatment is practically the same as for resection of the upper half of the diaphysis. As soon as the new bone has sufficiently formed to allow of the arm being flexed, passive movement is begun with the object of preventing stiffness at the elbow. It may be necessary to administer an anæsthetic on the first occasion this is done, and care must be taken not to fracture the new bone.

Results. In the four cases in which the humerus was operated on, from the lower third to the lower two-thirds of the diaphysis was resected. In all the cases there were tuberculous lesions in other bones. Primary union was obtained in three cases. One case healed slowly by second intention, but five years later the child was found to be in the best of health with no trace of tuberculous disease. In this case the humerus had re-formed unevenly and the arm was somewhat flail-like, though quite useful. In another case there was some angling at the junction of the old and new bone, which, however, was easily remedied by fracturing and splinting; six years later the functional result was found to be excellent, and the resected bone perfectly re-formed. In a third case where primary union was obtained, the child died about a year later, the cause of death being unknown. In the fourth and most recent cases the humerus is re-forming well, and the result promises to be good.

OPERATIONS FOR TUBERCULOUS OSTEOMYELITIS OF THE DIAPHYSIS OF THE RADIUS

Cases requiring resection are more frequently met with in the bones of the forearm than in the humerus. Resection of the *lower third* or so of the radius ranks amongst the commonest of these operations. The incision is commenced a finger's breadth below the dorso-radial tubercle on the back of the lower end of the radius,—a tubercle which separates the groove for the extensor carpi radialis brevior from that for the extensor secundi internodii pollicis (pollicis longus)—and is carried vertically

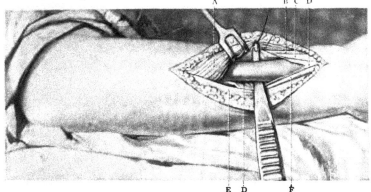

FIG. 58. RESECTION OF THE LOWER THIRD OF THE DIAPHYSIS OF THE RADIUS. The extensor pollicis brevis has been retracted upwards and outwards; the extensor minimi (quinti) digiti and extensor pollicis longus have been retracted inwards; the periosteum has been split, and the instrument for passing the wire saw has been introduced between the anterior aspect of the bone and the periosteum. A, Extensor pollicis brevis; B, Extensor carpi radialis longior; C, Extensor carpi radialis brevior; D, D, Periosteum; E, Extensor minimi digiti; F, Extensor pollicis longus.

up the middle of the lower half of the back of the forearm. After ligaturing the divided ends of the commencement of the radial vein, the deep fascia, along with the upper part of the posterior annular (dorsal carpal) ligament, is divided, and the outer border of the extensor digitorum communis is identified and freed. Appearing from beneath this muscle are the fleshy fibres of the extensor ossis (abductor pollicis longus) and the extensor primi internodii pollicis (extensor pollicis brevis), which pass obliquely downwards and outwards over the back of the radius and the radial extensor of the wrist. To expose the radius the extensor digitorum communis is retracted inwards, while the fleshy bellies of the extensor ossis and extensor primi internodii pollicis are retracted well

A   B C   D   C   EEE

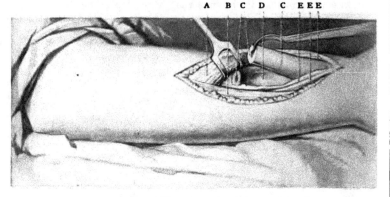

FIG. 59. FURTHER STAGE OF RESECTION OF THE LOWER THIRD OF THE DIA-
PHYSIS OF THE RADIUS. The diaphysis has been divided and hooked upwards
to enable the periosteum to be separated from the anterior aspect of the bone.
A, Extensor pollicis brevis; B, Extensor minimi digiti, C, C, Radius; D, Periosteum;
E, E, E, Extensor pollicis longus.

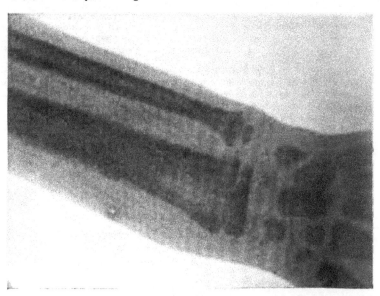

FIG. 60. SKIAGRAM SHOWING DIFFUSE TUBERCULOUS OSTEOMYELITIS OF THE
LOWER HALF OF THE DIAPHYSIS OF THE RADIUS. From a child aged 7 years.
Note the thickening of the bone. The disease has commenced to invade the
epiphyseal cartilage. (By Dr. H. Rainy.)

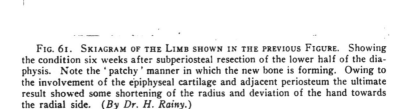

FIG. 61. SKIAGRAM OF THE LIMB SHOWN IN THE PREVIOUS FIGURE. Showing the condition six weeks after subperiosteal resection of the lower half of the diaphysis. Note the 'patchy' manner in which the new bone is forming. Owing to the involvement of the epiphyseal cartilage and adjacent periosteum the ultimate result showed some shortening of the radius and deviation of the hand towards the radial side. (*By Dr. H. Rainy.*)

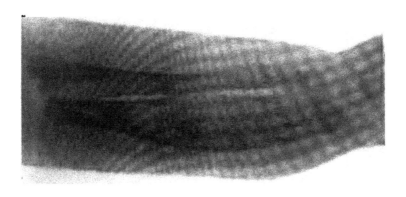

FIG. 62. SKIAGRAM SHOWING DIFFUSE TUBERCULOUS OSTEOMYELITIS OF THE LOWER THREE-FOURTHS OF THE SHAFT OF THE RADIUS. From a child aged 1 year and 4 months. Note the great thickening of the bone, in the interior of which a large sequestrum is seen. (*By Dr. H. Rainy.*)

upwards and outwards.   The fibres of the latter muscle are partly
detached from their origin from the back of the radius.   The periosteum
is now divided longitudinally as far upwards as is necessary.   The
terminal branch of the posterior interosseous (deep radial) nerve dips
beneath the extensor secundi internodii pollicis, and is therefore left uninjured at the ulnar edge of the wound.   The terminal branch of the posterior interosseous artery may require to be ligatured.   After dividing the
radius and hooking it up into the wound, the periosteum is separated from
the anterior aspect of the bone, and the latter is wrenched away from the

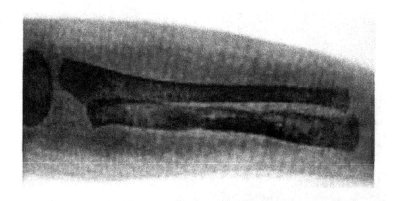

Fig. 63. Skiagram from the same Case as shown in Fig. 62. Showing
the condition four months after subperiosteal resection of the greater part of the
diaphysis. Note the rapidity with which new bone has formed; also the perfect
junction (represented by the dark transverse linear shadow) between the old and
the new bone towards the lower end of the diaphysis. (By Dr. H. Rainy.)

lower epiphysis. If the bone fractures across where it has been weakened
by the disease, the lower portion can easily be shelled out separately.

In some cases operated on by the writer, the disease had involved *the
greater part of the diaphysis of the radius* so that the bone had to be
divided immediately below the bicipital tuberosity. In these cases the best
plan is to resect the lower half or so of the bone in the first place, and
then to complete the operation by continuing the dissection upwards until
the bone is reached above the level of the disease. For this purpose the
incision already described is continued upwards along the outer border
of the extensor digitorum communis, so as to open up freely the inter-

muscular septum between it and the extensor carpi radialis brevior. In the floor of the wound there are exposed, from below upwards, the extensor primi internodii pollicis, the extensor ossis metacarpi pollicis, and finally the supinator brevis. The posterior interosseous vessels emerge between the two latter muscles, while the nerve pierces the supinator brevis a little above its lower border. Forceps are applied to the divided branches of the artery, but care is taken not to injure the nerve.

To expose the radius above the middle of its shaft, the fleshy belly

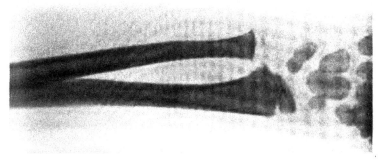

FIG. 64. SKIAGRAM FROM THE SAME CASE AS SHOWN IN THE TWO PREVIOUS FIGURES, SIX YEARS AFTER OPERATION. Note the perfect re-formation of bone. (*By Dr. E. Price.*)

of the extensor carpi radialis brevior is retracted well forwards and out-wards, while the extensor ossis metacarpi pollicis, previously retracted upwards and outwards, is now retracted in the opposite direction, namely, downwards and inwards. The periosteum is then incised longitudinally immediately external to the origin of the muscle, the incision being continued upwards so as to divide the lower fibres of the supinator brevis muscle parallel and external to the posterior interosseous nerve. The stump of the bone is now hooked upwards to enable the periosteum to be separated from the anterior aspect of the bone, which is then divided immediately below the bicipital tuberosity. In one case, where the disease extended still higher up, the writer was obliged to wrench the upper end of the bone away from the grasp of the orbicular (annular) ligament. When this had been done it was found that the upper epiphysis, which had not yet begun to ossify, had come away with the diaphysis.

The immediate result was satisfactory, but it is too early to say what the ultimate result will be as regards deformity and function. The operation is completed by suturing the periosteum, and after this has been done the adjacent edges of the extensor digitorum communis and the extensor carpi radialis brevior are united by a few catgut sutures so as to close the fascial envelope and repair the intermuscular septum.

If the disease be confined to the *middle third* of the radius, the bone may be more easily reached by placing the incision further outwards and passing between the fleshy belly of the supinator longus (brachio-radialis)

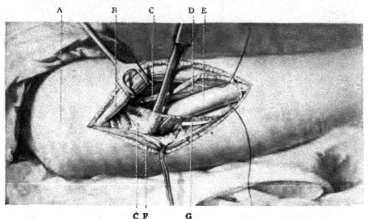

FIG. 65. RESECTION OF THE UPPER THIRD OF THE DIAPHYSIS OF THE RADIUS. The extensor carpi radialis brevior has been retracted forwards, the extensor digitorum communis backwards; the supinator brevis has been incised a little in front of the posterior interosseous nerve. The rugine separates the supinator brevis along with the periosteum from the upper third of the bone. A, External condyle; B, Extensor carpi radialis brevior; c, c, Supinator brevis; D, Periosteum; E, Radius; F, Extensor digitorum communis; G, Posterior interosseous nerve.

and the upper part of the tendon of the extensor carpi radialis longior. In the floor of the wound are the lower fibres of the supinator brevis, and immediately behind them the insertion of the pronator radii teres. The periosteum is incised immediately behind the latter tendon, and the incision is continued upwards through the lower fibres of the supinator brevis external to the posterior interosseous nerve.

After-treatment.   The important point in the after-treatment is to prevent shortening of the radius during its re-formation. Should this occur the hand will become deviated to the radial side. The best way to prevent this deformity is to keep the hand well adducted to the ulnar side until the bone has completely re-formed, that is to say, for about six months. This is most conveniently done by the application of a pistol-splint shaped out of a strip of aluminium.

Results. In the thirteen cases in which resection of portions of the diaphysis of the radius was performed the entire diaphysis was resected in three and the upper two-thirds in two, while the lower part of the radius to the extent of two-thirds to less than a half was resected in the other cases. As a rule the bone has re-formed well, and the functional results are excellent, but in some there is slight shortening of the radius with consequent deviation of the hand to the radial side.

OPERATIONS FOR TUBERCULOUS OSTEOMYELITIS OF THE DIAPHYSIS OF THE ULNA

Tuberculous osteomyelitis of the diaphysis of the ulna is frequently met with in the region of the olecranon and upper part of the shaft. As the bone is so superficial, the thickening and tenderness produced by the secondary periostitis soon become manifest. This is fortunate, as the operation should be undertaken before the focus has had time to produce an abscess followed by a sinus, and especially before the disease has had time to extend to the joint. As the greater part of the articular extremity is developed from the diaphysis, it follows that it is impossible to remove its upper end without opening into the joint. The surgeon is obliged, therefore, to fall back on gouging as the routine operation in dealing with the disease in the upper end of the diaphysis of the ulna.

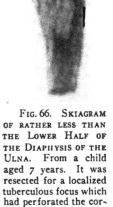

Fig. 66. Skiagram of rather less than the Lower Half of the Diaphysis of the Ulna. From a child aged 7 years. It was resected for a localized tuberculous focus which had perforated the cortex and produced a subperiosteal abscess. (*By Dr. E. Price.*)

Operation. The incision is carried down to the bone over the centre of the olecranon and along the posterior border of the shaft for a variable distance, depending on the extent of the disease. Care must be taken not to open into the joint at the upper end of the incision. In separating the periosteum the anconeus will be detached along with the outer flap, while the extensor carpi ulnaris will be partly detached with the inner flap. The bone is freely gouged into and the focus thoroughly scraped out. This is one of the situations in which a sequestrum is not infrequently met with. After introducing sublimated iodoform-bismuth paste or Mosetig-Moorhof's iodoform-wax

filling into the bony cavity, the periosteum is sutured with catgut and the
wound closed without drainage.

If an abscess exists, with the skin over it beginning to be involved,
it is better, instead of making a vertical incision through the damaged
skin, to make a longitudinal curved incision through the healthy skin
just beyond the abscess. The flap having been reflected, its deep surface,
which forms the superficial wall of the abscess, is carefully freed from all
tubercle, partly by scraping and partly by the aid of scissors curved on
the flat. If there be a possibility of the joint being involved, the above
curved incision is made along the outer margin of the abscess, so that,

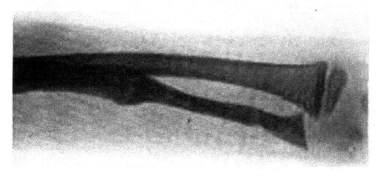

FIG. 67.   SKIAGRAM SHOWING NEW FORMATION OF BONE ELEVEN WEEKS AFTER
   RESECTION.   From the same case as the previous figure.   (*By Dr. E. Price.*)

should the joint require to be resected, the incision may be prolonged
upwards over the posterior aspect of the radio-humeral joint and behind
the external intermuscular septum. The entire incision is then practically
the same as that recommended by Kocher for excision of the elbow-joint.

It is not necessary to describe in detail the steps of the operation for
resection of the lower half or more of the diaphysis. The incision is of
course made along the posterior subcutaneous border.

After-treatment. In the after-treatment an aluminium pistol-splint
is applied so as to carry the hand as far as possible to the radial side.
When the wound is healed a plaster or starch bandage may be substituted
for the splint.

Results. Of the eleven cases in which a portion of the diaphysis of the ulna was resected, the lower part to the extent of one to two thirds was resected in eight cases. The upper end was scraped in two cases, while the upper half was resected along with the elbow-joint in another case. The bone re-formed well in all the cases that could be traced except in one, where the middle third of the ulna has not re-formed at all and the other third is too thin; the consequence is that the radius is a little bent where the ulna is deficient. A perfect functional result was obtained in three cases. In one case the elbow is completely ankylosed, pronation and supination being lost, but the patient's general health is good. The other cases have either been lost sight of, or have been too recently operated on to enable one to estimate the permanent result.

OPERATIONS FOR TUBERCULOUS OSTEOMYELITIS OF THE DIAPHYSIS OF THE FEMUR

The epiphyseal cartilage at the upper end of the femur is at the junction of the head and neck; it follows, therefore, that a juxta-epiphyseal lesion is situated in the intracapsular portion of the neck of the bone and that the joint is soon involved. If, by the aid of skiagraphy, the focus be detected before the joint is invaded, the treatment should be conservative rather than operative, as it is almost impossible to remove all the disease without opening into and damaging the joint.

When the tuberculous focus is situated in the greater trochanter, a free incision is carried vertically over it, midway between its anterior and posterior borders. After splitting the aponeurotic insertion of the gluteus maximus (and, if necessary, nicking it a little on either side so as to admit of its being more easily retracted), the outer aspect of the trochanter is exposed, overlapped above and anteriorly by the insertion of the gluteus medius, while immediately below its root is the upper part of the vastus externus (lateralis). If the lesion be a limited one this single vertical incision is sufficient for the purpose of separating the periosteum and muscular attachments, but if it be more extensive it is better to separate them by means of an inverted T-shaped incision. The superior perforating branch of the profunda artery is divided and ligatured. The chisel (or gouge) is now applied and the bone is sufficiently opened up to allow of the disease being removed under control of the eye. After applying sublimated iodoform-bismuth paste to the cavity, the periosteum and muscular attachments are sutured back into position. A second row of sutures unites the aponeurosis of the gluteus maximus, and the wound is closed without drainage. Should a sinus be present, it must be disinfected with pure carbolic acid, or, better still, excised, and part of the wound should be left open for the introduction of a strip of iodoform gauze.

After-treatment. The limb should be kept absolutely at rest for some months, and to avoid subsequent bending of the neck (coxa vara) no weight should be borne on the limb for about a year from the date of operation. The patient, however, may be allowed to get about by means

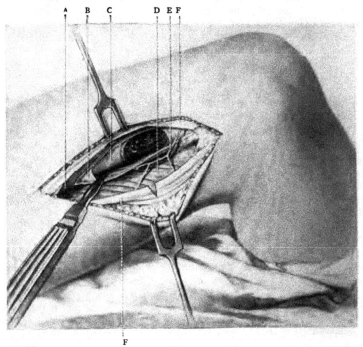

Fig. 68. EXPOSURE OF THE OUTER ASPECT OF THE LOWER THIRD OF THE DIAPHYSIS OF THE FEMUR. The ilio-tibial band has been split longitudinally and nicked transversely; the external intermuscular septum has been opened up, exposing the short head of the biceps and the anastomosis between the profunda artery and the superior external articular branch of the popliteal; the rugine separates the split periosteum from the posterior aspect of the diaphysis of the femur; the bone is opened into. The focus of disease is usually situated nearer to the condyle. A, Vastus externus; B, Periosteum; C, Femur; D, Biceps; E, Anastomosis between profunda and popliteal arteries; F, F, Ilio-tibial band.

of a Thomas's hip-splint, a patten being added to the boot of the sound limb.

It is advisable to have a skiagram of the hip taken every two or three months so that the progress of the repair may be watched.   By this means the surgeon is able to form a correct estimate as to when the patient should be allowed the free use of the limb.

Tuberculous osteomyelitis is comparatively common in the *lower end of the diaphysis of the femur* in the region of the trigone, and in the early stage it generally occurs as a more or less circumscribed focus limited to one or other supracondyloid region.   As the disease advances the trigone becomes perforated, with the result that sooner or later a deep-seated

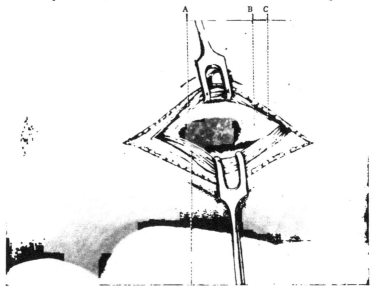

FIG. 69.   EXPOSURE OF A TUBERCULOUS FOCUS IN THE INTERNAL SUPRA-CONDYLOID REGION OF THE FEMUR.   The vastus internus (medialis) and periosteum have been split and the edges of both retracted; the bone has been opened into.   A, A, Vastus internus; B, Femur; C, Periosteum.

abscess forms in the popliteal space.   It is due largely to the readiness with which the focus makes its way through the trigone above the attachments of the capsular ligament, that the knee-joint itself owes its escape.

When the focus involves the *external supracondyloid region* an incision is carried from the posterior part of the outer surface of the external condyle upwards along the line of the external intermuscular septum, which separates the vastus externus from the biceps.   By deepening the incision in the plane of the septum and forcibly drawing apart the adjacent muscles by suitable retractors, the bone is at length reached. In dividing the periosteum care must be taken not to injure the superior external (lateral) articular artery, which lies close to the bone just above the external condyle. To enable the periosteum to be sufficiently stripped off the trigone it is generally necessary to make two short transverse incisions through the membrane at each extremity of the vertical incision. The lower transverse incision should be placed just above the superior external articular artery, which is displaced downwards along the periosteum.

When the disease is in the *internal supracondyloid region*, the dissection-down to the bone is made either in front of or behind the tendon of the adductor magnus, depending upon the exact position of the focus.

In the first method the incision is begun over the middle of the internal condyle, and is carried upwards a little in front of the sartorius. In the floor of the wound the oblique fleshy fibres of the vastus internus (medialis) are exposed and divided a little in front of the tendon of the adductor magnus so as to avoid wounding the deep branch of the anastomotic (genu suprema) artery. The loose cellular tissue between the vastus internus and the femur is opened into, and by retracting the edges of the divided muscle the bone is freely exposed. The superior internal articular artery is avoided, if possible.

To expose the trigone behind the tendon of the adductor magnus, an incision is carried upwards from the adductor tubercle between the sartorius and gracilis anteriorly, and the semi-tendinosus and semi-membranosus posteriorly. Retractors are now introduced and the dissection is deepened until the tendon of the adductor magnus is reached. By retracting it forwards and inwards along with the sartorius and gracilis (the semi-tendinosus and semi-membranosus along with the popliteal vessels being retracted backwards and outwards), the bone is freely exposed. The periosteum is incised immediately behind the internal intermuscular septum, which passes from the tendon of the adductor magnus to the internal supracondyloid ridge.

In chiselling the bone and gouging out the focus, care should be taken not to injure the epiphyseal cartilage unnecessarily. Should the bone focus be complicated by an abscess, either in the popliteal space or under the vastus internus, it must be thoroughly curetted, and, if possible, excised completely, the incision being enlarged for the purpose. The wound may generally be closed without drainage.

After-treatment. A Thomas's knee-splint is worn for some months so as to prevent the patient bearing any weight on the limb. If this precaution be not taken, the leg is liable to become deviated in consequence of unequal growth of the two supracondyloid regions.

In dealing with tuberculous osteomyelitis of the *shaft of the femur*, instead of resecting a complete segment of the bone, it is wiser to perform the less radical operation of gouging. In doing this, however, the medullary cavity should be very freely opened up.

The *lower half of the shaft* is best reached by dividing the vastus internus in the interval between the rectus muscle and Hunter's canal. For this purpose the incision is made in a line directed from the middle of the internal condyle towards the anterior superior spine of the ilium. No important vessels or nerves are injured. The incision is in front of the large nerve to the vastus internus. As this muscle merely covers, instead of arising from, the inner surface of the femur, there is no difficulty in retracting its divided edges so as to obtain sufficient room to incise and separate the periosteum.

To reach the *upper half of the shaft* an incision is carried down to the bone in the plane of the external intermuscular septum, which separates the vastus externus from the outer head of the biceps. To allow of sufficient retraction of these

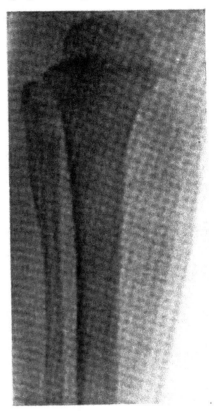

Fig. 70. Skiagram showing Tuberculous Osteomyelitis of the Upper End of the Diaphysis of the Fibula. From a boy aged 2 years. Note the sheath of new subperiosteal bone extending as far down as the junction of the upper with the middle third of the shaft. (*By Dr. H. Rainy.*)

muscles the divided edges of the strong fascia lata must be deeply notched transversely. One or two perforating branches of the profunda artery will require to be ligatured.

In a boy aged twelve years, on whom the writer adopted this method for a focus which occupied the upper third of the medulla, half the circumference of the shaft was removed for the extent of 3 inches. There was a small abscess at the bottom of the external intermuscular septum. In dealing with this the diseased portion of the septum and periosteum was excised, the remainder being united with buried sutures. Sublimated iodoform-bismuth paste was applied to the cavity, which was then lightly stuffed with iodoform gauze. The wound healed well, leaving, however, a sinus which closed two months later. The patient had been treated for some months for hip-joint disease. A skiagram was found to be a great help in revealing the exact nature and extent of the disease.

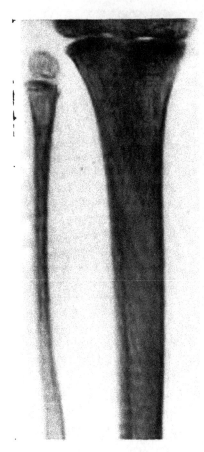

Fig. 71. Skiagram from the same Case as the previous Figure. Taken four years after resection of the upper third of the diaphysis of the fibula. (*By Dr. E. Price.*)

OPERATIONS FOR TUBERCULOUS OSTEOMYELITIS OF THE DIAPHYSIS OF THE FIBULA

To reach the *shaft of the fibula* the dissection should be made along the intermuscular septum (posterior peroneal), which separates the peroneal from the flexor group of muscles, so as to avoid injuring the musculo-cutaneous (superficial peroneal) nerve, which occupies the septum (anterior peroneal) between the peronei and extensors. The first-mentioned septum corresponds to a line drawn from the outer side of the head of the fibula to the posterior border of the external malleolus.

In resecting the *upper third of the diaphysis* care must be taken not to injure the external popliteal (common peroneal) nerve, which passes obliquely downwards and forwards behind the head of the fibula to pierce the peroneus longus an inch below it. After dividing the integuments in the line of the septum, the outer border of the gastrocnemius is defined and retracted inwards. The fibular origin of the soleus is now exposed, and the intermuscular septum between it and the peroneus longus is incised down to the bone, the popliteal nerve having previously been freed and retracted forwards. After separating the periosteum, the bone is divided well below the disease and either wrenched away from the upper epiphysis or snipped across at its neck. The periosteal tube is closed by catgut sutures, which should include the adjacent muscles, namely, the soleus and peroneus longus.

To resect the *middle third of the fibula,* the gastrocnemius and soleus are retracted inwards and the periosteum is divided between the flexor hallucis longus and the peronei.

The *lower third of the shaft* is resected through an incision passing between the peroneus brevis and tertius muscles. Care must be taken to keep below and external to the cutaneous termination of the musculo-cutaneous nerve.

After-treatment. After the wound has healed the limb should be put up in plaster for three months, or a Thomas's knee-splint may be worn instead.

OPERATIONS FOR TUBERCULOUS OSTEOMYELITIS OF THE DIAPHYSIS OF THE TIBIA

The diaphysis of the tibia is a comparatively frequent seat of diffuse tuberculous osteomyelitis. The disease may attack any part of the diaphysis, and occasionally the whole medullary canal is involved. The bone being superficial, its thickening is easily made out, and the disease is, fortunately, generally recognized before either the periosteum or the tissues outside the bone become involved.

The skin incision is carried down to the bone along the middle of its subcutaneous surface, the length of the wound depending, of course, on the extent of the bone to be resected. When the resection includes the *upper end of the diaphysis,* the incision is continued upwards on to the internal tuberosity in front of the insertions of the sartorius and inner hamstrings. In separating the periosteum it is important to keep close to the bone along the line of attachment of the interosseous membrane. The membrane is rather more firmly adherent also at the ends of the diaphysis, and in these regions it should be separated as far as possible with a suitable elevator before attempting to wrench out the diaphyseal extremity.

The manner in which the bone is divided and shelled out has been fully described on p. 124. It is in the case of the tibia that the instrument shown in Fig. 52 is particularly useful.

If the greater part of the diaphysis of the tibia has been removed it may be necessary to insert a drain into the interior of the periosteal

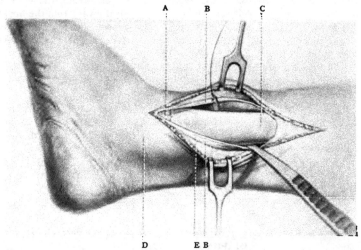

FIG. 72.   RESECTION OF THE LOWER THIRD OF THE DIAPHYSIS OF THE TIBIA. The integuments and periosteum have been divided; Gigli's wire saw is hooked on to the separator, which has been passed between the periosteum and the posterior aspect of the bone. A, Epiphyseal cartilage; B, B, Periosteum; C, Tibia; D, Internal malleolus; E, Fascia.

tube for a few days, so as to drain off the serum from the blood-clot with which it becomes filled.

After-treatment. The limb should be placed either in a box-splint or on a suitable posterior splint, care being taken to keep the foot in good position. In about six weeks plaster of Paris is substituted for the splint; the bandage should extend well up the thigh, and during its application it is important to see that the foot is held in good position. The plaster case is changed at the end of two or three months, and a skiagram is taken to ascertain to what extent the new bone has formed. In the case of young children it is generally necessary to renew the plaster for another three months, but in an older patient a Thomas's knee-splint may often be substituted at this stage.

It was in consequence of the excellent results obtained from resections of large portions of the diaphysis of the tibia that the writer was induced to adopt the same radical treatment in dealing with all the other long bones except the femur.

When there is reason to fear shortening of the new tibia, as for example in cases where the focus has involved the epiphyseal cartilage, or the periosteum in its neighbourhood, extension should be employed; and it is a good plan to fracture the fibula at the same time that the tibia is operated on. By this means compensatory shortening of the fibula can take place by overlapping of the fragments. Deviation of the foot may thus be prevented.

Result. In the nine cases in which resection of a portion of the diaphysis of the tibia was performed, the amount of bone removed varied in extent from a third to the entire diaphysis. In almost all the cases the tibiæ have re-formed well, and the functional results

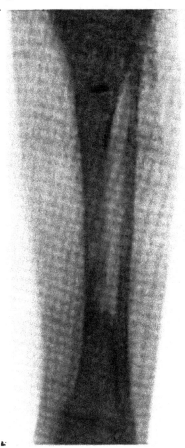

Fig. 73.   Skiagram showing New Formation of Bone. Eleven weeks after resection of the middle two-fourths of the diaphysis of the tibia for tuberculous osteomyelitis in a child aged 4 years. (*By Dr. H. Rainy.*)

are on the whole excellent. In one case where the greater part of the diaphyses of both tibiæ was removed six years ago, the bones have re-formed so completely that their skiagraphic appearances are practically normal (see Fig. 74). In some cases there is slight shortening along with some inwards deviation of the foot.

Fig. 74   SKIAGRAMS FROM SAME LIMB AS THAT IN THE PREVIOUS FIGURE. Taken six years after operation. Note the perfect re-formation of bone.

CHAPTER II

OPERATIONS FOR TUBERCULOUS OSTEOMYELITIS OF THE SHORT LONG-BONES

TUBERCULOUS osteomyelitis is very commonly met with in the short long-bones of the hands and feet, and it is very frequently associated with tuberculous bone and joint lesions in other parts of the body.

These short long-bones differ from the long bones proper, in that they have only one epiphysis, so that at one end of the bone the diaphysis forms the articular extremity, and it is through this extremity that the adjacent joint is liable to be infected. Owing to this peculiar mode of development, the shaft of the short long-bones cannot always be completely resected without opening into the joint at the anti-epiphyseal end of the bone, and, moreover, the operation of complete removal of the diaphysis is followed, comparatively, by more shortening of the digit than is the case with the long bones proper.

OPERATIONS FOR TUBERCULOUS OSTEOMYELITIS OF THE PHALANGES OF THE HAND

If rest and constitutional measures fail to bring about improvement, operation should be resorted to, otherwise one or other of the adjacent joints, or the flexor sheath, is liable to become involved.

Operation. The phalanx is exposed by two dorso-lateral incisions placed between the extensor tendons and the digital vessels and nerves. As pointed out by Kocher, the object of the bilateral incision is to prevent the lateral bending of the finger which would result from the cicatrization of a unilateral incision. The periosteum is separated first on one side and then on the other; the separation is then continued distally under the capsular ligament as far as the neck of the bone, which is then snipped across with a small pair of bone-forceps. The divided end is grasped with necrosis forceps and wrenched away from the epiphysis at the proximal end. One or two buried catgut sutures are introduced at either side to bring together the tendinous expansion of the extensor tendons along with the periosteum. When the wound has healed extension should be applied to the finger with the object of diminishing shortening.

OPERATIONS FOR TUBERCULOUS OSTEOMYELITIS OF THE INTER-PHALANGEAL JOINTS

This condition is rarely primary, but should it occur, amputation of the finger would be much more frequently called for than excision of the joint. The latter operation is done through two dorsal-lateral incisions. If possible, the excision should be done by the extra-capsular method.

OPERATIONS FOR TUBERCULOUS OSTEOMYELITIS OF THE METACARPAL BONES

When the disease affects the *first metacarpal bone,* every attempt should be made to preserve the thumb, either by scraping out the focus or by subperiosteal resection of the disease, if possible without opening into the adjacent joints.

Operation. The incision is made along the whole length of the bone immediately to the radial side of the tendon of the extensor primi pollicis (extensor pollicis brevis). If the incision be made to the ulnar side of this tendon, its proximal extremity must be kept superficial to the radial artery, and, if possible, the branches of the radial nerve should be identified and drawn aside. The periosteum is then divided between the origins of the abductor pollicis brevis and the abductor indicis muscles, which are separated from the bone along with the periosteum. In a young child the best way to resect the shaft of the bone is to cut it across with a knife at the junction of the epiphysis and the diaphysis; the extremity of the latter is then hooked upwards and the periosteum is carefully separated downwards from its palmar aspect until the neck of the bone is reached, where it is snipped across with forceps. A little sublimated iodoform-bismuth paste is applied to the inner surface of the periosteum, which is then closed by a few buried catgut sutures.

If the disease has spread to the *metacarpo-phalangeal joint,* amputation is generally necessary, in which case as much as possible of the periosteum of the metacarpal bone should be saved, with the object of obtaining a movable thenar eminence capable of approximation to the fingers.

In excising portions of the other metacarpal bones, the incision is made over the ridge separating the dorsal interosseous muscles, which are detached along with the periosteum. After dividing the skin the extensor tendon is exposed, freed, and drawn aside. The bone is dealt with in the manner above described, the epiphysis, however, being at the distal instead of the proximal end of the bone. If the disease be extensive, it may be necessary to disarticulate its carpal extremity, and an attempt should be made to do this by the subcapsular method.

If the disease has spread to the metacarpo-phalangeal joint, and if the flexor sheath and the soft parts be extensively diseased, amputation of the finger along with the metacarpal bone will be called for.

In resecting the *second metacarpal bone*, the incision is made along its dorsal ridge, between the abductor indicis and the long extensor tendon. If it be found necessary to remove the carpal extremity along with the shaft, the proximal end of the incision must be kept internal to the radial artery, and the insertion of the extensor carpi radialis longior should be separated subperiosteally.

When the *fifth metacarpal bone* is diseased, the incision is made immediately to the ulnar side of the tendon of the extensor minimi digiti (digiti quinti proprius). The proximal end of the incision is kept superficial, so as not to divide the dorsal branch of the ulnar nerve which winds to the back of the wrist round the cuneiform (triquetral) bone. If the carpal extremity of the bone be also involved, the tendon of the extensor carpi ulnaris should be separated subperiosteally before completing the disarticulation.

After-treatment. The after-treatment consists in keeping the hand and wrist quiet for a considerable time by means of an anterior splint. In a young child, after the wound has healed, a convenient way of doing this is to apply a strip of aluminium, covered with boric lint, to the palmar aspect of the hand and the forearm from a little beyond the fingers almost to the elbow. This splint must be secured to the limb, not by a bandage, but by means of strips of plaster, applied directly to the skin, which should be previously disinfected and rubbed over with boric powder. A strip of boric lint should be placed between each of the fingers. Over the strapping a narrow bandage is applied, partly to ensure thorough adhesion, and partly to keep the plaster clean.

OPERATIONS FOR TUBERCULOUS OSTEOMYELITIS OF THE PHALANGES OF THE FOOT

With the exception of the first phalanx of the great toe, tuberculous affections of the phalanges of the foot are best treated by amputation at the metatarso-phalangeal joint.

The *first phalanx* is treated in the same way as in the hand, except that a single incision, made to the inner side of the extensor tendon, is preferable to a bilateral incision. The operation should be done before either of the neighbouring joints become involved. If the metatarso-phalangeal joint be allowed to become involved, the head of the metatarsal bone will generally have to be sacrificed, and this means serious damage to the foot. Fortunately the presence of the epiphysis serves head of the bone.

Tuberculous disease of the other metatarsal bone
a similar manner to the corresponding bones of the h

CHAPTER III

OPERATIONS FOR TUBERCULOUS OSTEOMYELITIS OF THE BONES OF THE VAULT OF THE SKULL

OPERATIONS FOR TUBERCULOUS OSTEOMYELITIS OF THE SKULL

THIS is a rare affection, occurring generally in children and young adults, and usually along with other osseous lesions.

Operation. To illustrate the operative treatment, we shall take as an example the commonest condition met with, namely, a soft caseous focus in the region of the frontal eminence, with a secondary abscess beneath the pericranium. A horseshoe incision is carried at once down to the bone a little beyond the upper three-fourths of the limit of the swelling. The flap, which should include the periosteum, is rapidly dissected downwards, forceps being applied to the more important bleeding points in the scalp. The anterior wall of the abscess, which is exposed on the deep surface of the flap, consists of the pericranium covered by caseous granulations. These are thoroughly scraped away with a sharp spoon, the membrane being held taut with artery forceps to facilitate the process. If the tubercle has eaten into the pericranium it is better to dissect this portion away completely. Attention is now turned to the bone. If an area of the outer table has already been destroyed and replaced by a cheesy focus, it is scraped away, and if the inner table has also been destroyed, a sharp spoon is applied to the dura. The surrounding tuberculous bone is then removed by snipping it away with a suitable pair of skull forceps, care being taken to see that the removal is carried well into the surrounding healthy bone. To enable this to be done the skin incision should, as mentioned above, be made some distance beyond the outline of the swelling; if this be not done, one, or it may be two, additional incisions will have to be made at right angles to the original incision. In those cases in which the disease has extended downwards towards the orbital margin, it must be carefully and persistently followed up. If complete removal of the disease cannot be effected without opening the frontal sinus, this should be done without hesitation. The writer found it necessary to do this on two occasions, and in neither instance did the procedure interfere with the normal healing of the wound.

If all the disease in the bone be not removed, a persistent sinus is almost certain to result, and a second, and still more severe, operation will generally be necessary in order to bring about permanent healing.

Not infrequently, however, a cheesy abscess forms beneath the pericranium before the outer table has become destroyed. In such cases the bone subjacent to the disease has a more vascular and porous appearance than normal, and sometimes tiny buttons of granulation tissue can be seen projecting from its surface. These appearances afford sufficient indication that the diploë is diseased, but even if the above appearances are wanting, the diploë should be explored. This may be done either with a hammer and chisel, or by means of a trephine. If diploic disease be revealed the opening should be enlarged with forceps as above described.

When the disease produces a diffuse tumour-like thickening of the bone a large flap of scalp should be turned down, and the diseased bone removed either with a skull saw aided by the hammer and chisel, or, if preferred, by a circular saw driven by an electro-motor. Great care should be taken not to wound the dura. As long as this membrane is left intact, cerebral complications need not be feared.

The diseased bone having been removed, all cheesy matter and fungating granulation tissue is thoroughly scraped off the dura, which is then smeared over with a little sublimated iodoform-bismuth paste. The operation is completed by suturing the flap back into position. Drainage is seldom necessary.

OPERATIONS FOR TUBERCULOUS OSTEOMYELITIS OF THE LOWER JAW

This is a less common affection than is generally supposed. It occurs especially in the children of phthisical parents, and Stockman has shown that it is almost invariably the primary lesion in phosphorus necrosis of the jaw. The tubercle generally gains access to the bone through the alveolus of a tooth, but the writer has operated on a child with a large focus of tubercle in the ramus of the jaw in whom all the teeth were perfectly sound.

Operation. The operative treatment consists in subperiosteal resection of the portion of the jaw affected. If possible, this should be done before a cold abscess has developed, and especially before the stage of sinus formation followed by mixed infection.

When the ascending ramus only is involved, an incision is carried from immediately in front of the lobule of the ear downwards along the posterior margin of the ramus, round the angle, and thence for a variable distance forwards into the submaxillary region a little below the lower margin of the jaw. While the upper part of the incision is kept superficial so as to avoid injury to the facial nerve, the remainder is carried deeply down to the bone. The facial vessels are divided and ligatured, and forceps are applied to one or two veins in the substance of the parotid. After dividing the periosteum along the margin of the bone, the upper flap, together with the masseter and periosteum, is raised from the jaw with the aid of a periosteum elevator, and the same instrument is used to separate the internal pterygoid and periosteum from the inner surface of the bone. When the bone has been sufficiently laid bare, the saw is applied well in front of the disease and the division is completed with bone-forceps. The angle of the jaw is now grasped with lion forceps,

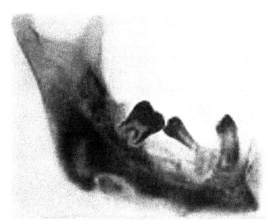

Fig. 75. Skiagram of Half the Lower Jaw. Taken after subperiosteal re-section for tuberculous disease. Note the small sequestra, the slight carious excavations of the surface, and the displacement and loss of the teeth.   (By Dr. E. Price.)

and, by applying torsion, both the condyle and the coronoid process may be wrenched away subperiosteally without opening either into the mouth or the temporo-maxillary joint. If the disease be advanced, the bone may break across during the twisting-out process, in which case the upper portion must of course be removed separately by the same manœuvre. The end of the torn inferior dental artery may sometimes be seen dangling from the inside of the periosteal tube; the bleeding from it is usually arrested by the torsion, but, if not, the vessel is easily ligatured. The operation is completed by suturing the wound with silkworm-gut, an opening being left for the insertion of a gauze drain into the periosteal cavity.

In the cases in which the adjacent lymphatic glands are tuberculous and complicated with abscess and sinus formation, the incision may have to be modified somewhat so as to include the sinus, while to give access to the glands it will be necessary to prolong the incision further down into the neck as well as further forwards into the submaxillary region. After dissecting away the sinus and glands the bone is dealt with in the manner already described.

When the disease is limited to the *portion of the mandible between the angle and the symphysis,* the subperiosteal resection of the focus is a comparatively simple procedure. A straight incision is made parallel to, and a little below, the margin of the jaw. After detaching the periosteum along with the muscles from both aspects of the bone with a suitable rugine, the mouth is freely opened into by continuing the separation until the gums are also detached. The jaw is then divided in front of the lesion, after which it is seized with lion forceps and levered downwards and outwards so as to facilitate the more complete separation of the soft parts behind the lesion, where the bone is again divided. In the young child the division of the bone may be done with bone-forceps, while in the adult Gigli's wire saw is the better instrument.

After removing the bone, any remains of a sinus, or suppurating pocket, must be carefully disinfected, or, still better, dissected away altogether; care should be taken, however, not to remove more of the periosteum than is absolutely necessary. If by mixed infection the wound has been rendered very unhealthy, it should be swabbed with turpentine. This is probably the best antiseptic for the purpose, as, in addition to being a powerful antiseptic and deodorizer, it is also a valuable hæmostatic; it produces no sloughing, nor does it interfere in any way with the healing of the wound.

In addition to the skin sutures, it is an advantage to partially close the wound in the mouth by uniting the raw edges of the gums with sutures introduced from within the mouth. Drainage of the wound is provided for by the introduction of a rubber tube, one end of which is stitched to the skin wound, while the other just projects into the cavity of the mouth.

When the disease involves the greater part of the horizontal ramus, including the symphysis, tracheotomy should be performed at the same time that the bone is removed. If this precaution be not taken, the patient is very likely to become asphyxiated during sleep from the tongue falling back into the pharynx. Advantage may be taken of the tracheotomy to plug the pharynx so as to prevent any blood gaining access to the trachea during the operation. The writer has had two cases in children in which the tracheotomy tube had to be worn permanently. In one of the cases the child lost its life from asphyxia, owing to the tube, which had been removed during the day, not having been replaced at bedtime.

Results. The results of resection of the lower jaw for tubercle are, as a rule, very satisfactory, especially if the greater part of the periosteum can be preserved. Considerable re-formation of bone takes place, the mouth can be well opened, and the only deformity consists in slight deviation of the chin towards the affected side.

OPERATIONS FOR TUBERCULOUS OSTEOMYELITIS OF THE UPPER JAW AND MALAR BONE

In children the upper jaw is the commonest seat of osseous tuberculosis of the face. The disease begins in the cancellated tissue in the neighbourhood of the malar process and floor of the orbit.

Operation. In the early stage of the disease (the proper time to interfere), the operation consists in making an oblique incision from a little below the middle of the infra-orbital margin outwards and slightly downwards over the malar bone for a variable length depending on the extent of the disease. This incision, which lies immediately above the infra-orbital foramen and the origin of the levator labii superioris muscle (caput infraorbitale), possesses the double advantage of running parallel to the natural folds of the skin as well as to the branches of the facial nerve. Should an abscess be present, its wall is dissected away, after which the periosteum is separated from the bone, and the tuberculous focus is removed either with a sharp spoon aided by a gouge, or by the hammer and chisel. The infra-orbital vessels and nerves should be avoided if possible, but it will often be necessary to open into the antrum. After applying sublimated iodoform-bismuth paste to the cavity, the wound is carefully sutured. An opening is left for the introduction of an iodoform-gauze plug.

When the alveolar process is involved, one or more of the permanent as well as the temporary teeth will almost certainly have to be sacrificed. After separating the gum and periosteum with a suitable elevator, the diseased portion of the jaw is snipped away with cutting forceps, the most suitable being a small pair of curved bone-forceps. In aggravated cases the greater portion of the upper jaw may have to be removed. The cavity left in the jaw is packed with a strip of gauze wrung almost dry out of turpentine.

CHAPTER IV

OPERATIONS FOR TUBERCULOUS OSTEOMYELITIS OF THE SPINE AND RIBS

TUBERCULOUS OSTEOMYELITIS OF THE SPINE

ABSCESSES secondary to tuberculous disease of the spinal column may occur in a variety of situations depending on the part of the spine involved. The course which the pus takes as the abscess enlarges depends partly on whether the patient is going about or recumbent during its development, and partly on the arrangement of the adjacent fascial planes.

ALBEE OPERATION FOR POTT'S DISEASE

The perfected technique of the Albee operation for Pott's disease is as follows:

With the patient in the ventral position, the tips of the spinous processes are reached by a curved incision and turning up of a flap of the skin and subcutaneous tissues. With a scalpel the periosteal tips of the spinous processes are split in the centre, also the supraspinous ligament. The interspinous ligaments are next split into approximately equal parts, to a depth of about ½ inch (12.70 mm.), varying with the age and size of the patient, without disturbing their attachments to the spinous process. Very little hæmorrhage results, because only dense ligamentous tissues are incised, which is in considerable contrast to the hæmorrhage resulting from the separation of the muscles from the spinous processes in a deeper operation, such as a laminectomy. With a thin, sharp chisel or osteotome and mallet each process is split longitudinally into equal parts for a depth of about ½ inch (12.70 mm.), care being taken that greenstick fractures are produced on one and the same side of all the spinous processes so split. The unbroken halves preserve intact the leverage of these processes. A separation of the halves of each spinous process produces a gutter into which the transplant is later placed. In all cases the full thickness of the tibial cortex is included with the periosteum, endosteum, and attached marrow substance, thus producing a transplant with approximately a rectangular cross-section.

It has been found advisable for bone-grafts for all purposes to include periosteum and endosteum, as it is through these media that cortical bone largely receives its nourishment. Thus the graft approximates a complete organic structure, with its normal means of distribut-

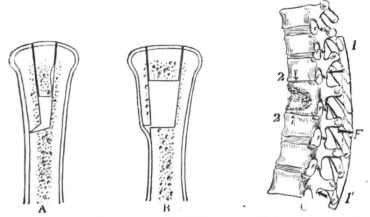

F‍IG. 76. ALBEE OPERATION FOR POTT'S DISEASE. A illustrates a cross-section of a spinous process split in half and fractured at its base. The deep, thin graft in cross-section has been removed from the crest of the tibia having its periosteum attached to two sides. The side in contact with the unbroken half of the spinous process is the saw-cut or the medullary surface of the graft.

B illustrates a cross-section of a spinous process which has been split and one-half has been set over to produce a gap sufficient to receive a broad graft removed from the antero-internal surface of the tibia having periosteum on one surface only; the medullary surface of the graft lies nearest the base of the spinous process in the gap.

C illustrates a lateral view of the spinal column. Each vertebra is a lever with its fulcrum point at small F. The arrow on the vertebral bodies at 2, 2, indicates lines of force from weight bearing, involuntary muscle spasm, etc., influencing crushing of vertebral bodies and progress of deformity by the approximation of the anterior lever arms, which is associated with an equal separation of the spinous processes or the posterior lever arms. This is prevented by a pull lengthwise on the graft, as indicated by the small arrows situated at each spinous process. The graft in respect to this direction of force is under a great mechanical advantage.

ing nourishment, and the early establishment of blood-supply is enhanced.

A graft of this thickness necessitates producing a full fracture of one-half of the spinous process and setting it over laterally in order to place it deep enough to be well covered with the above-mentioned ligaments. It is important that the spinous processes be split *in situ* with all the ligamentous and muscular insertion undisturbed, as in this way none of the natural supports of the spine are taken away and the ligaments afford, by means of strong ligatures, an excellent medium for firmly fixing the bone-splint in place.

The depth to which the spinous processes are split varies as to age, size of patient, and amount of pressure atrophy from former apparatus, etc., which may so reduce the spinous processes as to present mere tubercles on the posterior aspect of the neural arches and in certain instances can be split in depth only $\frac{3}{16}$ to $\frac{1}{4}$ of an inch (4.75 to 6.35 mm.), but this affords good bone contact, and as the graft is embedded into longer spinous processes at either end, it affords the usual efficient fixation. A hot saline pack is placed over the back wound until the bone insert is obtained.

With the patient still in the ventral position, the leg is flexed on the thigh and an incision over and down to the crest of the tibia is made. The fascia and subcutaneous tissues are carefully separated from the periosteum of the anterior-internal flat surface of the tibia. From its crest and anterior-internal aspect a strip of the tibia is removed with a motor saw. A motor saw affords a very rapid and exact method of securing the graft and is used exclusively for this purpose. The length of graft varies according to how many vertebræ are to be spanned, *i.e.* all those diseased and two healthy ones on each side if in the dorsal region, and one on each side if in the lumbar region, its breadth from $\frac{1}{4}$ to $\frac{5}{8}$ inch (6.35 to 15.85 mm.), its thickness from $\frac{3}{16}$ to $\frac{3}{8}$ inch (4.75 to 15.51 mm.), according to the size of the patient. The graft is inserted between the halves of the interspinous ligaments and the spinous processes with its edge anterior or innermost, and its cut side or marrow side in contact with the unbroken halves of the spinous processes. It is held firmly in position by interrupted sutures of heavy or medium kangaroo tendon, which are passed through the supraspinous ligament and posterior edges of the halves of the interspinous ligaments near the tips of the spinous processes, beginning at the centre of the graft. The ligaments are then drawn over the insert posteriorly by tense sutures placed closely together. Before tying the last sutures the posterior corners of the ends of the graft are removed by the rongeur forceps, and these fragments of bone, with others, are cut into small pieces and placed under and about each end of the graft; the ends of the graft are then drawn down and sutures tied. This is important, as it furnishes multiple foci for a rapid proliferation of bone, as, according to Macewen, the smaller the graft the greater the relative bone growth. If there is a moderate kyphosis of short duration, it is entirely obliterated; any kyphosis of a few years' or less duration becomes much diminished, either at the time of operation or during the first few days after, from the corrective effect of the lateral tension of the graft.

This sequence of the technique is important because, by preparing the back wound first and packing it with a hot saline compress, we secure hæmostasis, and control the blood clot about the graft, a condition to be desired.

Where a kyphosis is too great for implanting a straight splint properly in place in the spinous processes, the approximate contour of the knuckle is obtained by bending a silver probe over the tips of the spinous processes. The curved probe is then laid upon the anterior-internal aspect of the tibia as a pattern, and a graft of the desired shape, width, and thickness is outlined in the periosteum with a scalpel. The graft, however, is always straighter than the kyphosis and the spine is straightened by the usual pressure and drawn to the bone-splint by means of the heavy ligatures. When the deformity is too great, even for this method, the graft is placed with its wider diameter in a lateral rather than anterior-posterior plane, and then bent into place between the halves of the spinous processes and held with heavy kangaroo tendon, as above indicated.

This bending is accomplished by making numerous saw-cuts one-half to two-thirds the way through. These cuts not only shape the graft to the kyphosis, but also favour a rapid establishment of blood-supply and the throwing out of bone callus from the graft itself. The cross cuts, ⅛ to ⅜ inch (3.17 to 9.51 mm.) from each other, are always made on the marrow side. The transplants vary in size from 4 to 7½ inches (10.16 cm. to 19.05 cm.) in length, ¼ to ½ (6.35 to 12.70 mm.) in width, ¼ to ⅜ inch (6.35 to 9.51 mm.) in thickness. Care is taken that the insert has some bone marrow. The importance of this has been pointed out by several German investigators. Before placing the unbent graft in its bed, its periosteum is incised in many places, so as to allow the underlying osteogenetic cells exit for proliferation, and also an entrance of blood-supply to the graft. The graft, firmly imbedded under tension in the spinous processes and the dense intraspinous ligaments, affords immediate and excellent fixation of those vertebræ involved even before union takes place.

HIBBS'S OPERATION FOR POTT'S DISEASE

The technique of Hibbs's operation for Pott's disease is as follows:

A general preparation of the field of operation is made the night before, the back is thoroughly cleaned with soap, water, ether, and alcohol.

A sterile dressing is applied, which remains on until the patient is anæsthetized, and then it is removed and the back painted with full-strength iodine. This is sponged off with alcohol.

Instead of making an ellipitical skin incision, a straight one directly over the spinous process may be used, corresponding to the diseased vertebræ. The skin is turned back and hot laparotomy sponges control the hæmorrhage. The processes of one or two healthy vertebræ above and below the diseased ones are also included in the incision. The first knife is now put aside and a second knife is used to divide the muscle, ligament, and periosteum down to the tips of the spinous processes. These are broad and shelving, and in order to get the periosteum nicely lifted close to the tip, care must be used in denuding the end of the process. Hæmorrhage is controlled with very hot sponges, in the shape of a large cigarette. A special dissector is now placed under the tip and at the side of a spinous process and the periosteum and muscle dissected back in such a way as to free them and their laminæ. If the periosteum is cleanly.peeled down the hæmorrhage is less than when the muscle is torn and cut. When there is troublesome bleeding the hot cigarette sponges are packed in between the muscle and processes.

This procedure of denuding the spinous processes should include their lower and upper edges down to the articular processes, whose surfaces are cleaned away with a small curette or gouged out with a chisel with the design of destroying the joints and making for ankylosis. It must be remembered that in different regions of the spine the angle of entrance to the articular processes varies considerably, and this must be taken into consideration in attempting to enter them.

Practice enables one to feel along the inferior edge of a spinous process, travelling in the direction of the articular process and thus finding it by touch with the instrument. When the periosteum is peeled back and all edges and surfaces of the spinous processes and laminæ denuded and the articular processes destroyed, small bridges of bone from the lower edge of one spinous process and the upper edge of an adjoining one are shaved down to bridge over the space between the two vertebræ. The spinous processes are now split, and with a pair of special bone-cutting forceps are partly separated from their base. It is desirable to turn the raw surface down over the space between the vertebræ and in contact with the raw surfaces of the laminæ or bases of the spinous processes. This helps to complete the bridge between the vertebræ. Formerly an attempt was made to avoid complete detachment of the split processes. In most cases, however, it is impossible to prevent cutting the processes off. This does not lessen the efficiency of the bone plates to grow together and make a sheet of bone over the posterior aspect of the spine. When all processes and loose pieces of periosteum and shavings of laminæ have been thus welded together, a hot laparotomy sponge is placed over the fragments and they are pressed down as firmly and closely as possible. The strips of periosteum and ligaments are now drawn over the islands of osteogenetic material with catgut. The muscle is sutured with catgut and finally the skin is united with three interrupted catgut sutures, the needle being passed from in-out in each instance. The remaining closure is made with wound clips.

PREVERTEBRAL CERVICAL ABSCESS

The tuberculous process, after reaching the anterior surface of the diseased vertebra and perforating the periosteum, invades the prevertebral muscles and forms a collection of pus between the cervical vertebræ and the prevertebral fascia. Abscesses secondary to tuberculous disease of the retro-pharyngeal lymphatic glands are, on the other hand, situated in front of the prevertebral fascia, between it and the wall of the pharynx. As the spinal abscess enlarges, it strips the prevertebral fascia off the prevertebral muscles and at the same time extends laterally behind the carotid sheath and the posterior layer of the sheath of the sterno-mastoid, to approach the surface usually at the upper part of the posterior margin of that muscle.

Operation. The abscess should be opened not from the mouth but from behind the sterno-mastoid, a procedure which was first employed and advocated by Professor Chiene. The incision is made immediately behind the upper third of the posterior border of the muscle, care being taken not to injure the spinal accessory nerve. If the abscess be situated lower down in the neck, the nerve should be deliberately exposed and retracted out of the way before proceeding with the deeper part of the dissection. The posterior border of the sterno-mastoid is freed, and it is well to divide some of its fibres transversely a little below the mastoid process so as to allow of further retraction of the muscle forwards. Behind the sterno-mastoid are the fibres of the splenius and levator anguli scapulæ, which are traced to their origin from the transverse processes of the upper cervical vertebræ. These processes constitute the surest guide to the abscess, the wall of which may often be seen and felt immediately in front of them, while in front of the abscess again is the internal jugular vein covered by its sheath. Care must be taken not to mistake the sheath of the vein for the wall of the abscess. In opening the abscess the edge of the knife is directed towards the vertebræ. The opening should be enlarged with forceps. It is better to expose the wall of the abscess by careful dissection rather than to trust to entering it blindly with forceps through a small incision (Hilton's method).

The cavity is gently curetted to remove as much of the pyogenic membrane as possible. Evacuation of the cheesy pus and membrane is greatly assisted by pressure made from the opposite side of the neck with gauze pads. Occasionally a loose sequestrum may be removed. The final cleansing of the cavity is most conveniently done by repeated packing with fresh strips of gauze. Before closing the wound some sublimated iodoform-bismuth paste is introduced into the cavity and rubbed into the lining with the finger. The wound may either be closed completely, or, if the cavity be large and the pus less cheesy, an iodoform-gauze drain may be left in for a few days. If, as not infrequently happens, the abscess be bilateral as well as large, a counter-opening may be made behind the opposite sterno-mastoid; this is readily done by cutting carefully down on the blades of a long pair of dressing forceps pushed across the neck immediately in front of the vertebral column. Advantage may be taken of the counter-opening to flush out the cavity with normal saline solution.

After-treatment. The after-treatment consists in immobilizing the head by means of sand-bags, weight extension being added if need be. Permanent healing of the wound sometimes occurs, but a sinus is very liable to persist for a considerable time. A second curetting may be necessary before healing is finally brought about. The duration of the subsequent fixation treatment will of course vary in different cases. The writer has seen complete paraplegia disappear very rapidly after merely opening the abscess.

PREVERTEBRAL THORACIC ABSCESS

This condition is often revealed by skiagraphy when there are no symptoms indicating its presence. The pus, having reached the surface of the vertebral column on one or other side of the anterior common ligament, accumulates, in the first instance, under the periosteum. After perforating the periosteum, it forms an abscess between the mediastinal pleuræ and the bodies of the vertebræ.

Indications. Under the influence of prolonged recumbency and open-air treatment, the primary disease often heals, in which case the abscess generally becomes absorbed. If, on the other hand, the abscess enlarges, the tension may become so great that the œsophagus, the trachea, and the left recurrent laryngeal nerve may be pressed upon, or paraplegia may result from the pus finding its way into the spinal canal. If the above complications occur in spite of efficient rest treatment, operation becomes imperative.

Operation. The abscess in the posterior mediastinum is best reached by removing one, or it may be two, of the costo-transverse articulations on one or other side, preferably the right. This method of posterior mediastinotomy, which was first performed by Heidenhain, was brought into prominence in the treatment of thoracic spinal abscess by Ménard, who gave it the appropriate name of *costo-transversectomy*.

The advantages of costo-transversectomy over resection of ribs external to the transverse process are, firstly, that more direct access is got to the bodies of the vertebræ, and, secondly, that the pleura is less liable to be injured. Heidenhain employed a longitudinal incision close to the spines and separated the superficial and deep muscles outwards off the laminæ as far as the tubercle of the rib. He resected the transverse process first and then the head and neck of the rib. He showed that the removal of only one costo-transverse articulation was sufficient to enable the surgeon to introduce the finger and strip the pleura and endothoracic fascia off the lateral aspect of the diseased vertebra.

Kocher warmly recommends the principle of Heidenhain's operation, but prefers an oblique incision followed by transverse division of the muscles. He carries his incision from the most prominent spinous process involved in the curve downwards and outwards exactly in the line of the rib to be resected.

After dividing the integuments, the trapezius, and then the rhomboids, the cellular interval is reached between these muscles and the fascia covering the divisions of the erector spinæ (sacro-spinalis) muscle. The longissimus dorsi and accessorius (ilio-costalis dorsi) are divided in the line of the original incision. The cross division of the deep muscles is of no moment as they possess a segmental nerve-supply. The bleeding which occurs is, according to Kocher, much less than that which results from Heidenhain's method of separating the muscles longitudinally from the spines and laminæ.

The periosteum of the exposed rib is divided for a short distance external to its tubercle. The muscular attachments, along with the periosteum and the posterior costo-transverse ligament, are then separated from the transverse process and its base is snipped through with a pair of curved bone forceps. The divided process is seized with lion (or necrosis) forceps held in the left hand while the knife is used to free it from the remaining ligamentous attachments, namely, from the superior costo-transverse ligament passing from the neck of the rib below to its lower border, and from the middle costo-transverse ligament which passes between its anterior surface and the posterior aspect of the neck of the rib with which it articulates.

The next step consists in the removal of the head, neck, and tubercle of the rib. The periosteum is first separated from the posterior aspect of the neck, and a strong hook is then inserted into the end of the divided rib which is dragged backwards while the periosteum is detached from its anterior aspect, carrying with it the costal attachment of the anterior costo-vertebral (stellate) ligament. When this has been done the freed portion of rib is seized with necrosis forceps and twisted away from the spine. The pleura is not injured. Care must be taken not to wound the intercostal vessels which pass outwards a little below the lower border of the neck of the rib.

If the forefinger be now introduced into the bottom of the wound, it will enter the abscess cavity which occupies the cellular tissue of the posterior mediastinum. By directing the finger forwards and inwards the lateral aspect of the corresponding vertebra, and of the one above it, can be distinctly palpated, its surface scraped, or a sequestrum removed. Anteriorly and externally is the reflection of the posterior mediastinal pleura on to the ribs. When an abscess is present, this membrane, along with the intrathoracic fascia, is considerably thickened, so that with ordinary care the pleural cavity should not be opened into. If more room be desired in order to reach the upper of the two vertebræ with which the rib articulates, the upper edge of the wound must be retracted, and a second transverse process removed; this will generally suffice without removing the vertebral end of the corresponding rib, but there should be no hesitation in excising it if still more room be required.

If the mediastinal abscess be small, it may be gently packed with iodoform gauze for a few days, and the wound then allowed to heal. As a rule, however, if the cavity be large, and especially if paraplegia be present, a drainage tube should be inserted and kept in for a considerable time.

If the abscess has penetrated through an intervertebral foramen into the spinal canal, or if it has encroached on the canal after destroying the body of the vertebra, it can be drained more satisfactorily and with infinitely less danger by costo-transversectomy than by laminectomy. The latter operation is reserved for those cases in which the paraplegia is due to external pachymeningitis and thickening of the dura, and for those rare cases in which the compression is caused by narrowing of the osseous canal itself.

Results. The results of costo-transversectomy are very satisfactory, especially when compared with those of laminectomy, in which the mortality is from 40 to 50%. Of the twenty-four cases of costo-transversectomy collected by Ménard, nineteen recovered; two of these had a recurrence of the paraplegia, while four died subsequently of tuberculosis. The paraplegia generally begins to disappear within a few days of the operation, and it is often completely recovered from in a month or two. The same may be said of incontinence of urine. It is not uncommon, however, for a fistula to persist for several months. If the paraplegia recurs, the fistula must be opened up and free drainage re-established.

When the disease has already found its way along the posterior branch of an intercostal artery into the erector spinæ compartment, all that is necessary is to open the abscess freely, to search for the sinus in its floor, and, after enlarging it, to follow the abscess to its source. If the sinus be found to lead into the posterior mediastinum, it should be enlarged with forceps rather than the knife; and if an intrathoracic abscess be discovered, the operator should proceed to do a costo-transversectomy.

LUMBAR ABSCESS

This is a complication of tuberculous disease in the lower dorsal and upper lumbar regions. The pus is more liable to make its way into the loin if the abscess develops while the patient is kept recumbent. The pus generally reaches the loin through one or other of its two weak areas. The upper is situated at the angle between the outer border of the erector spinæ (sacro-spinalis) and the twelfth rib, where the internal oblique is aponeurotic; the lower is at Petit's triangle.

An abscess appearing in the angle between the erector spinæ and the last rib is opened by an oblique incision a little below and parallel to the twelfth rib. The abscess is reached after dividing the latissimus dorsi (possibly also the lowest fibres of the serratus posticus inferior), the outer fibres of the quadratus lumborum, and the middle layer of the lumbar fascia. Not infrequently the abscess will be found to have already perforated the quadratus and the aponeurosis common to the internal oblique and transversalis muscles. If the opening in these structures be small, it must be enlarged, and care should be taken to avoid unnecessary injury to the last dorsal nerve and its companion artery, or to the ilio-hypogastric and ilio-inguinal nerves. Occasionally one or other of these nerves can be felt crossing the cavity of the abscess.

When, on the other hand, the abscess is felt in the angle between the crest of the ilium and the outer edge of the erector spinæ (sacro-spinalis), the incision is made obliquely from above downwards and outwards, parallel to the posterior cutaneous branches of the lumbar nerves. The triangle of Petit is enlarged by dividing the outer border of the latissimus dorsi, and, beneath it, the quadratus lumborum and the middle layer of the lumbar aponeurosis. The abscess is now readily reached by blunt dissection carried inwards close to the front of the transverse process of the fourth or fifth lumbar vertebra.

In 1884 Treves advocated a more extensive dissection of the loin with the object not only of evacuating the abscess, but also of removing the osseous disease. Unfortunately, however, the nature and extent of the disease seldom admit of this being done, so that the operation has not come into general use. The tendency has been to confine operative treatment to the abscess alone, and to rely on prolonged rest and open-air treatment to bring about a cure of the osseous disease. The introduction of the Röntgen rays may possibly serve to revive the operation to some extent by enabling the surgeon to pick out those rarer cases in which the disease is limited to one vertebra, and especially when it is represented for the most part by a sequestrum.

The following is Sir Frederick Treves's description of the operation (*A Manual of Operative Surgery*, vol. ii, p. 772) : ' The patient's loin having been exposed, a vertical incision some 2½ inches in length is made through the integuments. The centre of this cut should lie about midway between the crest of the ilium and the last rib, and the cut should be so placed as to correspond to a vertical line parallel with the vertebral side of the outer border of the erector spinæ. . . .

' After cutting through the superficial fascia the dense aponeurosis is exposed which covers the posterior surface of the erector spinæ. . . . The dense aponeurosis with its attached muscular fibres having been divided in the full length of the incision, the erector spinæ is exposed. This muscle is at once recognized by the vertical direction of its fibres. The outer border of the muscle should now be sought for, and the whole mass drawn by means of retractors as far as possible towards the middle line of the back. In this way the anterior part of the sheath of the muscle, known as the middle layer of the fascia lumborum, is readily exposed. Neither in front nor behind has the erector spinæ any direct adhesion to its sheath at this part.

' The anterior layer of the sheath, as now exposed, is seen to be made up of dense white glistening fibres, which are all more or less transverse in direction. Through this sheath the transverse processes of the lumbar vertebræ should be sought for. The longest and most conspicuous process is that belonging to the third vertebra. It is readily felt. The erector muscle having been drawn as far as possible towards the middle line, the anterior layer of its sheath must be divided vertically as near to the transverse processes as convenient. By this incision the quadratus lumborum muscle is exposed. The muscle as here seen is very thin. It is composed of fibres which run from above obliquely downwards and outwards. Between the fibres are tendinous bundles which spring from the tips of the transverse processes. The muscle should be divided close to the extremity of a transverse process, and the incision cautiously enlarged until the muscle is divided to the full extent of the skin wound. It is at this stage that there is danger of wounding the abdominal branches of the lumbar arteries. The inner edge of the quadratus is overlapped by the psoas muscle, so that when the former is divided the latter is exposed. The psoas fibres, as now seen, take about the same direction as the posterior fibres of the quadratus—*i.e.* run downwards and outwards. The interval between the two muscles is marked by a thin but distinct layer of fascia, known as the anterior lamella of the fascia lumborum. Some of the tendinous fibres of the psoas having been divided close to a transverse process, the finger is introduced beneath the muscle, and gently insinuated along the process until the anterior aspect of the bodies of the vertebræ is reached. The incision in the psoas can be enlarged to any extent.

'With common care there should be no danger of opening up the subperitoneal connective tissue, much less of wounding the peritoneum. All risk on this score will be avoided by making the incision in the quadratus as near to the transverse processes as possible.

'Great care must be taken not to wound the lumbar arteries. The abdominal branches of these vessels run for the most part behind the quadratus lumborum. That, however, from the first vessel runs in front, and not infrequently those from one or two of the larger arteries follow its example. These vessels may be of large size—often as large as the lingual. They may be avoided, as well as the trunks from which they arise, by keeping close to a transverse process. The main vessel curves around the spine between the transverse processes, and between these processes also the division of the artery occurs. If, therefore, the rule be observed of always reaching the spine along a transverse process, the lumbar arteries and their abdominal branches need be exposed to no risk.'

ILIAC ABSCESS

Operation. An iliac abscess is best opened through an incision, about 2 inches in length, placed a finger's breadth internal to the anterior superior spine of the ilium. After splitting the external oblique the fibres of the internal oblique and transversalis muscles may be either separated by blunt dissection or divided in the direction of the original incision. The floor of the wound is formed by the fascia transversalis, close to its junction with the fascia iliaca. To reach the cavity of the abscess and at the same time to avoid opening the peritoneum, the operator should keep outside the transversalis fascia and close to the anterior superior spine, so as to get behind the fascia iliaca. Either the deep circumflex iliac artery itself, or its ascending branch, is generally seen in the course of the dissection; the former should be avoided, but the latter may have to be divided and ligatured.

When the abscess has extended below Poupart's ligament into the thigh, a second opening should be made into it. The incision for this purpose is made a little below the anterior superior spine of the ilium, along either the inner or the outer edge of the sartorius, according to the direction in which the abscess has become most superficial. The abscess wall, formed by the thickened fascia covering the ilio-psoas, is reached by retracting the sartorius and by deepening the dissection internal to the tendon of the rectus.

As soon as the pus escapes the finger should at once be introduced into the abscess cavity and the opening dilated. If the abscess be allowed to empty itself before the finger is introduced there may be some little difficulty in finding the cavity again. When the abscess has been evacuated, as much as possible of the pyogenic membrane should be removed, either with the finger-nail or with a Barker's flushing spoon. If the latter be used it must be applied cautiously, especially towards the abdominal aspect of the abscess. Moreover, too vigorous use of the sharp spoon is liable to cause an unnecessary amount of hæmorrhage as well as severe shock. The detached portions of membrane and caseous débris are removed by copious irrigation aided by compression applied to the abscess through the abdominal wall. There is no advantage in adding an antiseptic to the water used to irrigate the cavity. Normal saline at 100° F. is the best solution to employ. Before closing the wound, $\frac{1}{2}$ to 2 ounces (according to the size of the abscess) of glycerine containing 10% of iodoform in suspension may be injected into the cavity, as much as possible being squeezed out again before the wound is sutured. Or, instead of iodoform and glycerine, some iodoform-bismuth paste may be introduced into the abscess with a sharp spoon, and then rubbed over the wall with the finger. The same mixture should be smeared over the wound before it is sutured. Most surgeons now dispense altogether with drainage. In many instances the abscess does not re-form and the wound remains permanently healed. In other cases the abscess re-forms, the wound and scar become tuberculous, and, ultimately, a sinus results. The latter, however, often closes in the course of a few months. If not, the curetting should be repeated, after which the cavity may either be stuffed for a time, or the sinus and scar may be excised and the wound completely closed. If a mixed infection has occurred, a rubber drain must be introduced.

While many surgeons are in favour of treating spinal abscesses by curetting followed by the introduction of iodoform, there are others who employ neither, but trust merely to evacuation and irrigation. The writer has treated many abscesses successfully by the latter more simple method. Many surgeons, again, instead of opening the abscess, prefer to empty it by aspiration through a large trocar, and to inject iodoform and glycerine.

After-treatment. The after-treatment is all-important. It consists in keeping the spine quiet with the patient constantly recumbent (as much as possible in the open air) for at least a year, and generally longer. The bed-frame introduced by Bradford is probably the most convenient apparatus for the purpose. Extension must be applied if there be any spastic condition or tendency to paraplegia.

OPERATIONS FOR TUBERCULOUS OSTEOMYELITIS OF THE RIBS

Operation. While spontaneous cure of the disease rarely occurs, operative treatment is almost invariably followed by recovery, provided the bone focus be completely removed. Recurrence, on the other hand, is very prone to occur if, after opening the abscess, the surgeon trusts simply to scraping the rib. The proper course to adopt is to resect the diseased portion of the rib, and care must be taken that the bone or cartilage is divided well beyond the disease. The operative procedure in the case of a limited focus at the costo-chondral junction of one of the true ribs, with a secondary abscess under the pectoralis major, is carried out as follows: A horseshoe incision is made a little beyond the lower two-thirds of the circumference of the swelling, and a flap, consisting of skin and subcutaneous tissue, is dissected upwards off the pectoralis major. The fibres of this muscle are now divided along the circumference of the abscess down to its pyogenic wall, and the latter, along with the muscle, is then dissected off the chest-wall. By excising the abscess and the affected muscle *en masse* the risk of infecting the soft tissues is greatly diminished. A careful examination is next made of the diseased rib with a view of ascertaining the nature and extent of the mischief. Should a sinus be found leading into a small focus in the interior of the rib, a portion of the latter including the diseased focus should be resected subperiosteally. The operation is simplified by resecting the bone subperiosteally in the first instance and then dissecting away any disease which may be left behind in the periosteum and adjacent muscle. The intercostal vessels will generally have to be divided and ligatured. Care must be taken, however, not to injure the pleura.

Should an abscess exist between the pleura and the chest-wall, more of the rib, or it may be a portion also of the rib below, along with the intervening intercostal muscles, may have to be resected to enable the tuberculous lining of the abscess to be thoroughly dealt with. The intrathoracic fascia and the pleura are markedly thickened so that with ordinary care the pleural cavity need not be opened into. Before closing the wound sublimated iodoform-bismuth paste should be rubbed into the wall of the abscess. If the operation has been a limited one, and it be felt that no trace of disease has been left behind, the flap may be sutured back into position without drainage. If, on the other hand, the wound be of large size, it is well to introduce a drain for forty-eight hours or so, while in cases complicated with an abscess between the chest-wall and the pleura an iodoform-gauze tampon should be introduced for a week or so.

When the disease is situated at the costo-chondral junction of one of the lower ribs, the secondary abscess is in the neighbourhood of the lower margin of the chest, and not infrequently it gravitates downwards either between the lateral abdominal muscles external to the sheath of the rectus, or within the latter, between its posterior wall and the rectus muscle. When the abscess is situated within the sheath of the rectus, the pus collects as a rule behind the muscle in the first instance, and subsequently burrows through it. In a case of this kind a free longitudinal incision should be made into the sheath of the muscle, and after cleaning out and curetting the superficial portion of the abscess, the deeper portion should be laid open from end to end, by splitting the rectus and following the abscess upwards until its source from the diseased cartilage is reached. The diseased portion of the cartilage is then resected, a knife usually sufficing to divide it. The deep portion of the abscess should be dissected off the under surface of the rectus muscle as far as possible, and the floor of the abscess should be thoroughly curetted.

The same line of treatment is to be followed when the disease is situated in the abdominal wall external to the rectus. Here the deepest part of the abscess usually occupies the interval between the transversalis muscle and its fascia, the latter being considerably thickened to form the outer fibrous layer of the pyogenic membrane.

When the diseased focus is situated posterior to the costo-chondral junction, the abscess is situated under the serratus magnus, the external oblique, or the latissimus dorsi. In dealing with an abscess in any of these situations the operator should not hesitate to remove every particle of diseased muscle along with the abscess; if this be not done a tubercular sinus is almost certain to develop in the scar.

As pointed out by König, the operation for tuberculosis of a rib may be very troublesome when the disease is complicated with multiple sinuses which are both elongated and tortuous. Considerable patience and perseverance may have to be exercised before the disease can be satisfactorily removed. Not infrequently more than one operation will be necessary. In the female the mamma may have to be removed in order that the operation may be sufficiently radical.

When the abscess is situated in the axilla the surgeon must satisfy himself that there is no disease of the rib before deciding that caseous glands are alone responsible for the condition.

SECTION II

OPERATIONS FOR TUBERCULOUS AFFECTIONS OF THE BONES AND JOINTS

PART II

OPERATIONS FOR TUBERCULOUS AFFECTIONS OF THE JOINTS

BY

HAROLD J. STILES, M.B., F.R.C.S. (Edin.), Lieutenant-Colonel, R.A.M.C.(T.).

Surgeon to Chalmers Hospital, Edinburgh, and to the Royal Hospital for Sick Children, Edinburgh

CHAPTER V

OPERATIONS FOR TUBERCULOUS DISEASE OF THE WRIST-JOINT

UNDER the heading tuberculous disease of the wrist-joint there are included a group of lesions which are met with either singly or in various combinations depending on the site of origin of the disease and on the direction and extent of its spread.

Fortunately conservative treatment gives comparatively good results in the early stage of tuberculous disease of the wrist-joint, and in view of the somewhat unsatisfactory functional results following excision, the former treatment should be given a fair trial. Should it fail, however, operative measures must be undertaken. If the disease be allowed to run on until the synovial sheaths and tendons become involved, and if sinuses and mixed infection be allowed to occur, the functional result following excision will be unsatisfactory, owing to deficient movement of the fingers.

Operation. The nature of the operative interference will of course depend on the extent of the disease. By a complete excision of the wrist is meant the removal of the entire carpus (with the exception of the pisiform and the hook of the unciform) along with the adjacent articular extremities of the radius, ulna, and metacarpals. If the disease be confined to the carpus, the lower ends of the bones of the forearm may be left, and the same may be said of the proximal ends of the metacarpal bones when the disease has begun in the wrist-joint proper. The rule in operating on a tuberculous wrist should be to remove all the disease, but at the same time to sacrifice no more bone than is absolutely necessary; the greater the amount of bone removed the more are the flexors and extensors of the fingers left unnecessarily long, and the more is their action weakened.

Although a tourniquet is not essential, it has the advantage of expediting the operation and enabling the surgeon to obtain a clear view of the anatomy of the parts, which is rather more complicated than in the case of the other joints. The tourniquet should be applied to the lower third of the upper arm. Instead of placing the limb across the patient's body it will be found much more convenient to have the forearm and hand supported on a separate table of small size. The operator will find it an advantage to be comfortably seated while performing the operation.

Access to the diseased structures may be obtained either by a single dorsal incision (Langenbeck, Kocher) or by a dorso-radial incision, combined with an ulnar incision (Lister). Complete excision of the wrist by Lister's double incision has been dealt with by Mr. Burghard

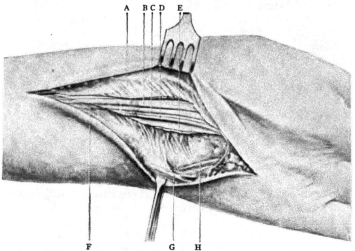

FIG. 77. EXCISION OF THE WRIST BY KOCHER'S SINGLE DORSO-ULNAR INCISION. The deep fascia and the posterior annular ligament have been divided, exposing the tendons of the extensor digitorum communis. The dorsal branch of the ulnar vein and nerve are seen at the inner border of the wrist. A, E, Posterior annular ligament; B, C, D, Extensor digitorum longus; F, Deep fascia; G, Posterior ulnar vein; H, Dorsal branch of ulnar vein.

in this volume, p. 9. This procedure should be reserved for cases in which the disease is especially advanced at the outer aspect of the wrist.

For the majority of cases the writer prefers the more conservative procedure recommended by Kocher. The incision, which is dorso-ulnar in position, is a modification of Langenbeck's straight dorsal incision; it passes from the middle of the fifth metacarpal bone to the middle of the back of the wrist, and thence for an equal distance up the middle of the back of the forearm, the entire incision measuring 4 to 5 inches.

After dividing the integuments and the posterior annular ligament, there is exposed, in the upper part of the wound, the inner edge of the extensor digitorum communis and the extensor minimi digiti (digiti quinti proprius), while in the lower part of the wound the dorsal branch of the ulnar nerve is seen, and, if possible, avoided.

The wound is now deepened so as to divide the thin posterior ligament of the inferior radio-ulnar joint; below it the dorsal ligaments are separated subperiosteally from the back of the cuneiform (triquetral)

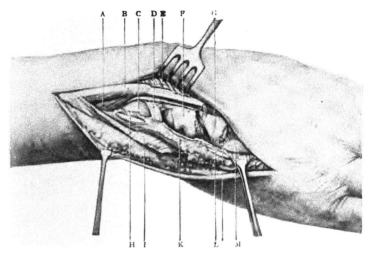

FIG. 78. FURTHER STAGE OF THE OPERATION SHOWN IN THE PREVIOUS FIGURE. The wound has been deepened, and the soft tissues, including the posterior ligaments and the periosteum, have been separated, exposing (from above downwards) the head of the ulna, the triangular fibro-cartilage, the cuneiform, unciform, and the base of the fifth metatarsal bone. The tendons of the extensor digitorum communis and the fibres of the extensor indicis are seen beneath the outer edge of the wound; the extensor minimi digiti and the extensor carpi ulnaris are seen at its inner edge. A, Extensor indicis; B, Extensor digitorum communis; c, Head of the ulna; D, Triangular cartilage; E, I, Posterior annular ligament; F, Cuneiform; G, Unciform; H, Extensor minimi digiti; K, Posterior ligament and periosteum; L, Tendon of the extensor minimi digiti; M, Base of the fifth metacarpal.

and unciform (hamate) bones, while still lower the tendon of the extensor carpi ulnaris is detached subperiosteally from the base of the fifth metacarpal bone. The inner flap, which contains the tendons of the extensor minimi digiti (digiti quinti proprius) and extensor carpi ulnaris along with the dorsal ligaments and periosteum, is now completely dissected off the head and styloid process of the ulna, the internal lateral ligament being divided. Below the ulna the flap is separated sub-

periosteally from the palmar aspect of the cu
until the joint between it and the pisiform
detached along with the insertion of the flex
down, the flap, along with the insertion of t

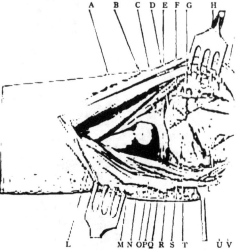

FIG. 79.   FURTHER STAGE OF THE OPERATION S
FIGURES. The extensor tendons, along with the pos
osteum, have been separated from the bones at the b
inwards. The soft parts at the ulnar edge have als
rated. The tendon of the extensor minimi digiti a
ulnaris have each been freed from its groove and re
the other soft parts, off the bones at the ulnar edg
indicis; B, Radius; C, Extensor digitorum communis;
annular ligament; F, II, Periosteal and dorsal ligame
num; K, Base of the third metacarpal; L, V, Extenso
carpi ulnaris; N, Head of the ulna; P, Triangular
R, Internal lateral ligament; S, Cuneiform; T, Pisifo
the fifth metacarpal; X, Base of the fourth metaca

is still further detached so as to expose the
metacarpal bone.
    Attention is next directed to the dorsal fl
wards by detaching the posterior ligament o
lower end of the radius; the extensor tendons,
are at the same time separated from the gr
bone. The separation is effected partly with

a sharp rugine. Lower down, the latter instrument is used to separate the dorsal ligaments of the carpal and metacarpo-phalangeal joints, and care is taken to separate the insertions of the extensor carpi radialis brevis and longus subperiosteally. In this way all the bones at the back of the wrist, except the trapezoid (lesser multangular), the trapezium (greater multangular), and the bases of the first and second metacarpals, are laid bare.

By removing the cuneiform (triquetral) bone, room is obtained for the finger to feel and identify the hook of the unciform (hamate), which is either chiselled off or snipped off with small bone-forceps. The operator should keep close to the bone so as to avoid injuring the deep branch of the ulnar nerve, which winds round its inner aspect. The inner flexor tendons are now exposed, and pulled aside, after which the anterior ligament of the wrist and the anterior carpal and metacarpal ligaments are separated from the palmar aspect of the bones. The parietal layer of the common flexor sheath is so closely related to the anterior ligaments that it is generally removed with the latter, but no harm is done as long as the wound is aseptic.

The operator now returns to the dorsal aspect of the wrist, and, after retracting the extensor tendons well outwards, the separation of the posterior ligament of the wrist is carried as far outwards as the styloid process of the radius, the periosteum and the two radial extensors being lifted out of their groove. While this is being done, the hand is forcibly flexed and dislocated to the radial side, so that the thumb comes in contact with the radial border of the forearm and the extensor tendons become dislocated to the outer side of the lower end of the radius. By this manœuvre the wrist-joint proper is freely opened up and the carpal bones are projected more into the wound; in short, a very free arthrotomy has been obtained.

The operator is now able to ascertain the exact distribution of the disease and to decide to what extent the resection must be carried in order to remove it completely. The carpal bones, with the exception of the trapezium (greater multangular) and the pisiform, are removed, either collectively, or, which is preferable, individually, by grasping them with necrosis forceps and partly cutting and partly wrenching them away from the remaining ligamentous attachments. Some little difficulty may be experienced in freeing the tubercle of the scaphoid (navicular) from the external lateral ligament and the trapezium (greater mult-angular) from the trapezoid (lesser multangular) bone.

If the disease has extended to the joint between the trapezium (greater multangular) and the first metacarpal bone, the former must be resected and the base of the latter removed, after separating the tendon

of the extensor ossis metacarpi pollicis (abductor pollicis longus). For
this purpose a short dorso-radial incision should be made to the outer

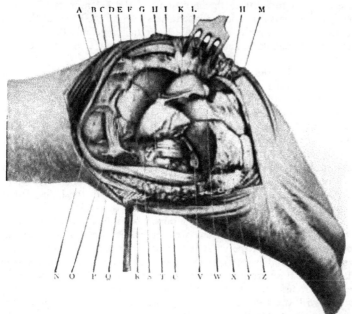

FIG. 80. FURTHER STAGE OF THE OPERATION SHOWN IN THE PREVIOUS THREE
FIGURES. The cuneiform bone has been removed, and the pisiform and the hook
of the unciform have been detached. The radio-carpal and intercarpal articulations have been opened up, and the hand has been flexed to the radial side. The
two radial extensor tendons are seen at the outer side of the dorsum of the wrist.
while the tendon of the extensor carpi ulnaris is seen at the inner side. In the
floor of the wound are the flexor tendons. A, Groove for the extensor minimi
digiti; B, Groove for the extensor digitorum communis and extensor indicis;
C, Extensor indicis; D, Groove for the extensor pollicis longus; E, Dorsal radial
tubercle; F, Radial articular surface for the semilunar; G, Radial articular surface
for the scaphoid; H, Extensor carpi radialis brevior; I, Extensor carpi radialis
longior; K, Scaphoid; L, Periosteal and dorsal ligaments; M, Base of the third
metacarpal; N, Head of the ulna; O, Triangular cartilage; P, Styloid process;
Q, Posterior annular ligament; R, Extensor carpi ulnaris; S, Anterior ligaments;
T, Semilunar; U, Flexor tendons; V, Cut base of the hook of the unciform; W, Os
magnum; X, Unciform; Y, Base of the fifth metacarpal; Z, Base of the fourth
metacarpal.

side of and parallel to the tendon of the extensor secundi internodii
pollicis (extensor pollicis longus). The radial artery and nerve are

exposed and drawn aside along with the soft parts before proceeding to remove the osseous disease.

The carpo-metacarpal joint, on account of its possessing a separate synovial membrane, is often free from disease, and when this is the case the trapezium (greater multangular) may generally be left, with the result that the movements of the thumb are not interfered with.

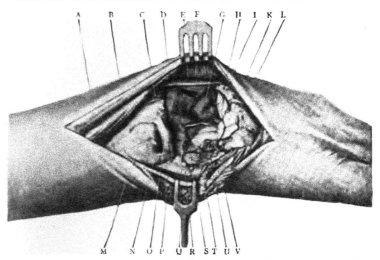

FIG. 81. FURTHER STAGE OF THE OPERATION SHOWN IN THE PREVIOUS FOUR FIGURES. All the carpal bones have been removed except the trapezium. The articular surfaces of the third, fourth, and fifth metacarpals are seen at the lower end of the wound. In the floor of the wound are the deep flexor tendons, and internal to them are seen the articular surfaces of the pisiform bone and the detached hook of the unciform. A, Extensor digitorum communis; B, Extensor indicis; C, Radius; D, Periosteal and dorsal ligaments; E, Extensor carpi radialis brevior; F, Extensor carpi radialis longior; G, Trapezium; H, Styloid process of the third metacarpal; I, Base of the third metacarpal; K, Base of the fourth metacarpal; L, Base of the fifth metacarpal; M, Head of the ulna; N, Styloid process; O, Triangular cartilage; P, Extensor carpi ulnaris; Q, Cut edge of the anterior ligaments; R, Dorsal ligaments; S, Pisiform; T, Flexor tendons; U, Cut base of the hook of the unciform; V, Extensor minimi digiti.

Unless the disease demands it, the bases of the metacarpal bones should not be sawn off; if on the other hand it be necessary to remove them, the periosteal connexions of the two radial extensors and of the radial flexor should be preserved as far as possible. If free from disease, the articular extremities of the radius and ulna along with the triangular fibro-cartilage should also be preserved. Should the disease have commenced in the wrist-joint proper it will, of course, be necessary to remove the lower ends of these bones along with the interarticular fibro-cartilage.

In removing the distal ends of the bones of the forearm and the proximal ends of the metacarpal bones, Kocher recommends that the saw should be applied so as to produce convex surfaces on a transverse axis, with the object of facilitating flexion and extension.

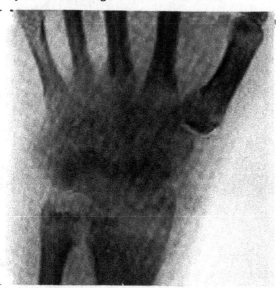

Fig. 82.   Extensive Tuberculous Disease of the Wrist. Skiagram from a female aged thirty-two. The carpo-metacarpal (with the exception of the joint between the first metacarpal and the trapezium) and wrist-joint proper were diseased along with the intercarpal joints. (By Dr. E. Price.)

On the removal of the carpal bones, the floor of the wound is seen to be occupied by the ligamentous structures and the remains of the periosteum separated from their palmar aspects. As a rule these structures are so invaded with tubercle that their removal is called for, along with the parietal layer of the common flexor sheath. The close relationship of the carpus to the parietal layer of the palmar sheath accounts for the frequency with which the latter is invaded by the disease. When this has occurred, the flexor tendons must be lifted well out of their tunnel, and the whole of the diseased sheath carefully dissected away.

It is advisable to operate before the palmar sheath has become involved, because the adhesions which follow its removal seriously interfere with the patient's ability to flex the fingers.

Cases complicated with abscesses or sinuses must be treated on the general principles already mentioned in dealing with the other joints. Fortunately the sinus is generally situated either at the radial or ulnar side of the wrist, so that in excising it the ellipse may be included in

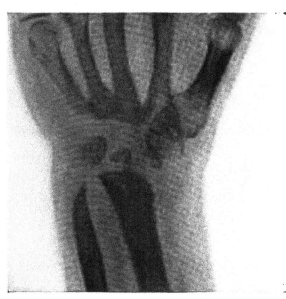

FIG. 83.   RESULT OF EXCISION OF THE WRIST.   Skiagram taken six months after excision by Kocher's single dorso-ulnar incision, from the same case as the previous figure.   Note the presence of the pisiform, the hook of the unciform, and the trapezium, also the healed condition of sawn surfaces of bones.   The patient had good use of the fingers and especially of the thumb.   (*By Dr. E. Price.*)

the main incision.   Before closing the wound sublimated iodoform-bismuth paste should be rubbed into the raw surfaces.   Drainage may be secured by pulling a rubber tube or strip of gauze through a button-hole opening made by cutting down on forceps projected from the main wound to the palmar aspect of the wrist just internal to the median nerve.   The advantage of the drain is that it allows the rest of the wound to be closely stitched, and so prevents any tendency to prolapse of the extensor tendons.

The advantages which Kocher claims for his
the incision avoids the dorsal branch of the
radial nerve is injured by the dorso-radial in
ment of the tendon of the extensor carpi u
disadvantage as has division of the radial ext
extensor has much less share in dorsiflexing
extensors. The extensor carpi ulnaris assists
flexion, a displacement which, due partly to th
partly to cicatricial contraction, is peculiarly lial
The division of this tendon is, therefore, rat
wise. (3) With the dorso-ulnar incision the e
tendency to protrude from the wound than in

After-treatment. The important point
treatment is to see that the hand is maintained i
with the thumb and fingers left free. For this
make use of Lister's anterior splint, which is thi
carpal region by means of a cork pad. In the
habit of using simply an anterior strip of alu
be bent backwards opposite the wrist so as tc
dorsiflexed position. The advantage of such
sterilized and applied inside the bandage whi

The chief drawback to excision of the wrist
of view is the difficulty the patient experienc
power of flexing the fingers. This difficulty i
tendons being too long after the bones have
to adhesion of the tendons. The former factor
the parts to consolidate with the hand dorsiflex
tendons as much on the stretch as possible,
combated by beginning massage and movement
as soon as the wound is healed.

CHAPTER VI

OPERATION FOR TUBERCULOUS DISEASE OF THE ELBOW-JOINT

Operation. Great difference of opinion still exists as to the relative merits of conservative and radical treatment in dealing with tuberculous disease of the elbow-joint.

In the early stage of the disease a skiagram should always be taken before giving a definite opinion as to whether conservative measures (including iodoform injections and Bier's congestion treatment) should be tried, or whether operation should be recommended. If a bone focus be revealed, the writer prefers to proceed to operation at once. If, on the other hand, there is reason to believe that the disease is purely synovial, conservative measures may be employed, but should no improvement manifest itself within a few weeks, radical treatment should be advised.

When operating in the early stage of the disease, instead of proceeding to do a stereotyped excision, the first step in the operation should be a free arthrotomy. For this purpose the writer prefers the external J-shaped incision of Kocher. This gives a good exposure of the interior of the joint and at the same time inflicts the minimum of damage to the muscles and their nerve-supply. The upper part of the incision, which begins about two inches above the external condyle, is carried downwards along the back of the external supracondyloid ridge through the fleshy fibres of the triceps external to its tendon; the middle part opens into the posterior aspect of the radio-humeral joint by dividing the posterior part of the external lateral and orbicular (annular) ligaments in the interval between the tendon of origin of the anconeus and the common extensor tendon; the lower part of the incision is continued downwards along the intermuscular space between the fleshy fibres of the anconeus and the extensor carpi ulnaris, and ends by curving inwards to reach the posterior border of the ulna about two inches below the tip of the olecranon.

The inner flap, including the insertion of the triceps and practically the whole of the anconeus, is detached subperiosteally from the back of the humerus and olecranon, partly with the knife and partly with a sharp rugine. Care is taken to preserve the continuity between the insertion of the triceps and the periosteum of the ulna below it. Kocher attaches

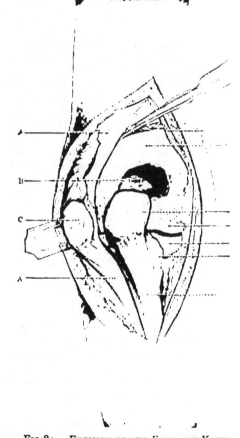

FIG. 84.   EXCISION OF THE ELBOW BY KOCH
EXTERNAL, SLIGHTLY J-SHAPED INCISION.   The
tensor flap, consisting of the tendon of the tricep
layer of cartilage detached from the olecranon, ¿
beneath it, of the anconeus, has been reflected
wards subperiosteally off the lower end of
humerus and the upper part of the ulna.   The orbi
lar (annular) ligament has been divided, expos
the head of the radius.   A, A, Periosteum; B, Olec
non fossa; C, Insertion of the triceps; D, Ul
E, Orbicular ligament; F, Radius; G, Capitell
H, Olecranon; I, Humerus; K, Triceps.

flection of the soft tissues off the external condyle and the head of the radius is a comparatively simple matter. The common tendons of origin of the flexor and extensor muscles, along with the upper attachment of the lateral ligaments, should, if possible, be preserved intact by detaching them either subperiosteally or along with a thin shell of bone. In the child the separation is easily effected by paring off a portion of the cartilaginous epicondyles along with the origins of the muscles; in the adult a strong sharp rugine should be used.

After the flaps have been completely dissected off the condyles, the assistant fully flexes the elbow and projects the lower end of the humerus well into the wound, so that the surgeon may clear it preparatory to applying the saw. Before doing so, however, the operator should carefully examine the olecranon fossa to ascertain the presence or absence of a small perforation leading into it from a limited bone focus higher up. If there be no visible focus of disease in the humerus, it should be sawn across at the level of the upper part of the epicondyles, and if no disease be detected on the raw surface, the sharp corners of the remaining portions of the epicondyles should be rounded off. It is well also to clip away the thin layer of bone forming the remains of the olecranon fossa, so as to leave a slightly crescentic extremity; this is done with the object of diminishing lateral movement subsequently. If, on the other hand, a well circumscribed focus of disease be revealed on the sawn surface, thorough curetting will generally suffice; if the focus be more diffuse it is safer to separate the periosteum and saw the bone at a higher level, well clear of the disease. In some cases it is impossible to remove all the disease without dividing the bone through the lower part of the medullary cavity. Fig. 60 is taken from a case in which the lower third of the humerus had to be resected subperiosteally at the same time that the elbow was excised. The periosteum was incised in the line of the original incision, which was prolonged further up the arm. The periosteal tube is closed by the same sutures which unite the triceps to the supinator longus (brachio-radialis) and the extensor carpi radialis longior.

Having dealt with the humerus, the operator next proceeds to clear the upper ends of the radius and ulna, the assistant meanwhile fully flexing the elbow and thrusting the bones of the forearm as far up into the wound as possible. To free the radius, the orbicular (annular) ligament should be completely removed, after which the neck of the bone is divided well below the head. The advantage of removing the greater part of the neck of the radius is twofold: (1) It ensures complete removal of the collar of diseased synovial membrane which occupies the recessus sacciformis—a diverticulum of the synovial cavity which surrounds the upper part of the neck of the radius below the level of the orbicular ligament.

(2) It diminishes the risk of firm union humerus, and thereby helps to preserve the supination.   To ensure still further the pres

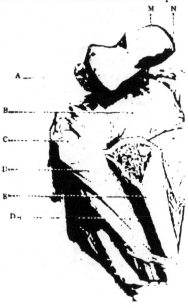

Fig. 85.   Further Stage of Excision of th
Both flaps, along with a portion of each epicondyl
on the condyles, and the lower end of the humeru
posteriorly.   The elbow is fully flexed, causing
olecranon has been snipped off with bone-force
from the portion of the ulna below it.   The orbi
and reflected outwards, exposing the head and n
the wound is occupied by the torn anterior ligame
is the A. Internal condyle; B. Anterior ligame
n.n. Periosteum; E. Ulna; F. Extensor carpi ulnar
of the radius; G. Orbicular ligament; K. Radius;
William; N. External condyle.

some of the fibres of the supinator brevis may be stitched over the stump of the bone. If the disease has perforated the thin part of the capsule below the orbicular ligament and burrowed downwards between the two bones, it may be followed up and removed either at this stage or after the ulna has been dealt with.

If there be no primary focus in the upper end of the ulna, the plan recommended by Kocher should be adopted, namely, to saw off the articular surface so as to leave a concave surface. For this purpose a fine bow saw is used; the section is made from before backwards. Before

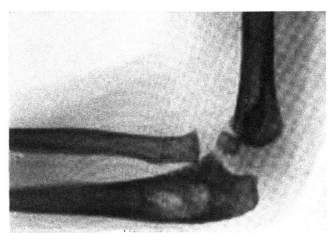

Fig. 86. SKIAGRAM OF THE ELBOW OF A CHILD AGED SIX YEARS. Shows tuberculous foci in the upper end of the ulna. (*By Dr. E. Price.*)

applying the saw, the anterior ligament, along with the insertion of the brachialis anticus, should be slightly separated subperiosteally from the front of the coronoid process.

If, on the other hand, the joint has become involved secondary to a primary focus in the olecranon, this process should be removed as soon as the extensor flap has been separated from it. By this means the joint is at once opened into and free access is obtained for the clearing and removal of the lower end of the humerus. After this has been done the operator returns to the bones of the forearm and completes the removal of their upper extremities, the ulna being sawn off below the disease.

When, as is not infrequently the case in young children, the disease

(2) It diminishes the risk of firm union between the radius and the humerus, and thereby helps to preserve the movements of pronation and supination. To ensure still further the preservation of these movements,

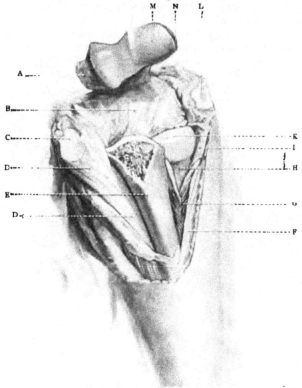

FIG. 85.   FURTHER STAGE OF EXCISION OF THE ELBOW BY KOCHER'S INCISION. Both flaps, along with a portion of each epicondyle, have been completely reflected off the condyles, and the lower end of the humerus has been cleared anteriorly and posteriorly. The elbow is fully flexed, causing the humerus to protrude. The olecranon has been snipped off with bone-forceps and the periosteum stripped from the portion of the ulna below it. The orbicular ligament has been divided and reflected outwards, exposing the head and neck of the radius. The floor of the wound is occupied by the thin anterior ligament covered by the synovial membrane. A, Internal condyle; B, Anterior ligament; C, Insertion of the triceps; D, D, Periosteum; E, Ulna; F, Extensor carpi ulnaris; G, Supinator brevis; H, Neck of the radius; I, Orbicular ligament; K, Radius; L, External epicondyle; M, Capitellum; N, External condyle.

some of the fibres of the supinator brevis may be stitched over the stump of the bone. If the disease has perforated the thin part of the capsule below the orbicular ligament and burrowed downwards between the two bones, it may be followed up and removed either at this stage or after the ulna has been dealt with.

If there be no primary focus in the upper end of the ulna, the plan recommended by Kocher should be adopted, namely, to saw off the articular surface so as to leave a concave surface. For this purpose a fine bow saw is used; the section is made from before backwards. Before

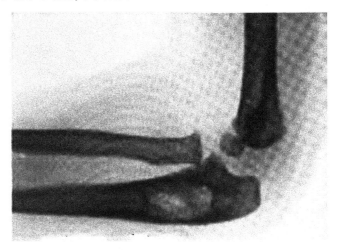

FIG. 86.   SKIAGRAM OF THE ELBOW OF A CHILD AGED SIX YEARS.   Shows tuberculous foci in the upper end of the ulna.   (*By Dr. E. Price.*)

applying the saw, the anterior ligament, along with the insertion of the brachialis anticus, should be slightly separated subperiosteally from the front of the coronoid process.

If, on the other hand, the joint has become involved secondary to a primary focus in the olecranon, this process should be removed as soon as the extensor flap has been separated from it. By this means the joint is at once opened into and free access is obtained for the clearing and removal of the lower end of the humerus. After this has been done the operator returns to the bones of the forearm and completes the removal of their upper extremities, the ulna being sawn off below the disease.

When, as is not infrequently the case in young children, the disease involves the upper part of the shaft of the ulna as well as the olecranon (Fig. 86), the bones of the forearm must be resected to a still lower level. After splitting the periosteum longitudinally the ulna may be shelled out, either from above downwards after opening into the joint, or from below upwards before the joint is opened into. The radius, whether diseased or not, should be divided at the same level as the ulna, care being taken not to injure either the biceps tendon or the posterior interosseous (deep radial) nerve. The edges of the split periosteum are united with buried catgut sutures before closing the skin wound.

Having dealt with the ends of the bones, attention is next directed to the disease in the soft parts. When the tuberculous mischief is still confined within the capsule, this is a very simple matter, as the arrangement of the synovial membrane is comparatively simple. The whole of the posterior ligament and the synovial pouch beneath the triceps is removed to a level well above the olecranon fossa. At the floor of the wound is the diseased synovial membrane covering the anterior ligament, in front of which is the brachialis anticus muscle, which excludes the brachial artery from the immediate field of operation. As a rule it will be found necessary to dissect the thin anterior ligament off the brachialis anticus along with the synovial membrane. Occasionally, however, the disease is so limited to the synovial membrane that the latter may be clipped or scraped away, leaving the ligament intact. As already indicated, it is important to make sure that no diseased synovial membrane is left in the recessus sacciformis which surrounds the neck of the radius below the orbicular (annular) ligament.

In more advanced cases, where the disease has extended through the capsule, involved the peri-articular structures, infiltrated the muscles around the joint, and, it may be, burrowed up the arm and down the forearm, the removal of all the infected tissues is a matter of considerable difficulty. Neither time nor perseverance should be spared in following up and removing them, as freedom from recurrence, and, which is more important, the avoidance of subsequent amputation, depend very largely upon the thoroughness with which this part of the operation is carried out. Every particle of tuberculous capsule and peri-articular tissue should be removed, no matter how extensive the infiltration, and all caseous pockets and abscesses should, whenever possible, be excised rather than curetted. If the ulnar nerve be in danger, it is better to ascertain its whereabouts by exposing it in the first instance above or below the disease, and then following it through the infiltrated tissue which surrounds it. The musculo-spiral (radial) and posterior interosseous (deep radial) nerves are less liable to be involved.

The presence of sinuses still further complicates the operation. They should be excised whenever possible. When situated towards the outer aspect of the joint they may be included in an ellipse which is made to form a part of Kocher's incision, while if they are situated upon the inner aspect of the joint, the openings made after excising them may be taken advantage of for drainage.

After the disease is all removed, the wound is sutured in two layers. The deeper sutures (interrupted catgut) unite the following muscles from above downwards: (1) The outer edge of the triceps to the external intermuscular septum, and to the muscles arising from it, namely, the supinator longus and the extensor carpi radialis longior; (2) the tendon of origin and outer margin of the anconeus to the common extensor tendon and to the inner edge of the extensor carpi ulnaris. The superficial sutures, consisting of silkworm-gut and intermediate horsehair, unite the skin and subcutaneous tissue. In the absence of mixed infection, drainage is often unnecessary, especially if no tourniquet be used at the operation.

After-treatment. Considerable difference of opinion exists among surgeons as to the best method of carrying out the after-treatment of excision of the elbow. Some prefer to place the elbow in the extended position for two or three weeks before flexing it, while others place it in the flexed position at the outset; some begin passive movement as soon as the wound is healed, while others wait for three or four weeks; some avoid passive movement if possible, but take special steps to encourage active movement. The fact, however, is that no single line of after-treatment is suitable for all cases. Much depends on the age of the patient, on the amount of bone removed, and on the extent to which the periarticular tissues and muscles have been interfered with. The ideal result to be arrived at is a freely movable, and at the same time a muscularly strong joint, without, however, any preternatural movement.

In the young child, in a case of average severity, the writer is in the habit of keeping the forearm extended and somewhat supinated for the first fortnight or so, complete rest being ensured by bandaging the limb to the side of the chest, which is thus converted into a splint. During the next fortnight the elbow is kept alternately flexed and extended for periods of forty-eight hours, the flexion being maintained by means of a rectangular aluminium splint. At the end of a month the arm is merely supported in a sling, and the child is encouraged to begin to use it. Should the patient refuse to do so, the opposite arm should be bandaged to the chest so as to encourage the child to play with its toys with the affected limb. If the disease has been more extensive than usual, the chances of a flail joint will be lessened if the limb be placed in the flexed position from the outset.

As a rule the after-treatment in the adult consists in keeping the elbow extended and somewhat supinated for the first two or three weeks, after which time the limb is massaged and active movement encouraged. If there be a tendency to stiffness, passive movements must be persevered with.   Pronation and supination may be begun almost from the first. If the joint shows signs of becoming flail, the limb should be fixed in plaster of Paris in the flexed position for some weeks.   If, on the other hand, it be evident that ankylosis is going to result, the patient's occupation must be taken into account in deciding as to the position in which the elbow is allowed to become stiff.   In well-to-do patients, and in almost all females, the limb should be fixed at an angle of about 70° or 75°, while in those whose employment entails the carrying and lifting of heavy objects, the elbow should be fixed at an obtuse angle.   In both instances the forearm should be in the mid-position between pronation and supination.   Kocher points out that on no account should the forearm be placed across the front of the chest in the flexed and adducted position.   He applies a splint which maintains the forearm in the supinated and vertical position, so that the ends of the radius and ulna may rest in the coronal plane against the lower end of the humerus.   He begins active movement after a few days, and maintains that plaster bandages are not needed.

Results. Of the forty-six primary excisions of the elbow which the writer has done during the last ten years, the disease was found to be primarily synovial in 29%.   In only one case was the radius primarily affected, in the others the primary disease occurred with almost equal frequency in the humerus and ulna.   Of the thirty-one patients subsequently traced, one died of broncho-pneumonia four days after the second elbow was resected, five of general tuberculosis, and two of an intercurrent disease.   Information as regards the functional after-result could only be obtained in sixteen cases.   Of these eight had a strong freely movable joint; in six there was lateral movement in addition to flexion and extension, and in some of these there was a tendency to a flail joint. In one the limb was ankylosed at a right angle with full pronation and supination, and in another at 145°.   In a little more than half the cases the child was under five years of age at the time of operation.   40% of the cases were complicated with either an abscess or a sinus.   In children a certain amount of shortening is inevitable, as all the epiphyseal cartilages about the elbow are removed.   In the cases operated on, the shortening of the upper arm varied from nothing to 2½ inches, and in the forearm from 1 to 4 inches.   Fortunately growth takes place to a less extent from the cubital epiphyses than from those of the shoulder and wrist.

CHAPTER VII

TUBERCULOUS DISEASE OF THE SHOULDER-JOINT

Except when associated with advanced pulmonary tuberculosis conservative treatment is not to be recommended in tuberculous disease of this joint, as it almost invariably results in ankylosis, a condition attended with great disability. By excision, on the other hand—especially if undertaken before the stage of abscess formation and involvement of the peri-articular structures—an excellent result with comparatively free movement at the shoulder may generally be looked for.

When the disease has begun in the upper end of the humerus, it is usual to excise the joint by the anterior method. When, however, the disease involves more especially the glenoid cavity, or when it is more advanced and diffused throughout the joint, Kocher prefers to resect the joint from behind.

With regard to the advantages of the posterior route, this author writes as follows: 'When the head has been thoroughly cleared, and especially if it be excised, an excellent view of the glenoid is obtained, much better than is possible by the anterior incision; and as it is most important to remove all the infected tissues in tuberculous disease, this complete exposure of all parts of the joint is the great advantage of the method. Moreover, this free exposure is obtained without interfering with the function of the deltoid or other muscles of the shoulder. Yet another advantage over the anterior method is, that when the disease in the head is limited or absent, only the posterior muscles require to be separated, while the anterior part of the capsule, the coraco-humeral band, and the subscapularis muscle are preserved intact, and in this way there is no tendency of the head of the bone to be displaced upwards towards the coracoid, which so frequently occurs as the result of the anterior operation.'

Both the anterior and posterior operations have been fully described by Mr. Burghard (pp. 34–40). It will suffice therefore in this article merely to draw attention to a few points regarding the operation as performed for tuberculous disease.

When the disease in the joint is secondary to a focus in the upper end of the humerus, the muscles attached to the tuberosities must be freely separated.   The capsule is slit up from the bicipital groove as far as the glenoid, and the tendon itself is freed and displaced to the inner side of the inner tuberosity.   The capsule, along with the rotator muscles, is then separated subperiosteally from the tuberosities by a strong rugine or, if preferred, a thin layer of bone may be detached along with the periosteum.   When a limited focus is situated in the great tuberosity, thorough curetting followed by the introduction of sublimated iodoform-bismuth paste will generally suffice.   If, however, the focus in the humerus be more diffuse, the periosteum must be still further separated and the bone sawn across immediately below the disease.   Care must be taken not to wound the circumflex vessels, and more particularly the circumflex nerve.   The saw is applied parallel to the anatomical neck.

In a case of primary synovial disease, there is no necessity to remove more than the articular surface of the humerus.   The bone is sawn obliquely along the line of the anatomical neck, and the sharp edge which is left is carefully clipped away with bone-forceps curved on the flat, so as to prevent injurious pressure on the axillary artery.

If the glenoid cartilage be diseased, or replaced by a carious surface, a thin slice of the bone must be removed, while if there be a primary focus in the neck of the scapula, the origin of the long head of the triceps must be separated subperiosteally, and still more bone removed.   It is in these cases that the posterior route recommended by Kocher is specially advantageous.

With regard to the soft parts, in order to obtain sufficient access for the removal of all the synovial membrane, it is important to lay open the capsule as widely as possible; hence the importance of carrying the incision along the line of the biceps tendon right up to the apex of the glenoid.   Transverse incisions into the capsule should be avoided, if possible, but any part of the ligament which is itself infiltrated with tubercle should be clipped away.   Fortunately the capsule is so redundant that the gap which is left in it can generally be closed with catgut sutures. Care must be taken to remove all diseased synovial membrane around the biceps tendon.   If the disease has invaded the bursa beneath the deltoid, the anterior part of this muscle should be divided close to the clavicle, so that, with the upper arm abducted (to relax the muscle), it may be everted as well as retracted.   If the bursa beneath the subscapularis be involved it also must be dissected away.

All suppurating pockets and sinuses must be carefully followed up, and, if possible, dissected out.   It is not uncommon to find a sinus extending down the upper arm from the bicipital groove.   To get at this, the original anterior incision must be prolonged downwards, and the upper part of the tendon of the pectoralis major may have to be detached from its insertion. Great care must be taken not to injure the circumflex nerve.

An abscess or sinus, the result of disease of the scapula, is generally found either in the axilla or in the region of the posterior border of the deltoid; it can be got at by prolonging downwards Kocher's posterior incision.

In the presence of sinuses and mixed infection, the wound should be only partially closed, plenty of room being left for the introduction of iodoform gauze. If necessary a drainage tube may be passed into the anterior wound and brought out through a button-hole opening opposite the posterior border of the deltoid. Even in the absence of infection, a rubber tube should be introduced from the lower part of the anterior incision down to, but not into, the sutured capsule.

In applying the dressing, a pad is placed in the axilla to prevent the upper end of the humerus being displaced inwards. The dressing is secured in position by a bandage which fixes the upper arm to the trunk, the forearm being lightly supported in a sling.

Cheyne and Burghard (*Manual of Surgical Treatment*, Part IV, p. 254) recommend the following after-treatment: 'As soon as the wound has healed, the arm may be fixed in proper position by a starch or water-glass bandage, and, after two weeks more, passive movement may be begun; the period at which this passive movement should be employed depends largely upon the amount of bone removed; if the whole of the upper end of the bone has been removed and the rotators divided, as was done in the old operation, the elbow should be supported and the arm fixed for four or five weeks, as otherwise a very lax joint is likely to result; if, on the other hand, the operation we have described is sufficient, passive movement should be begun after a fortnight. Special attention must be paid to preserving rotation, which is the movement most likely to be lost; abduction should also be carefully attended to. The axillary pad and the wrist-sling should be continued for six or eight weeks.'

CHAPTER VIII

OPERATIONS FOR TUBERCULOUS DI
AND ANKLE

OPERATIONS FOR TUBERCULOUS
TARSO-METATARSAL

THE disease is often secondary to a focus
metatarsal bones. Of the three synovial ca
tarso-metatarsal articulations, the inner is con
the first metatarsal and the internal (first) c
articulation between the fourth and fifth n
When the disease involves either of these syn
treatment will lie, according to the extent (
local excision and amputation of the involved
the adjacent tarsal bone.

To excise the joint between the base of tl
internal cuneiform, a semilunar flap is made to
extensor tendon, which is drawn aside. The
tibialis anticus (anterior) is either divided clos
separated subperiosteally. The base of the firs'
while the internal (first) cuneiform is either c
entirely, according to the extent of the dise
grasped with forceps and either wrenched or
of the peroneus longus.

The joint between the fourth and fifth me
excised in a similar manner to the above, but
flap directed outwards. The tendons of the p
are detached from their insertions, while that
by freeing it from the groove on the under sur
disease has commenced in the cuboid, the whol

COMPLETE ANTERIOR TA

When the disease involves the tarso-meta
regions more extensively, a complete anteri
performed. This operation, introduced by P
performed as follows: Two long dorso-later

200

inner extending from the middle of the first metatarsal bone to the neck of the astragalus (talus), the other from the middle of the fifth metatarsal to the outer aspect of the anterior process of the os calcis (calcaneus). These incisions should be carried down to the bone except in the case of the posterior extremity of the inner incision, which should be kept superficial so as to avoid opening either into the ankle or the astragalo-scaphoid (talo-navicular) joint.

After detaching the tibialis anticus (anterior) from its insertion, the extensor tendons, along with the vessels and nerves, are separated from

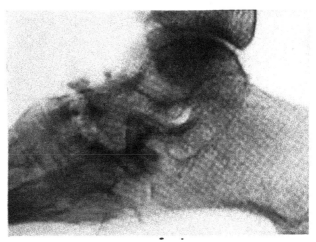

FIG. 87.   TUBERCULOUS DISEASE OF THE ANTERIOR TARSUS.   Skiagram taken before operation (anterior tarsectomy).   (*By Dr. E. Price.*)

within outwards from the ligamentous structures on the dorsum; the dorsalis pedis artery is divided close to where it passes through the first interosseous space.   Next, after freeing and retracting the upper border of the abductor hallucis muscle, the tendon of the tibialis posticus (posterior) is detached from its insertion into the tuberosity of the scaphoid (navicular), and the dissection is then continued as far into the sole of the foot as possible, care being taken to keep close to the bones.

The patient is now placed in the semi-prone position so as to give more comfortable access to the outer side of the foot.

The external incision passes down to the bones between the tendons of the peroneus brevis and tertius; it divides the outer attachment of the lower anterior annular (cruciate) ligament and some of the fleshy fibres of the extensor brevis digitorum. After detaching the insertion of the peroneus tertius from the base of the fifth metatarsal bone, the extensor tendons are separated from the outer side of the dorsum of the foot until the inner wound is reached; the separation is continued in an upward and downward direction until the bridge of soft tissues can be freely raised up from the bones. The soft structures are similarly separated from the plantar aspects of the bones, but before doing so the tendon of the peroneus brevis is detached from the prominent base of the fifth metatarsal and the tendon of the peroneus longus is freed from the groove on the under surface of the cuboid. The difficulty in separating the soft parts on the plantar aspect (due to the concavity formed by the transverse ridge of the skeleton of the foot) is to some extent diminished by snipping off the projecting base of the fifth metatarsal bone.

The remaining metatarsal bones are divided a little below their bases by a keyhole saw applied from the dorsum; the bridge of soft parts is meanwhile retracted well upwards. Posteriorly the saw is carried through either the scaphoid (navicular) and the cuboid bones, or further back through the head of the astragalus (talus) and the anterior process of the os calcis (calcaneus), according to the extent of the disease. Free drainage is provided for by passing through the tunnel one large or two smaller rubber tubes rolled up in a strip of iodoform gauze.

After-treatment. The chief point to attend to in the after-treatment is to keep the parts at rest with the foot maintained at a right angle. This is readily done by applying to the sole and lateral aspects of the limb a stirrup splint cut out of a sheet of aluminium.

By this operation the foot is of course considerably shortened, but if the tendons inserted into the metatarsal bones are separated as far as possible subperiosteally, the functional result is excellent.

OPERATIONS FOR TUBERCULOUS DISEASE OF THE OS CALCIS

Indications. A primary focus of tubercle is more frequently met with in the os calcis than in any other bone of the tarsus. It occurs quite frequently in young children and is not uncommon in adults. The lesion takes the form of a caseous deposit which may or may not contain a sequestrum. Occasionally the tuberculous mischief is more diffuse. The indications are to remove the focus before the surrounding soft parts, including the tendon sheaths, become infected, and especially before the disease involves the astragalo-calcanean joint. The situation and nature of the focus is best determined by skiagraphy.

Operation. *When the focus is small,* it may be treated by reflecting the soft parts, together with the periosteum, off the bone in the form of a flap. , The part of the cortex of the bone superficial to the focus is then chiselled away and the disease in the interior removed by gouging, which should extend well into the surrounding healthy bone. If the focus has given rise to local thickening at any part of the bone, the incision should be so planned as to expose that particular region. In dissecting a flap off the outer aspect of the bone the convexity of the incision should reach downwards well below the peroneal tendons, and these, along with the subjacent periosteum, should be dissected up along with the flap. In other cases a similar flap will have to be dissected up from the inner aspect of the heel, in which case care must be taken to avoid injuring the posterior tibial vessels and nerves or their plantar divisions.

When the disease is more diffuse, the best plan is to make a horseshoe incision a little above the borders of the heel opposite the insertion of the tendo Achillis.

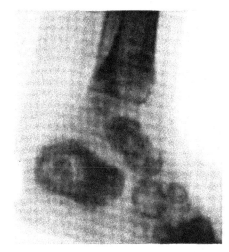

Fig. 88.   A Caseous Tuberculous Focus in the Os Calcis. Skiagram from a child aged two years. Note the sequestrum in the centre of the tuberculous focus. (*By Dr. E. Price.*)

Externally the incision may extend forwards as far as the base of the fifth metatarsal bone, while internally it should end a little behind the bifurcation of the posterior tibial vessels about a finger's breadth from the internal malleolus. In the adult, if the whole of the os calcis is to be removed, a second incision must be carried from the horizontal incision vertically upwards along the outer edge of the tendo Achillis for an inch or more. The details of the operation have been described by Mr. Burghard (p. 55). When the operation is being performed for tuberculous disease, however, it is important to remove the bone as far as possible subperiosteally.

In the child the operation is much simpler, so that the addition of a vertical incision is not necessary. In making the horizontal incision the knife is carried not merely through the periosteum, but also through the shell of cartilage which surrounds the cancellated tissue of the developing bone. The plantar portion of the cartilage is reflected off the osseous tissue along with the soft parts. By means of a gouge and sharp spoon the diseased focus, along with the whole of the surrounding cancellated bone, can readily be removed, leaving the cartilaginous shell intact. If desired, the cavity may be filled with Mosetig-Moorhof's iodoform-wax. The writer's experience, however, is that the new bone forms perfectly well if the cavity be allowed to fill simply with blood-clot.

A few catgut sutures are introduced posteriorly to unite the divided insertion of the tendo Achillis and the adjacent cartilage. No drainage is required unless a sinus exists, in which case the cavity should be stuffed with iodoform gauze. If the operation be performed before the articular cartilage has become infected, neither the calcaneo-astragaloid nor the calcaneo-cuboid joints are opened into. As the result of leaving the cartilage the bone is very largely re-formed.

After-treatment. The after-treatment consists in keeping the foot at right angles and avoiding pressure on the heel. In the adult this is best done by an anterior metal suspension splint, which is fixed to the limb above and below the wound by means of a plaster of Paris bandage. The splint is provided with hooks, to enable the limb to be suspended from a cradle. Though there is very little re-formation of bone in the adult the result is very satisfactory, especially if a pad be worn inside the heel of the boot.

OPERATIONS FOR TUBERCULOUS DISEASE OF THE ANKLE-JOINT

Operation. In tuberculous disease of the ankle-joint which has advanced in spite of rest and constitutional treatment, the writer almost invariably excises the joint by Kocher's method of dividing the anterior and external lateral ligaments of the ankle and then dislocating the foot inwards. A long J-shaped incision is made at the outer aspect of the ankle. The vertical limb of the incision extends well up behind the lower part of the fibula, while the curved portion, which reaches down to the peroneal tubercle, is carried up on to the dorsum, to end opposite the tendon of the peroneus tertius just external to the musculo-cutaneous (superficial peroneal) nerve. The external saphenous vein and nerve lie immediately below the incision.

The skin flap, along with the fascia and the periosteum covering the external malleolus, is dissected forwards off the peronei, the external malleolus, and the anterior ligament of the tibio-fibular articulation. Below and in front of the malleolus the flap is dissected off the origin of the extensor brevis digitorum, the outer attachments of the lower division of the anterior annular (cruciate) ligament, the broad anterior fasciculus of the external lateral ligament, and the outer part of the thin anterior ligament. It is through the latter structure that the disease in the joint is very liable to penetrate. The abscess which results is generally

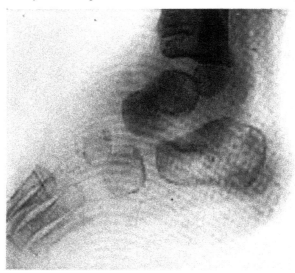

FIG. 89. A CASEOUS TUBERCULOUS FOCUS IN THE HEAD AND NECK OF THE ASTRAGALUS. This had given rise to secondary synovial disease of the ankle, the astragalo-calcanean and the astragalo-scaphoid joints. The skiagram was taken before operation from a child aged three and a half years. The astragalus was excised and the cartilages and synovial membrane of the adjacent joints removed. The foot was maintained in good position by a nail driven through the soft parts of the heel and the os calcis into the tibia. (*By Dr. E. Price.*)

covered by the flap, and is therefore easily dissected off its deep surface after it has been reflected.

The sheaths of the two peroneal tendons are next slit up, the tendons themselves are divided a little in front of the external malleolus, and the portions above are detached along with the periosteum from the groove behind the fibula.

The base of the flap, including the extensor tendons, is now retracted well forwards and inwards so as to allow of the detachment of the an-

terior ligament subperiosteally from the anterior border of the lower end
of the tibia as far inwards as the internal malleolus. The same ligament
is also detached from the neck of the astragalus (talus), but the astragalo-scaphoid (talo-navicular) joint is not opened into at this stage.

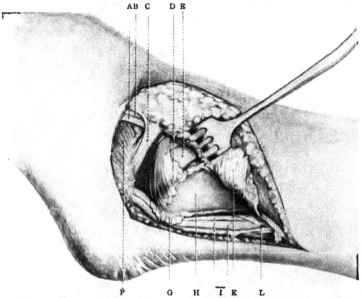

FIG. 90. EXCISION OF THE ANKLE BY KOCHER'S EXTERNAL J-SHAPED INCISION.
The flap, including the periosteum covering the external malleolus, has been
reflected forwards; the peroneal tendons with their sheath slit up are seen behind
the fibula; the body of the astragalus has been exposed by dividing the anterior
ligament immediately in front of the anterior fasciculus of the external lateral
ligament. The external tendons, the anterior annular ligament, and the origin of
the extensor digitorum brevis are exposed at the lowest part of the wound.
A, Peroneus tertius tendon; B, Extensor digitorum longus; c, Anterior annular
ligament; D, External lateral ligament; E, Astragalus; F, Extensor digitorum
brevis; G, External annular ligament; H, External malleolus; I, Peronei tendons;
K, Periosteum; L, Sheath of the peronei tendons.

The next step consists in dividing the bands of the external lateral
ligament by carrying the knife well upwards under cover of the external
malleolus. By wrenching the foot forcibly inwards, it can now be completely dislocated over the internal malleolus so that the sole looks
almost directly upwards. The upper surface of the astragalus (talus)
is thus thrust downwards and outwards into the wound, and a free

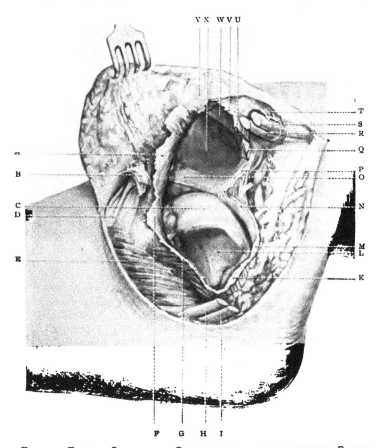

FIG. 91. FURTHER STAGE OF THE OPERATION SHOWN IN THE PREVIOUS FIGURE. The anterior, external, and posterior ligaments of the ankle have been divided, and the joint cavity fully exposed by forcible dislocation of the foot inwards. The peroneal tendons have been divided, also the outer attachment of the lower division of the anterior annular ligament. A, F, Anterior ligament of the ankle; B. Anterior annular ligament; C, Astragalus; D, Peroneus tertius; E, Extensor digitorum brevis; G, K, External lateral ligament of the ankle; H, Peroneus brevis; I. Peroneus longus; L, Astragalus; M, Q, Posterior fasciculus of the external lateral ligament; N, P, Posterior ligament of the ankle; O, Internal malleolus; R. S. Peronei tendons; T, External annular ligament; U, Middle fasciculus of the external lateral ligament; V, Anterior fasciculus of the external lateral ligament; W. External malleolus; X, Tibia; Y, Periosteum.

exposure of the joint is obtained. The internal lateral (deltoid) ligament is left intact as a hinge on which the foot rotates. It not infrequently happens, in forcibly dislocating the foot, that the periosteum, along with the internal lateral ligament, is either partly stripped from the internal malleolus or a portion of the latter is broken off; this is rather an advantage than otherwise, as it gives better exposure of the inner part of the joint cavity.

By detaching the posterior ligament, along with the transverse ligament, from the posterior border of the tibia, the foot can be so completely dislocated that every part of the joint cavity is brought well into view.

The next step in the operation consists in the removal of all the diseased synovial membrane, care being taken to clear out the recesses at the inner and posterior aspects of the joint. The thin posterior ligament of the ankle-joint had better be removed along with the synovial membrane; in doing this the deep flexor tendons and the posterior tibial vessels and nerve must not be injured. The internal lateral ligament may generally be left intact.

The stage is now reached when the operator decides as to whether it will be necessary to remove the whole of the astragalus. Some surgeons recommend its removal as a matter of routine whether it be diseased or not, the reason given being that unless the whole bone be excised, sufficient access is not obtained for the removal of the rest of the disease. This argument does not apply, however, if Kocher's dislocation method be adopted. If the astragalus itself be not diseased, the writer prefers simply to chisel off its articular surfaces. In doing this the raw surfaces left must be carefully shaped so that the remnant of the bone fits accurately into the tibio-fibular arch, which is also denuded of its cartilage. If, on the other hand, there be a primary focus in the astragalus, if it be the seat of extensive articular caries, or if the disease has invaded the astragalo-calcanean (talo-calcanean) joint, the whole bone must of course be removed. In looking for a primary focus in the astragalus the upper surface of its neck should be carefully examined, as it is in this situation that a small opening is not infrequently found leading into the joint.

To remove the astragalus the head should first be freed. This is done by dividing the outer attachment of the lower division of the anterior annular ligament and detaching the origin and posterior part of the extensor brevis digitorum. The peroneus tertius and extensor tendons are retracted well upwards and inwards. The posterior and outer part of the astragalo-scaphoid (talo-navicular) capsule is now exposed, and by dividing it in the coronal plane the head of the astragalus (talus) is

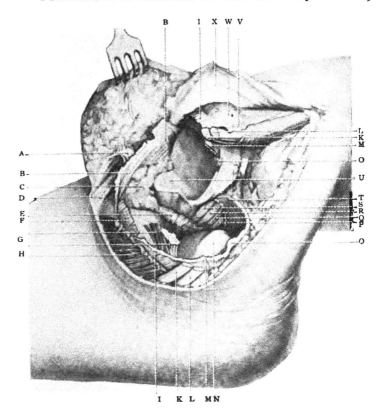

FIG. 92. FURTHER STAGE OF THE OPERATION SHOWN IN THE TWO PREVIOUS FIGURES. The astragalus has been removed, exposing the articular surfaces of the scaphoid and the os calcis. The internal lateral ligament has been partly detached subperiosteally from the internal malleolus; the posterior ligament of the ankle has been partly removed, exposing the deep flexor tendons along with the posterior tibial vessels and nerves. The extensor digitorum brevis has been divided at its origin from the os calcis. A, Anterior annular ligament; B, B, Anterior ligament of the ankle; C, Synovial membrane; D, Peroneus tertius; E, Internal lateral ligament; F, Astragalo-scaphoid ligament; G, Interosseous ligament; H, Extensor digitorum brevis; I, I, Anterior fasciculus of the external lateral ligament; K, K. Peroneus brevis; L, L, Peroneus longus; M, M, Middle fasciculus of the external lateral ligament; N, Os calcis; O, O, Posterior fasciculus of the external lateral ligament; P, Posterior tibial nerve; Q, Posterior tibial artery; R, Flexor digitorum longus; S, Tibialis posticus; T, Posterior ligament; U, Internal malleolus; V, External annular ligament; W, External malleolus; X, Periosteum.

laid bare. A sharp hook is then inserted into the astragalus, and while the bone is dragged upwards a knife is introduced beneath it so as to divide the strong interosseous ligament between it and the os calcis. To completely free the astragalus all that is needed is to detach it from the internal lateral (deltoid) ligament; to do this the foot is forcibly inverted so that a strong sharp hook may be inserted into the inner surface of the astragalus, which is dragged downwards and outwards, while the internal lateral ligament is divided close to the bone, or separated at its attachment with a strong sharp rugine. By keeping close to the bone the tendons at the inner ankle (especially the tibialis posticus) and the posterior tibial vessels and nerves escape injury.

Having removed the astragalus, the upper surface of the os calcis is freed from disease by removing the synovial membrane and chiselling away its articular surface. The synovial membrane of the astragalo-scaphoid joint is then examined; if it be found infected secondary to the focus in the astragalus, the whole of the astragalo-scaphoid capsule must be removed, and along with it the posterior articular surface of the scaphoid (navicular).

The removal of all disease having been effected, the next step is to see that the foot is accurately fitted into the tibio-fibular arch, and securely fixed there at a right angle, with no tendency either to inversion or eversion. The ultimate functional, as well as cosmetic, result depends largely on the care with which this part of the operation is carried out.

Reference has already been made to the careful shaping of the astragalus in removing its articular surfaces. When this bone has been completely removed it is generally necessary to reduce the breadth of the os calcis by chiselling off the sustentaculum tali. If this precaution be not taken permanent deformity results; the foot becomes displaced outwards and the internal malleolus projects unduly.

The articular surface on the upper aspect of the os calcis must be removed so as to leave a horizontal surface; this is attained by making the slice slightly wedge-shaped, the base of the wedge being directed posteriorly. If this point be not attended to, when the bones are brought into apposition it will be found that the foot is too much flexed towards the dorsum. Again, when the astragalus has been removed, the external malleolus must be shortened somewhat, and it is an advantage to gouge away part of the outer surface of the os calcis so as to leave a slightly hollowed out raw surface to receive it.

To keep the bones accurately and firmly in position during the healing of the wound the writer is in the habit of using a long, square, plated nail, which is driven through the skin of the heel, the os calcis (cal-caneus), and the remains of the astragalus (if not completely removed) up into the tibia for a couple of inches or so. Great care must be taken to see that the assistant holds the foot in the best possible position while the nail is being driven in.

Before closing the wound the divided peroneal tendons are sutured and replaced behind the external malleolus, and if possible secured there by stitching any remains of the sheath and deep fascia over them with buried catgut sutures. If the peroneal sheaths have become secondarily

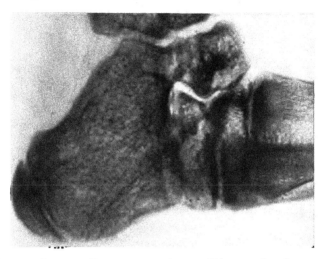

Fig. 93. RESULT OF EXCISION OF THE ANKLE. Skiagram taken six years after an operation performed when the child was nine years of age. The astragalus was not completely removed. There is no inversion or eversion, and no lateral displacement of the foot; the internal malleolus is a little more prominent than the external. The foot is shorter and narrower than its fellow. There is only very slight movement at the ankle itself, but this is partly compensated for by exaggerated movement at the mid- and posterior tarsal joints. The limb is ¾ inch shorter than its fellow. (*By Dr. E. Price.*)

infected they must of course be carefully dissected away. The same applies to the sheaths of the flexor tendons at the inner ankle.

Abscess formation in the region of the external malleolus has already been referred to. An abscess in the region of the internal malleolus does not, as a rule, call for a separate incision at the inner side of the ankle. After the bones have been dealt with, what remains of the abscess can readily be dissected away from within at the close of the operation.

If desirable, drainage may be provided for by passing a tube across the front of the ankle beneath the extensor tendon and bringing it out through a button-hole opening just in front of the internal malleolus. Drainage, however, is seldom necessary unless the disease has reached the stage of sinus formation.

After-treatment. The after-treatment is greatly facilitated by the use of the nail, which is kept in for three weeks or so. The patient is quite unconscious of its presence, and as it gradually becomes somewhat loosened, its removal is unattended with pain. The limb is placed in any convenient form of posterior splint which possesses a foot-piece. The wound is dressed in a fortnight to take out the stitches, and a week or two later the nail is removed and a plaster of Paris case applied.

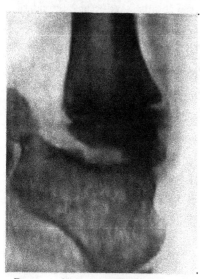

FIG. 94.   RESULT OF EXCISION OF THE ANKLE AND ASTRAGALUS. Skiagram taken nine years after an operation performed when the child was two years old. There is no inversion or eversion, and no lateral displacement of the foot; there is movement at the ankle in the direction of dorsiflexion to the extent of 15°. (*By Dr. E. Price.*)

Results. Of the sixteen excisions of the ankle performed by the writer in the last ten years, eleven have been traced. Three of these died of general tuberculosis. In the remainder there is no return of the disease and the wounds are all soundly healed. The functional result is good in all but one case in which both ankles were excised. In this patient both feet are displaced outwards and considerable discomfort exists from pressure on the prominent internal malleolus. In two others there is slight outward displacement of the foot, which, however, gives rise to no inconvenience. The remainder are able to walk well without irons or lateral supports of any kind. Two indulge freely in football. Osseous ankylosis is present in one case, and this is compensated for by the increased mobility of the anterior and mid-tarsal joints. In the remainder there is slight flexion and extension at the ankle. In one the peroneal tendons are displaced in front of the external malleolus.

The disease was purely synovial in half the cases; in the other half, with the exception of two, the primary disease was in the astragalus. An abscess or fistula was present in one-third of the cases. The average duration of stay in hospital before dismissal with the limb in plaster of Paris was four weeks.

MIKULICZ'S OSTEOPLASTIC RESECTION OF THE FOOT

This operation is indicated in tuberculous disease of the posterior tarsus when the soft parts above the heel are so involved that disarticulation at the ankle is out of the question. The procedure consists in the removal of the soft parts of the heel together with the astragalus and os calcis, and the approximation (after sawing off the articular surfaces) of the scaphoid and cuboid to the tibia and fibula, the foot being maintained in the extreme equinus position so that the patient walks on the heads of the metatarsal bones with the toes hyperextended.

With the patient placed in the lateral or prone position, a transverse incision is made across the sole from the tuberosity of the scaphoid to a little behind the base of the fifth metatarsal bone. A second transverse incision is made behind the ankle between the centre of the bases of the malleoli. The extremities of these incisions are joined by two oblique incisions placed one on each side of the ankle. All four incisions extend down to the bone. The foot is forcibly dorsiflexed and the ankle-joint is opened from behind. With the foot still further flexed towards the leg, the ligaments of the joint are divided and the soft parts are dissected off the astragalus until the scaphoid and cuboid are reached. If the ankle-joint itself be free from disease, the dorsal bridge of soft parts should be separated as far as possible subperiosteally, while if the ankle-joint be diseased the anterior ligaments should be removed, care being taken not to wound the dorsalis pedis artery, which, through its anastomosis with the external plantar, is the main source of blood-supply to the remainder of the foot. If the mid-tarsal joint be diseased, the scaphoid and cuboid should be sawn across without opening into it, or, if necessary, the section should be made further forwards through the cuneiform bones and the cuboid; if, on the other hand, the mid-tarsal joint be healthy, the astragalus and os calcis may be removed before the articular surfaces of the scaphoid and cuboid are sawn off. The articular surfaces of the tibia and fibula are next sawn off horizontally, and, after ligaturing the vessels, the remainder of the foot is brought into a line with the leg and maintained in this position by wiring the bones. If the tarsal bones have been sawn vertically and the tibia and fibula horizontally, as they should be, the metatarsals will be in the same straight line as the leg.

The divided ends of the posterior tibial nerve should be sutured if possible, but if this cannot be done no great harm results, as the intrinsic muscles of the foot are of very little use after this operation. Rose dissects the nerve out beforehand and takes care to leave it intact (Cheyne and Burghard, *A Manual of Surgical Treatment,* vol. iv, p. 248).

When the wound is sutured, the soft tissues on the dorsum form a redundant fold opposite what was the centre of the lateral incision: this redundancy, however, gradually disappears. Drainage is seldom necessary, but if desirable a tube, or strip of iodoform gauze, may be passed across the limb beneath the redundant bridge of soft tissues.

A strip of strong aluminium, or malleable iron, should be applied to the posterior aspect of the limb and bent forwards at a right angle opposite the metatarso-phalangeal joints so as to keep the phalanges hyperextended. As soon as the wound is healed a plaster of Paris case is applied.

The disadvantages of this operation are (1) that should osseous ankylosis not occur, the functional result is very unsatisfactory; (2) it is often a long time before the patient is able to bear his weight on the limb; (3) the special boot which is required is difficult to make; (4) the limb is lengthened, consequently the sole of the opposite boot must be thickened.

The above operation may be converted into a *complete tarsectomy* by making the transverse incision across the sole a little further forwards, and by dissecting the tarsal bones off the tissues on the dorsum as far as the bases of the metatarsal bones, which are then sawn across.

CHAPTER IX

OPERATIONS FOR TUBERCULOUS DISEASE OF THE KNEE-JOINT

In all cases where a doubt exists as to whether conservative treatment should be tried in the first instance, a skiagram should be taken. If a bone focus be revealed, operation should be performed without delay. If, on the other hand, there be no bone disease, conservative treatment may be tried in the early stages of the disease, but should no improvement occur within three months operation should be resorted to; this applies especially to young children, as the disease generally runs a more rapid course in them than in adolescents and adults.

OPERATIONS FOR TUBERCULOUS DISEASE OF THE SYNOVIAL MEMBRANE

When the disease in the synovial membrane is primary, and forms a localized focus which has not yet perforated into the joint, excellent results are obtained by arthrotomy and removal of the affected area of synovial membrane. If the focus be limited, the joint may be opened by a longitudinal incision on one or other side of the patella, according to the seat of disease, or if preferred, the incision may be more or less curved so as to enable a flap to be dissected back. When the disease is less accessible, or affects a larger area, the joint should be more freely opened, either by dividing the patellar ligament by the lower curved incision of Textor, or by detaching the tubercle of the tibia and everting the quadriceps apparatus by means of Kocher's external J-shaped incision.

The diseased synovial membrane may either be clipped away after dissecting the divided capsule from its outer aspect, or the joint may be freely opened into first, and the diseased membrane then dissected off the capsule. In either case care should be taken not to cut into the tuberculous tissue.

When the disease occupies the suprapatellar pouch, a curved incision, with its convexity upwards, is made above the patella. The lower part of the quadriceps, along with the skin, is reflected downwards off the synovial pouch, and the latter is then dissected off the supratrochlear portion of the femur. Before closing the wound the quadriceps is united with buried catgut sutures. Passive movement is begun in about three weeks, and a fortnight later the patient is allowed to begin to use the limb.

In diffuse tuberculous disease of the synovial membrane when the disease is aggravated, and especially when it has extended to the periarticular structures, an H-shaped incision may be employed with advantage. Cheyne and Burghard recommend this as the best routine incision for arthrectomy. ' The vertical incisions should reach from the upper limit of the suprapatellar pouch well on to the anterior surface of the tibia, and should be from 1 inch to 1½ inches away from the edges of the patella. These are deepened until the tendon of the quadriceps extensor is exposed. Division of this displays the fibrous capsule of the joint covered by fat and loose cellular tissue ' (*Manual of Surgical Treatment.* Part IV, p. 209). The transverse incision which unites the vertical incisions crosses the centre of the patella.

In cases of average severity the writer prefers the external J-shaped incision of Kocher. The advantage of this procedure is that, in addition to giving sufficient access to the disease, it preserves the quadriceps apparatus intact. The operation is performed as follows:—

Incision. The incision, which is external and somewhat J-shaped, begins 3 to 4 inches above the upper border of the tibia, extends vertically downwards about a finger's breadth external to the patella, crosses the outer tuberosity of the tibia, and then curves inwards about 1 inch below the tubercle of the tibia to end a little to the inner side of the crest. The integuments and the fascia lata having been divided, the fleshy fibres of the vastus externus (lateralis) are exposed in the upper part of the wound, while below is its aponeurotic tendon, which forms that part of the capsular ligament of the joint known as the external lateral patellar ligament. These structures, along with the subjacent synovial membrane, are divided along the whole length of the wound, and the outer aspect of the joint is thus freely opened into (external arthrotomy of the knee).

Free exposure of the interior of the joint. The outer border of the patellar ligament is defined and followed to its insertion into the lower part of the tubercle of the tibia, below which the periosteum is divided downwards and inwards for a short distance. The insertion of the patellar ligament is now detached along with the tubercle of the tibia and the periosteum immediately below it, care being taken to retain the attachment of the latter to the bone lower down. In the adult the tuberosity is detached with the chisel, while in the child the knife alone suffices, as the tuberosity is cartilaginous. The interior of the joint is freely exposed to view by dislocating the whole of the lower part of the quadriceps apparatus over to the outer side of the knee, and at the same time turning it inside out, so that the cartilaginous surface of the patella becomes directed upwards. Before this can be accomplished, however, it is necessary to open the joint more freely from the front by hooking the patellar ligament forwards and outwards, and then separating the capsule and thick infrapatellar pad of fat from the anterior edge of the upper end of the tibia. If there be no strong intra-articular adhesions, and especially if the cavity of the joint contains a quantity of tuberculous

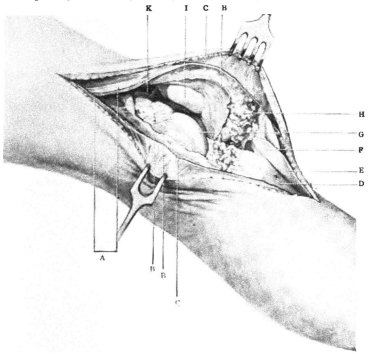

FIG. 95. THE ARTHROTOMY STAGE OF EXCISION OF THE KNEE BY KOCHER'S EXTERNAL, SLIGHTLY J-SHAPED INCISION. The joint has been opened by dividing the lower fibres of the vastus externus, the capsule, and the synovial membrane. The outer part of the infrapatellar pad of fat has been divided; below it is seen the cartilaginous tubercle of the tibia and the adjacent periosteum partly detached from the anterior surface of the tibia. A, Vastus externus; B, B, B, Synovial membrane; c, c, Capsule; D, Tibia; E, Periosteum; F, Tubercle of the tibia; G, External condyle; H, Infrapatellar pad; I, Patella; K, Suprapatellar pouch.

débris, the quadriceps flap can be dislocated without difficulty. To enable the interior of the joint to be still more freely exposed, the crucial ligaments are now divided, and, if necessary, the lateral ligaments may be more or less completely detached subperiosteally from the femoral condyles.

Before proceeding further, the interior of the joint is carefully examined and the extent of the disease ascertained. When, as is generally the case, the synovial membrane is diseased throughout, the crucial ligaments must be removed, otherwise sufficient access cannot be got for the removal of the synovial membrane lining the pouches behind the condyles.

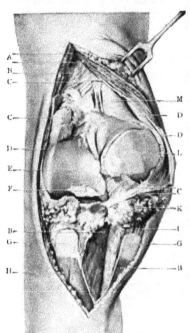

FIG. 96. FURTHER STAGE OF EXCISION OF THE KNEE BY KOCHER'S INCISION. The infrapatellar pad of fat, the synovial membrane covering its upper surfaces, the tubercle and adjacent periosteum have been more completely separated from the tibia so as to allow the lower part of the quadriceps, the patella, and the patellar ligament to be completely everted and displaced over to the inner side of the knee. The synovial membrane is well seen, as is also that lining the suprapatellar pouch. A, Vastus externus; B, B, B, Periosteum; C, C, C, Synovial membrane; D, D, D, Capsule; E, Femur; F, Ligamentum mucosum; G, G, Tubercle; H, Tibia; I, Patellar ligament; K, Infrapatellar pad; L, Patella; M, Rectus tendon.

Removal of the synovial membrane. This should be done by toothed forceps and knife dissection, aided by scissors curved on the flat. When the right knee is being operated on, the dissection is most conveniently effected from below upwards. The whole of the infrapatellar pad of fat and the synovial membrane covering its upper surface is first removed, then that lining the deep surface on the quadriceps on either side of and above the patella, including the anterior wall of the subcrureus bursa. When the summit of the pouch has been reached, its posterior wall, along with the subsynovial fat—often considerably thickened from chronic œdema—is dissected cleanly off the supratrochlear portion of the femur. The synovial membrane covering the lateral aspects of the condyles is more closely adherent to the bone. Care must be taken to see that all the membrane is removed from the inner side of the joint, where it is reflected from the internal condyle on to the adjacent portion of the capsule.

With the knee fully flexed and the assistant supporting the leg vertically, and at the same time drawing the upper end of the tibia forwards, the operator now detaches the semilunar cartilages from the upper surface of the tibia and dissects the crucial ligaments cleanly away from the intercondyloid notch; or, if preferred, he may simply clear the intercondyloid notch and leave the semilunar cartilages to be removed at the same time that the articular cartilage is sawn off the tibia.

The sawing of the bones. With regard to the articular surfaces of the bones, they may either be sawn off so as to leave two flat surfaces, or the operator may follow the advice of Kocher and saw the tibia so as to leave a concave surface, while the femur is sawn so as to leave a correspondingly convex surface. If the former plan be adopted, an ordinary amputation saw with a movable back will suffice. The latter method, which requires some little practice, necessitates the use of a bow saw so made that its blade, which should be narrow, may be fixed at any angle. In primary synovial disease only a thin slice should be removed from the tibia. The saw should be kept in a plane exactly parallel to the articular surface, and caution should be exercised when the posterior edge of the bone is approached.

In sawing the femur it must be remembered that the shaft of the femur does not occupy the axis of the thigh. The upper end is thrust outwards by its head and neck, but owing to the greater length of the internal condyle as compared with the external, the lower surfaces of both lie in the same horizontal plane when the patient stands erect. It follows, therefore, that the femur must be sawn in a plane at right angles to the axis of the limb and not to that of the femur, or, what comes to the same thing, in a plane parallel to the under surface of the condyles. Unless this rule be kept in mind, the inexperienced operator is liable to remove too much bone from the internal condyle, with the result that when the tibia is brought into position it is found to be misdirected inwards. Another error which is even more liable to be committed is the removal of too much bone from the front and too little from the back of the condyles, the result being that when the bones are brought into apposition the leg is tilted forwards so as to produce an angular genu recurvatum. It is not a bad fault, however, to err a little in the opposite direction and direct the saw a trifle upwards as well as backwards, so as to produce a few degrees of flexion, the cosmetic as well as the functional result of which is rather better than that produced by an absolutely straight limb.

When there is no osseous disease of the femur, there is no necessity to remove more than the lower third of the condyles, so that, laterally, the section should fall below the level of the attachment of the lateral ligaments. When, as in this operation, the patella is left, it is well to

saw off its articular surfaces. A corresponding flat surface is fashioned
for it on the femur by sawing off the remains of the prominent external
condylar portion of the trochlear surface of the femur.

The next step is the removal of the remains of the synovial membrane
from the back part of the joint, namely, that which covers the posterior
ligament as well as that which lines the pouches behind the remains of
the condyle. While this is being done, the knee should be flexed, and the
tibia and femur should be drawn as widely apart as possible so as to
stretch out the posterior ligament. Much assistance will be got by dragging the lower end of the femur upwards and backwards with a strong
double hook placed in what remains of the intercondyloid notch. The posterior ligament is freed from synovial membrane by means of scissors
curved on the flat. The azygos artery, which generally spurts, is secured
with forceps and ligatured. Unless the ligament itself is infiltrated with
tubercle, it should not be removed, as it not only protects the popliteal
artery from injury, but forms a barrier against tuberculous infection of
the popliteal space. Any tuberculous membrane about the sheath of the
tendon of the popliteus muscle should be followed up and removed.
Finally, a careful search should be made for a sinus leading through the
posterior ligament into an abscess in the popliteal space, or into the semi-
membranosus bursa. If necessary, a counter-opening should be made
posteriorly by cutting down on the blades of dressing forceps projected
backwards under the skin from the main wound so as to avoid the vessels.

Arrest of hæmorrhage and drainage. These may be with advantage
considered under the same heading. In the absence of sinuses and mixed
infection there is no necessity for drainage, provided (1) that no antiseptic solution be used to wash out the wound, and (2) that the bleeding
be carefully arrested before closing the wound. The best way to prevent
after-bleeding is not only to see that all the bleeding points are carefully
ligatured, but also to avoid using a tourniquet. It is far better that whatever bleeding occurs should take place during, and not after, the operation. The vessels forming the anastomosis about the knee are comparatively small, so that, with a good assistant, there should be no loss of
blood worth speaking about. In ligaturing some of the vessels, especially
those lying in or close to the periosteum, the catgut may have to be
carried under the vessel by means of a curved needle, otherwise the ligature will slip. Troublesome oozing may be arrested by the pressure of
gauze wrung out of hot saline solution. The great advantage of being
able to dispense with drainage is that the original dressing, always the
most secure, need not be changed for three weeks or even longer.

Fixation of the bones. Considerable difference of opinion exists as
to whether any step should be taken to secure firm approximation of the

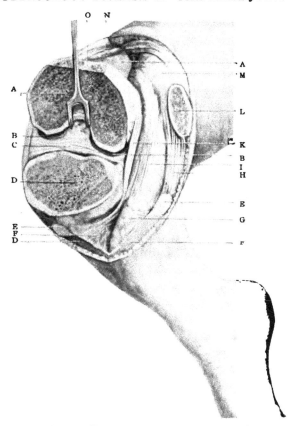

FIG. 97. LATER STAGE OF EXCISION OF THE KNEE BY KOCHER'S INCISION. The whole of the synovial membrane has been removed, with the exception of that lining the pouches behind the condyles. The articular surfaces have been sawn off the patella, the tibia, and the femur, and the upper part of the trochlear surface of the latter has been removed so as to leave a flat raw surface for the patella. Above the condyles the periosteum is seen covering the lower part of the shaft of the femur; between the patellar ligament and the internal lateral ligament appears that part of the capsule which forms the internal lateral patellar ligament; the floor of the wound between the femur and the tibia is occupied by the posterior ligament of the knee-joint, from which the synovial membrane has been removed. A, A, Femur; B, B, Synovial pouch; C, Posterior ligament; D, D, Tibia; E. E. Tubercle of the tibia; F, F, Periosteum; G, Infrapatellar pad; H, Patellar ligament; I, Internal lateral patellar ligament; K, Internal lateral ligament; L, Patella; M, Tendon of the rectus; N, Periosteum; O, Sawn trochlear surface of femur.

sawn surfaces beyond that afforded by careful external splinting.   O
the various artificial means which have been adopted to give additiona
fixation the best is undoubtedly by means of two long square nails, eac
driven from the tibia obliquely upwards into the femur.   While it cannc
be said that the introduction of the nails is essential, especially whe
the capsule, the lateral ligaments, and the quadriceps apparatus hav
been preserved practically intact, it must be admitted, on the other hand
that in cases in which the patella has been removed, and both latera
ligaments divided, the nails are a distinct advantage.   If properly intr
duced they certainly do no harm,—indeed, the patient is quite unconsciou
of their presence.   Not only do the nails ensure osseous union, but the
also render the after-treatment much easier.   The firm fixation afforde
by the nails does away with any necessity for complicated splints, an
plaster of Paris need not be employed until after the wound is soundl
healed.   For these reasons the writer makes frequent use of the nail
after excision in the adult, even by Kocher's method.   While introducin
them the surgeon should satisfy himself that the assistant is holding th
bones accurately and firmly in position.   After the quadriceps flap ha
been replaced, but not yet sutured, each nail is pushed through the ski
immediately below the tuberosity of the tibia and then driven obliquel
upwards into the opposite femoral condyle.   Care must be taken tha
the nails are kept sufficiently parallel to the bones to prevent their point
from penetrating into the popliteal surface of the femur.   In some case
the bones are found to have been so firmly united by the one nail that th
introduction of a second is unnecessary.   The nail should be of suc
a length that by the time it is passed well into the femur only about ½
inch is left projecting outside the skin: the advantage of this is that th
head of the nail may be covered by the dressing.

Closure of the wound.   Before closing the skin wound the tubercle o
the tibia is sutured into position with catgut (wire is seldom necessary
and interrupted sutures of the same material are used to close the incisio
in the vastus externus (lateralis) and subjacent capsule.   The skin woun
is united with silkworm-gut, in preference to silk and catgut, as it can
left in for a longer time without fear of setting up stitch suppuration
It is better not to use intermediate horsehair sutures, as it is well to en
courage the blood-stained serum to escape between the silkworm-gu
sutures.

An abundant sterilized gauze dressing should extend well above an
below the wound.   Plenty of wool, sterilized or sublimated, should
applied outside the gauze, taking in also the foot, and the whole is fix
in position with a domett bandage applied with some degree of firmness

The splint the writer prefers is the one used by Macewen after hi operation for knock-knee. This is practically a Liston's long splint, with the addition of a posterior support extending from just below the fold of the buttock to a little beyond the foot. An oval opening is cut out opposite the heel, and another opposite the external malleolus. The splint is well padded, and fixed to the limb with a roller bandage and to the chest with a binder. A figure-of-eight bandage should be placed separately round the foot, to keep it at a right angle. The posterior part of the splint, besides giving good support to the knee, prevents rocking and rotation outwards. It is an advantage to keep the hip quiet, at any rate until the wound is healed. As a rule the dressing need not be disturbed until the end of the third or fourth week, when the stitches and nails may be removed. A plaster of Paris case is substituted for the splint, and the patient is allowed to get about by the aid of crutches and a patten. This first plaster case should include the pelvis. Two or three months later the plaster should be renewed, but without including the hip. As a rule it is not advisable to allow the patient to bear weight on the limb without some support until six months have elapsed from the date of operation.

OPERATIONS FOR TUBERCULOUS DISEASE OF THE KNEE-JOINT SECONDARY TO A FOCUS IN ONE OF THE BONES

Unless the disease is so extensive that amputation is called for, the operation is practically the same as that above described, with the addition of one or two steps directed towards the removal of the disease in the bone. Small foci, whether situated in one of the condyles or tuberosities, are dealt with by thorough curetting, either before or after the articular surface of the affected bone has been removed. A sharp spoon generally suffices for the purpose, but if the adjacent bone be sclerosed, or if the focus invades the cortex, a gouge and hammer will be required. If the focus be larger and deeper, or if a sequestrum of considerable size be present, the affected condyle or tuberosity may be sawn through beyond the seat of the disease at a deeper level than its fellow. The opposite bone is dealt with in a similar, but converse, manner. The result of this manoeuvre is to produce two Z-shaped sawn surfaces, which must be so fashioned that when the limb is brought into good position they dovetail accurately, the one into the other. In other cases, instead of sawing the bones in the above zigzag fashion, an oblique section is made from before backwards or from side to side according to the position of the focus. The slice of bone removed is thus wedge-shaped, with the disease towards the base of the wedge. The extremity of the opposing bone is also sawn obliquely, and care must be taken that the surface which is left is in a plane exactly parallel to the first, otherwise when the tibia is brought into apposition with the femur it will be found to be misdirected. When it has been necessary to saw the bones obliquely they should be nailed into position to prevent the risk of a gliding movement between the two surfaces; one nail is sufficient.

In cases in which the whole epiphysis is destroyed, or in which a focus in the end of the diaphysis, either of the femur or of the tibia, has been allowed to run its course until first the adjacent epiphysis and then the joint has become involved, amputation will be called for. Such an unfortunate state of affairs is unlikely to occur in the case of the lower end of the femur, but the writer has met with it in neglected cases of tuberculous disease at the upper end of the diaphysis of the tibia.

OPERATIONS FOR PRIMARY TUBERCULOUS DISEASE OF THE PATELLA

This condition is probably not so rare as is generally supposed. The operator occasionally discovers it accidentally while excising a tuberculous knee. It is a good rule, therefore, always to saw off the cartilages of the patella in performing this operation. If a diseased focus be revealed, the whole bone had better be removed, but the periosteum and rectus tendon should be preserved if possible. This is easily done if Kocher's excision be performed. After everting the quadriceps flap, all that is necessary is to divide the periosteum around the margin of the patella, and then to peel the bone off the periosteum covering its anterior surface.

Cheyne and Burghard (*Manual of Surgical Treatment*, Part IV, p. 215) recommend the removal of the patella in most cases when excising the knee for tuberculous disease. After dissecting up a horseshoe-shaped flap from the front of the joint and directing the assistant to hold it well up out of the way, ' a vertical median incision is made through the quadriceps from the top of the suprapatellar pouch down to the tubercle of the tibia. This incision is very carefully deepened above until the muscular fibres are cut through, when the handle of the knife can be sunk between the muscle and the capsule and the two structures separated from one another. The periosteum over the patella is then turned off to either side with a raspatory, and the ligamentum patellæ is split longitudinally.'

When it is obvious, before operation, that the joint-disease is secondary to a focus in the patella, the technique of the operation is so planned as to include removal of this bone at an early stage of the operation. It is in cases of this kind that the method of excision of the knee recommended some years ago by A. G. Miller (*Transactions of the Edinburgh Medico-Chirurgical Society*, vol. xii, p. 16), and performed by him practically as a matter of routine, is particularly advantageous. The following is Mr. Miller's description of the operation:—

' 1. Incision from behind and above one condyle of femur to corresponding point of opposite side, brought down to near tubercle of tibia with a well-rounded sweep. Second cut straight across about middle of patella.

' 2. Flap of skin from upper incision (that across patella) reflected up till muscular fibres of vasti are seen. These carefully cut through. Tendon of rectus cut very carefully as it lies embedded in the thickened synovial membrane. Then muscles and tendon raised with handle of knife and fingers till upper border of thickened synovial membrane defined. Diseased mass of synovial membrane then dissected downwards off femur, mainly with handle of knife and fingers, till attachment at articular surface of femur is reached and cut through. Lateral attachments cut. Last of all, attachment to tibia and ligamentum patellæ cut through, and thus anterior portion of diseased synovial membrane removed *en masse,* with patella in centre and elliptical portion of skin attached.

' 3. All remaining visible synovial membrane scraped away in detail from lateral ligaments and anterior crucial ligament,—joint being flexed for this purpose. Semilunar cartilages removed, and joint made clean so far. Then lateral and anterior crucial ligaments cut, and the posterior ligaments scraped and cleaned thoroughly. All ligaments scraped when *in situ* and tense, or cut away.

' 4. Enough of bone removed from femur and tibia to thoroughly open the cancellated tissue to inspection, and all osseous tubercular foci dealt with.

' 5. After approximation of bones, tendon of quadriceps may be stitched to remains of ligamentum patellæ, and then skin flap brought down and stitched. Drainage provided from posterior ends of incision.'

In primary tuberculous disease of the patella without involvement of the knee-joint, J. B. Murphy (*Surg. Gyn. and Obstet.,* March, 1908) operates as follows:—

'(*a*) Preliminary preparation of the joint, which consists of producing a chemical inflammation in the joint by injecting 2 to 6 drams of 2 to 5% solution of formalin in glycerine (which is prepared twenty-four hours before needed), a week or ten days before the operation. We induce this chemical inflammation preparatory to all arthrotomies for patellar fractures, movable cartilages, &c. By the preparatory treatment of the joint, a local immunity is developed, through the infiltration of the tissues and the occlusion of all the lymph-spaces, induced by the chemical inflammatory reaction. Trauma, in the way of dissection or handling in these joints, will not produce a large quantity of effusion, as it does in non-immunized joints. They offer a much greater resistance against infection.

'(*b*) Open the knee-joint by a 7-inch incision in the outer side of the patella.

'(c) Make a subaponeurotic excision of the patella, leaving ends of quadriceps tendon and ligamentum patellæ exposed.

'(d) Prepare the flap, for the extension of the quadriceps tendon downward, by splitting the quadriceps tendon and vastus externus muscle from point H to point E, dividing the vastus externus transversely to F, and splitting it back to I; then turn the flap downward, with its fascial side to the joint, and approximate point H of the flap to C of ligamentum patellæ, and point F of flap to B of ligamentum patellæ. It may be united end to end, or may overlap the patellar ligament. The fascia and its fat should be turned toward the joint. This flap is used as a substitute for the patella, and is an extension of quadriceps tendon. The suture is done with kangaroo tendon, silk, or chromicized gut, or it may be accomplished with a figure-of-eight silkworm-gut suture, supporting the outer loop with a gauze pad, so that it does not cut into the skin. This is probably the most desirable, as well as the strongest, method of suture.

'(e) Suture the aponeurosis of patella securely to the divided edge of the deep fascia, and continue until the quadriceps tendon and muscle are entirely embedded. Close the rent left in the vastus externus by buried catgut sutures.

'(f) Insert a superficial drain from the joint surface to the lower angle of the wound.

'(g) Dress in a straight posterior splint.'

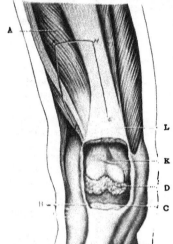

Fig. 98. Excision of the Patella. Anterior view of the joint with the patella excised. A, Quadriceps; B, Capsule; C, Ligamentum patellæ; D, Infrapatellar pad; E H F I, Flap from the quadriceps; K, Supratrochlear surface of the femur; L, Quadriceps tendon. (*After Murphy.*)

Results. As far as the certainty of curing the disease goes, excision gives better results in the knee than in any other joint, but unfortunately at the expense of loss of mobility. The preservation of the other functions, namely, stability and weight-bearing capacity, can practically be guaranteed. In diffuse tuberculous disease of the knee-joint, the writer has practically given up all operative procedures which do not aim at producing osseous anklyosis. Simple arthrectomy, better termed synovectomy, either alone or combined with division of the crucial and lateral ligaments, rarely gives satisfactory results. If the crucial and lateral ligaments be not divided, there is a great risk of recurrence due to incomplete removal of the disease at the posterior aspect of the joint, especially from the pouches behind the condyle; and if the patient escapes recurrence he is generally left with a more or less stiff and bent knee. If, on the other hand, the crucial and lateral ligaments be divided, an unstable

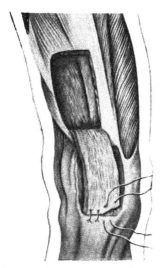
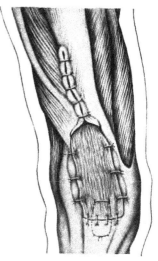

Fig. 99.   Excision of the Patella. Extension flap placed in position. (*After Murphy.*)

Fig. 100.   Excision of the Patella. Shows the line of suture for the flap and closure of the rent in the quadriceps muscle.   (*After Murphy.*)

knee generally results; hence the rule should be to remove enough of the articular surface to make sure of osseous ankylosis.

It is often stated that excision of the knee is contra-indicated in young children on account of the shortening which results. In primary synovial disease, however, there is no necessity to interfere with the epiphyseal cartilages. The following table prepared by Dr. W. L. Robertson, formerly House Surgeon at the Royal Edinburgh Hospital for Sick Children, gives the after measurements of as many of the writer's old cases of excision of the knee in children as could be traced. If we include the three cases in which cuneiform osteotomy was performed for bending subsequent to excision, the average amount of shortening was

1½ inches, of which the femur accounted ·
inch. Nearly all authors in referring to st
knee seem to agree that an amount which
easily compensated for that it is of little pr
noted that in four cases there was no sho
these the excision was performed during
the limbs were measured four years afte
nearly three years after. In compensatin
shortening the sole of the opposite boot n
extent of about ½ inch, the remainder bei
acted by slight drooping of the pelvis and s
both limbs be the same length, the patient
losed limb outwards in order to clear
ankylosed limb be allowed to be 1 inch sh
tient can advance the limb much more com
plished by heightening the sole of the boot
varying from ½ to 1 inch.

Age at Operation.	Age at Measurement.	Shortening.
1⁹⁄₁₂	8½	2½″ (after cun. resection)
2	9	¾″
2⁹⁄₁₂	8	0″
2¹¹⁄₁₂	6	0″
3	9	½″
4	11	2″
4¹⁰⁄₁₂	13	1½″
4¹⁰⁄₁₂	12	0″
4¹⁰⁄₁₂	12	1½″
5½₁₂	14	1¾″
5⁷⁄₁₂	15	0″

0–2

3–5

9–11 I I I I I

A more important bad result of excisio
is bending at or close to the seat of opera
gives rise to serious deformity, and great
Fortunately it is a rare complication. It
excision in children, and the rule is for it
or two years, after the operation.

Of the two forms of antero-posterior bending, the more common is the backward variety, in which the bending is due to the formation either of an angle at the junction of the two bones or to curvature of the lower part of the shaft of the femur.   In the other variety, namely, genu

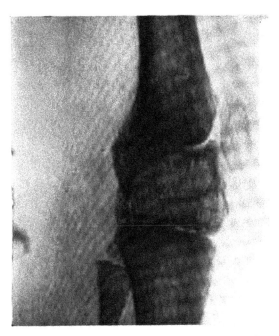

FIG. 101. SKIAGRAM FROM A CHILD AGED 8 YEARS, TAKEN TWO YEARS AFTER EXCISION OF THE KNEE BY KOCHER'S METHOD FOR DIFFUSE TUBERCULOUS INFILTRATION OF THE SYNOVIAL MEMBRANE. The lower end of the femur was pared, leaving a convex surface, the tibia leaving a correspondingly concave surface. The articular surface of the patella was removed, also a slice of cartilage from the femur opposite the patella. Note the complete osseous ankylosis, also how little the epiphyses have been interfered with. Amount of shortening = ½ inch. (*By Dr. E. Price.*)

recurvatum, the tibia may either be bent forwards at an angle at its junction with the femur or the upper part of the tibia may be curved. The angular deformities at the junction of the two bones are due either to faulty sawing of the bones, to their incomplete apposition, or to too early use of the limb. The deformity, on the other hand, which is pro-

duced by a curvature above or below the junction of the two bones is
a static condition due to bending of the growing bone at the end of the
diaphysis rather than to any error in the technique of the operation.
This latter deformity comes on more gradually and is later in its onset
than is the case with the angular bending at the seat of operation. No
attempt should be made to deal actively with the curvature until after it
has become stationary. In the case of the femur, the simplest plan is
to fracture the femur above the condyles by osteoclasis and to maintain
the corrected position by means of a plaster of Paris case. Failing this
a simple osteotomy should be performed. The operation of cuneiform
resection for ankylosis of the knee in the flexed position has been described by Mr. Burghard (p. 84).

OPERATION FOR ANKYLOSIS WITH GENU RECURVATUM

The principle of the operation is the same as that for ankylosis in the
flexed position, but the technique is a little more troublesome as access
cannot be got directly to the base of the wedge owing to its being directed
towards the popliteal space. The incision, which must therefore be made
over the concavity of the bend, may be planned with the object of dissecting upwards a single square flap, or, if preferred, two flaps may be
made by means of an H-shaped incision. If the patella be present, it had
better be removed. The remains of the quadriceps tendon and the subjacent periosteum are separated from the bone in the form of two short
flaps, a resection knife and a strong sharp rugine being used for this
purpose. In removing the wedge, the upper section is made first, the
edge of the saw being directed upwards as well as backwards. The
lateral soft tissues are well retracted backwards out of the way of the
saw, which is used cautiously towards the posterior aspect of the bone:
the latter is not completely divided for fear of wounding the popliteal
artery. The posterior cortex is fractured by using the leg as a lever, a
fulcrum being provided by placing a sand-bag behind the lower part of
the thigh. With the leg flexed so that the raw surface of the lower
fragment faces upwards, a wedge, with its base directed posteriorly, is
now removed by applying the saw to its anterior margin and directing
it downwards as well as backwards. The breadth of the base of the
wedge will of course be proportionate to the severity of the deformity.
As soon as the saw reaches close up to the posterior surface of the bone,
the latter is fractured across by levering the fragment upwards and backwards with the saw. In one instance, where the bone was considerably
sclerosed, the writer found it necessary to complete the section with an

osteotome. The wedge of bone is grasped with lion forceps and partly twisted and partly dissected away from the thickened periosteum, which protects the structures in the popliteal space. All sharp edges and irregularities are carefully trimmed away from the bones before they are brought into position. If the deformity has not been completely corrected, a second slice must be removed from whichever bone seems the more suitable for the purpose. When the limb has been brought into good apposition, it will generally be found that the divided quadriceps and periosteum have become too much drawn apart to admit of their approximation by buried sutures. The integuments, however, are sufficiently elastic to allow the skin wound to be closed. Drainage is not necessary. Here, as in a typical excision of the knee, the writer has found it an advantage to nail the bones together. The after-treatment is the same as for excision of the knee.

CHAPTER X

OPERATIONS FOR TUBERCULOUS DISEASE OF THE HIP AND SACRO-ILIAC JOINTS

OPERATIONS UPON THE HIP-JOINT

WIDELY different opinions have been expressed as to the relativ value of conservative and operative measures in the treatment of tuber culous arthritis of the hip-joint. It cannot be said even yet that th question has been definitely settled, but the prevailing view at presen seems to be that, in the early stage of the disease, appropriate mechanica treatment, aided by suitable constitutional and hygienic means, is gen erally capable of arresting the disease, and that the functional result i as a rule better than that which is to be obtained from an early excision

In hospital practice, unfortunately, by the time the surgeon see the patient the disease has often already advanced beyond the firs stage, and very commonly presents some of the following clinical fea tures: The region of the hip is swollen; the muscles of the thigh ar atrophied; the limb is more or less flexed and adducted; the trochante is thickened and frequently more or less elevated above Nélaton's line while if there has been erosion and migration of the dorsal margin o the acetabulum, the head of the femur can be felt to form a prominenc immediately above and behind the great trochanter. Deep-seate fluctuation may be felt beneath either the ilio-psoas or the tensor fasci femoris, in the adductor region, or posteriorly in the neighbourhood o the partially dislocated head of the bone. Any attempt to move th joint generally gives rise to more or less severe pain, and to reflex rigidit of the muscles guarding the joint. If the limb be examined while th patient is anæsthetized, the rigidity will largely disappear, and on rotatin the femur grating may be detected in the joint. Few will deny tha such cases as the above, especially among the poorer classes, are bes treated by excision.

Operation. Here, just as in tuberculous arthritis elsewhere while the chief aim of the operation is the removal of the disease, ever) endeavour should also be made to obtain as good a functional result a possible. Unfortunately the anatomy of the hip-joint is such tha these two indications can only be imperfectly fulfilled. By excising th head and neck of the femur we can remove the primary focus, but by the time the disease has advanced far enough to demand operation, the synovial membrane and the acetabulum will almost certainly be involved. It would appear, too, that the acetabulum is more frequently the primary

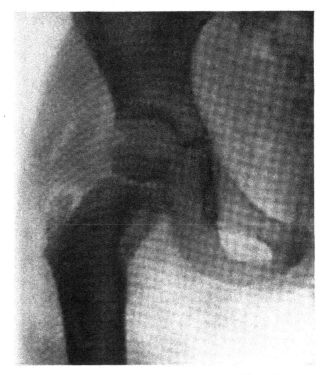

FIG. 102. TUBERCULOUS HIP-DISEASE. Skiagram from a child aged 5 years, showing an elongated and slightly wedge-shaped tuberculous focus in the under surface of the neck of the femur. The joint itself is not yet involved. This is a typical case for conservative treatment. (*By Dr. E. Price.*)

seat of the disease than was formerly supposed. It follows, therefore, that whatever incision be employed it should give access, not merely to the head and neck of the femur, but also to the acetabulum and to the synovial lining of the capsule.

The anterior route recommended by Hueter and Barker gives good access to the femur but not to the acetabulum, and for this reason it is not to be recommended for advanced cases. The conditions for which this operation would be most suitable are cases in which the disease in the head or neck of the femur has not yet given rise to secondary infection of the joint. Such cases, however, are best treated by conservative means.

The method of Langenbeck, namely, by the external vertical incision, is best adapted for those cases in which it is necessary to remove the trochanter as well as the head and neck of the femur.

In the opinion of the writer, the operative procedure recommended by Kocher is to be preferred to any other, as in addition to giving good access to the femur—trochanter as well as head and neck—it undoubtedly gives the best access to the acetabulum. Moreover, it has the great advantage of being applicable in practically all cases in which either arthrotomy or excision is indicated, and for this reason the writer has come to employ it almost exclusively.

Before describing the technique of the operation, one or two preliminary points are worthy of mention. The disinfection of the skin must not be confined simply to the buttock; it should include the lower part of the abdomen and back as well as the thigh. Special attention should be paid to the gluteal cleft and perineum. It is well also, as an additional precaution, to smear the anal region with sublimated iodoform. In arranging the sterilized sheets, it should be remembered that during the operation the affected limb has to be manipulated in various directions by an assistant; it must therefore be enveloped separately in an additional sheet from the toes up to a little below the buttock, while, to prevent it from slipping, a sterilized cotton bandage should be applied over it.

Supposing the right hip to be affected, the patient is placed on the left side in the semi-prone position, with the left thigh extended and the right flexed and adducted across it. The incision employed by Kocher is an angular modification of Langenbeck's external vertical incision. The upper half of the incision, which is placed obliquely, runs parallel to the fibres of the gluteus maximus, and practically also to the axis of the head and neck of the femur; it extends from the posterior superior angle of the great trochanter upwards and backwards towards the posterior superior spine of the ilium. The length of this portion of the incision will necessarily vary somewhat according to the obesity of the patient and according also to the amount of upward displacement of the femur. The lower half of the incision extends from the posterior superior angle of the great trochanter downwards in the axis of the femur to a short distance below the root of the trochanter. With the affected limb held in the flexed position the incision will be found to be more curved than angular.

Having divided the skin and subcutaneous tissue, the gluteus maxi-

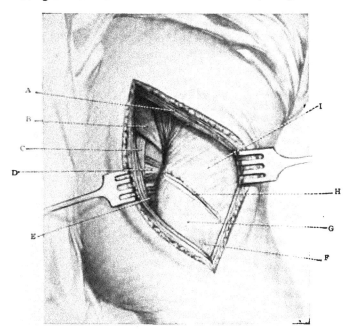

FIG. 103. FIRST STAGE OF EXCISION OF THE HIP BY KOCHER'S POSTERIOR ANGU-LAR INCISION. The gluteus maximus is split in the direction of its fibres; its edges are retracted, exposing the insertion of the gluteus medius into the outer surface of the great trochanter. The periosteum of the latter has been incised immediately below and parallel to the insertion of the gluteus medius. Above and behind the trochanter are seen, from above downwards, the pyriformis, the edge of the great sciatic nerve, the obturator internus with the gemelli, and the quadratus femoris. A, Gluteus maximus; B, Pyriformis; C, Great sciatic nerve; D, Obturator internus; E, Quadratus femoris; F, Vastus externus; G, Root of the trochanter; H, Incision; I, Insertion of the gluteus medius.

mus is exposed. The fleshy portion above and behind the trochanter is split in the direction of its fibres, while the aponeurotic portion, which covers the outer aspect of the trochanter, is divided vertically with the knife until the upper part of the glistening tendon of the vastus externus is exposed. A branch of the superficial division of the gluteal artery is secured in the fleshy part of the muscle, while in the aponeurotic portion forceps may have to be applied to the anastomosis between the transverse branch of the external circumflex artery and the first perforating branch of the profunda.   When the head of the femur is displaced

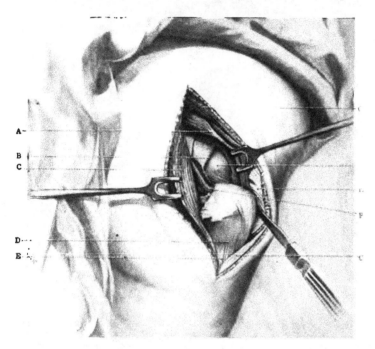

FIG. 104. ARTHROTOMY STAGE OF KOCHER'S EXCISION OF THE HIP. The insertions of the gluteus medius and minimus, and of the pyriformis, have been separated from the great trochanter subperiosteally and retracted upwards and forwards. The head and neck of the trochanter are exposed by dividing the posterosuperior portion of the capsule in the coronal plane. A, Pyriformis; B, Capsular ligament; C, C, C, Gluteus maximus; D, Root of the trochanter; E, Vastus externus; F, Obturator internus; G, Gluteus medius; H, Head of the femur.

upwards, the upper part of the incision may be made at the level of the upper border of the gluteus maximus, which is then freed and retracted downwards.   The same procedure may be adopted when the disease has spread from the acetabulum upwards into the ilium.

On retracting the edges of the gluteus maximus the following structures are exposed from above downwards: a layer of fatty tissue occupying the hollow above and behind the great trochanter, the insertion of the gluteus medius covering the upper and anterior part of the great trochanter, the periosteum covering its posterior and lower part, and, lastly, the upper part of the aponeurosis of the vastus externus (lateralis). After clearing away the fatty tissue above mentioned, and applying forceps to any divided vessels forming the anastomosis between the sciatic and internal circumflex arteries, the lower border of the gluteus medius is defined. Below it is the pyriformis muscle, the tendon of which cannot be followed to its insertion until after the gluteus medius has been detached from the great trochanter. Below the pyriformis are the obturator internus, the gemelli, and the upper fibres of the quadratus femoris. The sciatic vessels and nerves need not as a rule be exposed.

The next step in the operation consists in detaching the insertion of the gluteus medius. This is done by dividing the periosteum from the posterior superior to the anterior inferior angle of the trochanter, and then detaching the tendon upwards and forwards until the upper and anterior borders of the trochanter are exposed. In the child, this is readily effected by using a resection knife and including a slice of the subjacent cartilage along with the tendon; in adults, on the other hand, the operator must use either a strong sharp rugine (Farabeuf's), or he must apply the hammer and chisel and detach a layer of bone along with the tendon.

By retracting the separated insertion of the gluteus medius well upwards and forwards with a sharp double hook, the insertion of the gluteus minimus is reached and may, if necessary, be more or less completely detached from the anterior border of the trochanter. The tendon of the pyriformis, now freely exposed, is detached from the trochanter and retracted either upwards and forwards with the glutei, or downwards and backwards along with the obturator internus and gemelli. The former procedure is adopted when there is no displacement upwards of the femur, while the latter is preferable when the head of the bone is displaced upwards. The insertions of the obturator internus and gemelli are separated and retracted downwards. While the above muscles are being detached from the trochanter, a third assistant manipulates the thigh so as to render the individual tendons as accessible as possible.

The posterior part of the capsule is now fully exposed, and when there is marked flexion and adduction combined with upward and backward displacement of the femur, more or less of the head of the bone may be felt projecting outside the acetabulum, the posterior part of the capsule being stretched over it. In the cases where an abscess has formed, and is still confined to the cavity of the joint, tense fluctuation may be felt beneath the capsule. When there is little or no flexion and adduction deformity it is a good plan to break down any adhesions before commencing the operation. If this be done, the third assistant is generally able, by flexing, adducting, and rotating the thigh inwards, to cause a considerable portion of the head of the bone to project against the capsular ligament.

The posterior part of the capsule, after being fully exposed, is incised in the coronal plane over the projecting head of the femur parallel to the pyriformis, either immediately above or immediately below it. The opening is then extended right up to the margin of the acetabulum and well down to the trochanter. By rotating the limb inwards as fully as possible, and at the same time pushing the thigh well upwards and backwards, the head of the femur is made to project through the opening. Should the ligamentum teres still be present, it must be divided at its attachment to the femur either with a probe-pointed knife or by scissors curved on the flat. To bring the femoral attachment of the ligament into view the thigh should be flexed, adducted, and rotated inwards.

At this stage of the operation it is the duty of the operator to make a careful examination of the various components of the joint in order to ascertain the precise nature and extent of the tuberculous mischief. The head (epiphysis) and neck (end of the diaphysis) should be examined in the first place. A description of the various morbid conditions which may be met with is not within the scope of this article. Suffice it, therefore, to say that in cases of morbus coxæ which have reached the stage at which operation is justifiable, removal of the head and neck of the femur is almost invariably demanded. Perhaps the only possible exception to this rule is when the disease is confined to the synovial membrane, but even in these cases, if the disease be at all advanced, the removal of the head of the bone is generally necessary in order to give sufficient access for the removal of all the diseased synovial membrane. Another conceivable exception may be mentioned, namely, the presence of a primary osseous focus in the lower part of the neck of the femur which has not yet given rise to secondary infection of the synovial membrane. It is very unlikely, however, that such a localized morbid condition would give rise to symptoms calling for operation. In cases in which radiography has demonstrated such a condition, Huntingdon has advised that the focus should be removed without opening into the joint by tunnelling into the neck from the outer aspect of the great trochanter. The writer has performed this operation with advantage in the early stage of acute infective osteomyelitis of the neck of the femur, but it is doubtful if all the disease can be removed in tuberculous cases without the joint being opened into.

Most authorities are agreed that, whether the head of the femur be

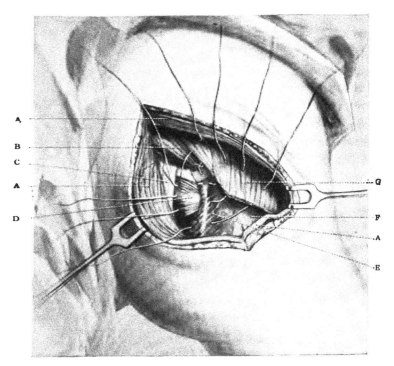

FIG. 105. LATER STAGE OF KOCHER'S EXCISION OF THE HIP. The head and neck of the femur have been removed. The upper end of the trochanter has been rounded off and placed in the acetabulum, with the limb in the abducted position. The capsule has been closed by two deep stitches. Four other stitches, not yet tied, are seen uniting the gluteus medius to the obturator internus, gemelli, and quadratus femoris. A, A, A, Gluteus maximus; B, Pyriformis; C, Great sciatic nerve; D, Obturator internus; E, Quadratus femoris; F, Vastus externus; G, Gluteus medius.

much diseased or not, it is wiser to remove it. The neck of the femur, especially the region of the calcar, is a common situation to meet with a primary osseous focus, and when this is present the whole neck should be removed along with the head. But even when the neck itself is free from disease it should be removed. The reasons in favour of this procedure will be evident when the after-treatment has been considered.

For dividing the neck of the bone the surgeon may use either Adams's saw, or, what is generally more convenient, a broad chisel (or Jones's gouge-chisel) and hammer. The whole of the neck should be removed. To include the lower part of the calcar it may be necessary to apply the chisel a second time. The cut surface of the femur is carefully examined to make sure that the disease has not extended into the trochanter. If it has, it is often possible to remove it with a gouge, or by curetting with a sharp spoon. Should the disease be still more extensive, the periosteum must be completely separated from the trochanter and the whole of the latter removed. The separation of the periosteum is facilitated by adding to the oblique incision already mentioned a transverse one at the level of the root of the trochanter. Unless, however, the disease has invaded the trochanter, the latter should not be removed. To remove the trochanter simply for the purpose of draining the joint is, in the opinion of the writer, as unnecessary as it is mutilating.

Having removed the head and neck of the femur, attention is next directed to the acetabulum. Any remains of the ligamentum teres, along with the adjacent synovial membrane and Haversian pad of fat, should be removed in the first place. If the cartilage be healthy it should be left with the object of obtaining a movable joint. Any pitlike or digital depression seen on the surface of the cartilage must be curetted with a sharp spoon, to ascertain if it be connected with a tuberculous focus in the subjacent bone; if so, the focus must be thoroughly gouged out. Should the cartilage be extensively eroded, or replaced by tuberculous granulations, the whole cavity, along with the superficial carious bone, must be vigorously curetted until the surface which is left is normal both in appearance and consistence. At this stage of the operation it is not uncommon to find that at some point the disease has perforated the acetabulum, and it may have given rise to a caseous abscess between it and the obturator internus muscle. When this is the case the opening must be enlarged so as to admit of the abscess being thoroughly cleaned out. Should a sequestrum be present, it must of course be removed.

When the acetabulum is involved, Bardenheuer has recommended that it should be completely excised. The severity of such a procedure, together with the disability to which it gives rise, is such that most surgeons prefer to trust to an extensive use of the hammer and gouge, assisted by the sharp spoon. A case sufficiently advanced to warrant excision of the acetabulum would almost certainly call for disarticulation at the hip-joint.

Attention is next directed to the diseased synovial membrane lining the capsule, and also to any infected pockets or abscesses extending from it. All tuberculous débris and fungus-like granulations should be got rid of in the first place by the sharp spoon aided by vigorous wiping out with gauze, while adherent clumps of synovial membrane and diseased portions of capsule are seized with toothed forceps (Kocher's artery forceps or Leedham Green's dissecting forceps), and clipped away with strong scissors curved on the flat. This part of the operation should as far as possible be done under direct inspection, and, if necessary, the opening in the capsule must be enlarged by an incision at right angles to the original incision.

The cavity of the joint and the wound may be douched out with sterilized salt solution, or, if preferred, a Barker's flushing spoon may be used for the curetting. Following this, some surgeons swab out the joint with a strong antiseptic, such as pure carbolic acid, followed by alcohol, or with chloride of zinc (40 grs. to the ounce). The disadvantage of this procedure is that drainage of the cavity becomes necessary. Instead of using any strong antiseptic, therefore, the writer prefers simply to rub some sublimated iodoform-bismuth paste over the interior of the capsule and the raw surfaces of the bones.

The upper border of the trochanter is now rounded off with a strong resection knife so as to make it fit into the bottom of the acetabulum when the limb is abducted. With the trochanter placed in this position, the patient is rolled gently back from the semi-prone position on to the sound side, the assistant keeping the affected thigh in the abducted and extended position. The operator now unites the deeper structures over the trochanter by means of interrupted catgut sutures, introduced either with a Doyen's handled needle or a suitable needle-holder. The deepest sutures close the opening in the capsule, the next layer unites the separated gluteus medius to the pyriformis and superior gemellus, while the third layer brings together the edges of the split gluteus maximus. The integuments are united with interrupted sutures of silkworm-gut. In children the silkworm-gut tends, after some days, to cut into the delicate skin. To prevent this, and to allow the stitches to be kept in for two or three weeks without disturbing the dressing, each suture, after it has been passed, but before being tied, is threaded at one end with a piece of fine rubber drainage tubing, about ¾ inch in length; when the suture is tied the tubing is left surrounding that portion of the loop which overlies the skin.

The question of drainage has been a good deal discussed in connexion with the operation of resection of the hip. Some writers have objected to Barker's anterior operation, on the ground that the drainage is unsatisfactory. The writer quite agrees with Barker that, in the absence

of sinuses, and provided also the wound ha
antiseptic, there is no necessity for drainage
the whole of the neck of the femur be re
thrust into the acetabulum there is no ne
there is no cavity left to drain.   If thought

FIG. 106. PHOTOGRAPH OF THE AUTHOR'S
(*Photograph by Dr. Lewis*

iodoform gauze may be passed down into
gluteus maximus.   In the majority of cases
pensed with altogether, so that the wound
is time to remove the stitches.

After-treatment.   Every precaution
the hip in the abducted position during th
treatment.   For this purpose the writer us
splint shown in Fig. 106.   It is in reality

long-splint (box-splint) introduced many years ago by Hamilton for treating fractures of the lower extremity in children. The cross-piece, instead of being placed at the very end of the splint, as in Hamilton's, unites the two portions posteriorly a little above the heels. The splint is padded with wool covered with jaconet waterproof. Besides giving a posterior support to the legs, this position of the cross bar is very

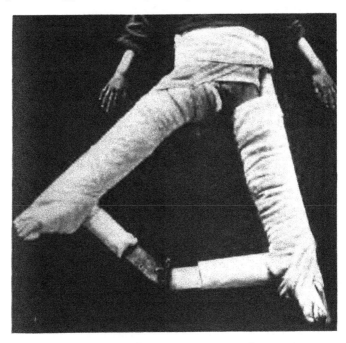

FIG. 107. PHOTOGRAPH OF A CHILD WITH ABDUCTION SPLINT APPLIED AFTER EXCISION OF THE HIP-JOINT. (*Photograph by Dr. Lewis S. Beesly.*)

convenient for lifting or carrying the patient while in the splint. To convert this simple splint into an abduction hip-splint, two modifications are necessary. The first is that the portion corresponding to the diseased side is sawn across opposite the hip, and the two parts united by a common hinge screwed on to the outer side of the splint; the other alteration is that the two halves of the splint are separate from each other, each with its own cross-piece. The cross portions are made long enough for their free extremities to overlap when the affected limb is abducted

to the desired degree.   To maintain the abduction all that is necessary
is to fix together the cross portions at the point where they overlap
with a common screw-clamp.   The upper portions of the splint are of
course secured to the chest by a broad binder.

Throughout the subsequent dressings care must be taken to keep
the limb in the exact position it occupied while in the splint, otherwise
there will be a great risk of the trochanter becoming displaced from the

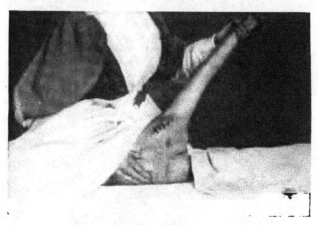

FIG. 108. THE METHOD OF MAINTAINING ABDUCTION DURING THE DRESSING AFTER
EXCISION OF THE HIP-JOINT.   (*Photograph by Dr. Lewis S. Beesly.*)

acetabulum.   The splint and dressings having been removed, the nurse,
whose duty it is to maintain the abducted position of the limb, stands on
the sound side of the patient, and, with one hand placed behind the child's
back and the other grasping the leg above the ankle, she gently turns the
child towards herself until it rests on its sound side (Fig. 108).   The
drain (or stitches) having been removed, and the wound dressed, the
patient is rotated back into the supine position and the splint reapplied.

When the wound has soundly healed, which is generally at the end of
three weeks, a plaster of Paris case is substituted for the splint, the limb
being maintained in the abducted position.   This first plaster case should
extend from the metatarsus to the level of the nipples, the patient afterwards being allowed to get about by the aid of crutches and a patten
added to the boot on the sound limb.   To prevent hyperextension of the
knee a special pad of cotton-wool should be placed under the popliteal
space.   From below the middle of the thigh downwards, the case should

be fairly thin, while in the region of the hip it should be strengthened by incorporating with it two strips of aluminium or Britannia metal, one placed anteriorly and the other externally. The addition of one part of dextrine to three parts of plaster of Paris makes the case much less brittle, and therefore less liable to crack.

After three months a Thomas's abduction splint may, in some cases, be substituted for the plaster, while in others it is easier to apply a second

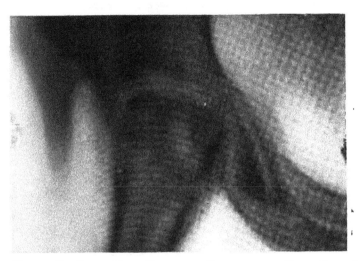

Fig. 109. The Result Three Years after Excision of the Hip by Kocher's Posterior Angular Incision. Skiagram from a child aged 9 years. Note how the upward displacement is prevented by the trochanter being placed in the acetabulum with the limb maintained in the abducted position. Absolute ankylosis. Shortening = 2 inches. (*By Dr. E. Price.*)

plaster case which need only envelop the pelvis and the upper two-thirds of the thigh. No attempt should be made to reduce the abduction. At the end of six months or so from the operation there is, as a rule, no longer any necessity for the patient to wear a splint; he should, however, continue to use the crutches and patten for two or three months, so as to prevent him bearing his weight upon the excised joint. Lastly, the patten is removed and the patient gradually begins to bear his weight on the limb.

Judging from the literature on the subject, considerable difference of opinion would appear to exist as to the best position in which to place the limb during the after-treatment; by some the straight position is preferred, by others the abducted; some advocate extension, while others disapprove of it. The writer is strongly in favour of the abducted position. The reasons for, and the advantages of, this position will be found clearly set forth in a paper by my former House Surgeon. Dr. Lewis S. Beesly (*Scottish Med. and Surg. Journ.*, Aug., 1907).

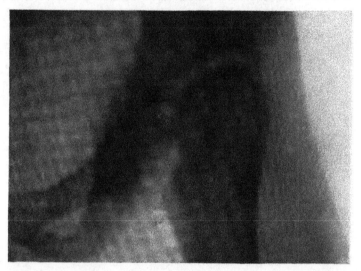

FIG. 110. THE RESULT A YEAR AFTER EXCISION OF THE HIP BY KOCHER'S POSTERIOR ANGULAR INCISION. Skiagram from a child aged 11 years. Trochanter placed in the acetabulum with the limb abducted. The joint is ankylosed; there is no displacement upwards of the trochanter. Two inches of shortening. (*By Dr. E. Price.*)

In the normal condition the weight of the trunk is not transmitted directly from the os innominatum to the shaft of the femur, but indirectly to it through the head and neck of the bone, which form an angle with the shaft varying from 160° in the new-born to 110° in the adult. By this arrangement the mechanical disability of the long axis of the os innominatum being practically parallel to the shaft of the corresponding femur is overcome, and the weight-bearing stability of the joint maintained. If the limb be kept in the straight position after the head and neck of the femur have been removed, the osseous stability of the joint is lost, for the pelvis on that side is then merely slung to the limb by the remains of the capsule and certain of the muscles which pass from the pelvis to the femur. If under such conditions the patient attempts to bear his weight upon the limb the trochanter becomes displaced from the acetabulum upwards and outwards on to the ilium. The result is progressive lameness and deformity owing to shortening combined with adduction and flexion.

By placing the limb in the abducted position, on the other hand, the pelvi-femoral muscles and the weight of the body cause the femur to be pressed upwards and inwards towards the acetabulum, which furnishes a stable surface for the femur to act against. Another advantage of the abducted position is, that by drooping the pelvis on the affected side to bring the limbs parallel for the purpose of progression, the patient not only compensates for the shortened condition of the limb but at the same time maintains the abduction at the hip, and in this way prevents the tendency to upward displacement of the trochanter. The obliquity of the pelvis is of course compensated for by a secondary curvature of the spine. Instead of drooping the pelvis on the sound side, the shortening might be compensated for by providing the patient with a high boot on the affected side; but unless the operation has resulted in either osseous or firm fibrous union, the danger is that the high boot, by doing away with the necessity for the drooping of the pelvis, would favour upward displacement of the femur. It must be admitted, however, that the abducted position predisposes to ankylosis, either complete or partial. But there can be no doubt also that an ankylosed hip in good position is preferable to the progressive deformity and lameness associated with displacement upwards of the femur. For this reason the writer is not in the habit of applying extension after excision of the hip. The best position for an ankylosed hip is with the limb abducted, slightly flexed, and a little rotated outwards. The advantage of slight flexion is that the patient is able to sit with greater comfort.

OPERATIONS FOR THE CORRECTION OF DEFORMITIES RESULTING FROM TUBERCULOUS HIP-JOINT DISEASE

TENOTOMY OF THE ADDUCTOR MUSCLES

Indications. This operation is called for—

(i) As a preliminary to excision of the hip in advanced cases of tuberculous disease in which there is marked adduction combined generally with flexion, internal rotation, and upward displacement of the femur. In such cases, without dividing the adductors, it is often impossible after excising the head and neck of the femur to place the limb in the abducted position. A further advantage of dividing these muscles is that, if the joint should become unstable, the division of the adductors, by preventing adduction of the thigh, diminishes the tendency to upward and backward displacement of the femur. The operation may be performed at the same sitting as the excision.

(ii) In old quiescent, or healed, cases of hip-joint disease in which the limb, without being ankylosed, has become markedly adducted. In some of these cases the limb can be straightened either gradually or by

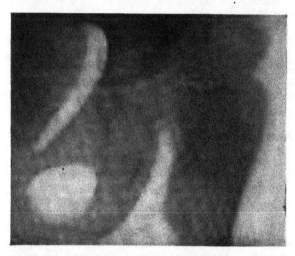

FIG. 111. QUIESCENT TUBERCULOUS DISEASE OF THE HIP. Skiagram from a child aged 6 years. The limb is slightly flexed and adducted. Note the upward displacement of the femur. The adductors were divided by the open method and the limb was put up in an abduction splint, and subsequently in the same position in plaster of Paris. (*By Dr. E. Price.*)

stretching the muscles under an anæsthetic, but, unless the patient continues to wear some form of splint or retention apparatus, the adduction is very liable to recur. Division of the adductors, followed by the placing of the limb in the abducted position, is, in many instances, the surest and best method of treating the deformity, along with the aggravated lameness to which it gives rise.

(iii) At the close of the operation for ankylosis with adduction.

Operation. The operation is performed as follows :—

Careful attention should in the first place be paid to the disinfection of the skin, not only in the groin, but also in the perineum, and especially in the deep cleft between it and the adductor region.

While the assistant attempts to abduct the thigh so as to put the adductors on the stretch, the surgeon makes a longitudinal incision from the origin of the adductor longus downwards along its prominent margin for two or three inches. After dividing the skin and subcutaneous fat, the deep fascia forming the sheath of the muscle is also divided longitudinally. The muscle itself is divided a little below its origin. Next, the inner edge of the skin wound is retracted so as to expose the anterior border of the gracilis, which is divided right back to its posterior border. The whole thickness of the adductor brevis is now divided, care being taken to avoid injuring the superficial and deep divisions of the obturator nerve, the former lying superficial to the muscle, the latter behind it upon the adductor magnus. In some cases the inner border of the pectineus may also require division. The best method of dividing the muscles is to isolate each one separately by a blunt dissector (Kocher's or Cheyne's) and then, while the muscle is put on the stretch, to cut it across with straight blunt-pointed scissors. The dissection scissors of C. H. Mayo answer both purposes admirably.

Any intervening bands of fascia which are felt to be stretched must also be divided, care being taken to avoid the internal circumflex artery and its branches. All bleeding points which can be detected on the cut surfaces of the muscles should be carefully ligatured so as to allow the wound to be closely sutured without drainage.

From the position of the wound it is obviously not advisable to apply an ordinary dressing fixed with a spica bandage. The writer is in the habit of treating the wound by simply smearing it over with sublimated iodoform-bismuth paste and taking precautions to prevent either the hands or the clothing from reaching it. Or, if preferred, the wound may be covered with one or two strips of iodoform gauze over which is applied a larger piece of gauze, the whole being secured in position by the free use of collodion. The advantage of avoiding a collodion dressing, at any rate during the first forty-eight hours, is that if any tension should occur within the wound it is relieved by the escape of the serum between the stitches. At the end of forty-eight hours, when the wound is perfectly dry, a collodion dressing may be applied. In the female great care must be taken to prevent the wound being soiled during urination.

After-treatment. For the first three weeks or so the patient is placed in an abduction splint similar to that used after excision of the hip; after this a Thomas's abduction hip-splint is applied and the patient allowed to get about on crutches. Should there be a tendency for the limb again to become adducted, the splint must be worn for a considerable time; and the more tendency there is to shortening and upward displacement the more should the limb be abducted.

The benefit derived from free open division of the adductors in old healed cases of hip-disease with marked adduction is very striking: the child, in place of being a pronounced cripple, is able to get about with comparative comfort.

TENOTOMY FOR FLEXION DEFORMITY

Any flexion deformity which remains after dividing the adductors can generally be got rid of by manipulation under an anæsthetic followed by subsequent weight extension. Should these means fail to correct the flexion, it will be necessary to divide the sartorius, the tensor fasciæ femoris, the fascia lata, and, in more aggravated cases, also the rectus. For this purpose a longitudinal incision is carried downwards from the anterior superior spine of the ilium in the interval between the tensor fasciæ femoris and sartorius muscles. After dividing these a little below their origin, the edges of the wound are retracted and the tendon of the rectus is divided. A branch of the external circumflex artery may require to be ligatured, while the external cutaneous nerve should, if possible, be avoided.

OPERATIONS FOR OSSEOUS ANKYLOSIS FOLLOWING HIP-JOINT DISEASE

Indications. Osseous ankylosis of one hip in the straight position is of very little consequence unless it is combined with flexion and adduction. A slight amount of flexion is rather an advantage than otherwise, as it allows the patient to sit with greater comfort. If the flexion be at all marked, and more especially if it be combined with adduction, the disablement becomes very great, and, unless there are weighty reasons to the contrary, operation should be urged. The adduction adds greatly to the lameness as well as to the deformity, as, in order to bring the limbs parallel for the purpose of progression, the patient is obliged to elevate the pelvis on the affected side and thereby to increase the shortening.

Various forms of osteotomy of the femur have from time to time been recommended for the treatment of ankylosis with malposition. The earlier methods took the form of a simple transverse subcutaneous osteotomy, the femur being divided either through the neck (Adams) or a little before the trochanter (Gant).

OPERATION FOR THE PRODUCTION OF PSEUDO-ARTHROSIS OF THE HIP WITHOUT DISARTICULATION OF THE HEAD

This operation, which we owe to Mr. Robert Jones, is indicated in those cases of tuberculous disease of the hip-joint in which ankylosis has occurred in a bad position without destruction of the head of the femur. The operation consists in 'removing a slice of the great trochanter, chiselling through the neck and screwing the separated portion of the trochanter to the proximal end of the neck in order to avoid union of the fragments. The neck may be chiselled close to the head or at a little distance, or the neck may be completely removed, or, where there has been destruction from disease, additional bone may be removed.'

The following is Mr. Jones's description of the operation :—

' A longitudinal incision is made about 6 inches in length with the upper border of the trochanter in its centre.

' An incision is made across the base of the trochanter just below the insertion of the gluteal muscles.

' A slice of the trochanter from this point to its junction with the neck above is sawn or separated by a very wide osteotome and retracted upwards. The capsule is now opened and the head separated from the neck with an osteotome.

' Extension is next put on the femur, and the trochanter with its muscles attached is screwed on to the head of the femur, which remains in the acetabulum.

' Deep and superficial sutures complete the operation.

' In the case of a tender joint, to avoid impinging, it may be necessary to remove a portion of the neck. In the case of an ankylosed sound joint following sepsis, it may be advisable, instead of dividing the neck near the acetabulum, to divide it near the trochanter.'

Mr. Jones commends the operation as a ' very suitable to those advancing in years. It saves the shock of disarticulation, an all-important consideration.

' In bony ankylosis, where disarticulation has to be made with a chisel, the time saved is great, and the result is more reliable than where a flap of tissue intervenes, unless the piece of bone removed is considerable, while the removal of much bone involves the sacrifice of muscle and some control of movement. The femur remaining is well supplied with muscles for useful movement, and no stitching of capsule is needed for the prevention of displacement upwards.'

Kocher divides the bone obliquely immediately below both trochanters (oblique subtrochanteric osteotomy). This method possesses the advantages of leaving two broad osseous surfaces and of preventing the lower fragment from being displaced inwards when the limb is forcibly abducted. Cheyne prefers a cuneiform osteotomy at the junction of the neck with the trochanter, the base of the wedge being placed either superiorly or superiorly and posteriorly, according to whether the limb is simply adducted or flexed as well. He makes a free incision down to the bone between the sartorius and the tensor fasciæ femoris muscles.

In ankylosis following tuberculous disease of the hip, however, the head of the femur is often more or less absorbed, or the neck is abnormally short and thick. For this reason Adams's operation is seldom feasible, and Cheyne's may be unnecessarily difficult. The operation which the writer is in the habit of performing is a cuneiform osteotomy, the wedge being removed immediately above the lesser trochanter (Volkmann) if the bone be not specially thickened; if it be, the wedge is removed immediately below both trochanters. The base of the wedge is directed externally if the ankylosis be attended with adduction only, while if there be flexion as well the base of the wedge is directed backwards as well as outwards.

The incision may be placed either transversely across the outer aspect of the root of the trochanter or longitudinally over the middle of its outer aspect. After dividing the skin and subcutaneous tissue, the aponeurotic insertion of the gluteus maximus is exposed and divided transversely. Beneath it is the great trochanter with the glistening tendon of the vastus externus lying immediately below it. The periosteum is now divided transversely across the outer aspect of the root of the trochanter, and, after separating it upwards and downwards with a strong sharp-edged rugine (Farabeuf's), the wedge is removed with the hammer and a broad, highly tempered chisel. The more the limb is shortened, the broader should be the base of the wedge so as to allow of the limb being well abducted. In removing the wedge it is well not to sever the bone completely until both sides of the wedge have been cut. During the operation the patient should be placed on the sound side, and a sand-bag (not too tightly filled) should be placed between the thighs so as to provide a firm and steady bed for the affected limb to rest upon. The sand-bag is covered with jaconet and completely enveloped by at least two layers of sterilized cotton sheeting. After the wedge has been removed, the periosteum and the fascia lata are united with buried catgut sutures. The skin wound is closed without drainage.

The limb is maintained in the abducted position by means of the splint already described. Before this can be done it will be necessary either to forcibly stretch or divide the adductor muscles.

After-treatment. There is no necessity to apply weight extension to the limb, as there is no fear of the osseous surfaces becoming displaced. Osseous union is aimed at, and the after-treatment is therefore conducted on the same lines as for simple fracture, care being taken that the limb is not allowed to become everted. The patient may be kept in the abduction splint for six weeks, but if desired a Thomas's abduction splint (or a plaster of Paris case) may be applied at the end of three weeks and the patient allowed to get about on crutches with a patten to raise the opposite limb. Two months after the operation the patient may begin to bear his weight upon the limb.

OPERATIONS FOR ANKYLOSIS WITH SINUSES

It is by no means uncommon to meet with old-standing cases in which the ankylosis with flexion and adduction is complicated with one or more sinuses which have persisted in spite of repeated attacks on them by the ordinary method of laying them open and curetting, followed by the application of a powerful antiseptic and gauze packing or drainage. In many of these cases the sinuses are prevented from healing by the presence of foci of osseous disease—often containing a sequestrum—imbedded in the region of the ankylosed joint, either in the innominate bone, in the remains of the head or neck of the femur, or in the trochanter. While amputation may be called for in exceptional cases, there are many cases in which by excising the joint the disease can be removed and the limb at the same time straightened.

Operation. The operation is carried out on the following lines: In the first place the sinuses are laid open, curetted, and disinfected either with pure carbolic acid or turpentine; those that lie in the region of the main operation wound may often be completely excised. Free access must be got to the ankylosed joint, and in the presence of adduction and flexion this is best effected by means of Kocher's postero-external incision. If the sinuses be carefully probed, one or more of them will be found to lead, either directly or indirectly, to the diseased focus in the bone, and whatever be its situation, this should be thoroughly gouged away, and, if necessary, the wound should be enlarged to give sufficient access to do this thoroughly. The next step consists in chiselling across the neck of the femur, and then gouging out the remains of the head of the bone from the acetabulum. Should the bone be dense this may be rather a laborious process. The writer has found the highly tempered gouge-chisels made by Weiss of London for Mr. Robert Jones very helpful for this purpose.

Should a focus of disease be discovered in the root of the neck or in the trochanter, it must be removed, after which the end of the latter should be so fashioned that it can be implanted into the gouged out acetabulum, the adductors being stretched, or if necessary divided, to allow the limb to be placed in the abducted position. A drainage tube should be introduced into whichever sinus leads most directly down to the joint, the others being packed with iodoform gauze. The after-treatment is the same as that described for excision of the hip.

Operations for treatment of ankylosis of the hip-joint where it is designed to produce a mobile joint are described in Vol. I. They will seldom be used, however, where the ankylosis follows tuberculosis.

OPERATIONS FOR ABSCESSES AND SINUSES, THE RESULT OF TUBERCULOUS DISEASE OF THE HIP-JOINT

Although these complications are frequently met with, their treat-ment is so much a matter of general principles that the operative details need not be fully discussed in a work of this description.

Should a small abscess form with the patient going about in the early stage of the disease, it will occasionally absorb if the limb be kept at rest. If, on the other hand, it should continue to enlarge it must be opened and curetted. While there are some cases in which the joint may be left untouched, it is usually wiser to make the incision of such a size and so to place it that the joint may be investigated in order that a definite decision may be come to as to whether radical measures should be pro-ceeded with. When the abscess is situated posteriorly, excision may be proceeded with by Kocher's method.

Sometimes after opening an anterior abscess along the inner border of the sartorius a suppurating track may be followed underneath the iliacus to its origin from a small primary bone focus at the margin of the acetabulum close to the anterior inferior spine of the ilium. In such a case it not infrequently suffices to curette the bone without incising the capsule. When, however, the abscess communicates with the joint, the latter should be explored. In other cases the abscess is confined within the capsule of the joint, and is then treated either by simple arthrotomy or by excision, according to the extent of the disease. In cases where ex-cision was deemed advisable the writer was formerly in the habit of employing Barker's method; more recently, however, he has abandoned it in favour of the posterior operation.

In the case of a large abscess extending down the thigh under the fascia lata, it is sometimes advisable, on account of the debilitated state of the patient, to defer the excision until some time after the abscess has been dealt with. Should the general condition of the patient seem equal to it, however, it is better to proceed at once to excision; if the disease in the joint be left it only serves to reinfect the abscess cavity.

The incision used to excise the joint should be prolonged down the thigh sufficiently to allow the whole abscess cavity to be laid open and thoroughly cleaned out. The whole wound should be sutured, except at its lowest part, where a rubber or gauze drain should be introduced, and a second drain should be introduced opposite, and down to, the joint. A counter-opening may be made if necessary. The shock, although considerable, may be counteracted by the introduction of large quantities of normal saline into the rectum by the drop method introduced by Murphy.

After opening and removing the tubercular lining of the abscess by curetting, followed by vigorous scrubbing out with dry gauze, it is customary to introduce some antiseptic with the object of destroying the few bacilli which have almost certainly escaped removal. A 10% emulsion of iodoform and glycerine has been most commonly employed for this purpose. More recently Murphy has made use of a 2% solution of formalin in glycerine. The writer uses the sublimated iodoform-bismuth paste in the proportion of one part of the former to two or three of the latter, according to the size of the abscess.

While the presence of sinuses renders the results of excision less favourable on account of their liability to set up a general infection of the wound, their presence should not *per se* be regarded as contra-indicating excision; indeed their persistence is often an argument in favour of excision, as in the majority of cases it is only by removing the joint lesion that they can be got to heal.

TUBERCULOUS DISEASE OF THE SACRO-ILIAC JOINT

The disease is generally secondary to a focus in the sacrum or ilium, and in adults it is frequently accompanied by pulmonary tuberculosis. In children it is often secondary to disease in the lower lumbar spine.

Skiagraphy is of the greatest assistance to the surgeon in enabling him to localize the situation of the bone focus at a comparatively early stage of the disease. In the absence of advanced pulmonary tuberculosis, the operation should be advised, and, if possible, it should be performed before suppuration occurs.

Operation. The joint is best exposed by a semilunar incision placed internal to the articulation. The size of the incision will, of course, depend on the extent of the disease. After retracting the flap outwards, the periosteum is incised over the back part of the crest of the ilium, while below the level of the posterior superior spine the knife is carried down to the back of the sacrum between the origin of the gluteus maximus and the lumbar aponeurosis. The posterior fibres of the gluteus medius, the upper fibres of origin of the gluteus maximus, and the upper part of the great sacro-sciatic ligament and the subjacent periosteum are separated from their attachments and retracted well outwards. The inner flap, consisting of the lower part of the erector spinæ, is detached inwards. The posterior superior and posterior inferior spines of the ilium are removed with a chisel. If the disease be limited to the ilium, little more requires to be done except perhaps to scrape and clip away some disease which has invaded the posterior ligament and adjacent soft parts. If, on the other hand, the sacrum be involved and the joint more extensively diseased, more of the ilium may have to be removed before sufficient access can be got. The strong interosseous ligament, along with the diseased portion of the sacrum, is then removed with a chisel or gouge. If possible, the periosteum and ligaments covering the anterior aspect of the joint should be left intact, and the important structures immediately in front of it, namely, the internal iliac vessels, the ureter, and the lumbo-sacral cord, must be kept in mind.

An abscess or sinus confined to the posterior aspect of the joint is easily dealt with, but considerable difficulty may arise in following up suppurating tracks and collections of pus which have burrowed into the pelvis. In the presence of such complications, in order that free through and through drainage may be established, it will generally be necessary to make a counter-opening either in the iliac region, the buttock, the upper and inner aspect of the thigh, or the perineum, according to the route taken by the abscess.

After-treatment.   The after-treatment consists in prolonged re-cumbency, as much as possible in the open air. To ensure rest sand-bags may be used, or the patient may be fixed to a Bradford's bed-frame.

Results.   The results are often very unsatisfactory; the patient not infrequently dies of meningitis or general tuberculosis. Sinuses are very liable to persist indefinitely, and to lead to waxy disease.

SECTION III

OPERATIONS UPON THE LIPS
FACE AND JAWS

PART I

OPERATIONS FOR HARE-LIP AND
CLEFT-PALATE

BY

EDMUND OWEN, F.R.C.S. (Eng.), D.Sc.(Hon.)

Consulting Surgeon to St. Mary's Hospital and to the Hospital for Sick
Children, London

CHAPTER I

OPERATIONS FOR HARE-LIP

Indications. As is shown later on in this article, if a child has a hare-lip and a cleft-palate, the palate should be operated on before the lip. But if an infant has a hare-lip and no cleft-palate, the sooner the lip is operated on the better; it may be done any time after the tenth day—and earlier still, if need be—but it should not be done without an anæsthetic, for which purpose chloroform answers best.

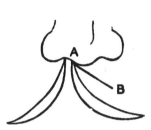

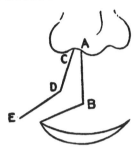

FIG. 112. THE OPERATION FOR HARE-LIP. *First stage.* The mucous border of the right side of the gap is to be peeled off, and the flap on the left side which is set free by the incision A B is to be brought across below the right side of the lip.

FIG. 113. THE OPERATION FOR HARE-LIP. *Second stage.* The left side of the lip being drawn well across, the incision A B becomes vertical, and a full prolabium is obtained.

Operation. One of the most important points in the operation is to detach the lip and cheek freely, so that the vivified edges may meet across the gap without any tension. The bleeding vessels can be caught by clip-forceps, and all blood thus prevented from entering the mouth.

After the labial flaps have been fully detached, the incisions are made for obtaining the raw edges. By one of the old methods of operating the mucous membrane was dissected from each side of the gap, and, thus, when the raw surfaces were drawn together, an unsightly notch was apt to be seen on the free border of the lip. The border of the lip should be vivified by a very sharp scalpel; an old scalpel which has been worn thin by grinding does excellently for the purpose. The mucous membrane is peeled from one side of the cleft and from along a good deal of the free border of the smaller side of the lip, while from the other side a bold flap is cut as is shown in Fig. 113. c D E. This flap is afterwards brought across to the denuded border of the lip from the other side. Of its thickest part a prolabium is formed, while the part which before had been the mucous border of the vertical cleft becomes the horizontal border all along the rest of the lip. The piece thus brought across is a thick, wedge-shaped flap, which is boldly tilted down so as to leave an angular space into which the opposite side of the lip, also vivified, may be dove-tailed.

The right side of the lip having had its mucous membrane carefully

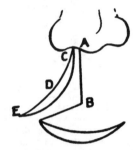

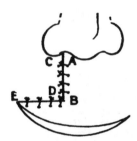

FIG. 114. THE OPERATION FOR HARE-
LIP. *Third stage.* The mucous border
has been removed from the right side
and a flap cut from the left side.

FIG. 115. THE OPERATION FOR HARE-
LIP. *Final stage.* The flap from the
left side has been adjusted along the
right half of the lip.

pared off up to the curved line C D E (Fig. 114), the lateral halves of the lip are drawn together in the middle line. When the left half of the lip has been thus brought to the middle line, the incision A B, which had been made obliquely into the lip (Fig. 112), becomes vertical, the thick flap, which had previously been vertical, becoming horizontal and ready to form the mucous border of the restored lip. The right side of the lip being drawn inwards, some of its freshened border, C D, is placed vertically, whilst the rest of it, D E, becomes horizontal, and to it the deflected flap from the left half of the lip is adjusted, the middle part, D, being fitted into the angle on the left side as at B in Fig. 115. The mucous membrane must be entirely removed in order that primary union may be complete, and it should be removed from around the whole thickness of the lip. Not a particle of the skin, however, should be sacrificed.

The flap thus described is not the same as in Mirault's operation. His method entailed the cutting with a pair of scissors merely of a ¼-inch flap from the lower border of the lip which was to be arranged to form a normal prominence for the lip, as a sort of pedicle.

Sutures. For the thorough adjustment of the flaps stitches should be inserted not only down the front of the lip, but also on the dental aspect, and some of them should be placed very deeply, so as to prevent the halves of the orbicularis and the associated muscles dragging upon the wound. Prepared horsehair may be used for adjusting the edges of the skin and for securing the transplanted flap along the opposite half of the lip; silk is not suitable as it swells and becomes septic. The vivified surfaces must be kept in close contact by passing some of the posterior stitches deeply and boldly with a curved needle, the needle being brought almost through to the skin, but just missing it; these stitches are of great use in steadying the flaps. The old-fashioned hare-lip pins should never be used; they are not needed even in cases of the worst kind. The spots at which they traversed the skin were apt to be permanently marked by white scar-tissue. A great advantage of the deep sutures at the dental aspect of the lip is that they leave no mark; they also arrest bleeding, and they adjust the surfaces and edges of the wound so well, that possibly only a few stitches may be required for the front. None of the stitches should be tied very tight or they will cut their way out by ulceration; they are wanted merely to hold the surfaces gently together. Their ends should be left about ¼ inch long, so that they can be easily seized by the forceps when the time comes for their removal.

If, as often happens, the nostril be wide and flat, it should be made shapely, and fixed in the approved position; some of its cartilaginous ring may have to be cut away so as to reduce its size and round it off. It may need also to be separated from the bone, and it may be advisable to hitch up its lower and outer part by a silver-wire suture. In some cases it is well to turn up the mucous membrane from the projecting ring of the nostril, and then, having shaved off a thickish slice of the cartilage, to bring down again and suture the membrane.

Dressings. When the last stitch has been inserted, and the face has been washed and thoroughly dried, the assistant should purse up the lip with the finger and thumb whilst the surgeon applies a dressing of gauze dipped in collodion and long enough to reach well on to the cheeks. Next day this had better be removed, and it is often advisable to do this first dressing under chloroform. The nurse gently holds the slack of the cheeks towards the middle line, and the surgeon peels off the gauze by pulling the ends *inwards,* being careful not to drag upon the sutures; then, when the part has been cleaned, he may decide to remove, perhaps, every other stitch, as the edges of the wound are closely adhering. If a thick stitch has been deeply inserted from the front, it certainly ought to be removed, lest it should leave a scar. The sutures at the top end of the vertical wound may also be ready for removal. A gauze and collodion dressing is applied as before, and next day, or the next day but one, the wound should be dressed again, a few more of the anterior stitches being removed, the posterior stitches still being left. Thus, within four or five days all the visible sutures are removed, those at the tail end of the flap and at the free border of the lip being last taken out. For ten days or a fortnight after this the lip must be kept from disturbance by gauze and collodion or by waterproof strapping. If the surgeon does not think it necessary to have chloroform administered for the dressings, the nurse should be sitting in a chair opposite to him with the child lying on her lap, whilst the surgeon grips its head firmly between his knees, so as to keep it quite steady.

If the case be one in which the intermaxillary bone and the prolabium have been sacrificed and the new lip is very small, the removal of a wedge-shaped piece from the middle of the lower lip may improve the appearance, a prominent lower lip being very unsightly.

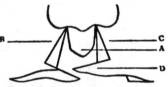

FIG. 116. OPERATION FOR DOUBLE HARE-LIP. A, Prolabium with borders denuded; B, Right side of lip denuded and flap brought down; c, Left side of lip denuded; D, Flap brought down and vivified on lower border, ready for being tucked round between the right side of the prolabium and the right labial flap.

Double hare-lip. If in the case of a double hare-lip the prolabium can be used, it may need to be lowered somewhat before it can be made available for the new lip. This being done, the mucous membrane should be thinly and cleanly dissected off its borders, and the two sides of the lip should be arranged for blending with it. Probably one side of the lip is larger than the other; this, therefore, should be chosen to build up the mid-part and the lower border of the new lip. A flap is also cut from the other side of the lip, but before this is done, the mucous membrane is peeled from its free border, so that the flap can be dove-tailed in between the vivified border of the median bud and the fresh-cut surface of the other flap, as shown in Fig. 116.

If this flap, which is denuded on both its upper and its lower surfaces, be long enough, it may be bent around the border of the median bud towards the opposite side, lying between the median bud and the large flap, and in this position it is duly secured by a few deep sutures, as already described, and by superficial ones of horsehair.

Sometimes the closure of the cleft in the lip causes a great difficulty of breathing, for whereas the air-way had been unusually free, the infant is subsequently obliged to breathe only through the nose and mouth, and the nostrils are, perhaps, a good deal blocked by dry blood and mucus. In these circumstances the nurse has to guard the child from the risk of suffocation by gently depressing the lower lip. If the difficulty of breathing be very marked, the surgeon may feel inclined to pass a suture through the back of the lower lip and bring the two ends round the border of the lip, fixing them to the chin by a piece of waterproof strapping. The sucking in of the lower lip and the difficulty of breathing are thus done away with, and as there is no tension on the suture it does not hurt the lip.

It sometimes happens that the lower border of the lip is marked by a notch, either with or without an operation having been performed; this may be effaced by making a horizontal incision into the substance of the lip a little above the notch, and then closing the wound in the vertical manner. This operation is on the principle which is adopted for widening a short constriction in the alimentary canal, an incision being made in the length of the bowel and closed at right angles to it.

If after operating on a hare-lip the surgeon sees in a day or two that the line of sutures is 'breaking down,' and that there is no longer any chance of obtaining primary union, he may still look for a good result by the fusing together of the two layers of granulation tissue. If, therefore, the flaps fall apart, the sutures should be removed, and the lip should be bathed in warm boric lotion and covered with wet boracic gauze. So long as the tissues are acutely inflamed, nothing can, of course, be done with a view to bringing the parts together again; but as soon as the inflammation has subsided, and healthy granulations begin to cover the raw surfaces, the sides of the lip should be readjusted by gauze and collodion, or by strips of waterproof strapping. In this way a very excellent result may often be obtained for an operation which had at one time threatened a complete failure—a good example of healing by granulation.

ROSE OPERATION

Blair, in the *International Clinics*, has described this operation in detail as follows:

Restoration of the Lip and Nostril. Of the numerous plans which have been proposed for this purpose a 'Rose' type of operation is the simplest to plan and execute and is capable of giving the best anatomic results. Last but not least, disappointing results which will occur are more easily corrected after this plan of operating than any other. Many operators use an angular in place of the curved incision of a typical 'Rose' operation, but the principle is the same. For complete double hare-lip the author prefers the plan that somewhat resembles a 'Maas' operation (Fig. 117), but even in the double cleft the 'Rose' operation

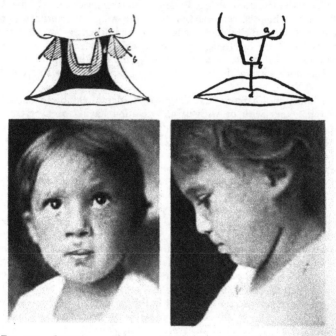

Fig. 117. Showing a Modified Maas Operation for Double Hare-lip which for want of a better designation we have called the Washington University Operation. The child shown below had this operation done in early infancy. Notice the beautiful development of the nose that has taken place spontaneously. The defect in the middle of the lip is due to inadvertently leaving a slight bit of the vermilion border of the prolabium. (Blair, *International Clinics.*)

is efficacious and, unless one has special skill, is apt to be more satisfactory in the result (Fig. 118).

Operation for Single Hare-lip. If this is accompanied by a complete palate cleft, the alveolar portion is to be dealt with according to one of the plans already given. In a simple alveolar cleft, without complete separation, the alveolar process needs no special treatment. Whether a lip cleft is complete or only a notch, the plan of operating is the same, for incomplete clefts are accompanied by a spreading of the nostril on

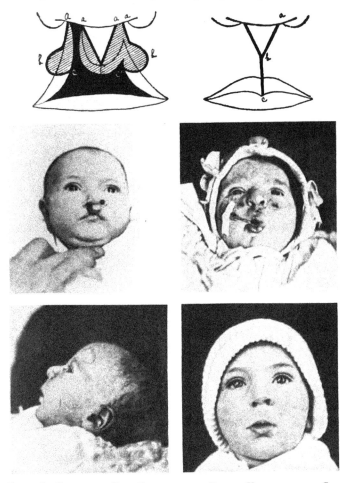

FIG. 118. SHOWS THE ROSE OPERATION FOR DOUBLE HARE-LIP AND A CASE SO TREATED. The second picture in the series shows the distortion that immediately resulted, but the other two show the good later results. The only fault here is that the upper lip was made a little too long, a mistake very easy to make. (Blair, *International Clinics.*)

that side which should be remedied (Fig. 120). The following points should receive special attention during the operation:

(*a*) Incision should be carefully planned and then plainly outlined with the point of a knife.

(*b*) Unless varied for some special adjustment, the cuts should ex-

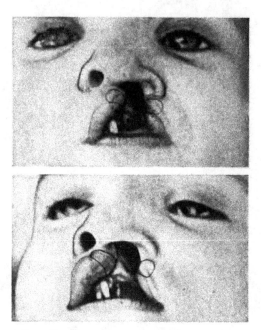

FIG. 119. TWO PHOTOGRAPHS TAKEN AT SLIGHTLY DIFFERENT ANGLES SHOWING ROSE INCISIONS FOR SINGLE COMPLETE HARE-LIP. These are depicted here chiefly to show the relation of the upper portion of the incisions to the nostril. On each picture the head is tilted back somewhat, which causes a foreshortening of the incisions. (Blair, *International Clinics.*)

tend squarely through the full thickness of the lip. A sharp, long, straight bistoury is preferable for the purpose.

(*c*) On neither side of the cleft does the incision really enter the nostril, but it should end at the level of the junction of the columella with the lip on the mesial side and of the ala with the lip on the lateral side; the upper ends of the incisions run almost transversely (Fig. 119). One is rather apt to run the incisions somewhat upward along the inner surface of the ala or septum, which will cause an internal obstruction of the nostril most difficult to correct. Just at the entrance of the nostril the incision should run sufficiently close to the ala on one side and the columella on the other, so as to bring them close enough together to make a nostril of a proper size (Fig. 119).

(d) In doing a 'Rose' operation the convexity of the curved incision should extend laterally to the fullest width of the cleft defect,

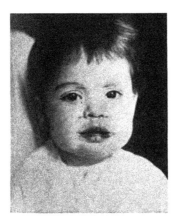 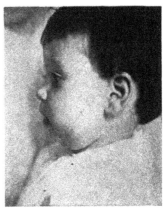

FIG. 120. THE CHILD'S UPPER LIP IS NORMALLY A PYRAMID WITH THE APEX AT THE CENTRE OF THE VERMILION BORDER. In correcting a hare-lip, this pyramidal form should be preserved. This is best accomplished by the 'Rose' operation. (Blair, *International Clinics*.)

and each curved out, if drawn out straight, should be of the same length as its fellow of the opposite side.

(e) The length of the cut within the vermilion border should correspond to the width that it is desired the vermilion border should be at the completion of the operation (Fig. 120).

(f) The ala is approximated to the columella by a deep suture of paraffined silk, placed just below the ala and the columella; this includes the full thickness of the lip and a superficial stitch that accurately approximates the skin. These are best combined in an inverted figure-of-eight suture, that is drawn up tentatively, first observing whether the ala is brought to a level symmetrical with its fellow of the opposite side. If this is not the case the suture is removed and replaced; then it is necessary to see that the cut edges of the skin in the floor of the nostril abut fairly and do not overlap. If this should not be the case, a superficial stitch of silk or horsehair is placed in the skin above the figure-of-eight stay suture and immediately tied; the figure-of-eight suture is then tied, the ends being cut short.

(*g*) A somewhat superficial suture is put exactly through the muco-cutaneous border and before tying this gentle traction is made downward to see that both freshened borders of the cleft are of the same length (Fig. 121).

(*h*) The skin and mucosa of both surfaces are now accurately ap-

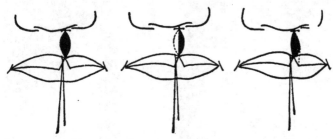

FIG. 121. AFTER PLACING THE FIGURE-OF-EIGHT SUTURE AT THE ENTRANCE OF THE NOSE AND A SIMPLE SUTURE AT THE MUCO-CUTANEOUS BORDER AND THEN DRAWING, GENTLY, DOWNWARD UPON THE LATTER, THERE SHOULD BE AN ELLIP-TICAL GAP, WITH SYMMETRICAL BORDERS, THAT IS TO BE CLOSED BY CUTANEOUS SUTURES. If it is found that one border is shorter than the other, first it is determined if one is too short or the other too long and then dealt with as suggested in the other two figures; cutting along the dotted line through the full thickness of the lip. The central figure shows the method of lengthening the short segment of the lip, while a cut made through the dotted line, in the figure to the right, will shorten the lateral part of the lip. Both sides may be shortened or lengthened in the same way. (Blair, *International Clinics*.)

proximated by several superficial interrupted sutures of horsehair or fine silk, the ends of all being cut very close to the knots.

If the ala has been brought into proper relation to the columella, any present kinking of the nostril had best be disregarded, for it is rapidly and more accurately corrected by growth than by a plastic on the ala. When finished, the two halves of the lip should be symmetrical, with neither a notch nor a protrusion at the line of union. It has been the writer's observation that a lip which is slightly short at the suture line tends to correct itself with growth; that if it is made too long, or with a protrusion, these faults tend to persist. With this type of operation, either a moderate notch or a protrusion are easily corrected at a subsequent operation. After the superficial suturing is completed, two deep stay sutures are placed, one on the mucous surface of silkworm-gut

(Fig. 122), a little above the muco-cutaneous border, its ends being left free and 4 inches long; the other of No. 26 silver wire is placed through the upper part of the lip and shotted over lead plates that rest on the skin. If no infection takes place, these are sufficient. The lower part of the lip usually holds; in but two instances in the writer's practice have infection and tension combined been sufficient to cause a separation

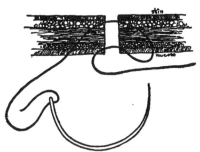

FIG. 122. AFTER BOTH THE CUTANEOUS AND MUCOUS SURFACES OF THE LIP ARE ACCURATELY APPROXIMATED BY FINE INTERRUPTED SUTURES, THEN IN THE FLESHY PART OF THE LIP ARE PLACED ONE OR POSSIBLY TWO OF THESE MODIFIED LANE SUTURES OF SILKWORM-GUT, TIED ON THE MUCOUS SURFACE. This suture ensures the accurate approximation of the muscular surfaces, controls bleeding and bears the brunt of the strain; the two ends are left four inches long so as not to fall into the mouth and are not knotted together, otherwise the child might catch its finger in the loop. Care must be exercised in removing this suture; the knot might be cut off and the loop left in the lip. (Blair, *International Clinics.*)

here. The greatest tension is in the upper part, the silver wire suture having a tendency to cut, thus allowing one or both nostrils to spread. For this reason it is advisable to further support the face by adhesive strapping.

Double hare-lip, complete or incomplete, is almost as well treated by the ' Rose ' operation as the modified ' Maas ' operation used by the writer (Fig. 117) and its execution is more simple. The prolabium is cut to a point and the curved incision is made in each lateral piece of the lip, after adjusting both nostrils as described in taking care of a single hare-lip. The muco-cutaneous border suture is placed, the lip is drawn down to the proper length, and the remaining sutures put into place. The same precautions are observed as in repairing a single hare-lip, and what should be remembered is that a double operation is much more of a strain on the child, and possibly more so on the operator, than the single cleft operation. Both operations are completed by putting a modified 'Lane' suture in the lower third of the lip and a lead plate suture below the level of the nostril, and then strapping the face.

The figure-of-eight suture placed at the entrance of the nostril is not sufficient to prevent the subsequent suturing of the ala. Garretson devised the plan of placing a silver wire suture through the lip, shotted at each end for a lead plate. If there is no infection, this may be effective, but in the presence of infection, the wire rapidly cuts through the flesh. We first supplanted the use of this wire by the use of adhesive straps brought around the cheeks and crossing at the root of the nose and under the chin. We now in addition put in a deep suture from

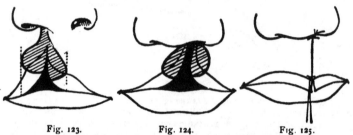

Fig. 123. Fig. 124. Fig. 125.

FIG. 123. OUTLINES OF INCISIONS IN A ROSE OPERATION FOR PARTIAL LIP CLEFT, IN WHICH THERE IS ALSO A SPREADING OF THE NOSTRIL OF THAT SIDE. By the vertical dotted lines it is seen that the incisions extend laterally as far as the widest part of the cleft. It will also be seen that the length of each cut within the vermilion border of the lip is the same. If the lengths of the two curved incisions were measured, it would be found that they were of the same length on each side. These are the three important points in designing the incisions of a Rose operation. (Blair, *Oral Surgery*.)

FIG. 124. INCISIONS FOR ROSE OPERATION OF A COMPLETE SINGLE CLEFT. (Blair, *Oral Surgery*.)

FIG. 125. AFTER MAKING THE INCISIONS FOR THE ROSE OPERATION, THE ALA IS REPLACED WITH ONE SUTURE, AND THE NEWLY PARED BORDERS ARE APPROXIMATED AND PUT ON THE STRETCH BY A TENSION SUTURE PLACED AT THE MUCO-CUTANEOUS BORDER. (Blair, *Oral Surgery*.)

within the mouth of heavy silver wire at the level of the ear: this to be removed later. Any support or any dressing resting on the suture line is very objectionable. Prominent scars are almost always due to infection and the only effective way of controlling this that we have found is the immediate and continuous removal of all crusts or scabs as rapidly as they form.

CHAPTER II

OPERATIONS FOR CLEFT-PALATE

ON THE EMPLOYMENT OF PRESSURE IN THE TREAT-MENT OF CLEFT-PALATE

In the *Medical Record* of Australia for June 15, 1861 (Melbourne), is an article by the editor, Dr. Reeves, which is apparently the first recommendation of the pressure-method of dealing with cleft-palate. Dr. Reeves was led to try it on the dead body of a child who had died three weeks after birth. The fissure was complete, and large enough to admit the end of the little finger. By means of a pair of clamps the sides of the fissure were readily brought together. The gums of the upper jaw were then found to be within those of the lower jaw, but Dr. Reeves formed the opinion that Nature would be able to remedy that defect as the living child grew up. Dr. Reeves insisted that *the operation for cleft-palate should be performed as early as possible after birth, when the bones were in their softest condition.* He suggested that the edges of the fissure should be pared, and that by the padded blades of the horseshoe-shaped clamp the maxillary bones should be slowly brought together. He does not appear to have performed this operation on a living infant, and his suggestion seems to have been lost sight of, but if, as is probable, this treatment of congenital cleft-palate is to be adopted, it is right that his suggestion should have due acknowledgment.

It was through the published works of Dr. Brophy of Chicago that my attention was first called to the method, and I have every reason for speaking well of it.

Time for operating. Inasmuch as cleft-palate is an arrested development, the gap ought to be closed at the earliest possible moment, and the most favourable time for operating upon it is between the age of two weeks and three months. Brophy is probably right in affirming that at this age there is less shock from the operation because the nervous system is in a rudimentary condition; and, certainly, the sooner the muscles of the soft palate are enabled to work with a definite scheme of vocalization in view the more perfect will the voice eventually become. It is a generally recognized and disappointing fact that when operation is undertaken at a later age, though the gap in the palate may be completely closed, only a slight improvement in vocalization may take

271

place. Still, if a new-born infant be badly nourished and ill-suited for the struggle for existence, it would be wrong to submit him to any operation. He should be wrapped in wool, rubbed daily with cod-liver oil, and brought into a satisfactory state of health before the cleft is dealt with.

Once more, therefore, if it be admitted that distinct vocalization depends upon the anatomical integrity of the soft palate, the earlier that a cleft is repaired the better: it should certainly be done before the hare-lip is operated on.

Some surgeons are still in favour of postponing operation upon the palate until the child has passed the age of infancy. But the earlier the cleft is closed the better will be the voice, and if the hare-lip be dealt with before the palate the surgeon has less room for operating on the palate. One argument raised in favour of operating first on the lip is that the mother may not be subjected to the constant grief of seeing her child's serious disfigurement. But if it be explained to the mother that the delay in operating on the lip is advised in the child's interest, she will be likely to take a reasonable view of the question. The physical well-being of the child must not be sacrificed to the sentiment of the mother. Certain it is that if the lip were closed the infant would still have to be brought up by a large-teat bottle or by spoon-feeding. It is further advised by some who are in favour of doing the lip-operation first that if, when the child has attained the age of two years or so and the surgeon is about to deal with the palate, the mouth is so small that there is not room for the gag, the lip can be divided so as to get rid of that difficulty. But those who have made themselves familiar with the operation on the palate by thrusting the maxillæ together, will be able to appreciate the great help which is given in the subsequent repair of the lip when the maxillæ and their labial coverings have been brought together. It is all in favour of a good appearance being given to the hare-lip if the cleft-palate be dealt with by first approaching the maxillæ to each other.

Blair states that it is very essential that the surgeon should cover his mouth and nose with thick gauze to protect the patient from the breath and mucus cast off during speech.

Operation. The operation by pressure consists in thrusting the two superior maxillary bones together and then adjusting with sutures the vivified edges of the cleft. Brophy maintains that in cleft-palate cases the roof of the mouth is excessive in diameter by just the width of the cleft, and that after the maxillæ have been thrust together and the palatine processes united, the development of the alveolar processes becomes normal, and that when the teeth of the superior maxillæ which have been shifted inwards by the radical operation are erupted they will exactly meet those of the lower jaw. One of the important features of

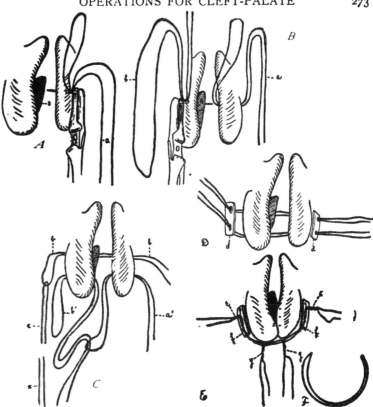

FIG. 126. APPROXIMATING THE MAXILLÆ BY THROUGH-AND-THROUGH WIRES.
A, first step, placing a heavy silk loop through one maxilla posteriorly. B, second
step. placing a heavy silk loop through the other maxilla posteriorly. C, anteriorly is shown how one loop (a) is passed over the ends of a second loop (b).
By drawing on the (a) loop, the (b) loop is made to traverse both maxillæ; (b)
shows loop in position with wire; (c) ready to be drawn in place. D, showing
two double wires in position, threaded at each end on a lead plate (d). If single
wires are used, No. 20 is the proper size, while No. 22 or 24 is used double. E,
this shows the maxillæ approximated. This is done by pressing the bones together
and taking up the slack by twisting appropriate wires. The approximation of
the alveolar part of the cleft is made more sure by bringing two of the wires
around the intermaxillary bone and twisting them at (g-g). The extra posterior
wire is discarded if not needed. F, the needle used in piercing the maxillæ is
what is known as ⅝ circle, reverse-eyed Hagedorn. Two sizes are used; one of
a circle the size of a nickel and the other of a circle the size of a quarter.
Usually some of the broad cutting point is ground off. (Blair, *International
Clinics.*)

this operation is that the halves of the soft palate so brought together can be sutured without interference with the muscles of the palate, the prospects of securing a natural voice being thereby greatly increased. And just as the approximation of the hinder part of the maxillary processes gives assistance in the repair of the soft palate, so does the ap-

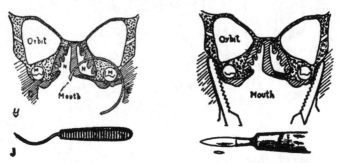

Fig. 127. G, An accurate diagrammatic Reproduction of a Section of a Frozen Head of an Infant with a Single Cleft of the Palate. This illustrates how a ⅝-circle needle can be made to pass from the upper buccal fornix, through the jaw-bone, along the floor of the orbit and into the cleft. H, showing position of the jaws of the forceps in forceful approximation of the maxillæ. I, Brophy needle. Dr. Brophy has two of these made, right and left. The shank of this needle is shorter than the original instrument. The use of Brophy's needle is simpler than the author's method, but the latter insures placing the wires at a higher level in the jaw, *i.e.*, above the tooth buds. J, double-edged knife occasionally used in cutting the maxilla. The knife is thrust high into the body of the bone through a small mucous opening, and moved forward and backward in the bone. (Blair, *International Clinics.*)

proximation of their anterior part simplify the subsequent operation on the hare-lip.

The operation is begun by raising the cheek. A strong needle on a handle is then thrust through the maxilla just behind the malar process of the superior maxilla, and above the level of the horizontal process of the palate bone. This needle carries a thick silk pilot-suture through to the cleft, and its loop is pulled down towards the mouth. Then the needle is similarly passed through the opposite maxilla, the loop being brought down as before. This second loop is passed through the first, which, being drawn upon, is made to bring the second loop out through the maxilla and across the nasal fossa. The suture then is horizontal. The sharply-bent end of a thick silver wire is then hooked on to this loop, and, by pulling on the latter, the wire is made to take its place.

The wire suture thus lies above the horizontal processes of the palate bones, where it can be seen through the cleft. Similarly, a wire suture is taken through the maxillæ above the front part of the cleft. Two small, oblong leaden plates, with a hole drilled near each end, are then laid along the outside of the right maxilla, under the cheek, the end of the hinder wire being passed through the posterior hole and the end of the front wire through the anterior hole. The right ends of the wires are then twisted together from left to right, the plates being closely applied against the maxilla, and after this the twisted ends of the wires are pressed flat. The ends of the wires under the left cheek are then similarly treated, and as they are being twisted up the maxillæ are firmly squeezed together. If, however, they are too solidly fixed to be moved towards each other, the bones themselves must be divided by a scalpel sufficiently to enable the surgeon to force their palatine processes into the middle line. In this way the width of the gap in the lip is greatly reduced and the lateral halves of the soft palate come together. Fine sutures are then passed through the freshened borders of the entire cleft. After the maxillæ have been thrust together, the wires extending between the leaden plates have to be tightened up. These wires and plates are not disturbed for three or four weeks. Some superficial ulceration may take place beneath or against the borders of the plates, but it is not of importance. The wires and plates may be removed after about the third week.

When the prolabium and the incisive bone are so advanced and isolated that the surgeon is unable to make use of them, he must remove them; but it should always be his endeavour to save them. Sometimes the projection can be thrust into position only by bending down the tip of the nose, and when it has become firmly attached in its new position the connexion with the nose may be divided; or it may be found that after the removal of a triangular piece from the septum the prolabium comes easily into position.

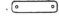

Fig. 128. Lead Plate for supporting Wire Sutures. Actual size.

It is not desirable to free the maxillæ by cutting into them, and fracture of the alveolar process is to be avoided. For these reasons the operation is seldom advisable after three months. In doing this operation the writer now makes no attempt to close completely, or even materially to narrow, the posterior part of the cleft in the hard palate, since it is unnecessary, and a strenuous effort to do so is hazardous. In this adjustment of the palate, whether it is for a single or double cleft, the premaxillary part should be placed well in front of and not to the mesial side of the maxillary portion of the alveolus. In a single cleft the maxillary bones are to be pushed toward each other and the protruding premaxilla brought to lie somewhat in front of the short maxillary process. No bone-cutting is required. In the double, complete cleft, where the premaxilla stands out on the end of the nasal septum, it is usually advisable to make an oblique, single, submucous cut, or a submucous removal of 5 mm. of the lower border of the septum, so as to allow the premaxilla to drop back into contact with the maxilla. However, this cut in the septum should not be made until it is determined that the anterior end of the maxillary processes can be sufficiently approximated to ensure the premaxilla of resting in front of the maxillae and not dropping back into the cleft. If this cannot be done, then it is probably better practice not to cut the nasal septum but, after pushing the premaxilla as far back as possible with thumb pressure, to free the cheeks and alæ of the nose from the maxillary bones by undercutting and to make the repair of the lips over the cleft.

After three months the Brophy operation is seldom advisable. The lip may be repaired over the alveolar cleft, but as Blair has shown after operation the alveolar cleft may close rapidly from the lip pressure or it may remain open indefinitely. Better results are obtained where teeth are present by approximating the maxilla and the premaxilla by orthodontic appliances. Considerable tissue may be gained in a single cleft-palate by including some of the muco-periosteum of the septum with the palate flap.

Mr. Arbuthnot Lane is also an advocate of the palate being operated on before the lip, and he prefers to operate on the palate when the infant is five weeks old. He raises a flap of muco-periosteum, and, turning it over like a page of a book, tucks its free border in between the bone and the muco-periosteum of the other side, having previously made ready the groove for its reception by detaching the muco-periosteum for about a quarter of an inch. The soft palate he treats in like manner, splitting it and turning it over, and suturing it to the other side, which he has already vivified by a little splitting and unfolding. The splitting and suturing of the flaps are done with special knives and needles.

STAPHYLORRHAPHY AFTER INFANCY

Preparation. In the case of a child with cleft-palate who has passed beyond infancy, the sooner that the operation is undertaken the better. But before this is done the child must be duly prepared. Carious teeth should be extracted, or cleaned and filled; enlarged tonsils should be amputated, and adenoids cleared away, and the mouth made as healthy as possible. And it may be well for the nurse to wash the mouth with a hand-spray of some mild antiseptic, so that after the operation, when its use is highly desirable, the child may not be alarmed by it.

Operation. The operating-table should be between 3½ and 4 feet high (inclusive of a firm mattress), and quite narrow, so that the assistant may also be able to see into the mouth. The instruments should be laid on another table of the same height, and should be arranged upon an aseptic cloth from left to right in the order in which the surgeon is likely to use them. They should not be placed in any lotion. The most convenient anæsthetic is chloroform, given on a flannel mask, which, later on, is changed for a Junker's apparatus. The chloroformist should not be called upon to help in the operative work; he has enough to occupy his thoughts and his hands. The child ought to be only just 'under'; the anæsthetist should be able to feel that at any moment, if need be, he could wake him up. The operator should not object to the child making purposeless movements from time to time, as he then knows that his patient is 'upon the safe side.' If the breathing becomes embarrassed the surgeon should stop and see if a change in the position of the head, or of the gag, may improve matters.

The best position for the child during the operation is upon the back, with the head hanging over the end of the table, so that the blood may escape by the mouth or nostrils. This position, however, sometimes hinders the breathing; still, it should be tried in every case. It often happens that after the operation the child vomits blood; and sometimes when there has been little or no vomiting, the first motion passed after the operation is tarry, some blood having found its way into the alimentary canal in spite of the child having been kept inverted during the operation.

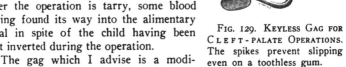

FIG. 129. KEYLESS GAG FOR CLEFT-PALATE OPERATIONS. The spikes prevent slipping even on a toothless gum.

The gag which I advise is a modification of Sir Thomas Smith's (Fig. 129).

The raspatories, which should be slender, are made of steel, and about eight inches long, with the ends in different curves for suitable or variously pitched arches. The ordinary steel aneurysm needle makes a very useful raspatory. The swabs can be made of tufts of absorbent cotton-wool loosely tied up in gauze. They should vary in size from a cherry to a plum. They should be used dry.

The most convenient needle for a cleft-palate operation is the tubular one, with a reel containing an abundant supply of fine silver wire. At the end of the needle is an arrangement by which one of the curved, sharp points can be rigidly fixed; the wire is made to run through it by the movement of a small wheel upon the handle. The points are of various curves and sizes, and, being round, do not cut the flaps (see Fig. 130).

As already stated, the best time for operating on a cleft-palate is within the first few weeks after birth. But it may happen that the child has passed that age when he is brought for operation. Assuming, then, that he is in a good state of health and that his mouth is clean, he is placed upon the table for operation. The child being under chloroform, the surgeon passes a long suture through the tip of the tongue and gently pulls it forward, so that when the gag is fixed the tongue may not block the air-way.

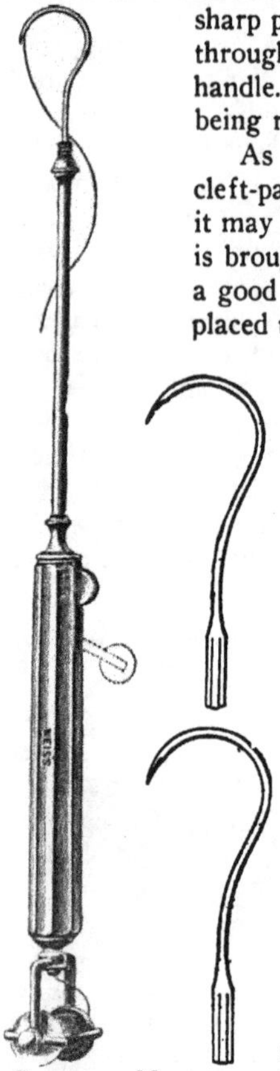

A strip of mucous membrane having been removed from each side of the cleft, incisions are made close near the teeth, passing down to the bone, as shown in Fig. 131.

Some children bleed much more than others. Bleeding may, as a rule, be quickly stopped by firm pressure with a dry swab. The closer that these incisions are made to the teeth the less t h e chance of wounding branches of the descending palatine artery, the broader will be the flaps, and the less

FIG. 130. MECHANICAL NEEDLES FOR CLEFT-PALATE OPERATIONS.

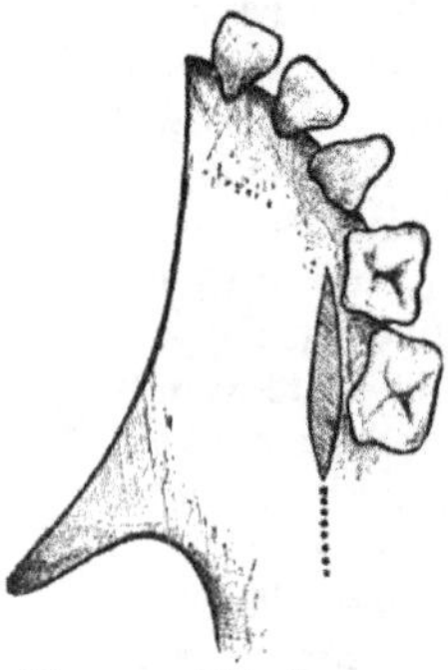

FIG. 131. THE INCISION MADE NEAR THE ALVEOLAR PROCESS THROUGH WHICH THE FLAP OF MUCO-PERIOSTEUM IS DETACHED.

the likelihood of their blood-supply being seriously interfered with. Then, by raspatories introduced through these incisions, the muco-periosteum is detached from the hard palate. The higher the pitch of the roof the greater is the probability of the flaps being brought together without tension. Indeed, in some cases of high roofs, the flaps are so slack that not only their bare edges but some of their raw upper surfaces can be brought together, which much increases the chance of securing prompt union. But they do not often come together without some tension; this is because they are continuous with the velum which is firmly connected with the hard palate. In the velum is an aponeurosis which, attached to the border of the hard palate, receives part of the insertion of the tensor palati and the levator palati. and this aponeurosis must be detached before the velum can be moved inwards. Success largely depends upon the thoroughness with which the disconnexion of the aponeurosis is made. It is best done by passing one blade of a pair of scissors (bent on the flat almost to a right angle) between the detached muco-periosteum and the under surface of the back of the hard palate, and the other through the cleft and over the back of the velum, as shown in Fig. 132. Thus between the blades are placed the mucous membrane which is continued from the floor of the nasal fossa and the aponeurosis of the soft palate, together with that part of the tendon of the tensor palati which is inserted into the palate bone. When this scissor-cut has been made, the muco-periosteum and velum hang loose, and the flaps are ready for suturing. When the surgeon has

passed the sutures through the flaps, he may find so much tension upon the edges of the flaps that he deems it best to twist up the sutures only loosely. Later, when he has increased the length of the lateral incisions, he may tighten them up permanently with torsion-forceps. And so that he may know in which way he should twist to tighten, he should make it a rule always to twist from left to right, as in dealing cards. If it be found that, as the flaps are drawn together, there is still so much tension that. if the silver sutures were fully twisted up, either the wire

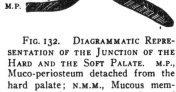

FIG. 132. DIAGRAMMATIC REPRESENTATION OF THE JUNCTION OF THE HARD AND THE SOFT PALATE. M.P., Muco-periosteum detached from the hard palate; N.M.M., Mucous membrane passing on to the floor of the nares; P.A., Aponeurosis of the soft palate; s, Blade of curved scissors about to cut through the aponeurosis and the membrane.

would break or cut its way through the flap, he must prolong the incisions backwards well into the halves of the velum, as is indicated by the dotted line on Fig. 131. The incisions thus made sever the aponeurotic insertion of the tensor palati and the chief part of the insertion of the levator palati.

Experience shows that however wide a cleft of the hard and soft palate may be, it is advisable to operate upon the entire cleft at one time rather than divide the operation into two parts, one for the hard palate and one for the soft. In certain cases of wide cleft of the hard palate of a grown child, the bone may be cut about ¼ inch from the gap on each side and the flaps of bone and mucous membrane shifted together, the vivified edges being adjusted by sutures. After the operation, and before the gag is removed, it is a good plan (the head still being dependent) to send several syringefuls of warm water up the nostrils. This clears away all clots and gives a free air-way.

In those cases in which the muco-periosteal flaps have been destroyed completely by previous operation, the roof of the mouth may

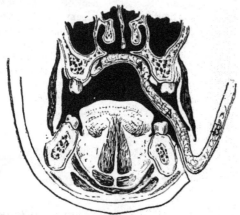

Fig. 133. Diagram illustrating a Flap (aaa), which has been raised from the Side of the Neck and, still attached to the Cheek (b), can be brought through an Incision in the Lower Buccal Fornix and laid in a Palate Defect. It can be seen that this flap could be used for lining a cheek, instead of a palate defect. Flap is cut after union has taken place. (Blair, *Oral Surgery*.)

be restored by a flap from some extraneous source, *e.g.*, cheek, forehead, neck or finger (see Figs. 133 and 134).

After-treatment. When this is all done, and the gag and the tongue suture are removed, the child should be so placed that the saliva, blood, and mucus may dribble out of the mouth without having the chance of entering the larynx or œsophagus. In the case of an infant, the nurse had better keep him in her arms for a while, with the face directed downwards. But if he is too heavy to be thus nursed, he should be put in the half-sitting position, and partly turned to one side, with the head bent down, so that the discharges may dribble into a towel

If the child be collapsed it may be necessary to keep his head low and to give an enema of hot water with a little brandy. He should have nothing by the mouth for several hours, but when the nausea has apparently passed off, small quantities of beef jelly may be given in a teaspoon: jelly slips down easily and is preferable to milk; it does not form curds in the stomach and it is easily absorbed. This should be supplemented by rectal feeding. In the course of a day or so a little sweetened orange-juice, pulped strawberries or peaches, chicken or meat which has been run through a fine sieve, bread and milk, or soft custard pudding may be given. Fresh, home-made beef jelly, broth, and all

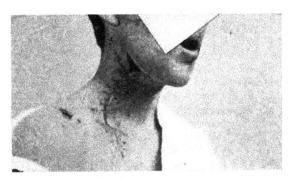

FIG. 134. SHOWS NECK DEFECT ALMOST ENTIRELY OBLITERATED BY DRAWING THE SKIN EDGES TOGETHER. The upper triangular defect still remaining is closed with the pedicle of the flap, after it is cut and withdrawn from the mouth. (Blair, *Oral Surgery*.)

other foods for children are far better than the various meat essences, extracts, and juices supplied by the shops.

Possibly the child will allow the nurse to use a mild antiseptic spray for the mouth, but it should not be persisted in if it frightens him. As regards the fluid for irrigation, sanitas and water, a very mild solution of Condy's fluid, or a solution of boracic acid with glycerine and eau-de-Cologne, answers well. It is unnecessary for the surgeon to remove the sutures; they will quietly ulcerate their way out. This refers, of course, only to the fine wire and horsehair sutures, not to those more solid ones of silver wire which pass through the maxillæ and the lead plates in the radical operation of infancy as described on p. 272.

Complications. If, by chance, severe hæmorrhage should set in, the gag must be reintroduced and search made for the bleeding vessel. All clots should be removed, and the mouth and naso-pharynx should be syringed out with warm water, the head being in the over-extended position. This might suffice to arrest the bleeding. If it does not, and the bleeding is seen to be from one of the lateral incisions, a long strip of gauze dipped in a solution of adrenalin should be gently stuffed through the gap, and to the back of the velum, and the soft palate should be gently thrust up against this packing by means of a dry pad of gauze on a holder. Chloroform may be again required.

Sometimes, in spite of every precaution, septic inflammation attacks the mouth. The child then looks ill and yellowish, his temperature goes up, and his breath becomes foul. But with all this against it the operation need not prove a failure. Some part of the cleft generally remains closed, and granulation-tissue in due course fills up more of it; and as soon as healthy granulations cover the surfaces (which will be in about a fortnight) the child will probably have undergone auto-immunization, and the operation may have some final touches given to it with a good prospect of a complete success being obtained. A perforation remaining after a not entirely successful operation may of itself close with time; at any rate, it will become much smaller. A hole as large as a pea may, perhaps, be seen at the junction of the hard and soft palate after the performance of an otherwise successful operation. If so, after some months, the introduction of the slender blade of a thermo-cautery will be likely to complete its obliteration.

Results. As already insisted on, the narrower the cleft and the earlier the date at which it is closed the more perfect will be the speech; the closure of a wide cleft in late childhood brings but slight improvement to the voice. Subsequent improvement depends to a large extent upon the attention which the parents devote to teaching the child to pronounce distinctly. The child should be shown the movement of the lips and tongue of the teacher when the difficult words are being pronounced, and he should be made to imitate them over and over again. A person accustomed to teaching deaf-mutes would give very helpful instruction.

If, after the performance of the pressure operation, the maxillary arch did not widen out sufficiently, this could be easily made right by a practical dentist. But even if it remained small, that defect would be more than counterbalanced by the fact that, owing to the approximation of the hinder ends of the maxillary processes, the surgeon had been enabled to form a soft palate without tension, and without interfering with the tensor and levator palati. One constantly found, after operating by the old method, that the velum was extremely tight and ill-adapted for the purpose of vocalization; but, of course, it was not left in that condition. It was relieved of tension by the method of Fergusson or Pollock, or in some other way. My own plan is to make a free incision from before backwards, with a very slender scalpel, through the velum near its lateral attachment, in fact by extending still further backwards the incision indicated by the dotted line in Fig. 131.

SECTION III

OPERATIONS UPON THE LIPS
FACE AND JAWS

PART II

OPERATIONS FOR CANCER OF THE
LIPS AND FACE

BY

G. LENTHAL CHEATLE, C.B., F.R.C.S. (Eng.),
Surgeon General, R.N.
Surgeon to King's College Hospital and to the Italian Hospital

CHAPTER III

OPERATIONS FOR CANCER OF THE LIPS AND FACE

GENERAL CONSIDERATIONS

In planning incisions for the excision of cancer from the front of the face there are four things to be considered:—

1. The writer has shown that a cancer originating in any part of the lips, angle of the mouth, or skin over the cartilaginous part of the nose, will always spread directly into the nasal and labial regions before it progresses in any other directions.

2. Wherever squamous epithelioma or rodent ulcer exists the growth has spread under the normal epithelium which surrounds the malignant ulcer; therefore the area of disease is greater than the size of the ulcer.

3. The cutaneous striated muscles of the face are in close anatomical relation to the dermic glandular structures and almost touch the basal layer of the epidermis. The relationship of these muscles to the skin is closest round the eyelids and mucous membrane of the lips. Not only will cancer invade these muscles in its earliest stages, but the writer has seen one particular muscle, the levator labii superioris alæque nasi (caput angulare), picked out as its only path of spread.

4. There are lymphatic glands on the face, in the submental, submaxillary, and anterior triangle regions, which must be removed; and where possible it is wise to remove *en bloc* the tissue which connects the lymphatic glands with the primary growth. To this necessity particular attention has been paid in describing the following operations.

In most cases of squamous epithelioma in the region of the lips, it is generally late in the disease that the lymphatic glands contain cancer-cells. The lymphatic glands may become enlarged quite early, but then their enlargement is generally due to a great proliferation of their endothelial cells, masses of which can be seen arranged among, and isolating patches of, the normal lymphoid tissue of the glands. Therefore, although glands may be enlarged in lip cancer, they are not necessarily cancer-bearing.

With regard to the group of lymphatic glands on the face there is no doubt that their presence is exceedingly variable. In the cases from which the writer excised cancer in the angle of the mouth, and removed with it the specified site of the buccinator group of lymphatic glands, he could not find any trace of a lymphatic gland during a most careful dissection of the excised parts. In one case a microscopical examination was made of the whole parts removed; it revealed total absence of lymphatic glands in this region.

The question will have to be considered whether it is advisable to remove the glands at the time the main lesion is excised. The benefit gained by removing the growth and its attached lymphatic glands at one operation is that it is possible to excise the diseased skin with its lymphatic vessels and glands *en bloc,* and hence to occasion less risk of cell-transplantation. The disadvantages are that the tissues, in which lie the lymphatic glands, are opened during the course of a septic operation.

The writer has come to the conclusion that if great care in the details of antiseptic work be observed and good drainage be subsequently provided, no great harm can occur should both stages be done at the same operation. This statement also applies to that state of affairs when the growth and the glands cannot be removed *en bloc.*

However, should it be decided to do one part first, it would be better to remove the glands first, and, later, to attack the main disease, because the glandular parts of the operation heal by first intention and no valuable time would be lost before removing the primary focus. On the other hand, should the primary focus be removed first, the period of healing would be longer in certain cases because it would remain septic for a longer period, which would delay the completion of the work.

The operations for cancer of the lips will be described first.

Preliminary measures. To avoid repetition of precautions common to all cases it is necessary to state that (1) the mouth must be cleaned with a carbolic mouth wash, 1–60 carbolic acid lotion, or some antiseptic solution daily for a week before operation. All decayed teeth must be stopped and stumps extracted. This is easily done in cases of small cancer, but in advanced cases in which the teeth cannot be cleaned nor the mouth opened, except by inducing exquisite pain, no great antiseptic preparation can be made until the anæsthetic has been administered and the diseased parts removed; then it is quite worth while to interrupt the operation to scrape and clean the teeth and to extract stumps. Before proceeding with the removal of lymphatic glands and formation of skin flaps, care should be taken to remove all soiled instruments, towels, sponges, and gloves which have been used in this part of the preparation, and to protect raw surfaces from septic contamination.

(2) When practicable, before beginning the operation, the writer advises that the ulcerated part of the cancer should be cauterized by a suitable cautery at a dull red heat until the surface of the ulcer becomes of a leathery consistence and all hæmorrhage stops. This is a precaution

taken against the possibility of transplanting malignant cells of the tumour upon the fresh cut surfaces of the normal parts. The danger of transplantation is further diminished by treating the parts to be removed with the utmost gentleness, so that cancer-cells are not squeezed from their positions on to other parts, and care should be taken that the ulcer does not touch the cut surfaces of the normal tissues during the manipulations which are necessary for its removal. Each operation will be described as far as possible in three stages: (1) the removal of the growth; (2) the removal of the lymphatic vessels and glands; (3) the plastic stage.

OPERATIONS UPON THE LOWER LIP

Cancer usually spreads along the margin of the lip, but more rarely it spreads downwards to a greater degree than usual before it eventually curls round the angle of the mouth to reach the upper lip. The importance of this observation is that in early cases it is impossible to say in which of the two directions the cancer is mainly spreading. Hence it is advisable that the incisions should be so planned as to include both paths of spread.

First stage. If a small cancer be situated midway between the angle of the mouth and the centre of the lip (see Fig. 135), two incisions should be made, one external to it and the other internal. The incisions should begin at least three-quarters of an inch away from the edge of the ulcer. The external incision is carried downwards and slightly outwards through all the

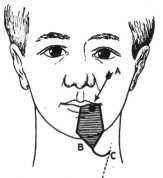

FIG. 135. INCISIONS FOR THE REMOVAL OF A SMALL CANCER, A, MIDWAY BETWEEN THE ANGLE OF THE MOUTH AND THE CENTRE OF THE LOWER LIP.

structures of the lip down to bone, and ends at the lower margin of the inferior maxilla. The internal incision is carried downwards and slightly inwards through all the structures down to bone, and ends at the lower margin of the inferior maxilla. The ends of these two incisions are united by two converging incisions which meet at a point midway between the lower margin of the inferior maxilla and the hyoid bone, and are only skin deep (see Fig. 135). The mucous membrane and muscles included in the lip incisions are cut away from the jaw as close as possible to the bone.

The cancer-containing tissue is not cut away from its fascia and platysma attachments, which will be taken away *en bloc* with the lymphatic glands. But before passing on to the next stage it is completely enveloped in a thick layer of cyanide gauze which has been wrung out of a 1–20 solution of carbolic acid.

Second stage. The lymphatic glands are then dealt with by undercutting the internal flap as far as the submental glands on each side so that all the glands in this region can be removed. The submaxillary and anterior triangle regions are exposed by means of a curved incision with its convexity downwards, and which starts at B (see Fig. 135), that is to say, from the point at which the converging incisions meet, and ends at the anterior border of the sterno-mastoid muscle, C (see Fig. 135). The flap is held upwards and backwards and the submaxillary lymphatic glands are removed, a process which is rendered easier by the removal of the submaxillary salivary gland with the facial artery and vein. If sufficient room has not been obtained for the efficient removal of lymphatic glands in the anterior triangle, an incision is made which extends downwards as far as necessary from the point C (see Fig. 135).

Third stage. In order to join the lip without tension on the stitches, the internal and external flaps must be freely divided from their attachments to the lower jaw. The parts are then stitched together and two drainage tubes are inserted, one at B and the other at C (see Fig. 135).

When a small squamous epithelioma is growing on the middle of the lower lip, the incisions are lateral and must begin at least three-quarters of an inch away from the edge of the ulcer. They are carried through all structures downwards and slightly outwards to the inferior margin of the lower jaw, and are ended in the same way as those just described in the first operation, and instead of removing the lymphatic glands from one side only, this is done on both sides by means of incisions similarly planned.

Results. The resulting deformity is not so great as would be imagined from so extensive a removal of tissue; in any case the importance of removing cancer is greater than that of leaving a picturesque appearance.

It will be observed that the V-shaped incisions, which are up to the present usually adopted for the removal of cancer from the lower lip, are not advised in this article, because they converge towards the cancer and cut across the possibly cancer-bearing tract which leads from the cancer to the lymphatic glands. The writer considers that the so-called recurrence of cancer in the lip is due to the dangerous positions of these V-shaped incisions.

That the writer is justified in attempting to expel the V-shaped incisions from surgery in connexion with cancer in this region can be seen in the figures published by Mr. C. W. Rowntree which he collected from the records of the Middlesex Hospital. Mr. Rowntree noted 126 cases of cancer of the lower lip. In the majority of instances the growth had been removed by means of the simple V-shaped incision. There were seventy cases of recurrence, in forty of which the growth had recurred in the lip.

OPERATIONS UPON THE ANGLE OF THE MOUTH

First stage. To remove a small cancer from this part the first incision is made internal to the tumour and through the lower lip; it begins at least three-quarters of an inch from the edge of the ulcer and is continued downwards and slightly inwards as far as the lower margin of the inferior maxilla, and must cut through all structures down to bone (see Fig. 136). From this point the incision is carried through skin only, horizontally backwards along the lower margin of the inferior maxilla until it nearly reaches the anterior edge of the masseter muscle.

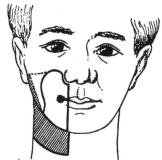

The incision in the upper lip begins at least three-quarters of an inch from the ulcer's edge and is carried vertically upwards through all structures as far as the nose, around the ala of which it curves (see Fig. 136). It is not necessary to remove any part of the ala. It is then carried in a semicircle, the convexity of which is upwards, through

FIG. 136. INCISIONS FOR THE REMOVAL OF A CANCER AT THE ANGLE OF THE MOUTH.

all the structures of the cheek down to the bone, and at least three-quarters of an inch from the periphery of the ulcer until it reaches the anterior border of the masseter muscle.

The terminations of these two incisions are then joined by a curved incision, the convexity of which is directed backwards (see Fig. 136). The attachments of the parts enclosed within these incisions are then divided, care being taken not to cut through the parts left adherent to the structures below the jaw, so that they may be removed with the lymphatic vessels and glands when they are taken away.

Before proceeding with the next stage, the disease-containing flap (which has been detached everywhere except at its lower margin) must be wrapped in thick layers of cyanide gauze wrung out of 1–20 solution of carbolic acid.

Second stage. The next step is to remove the lymphatic glands *en bloc* and at the same time to keep in view the formation of a flap to cover the gap that has been created. The submental, submaxillary, and anterior triangle lymphatic glands are easily exposed as follows: Continue the vertical incision in the lower lip downwards to the level of the hyoid bone, and carry it back to the middle of the sterno-mastoid. Turn back the flap thus marked out, and keep it protected in cyanide gauze. The region which contains the submaxillary and anterior triangle lymphatic glands is thus exposed, but to remove the submental glands of both sides the skin covering the chin and upper parts of the neck must be undercut past the middle line and held there by a retractor. It will be seen that these incisions will include the supramaxillary and buccinator groups of lymphatic glands on the face.

Third stage. The final stage is to cover the gap left by the removal of so much of the cheek tissues.

This is easily performed by sewing the flap (marked by the shaded area in Fig. 136) up to the cheek, the mucous membrane and the skin of the normal lower lip. The raw surface of the upper lip is sewn to the side of the cheek near the ala of the nose. In order to prevent puckering, and to make the flap lie nicely in its new position, it will be necessary to excise the V-shaped piece of skin from the cheek, which is marked by dots in Fig. 136, before attempting to place the flap in its final position. The flap must be well attached to the cheek and lip of the opposite side by many closely-placed interrupted stitches. The writer has never seen a salivary fistula result from this operation.

It is hardly necessary to point out that the transplantation of the flap leaves a raw surface on the neck below it. If the skin of the neck be undercut it can be brought up and stitched to the inferior margin of the flap without fear of undue tension.

Two tubes should be inserted, one at the lowest part of the wound in the middle line, and one at the posterior and inferior angle of the wound.

OPERATIONS UPON THE UPPER LIP

There are four anatomical conditions which complicate the spread of cancer in this region, and which do not concern cancers in the lower lip or angle of the mouth.

1. The early spread along the alveolar margin of the upper jaw, particularly when the disease begins in, or spreads into, the central part of the lip. The upper lip at this part is naturally shorter than elsewhere.

and the lip is made smaller by the contracting newly-formed connective tissue which encircles and pervades cancer. Atrophy of the normal tissue will also accentuate the diminution in the natural size of the lip.

2. The relation of the disease to the alæ nasi and columella. When cancer begins in the upper lip, the columella is more invaded than the alæ nasi. The septal origin of the orbicularis oris forms an easy pathway by which the disease reaches the columella.

3. The extensive area and importance of the tissues that intervene between the lymphatic glands in the parotid and submaxillary regions render it necessary to run the risk of not removing the area and glands *en bloc,* as has been advised in the two operations just described.

4. Until more trustworthy evidence is available the writer advises that the parotid glands should be left out of the question in removing small cancers from the upper lip, that is to say, unless these glands are enlarged; then of course it would be wise to remove them.

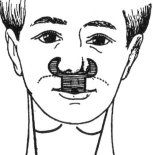

FIG. 137. INCISIONS FOR THE REMOVAL OF A CANCER IN THE CENTRE OF THE UPPER LIP. The thick lines in the neck show the incisions for removal of the glands.

The necessary steps to remove a small cancer in the centre of the upper lip are as follows: First make two lateral incisions, which must include all the structures of the lip and which start at least three-quarters of an inch away from the edge of the ulcer and are carried vertically upwards from these points to the level of the ala nasi of each side. The ends of these two incisions are then continued into the cheek, by curving them outwards; these outwardly curved incisions are to terminate at the groove which marks the junction of the ala with the side of the nose (see Fig. 137), and all the structures must be included. The two incisions are then joined by a cut, which becomes transverse after curving round the grooves formed by the junction of the cheek with the ala nasi of each side. In the transverse part of this incision, the base of the columella should be also removed and the septal origin of the orbicularis oris must be detached. By adopting these measures the shaded part of the diagram (see Fig. 137) will be removed; the levator labii superioris alæque nasi (caput angulare) does not come into important relation with a small cancer of this part of the lip. A new upper lip can be formed as follows: Make on each side an incision an inch and a half long which starts from the lateral incision at a point where the upward direction of it ceases and the curved portion begins (see dotted lines in Fig. 137), and carry it downwards and outwards through all the structures, and end when it reaches the centre of the buccinator muscles. This incision must not involve Stenson's duct, the orifice of which can be seen in the mouth and easily avoided. These lateral incisions, besides forming half a new lip, will also enable the surgeon to look for, and remove, if present, the buccinator group of lymphatic glands. The free ends of the new lip thus formed can be sutured across the middle line, and finally the cheeks can be sutured to the alæ nasi. These steps are rendered easy by thoroughly and extensively undercutting the attachments of the cheeks to bone. It will be necessary to remove the submaxillary and the supramaxillary lymphatic glands of both sides; this can be done by making suitable incisions in the submaxillary and anterior triangle regions on both sides (see Fig. 137).

The necessary steps to excise a small cancer growing in the centre of one side of the upper lip are as follows (see Fig. 138) :—

An internal incision, which begins at least three-quarters of an inch from the edge of the ulcer, is made vertically upwards, as far as the columella or nostrils as the case may be, through all structures down to the bone. An external incision is carried through all structures down to the bone obliquely upwards and outwards from a point at least three-quarters of an inch from the edge of the ulcer towards the external canthus of the eye, but ends when it reaches the level of the groove which marks the junction of the ala with the side of the nose. This incision is made obliquely outwards to include the zygomaticus minor muscle (caput zygomaticum). The third incision joins the two previous ones by passing transversely inwards through all structures down to the bone, and extends from the end of the second incision to the junction of the ala with the side of the nose. This must be made to include the attachments to bone of the levator labii superioris (caput infraorbitale), the levator anguli oris (caninus), and the zygomaticus minor (caput zygomaticum) muscles; it cuts across the continuity of the fibres of the levator labii superioris alæque nasi (caput angulare). It will also include the lymphatic glands which may be found in the naso-genial groove. The incision is then continued downwards in the groove formed by the junction of the ala with the cheek, and ends by cutting across the junction of the upper lip with the nose, so as to include half the base of the columella and the septal origin of the orbicularis oris. The incisions include the shaded portion in Fig. 138. The remaining half of the lip must be the great source of supply for the tissues which are to cover the gap thus made; all its attachments to bone and to the base of the nose must be divided, and, to render it more adaptable, an elliptical piece of skin must be removed

from around the ala of the normal side (see Fig. 138). These proceedings will enable the remaining half of the lip to be drawn across the gap,
without interfering with the appearance of the nose. The upper lip can
be formed, and the buccinator glands can be sought for, and (if present)
removed, by making an incision, which includes all the structures of the
cheek and which starts from the external incision at the level of the junction of the ala with the lip, and ends, after running in a downward and
outward direction, over the centre of the buccinator muscle (see Fig.
138). This flap is then stitched to the opposite lip and, in order to prevent undue puckering at the angle of the mouth, it may be necessary to
make an incision into the cheek which is directed downwards and outwards from the angle of the mouth, parallel with the last incision (see
Fig. 138). In order to cover the interval between the nose and the cheek,
a third incision, parallel with the two just described, must be directed
backwards in the cheek from the top angle of the gap (see Fig. 138); the
tissues of the cheek thus separated must then be brought inwards and
stitched to the ala. These steps can be performed without undue tension
by extensively undercutting the attach-
ments of the cheek to the bone.

The lymphatic glands which can
always be found are the submaxillary
glands, into which lymphatics from the
upper lip drain, but before reaching
them the lymph-stream from the upper
lip may pass through the buccinator
and the supramaxillary groups.

The buccinator group has been
dealt with in describing the necessary
steps in the formation of the new lip
(see p. 293). The submaxillary group
is reached through an incision made
below the inferior border of the lower
jaw from below the symphysis to the
anterior border of the sterno-mastoid.

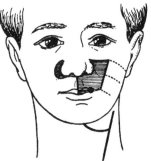

Fig. 138. Incisions for the
Removal of a Small Cancer in
the Centre of one Side of the
Upper Lip.

The supramaxillary glands can be
reached by dissecting up the upper edge of this incision, and exposing
them on the horizontal ramus of the jaw in front of the attachment of
the masseter. In cancers on one side of the upper lip the supramaxillary
and submaxillary glands of the same side must be removed. If the
glands of the normal side be enlarged they also must be excised.

In removing large cancers from the lips a combination and modification of these incisions and flaps can be easily planned. For instance,

when a cancer occupies the whole of the lower lip and the angles of the mouth, it means that the operation which has been described for the removal of cancer at the angle of the mouth is necessary, only it must be done on both sides, and one broad flap must be raised from the neck to take the place of the cancerous lower lip. This flap requires more support than is given it by the stitches which connect it with the sides of the cheeks, and the writer has successfully kept this large flap *in situ* by four tin-tacks hammered into the lower jaw. The operations upon large cancers of the lower lip and angle of the mouth which do not involve the inferior maxilla are more favourable from the point of view of cure than are those which occupy the upper lip, as the latter soon involve the nose and superior maxilla extensively; in the case of the lower lip the disease remains so localized that even when the lower jaw is affected its removal undisturbed within the areas of incision has resulted in cure in two of the writer's cases, that is to say, if six years and ten years respectively can be justly accounted cures.

OPERATIONS UPON THE FACE

Cancers at the inner or outer canthus of the eye must be removed on the lines described for excision of cancer at the angle of the mouth; in fact the distribution of cancer of the lower lid and angles of the eyelids very much resembles the spread of cancer in the lips. For instance, a cancer beginning in the lower lid near the free margin, or at the internal or external canthus, will occupy the area around the eyes and will include the upper lid before spreading to other parts; for this reason the writer advises diverging lines as in the mouth operations, if the edge of the lid must be removed. When the cancer occurs elsewhere on the eyelids it is essential to keep the incisions at least three-quarters of an inch away from the periphery of the growth, and to perform plastic operations according to the circumstances of each case.

When cancer appears in the forehead or sides of the face it is a wise plan to first excise the disease widely, that is to say, never to allow an incision to approach nearer the disease than a point three-quarters of an inch from its edge. All the incisions should go down to bone and all the soft structures must be removed. After the cancer has been taken away it is time to settle the best plan for covering the raw surface thus made.

The operator can get a good idea from where he can form his flap or in which direction he can sew up the wound, by picking up the skin, of the normal side, in various directions, and by so doing he can estimate where there is most available skin for his purpose, on the diseased side. (See Plastic Operations, Vol. I.)

With regard to the lymphatic glands which ought to be removed when cancer occurs in the regions of the forehead and eyelids, it may be stated that the lymphatic glands in the parotid region are the most usually affected. According to Sappey and Küttner the lymphatic vessels of the skin near the inner canthus of the eye drain directly into the submaxillary region.

SECTION III

OPERATIONS UPON THE LIPS
FACE AND JAWS

PART III

OPERATIONS UPON THE JAWS

BY

C. H. FAGGE, M.S. (Lond.), F.R.C.S. (Eng.),
Major, R.A.M.C.(T.)

Assistant Surgeon to Guy's Hospital

CHAPTER IV

OPERATIONS UPON THE UPPER JAW

COMPLETE REMOVAL OF THE UPPER JAW

Indications. (i) **Malignant new growths of the maxilla.** This operation is most commonly required when the bone is involved by a malignant growth, either primarily or secondarily; that is, one which in the former case arises from the periosteum, whereas in the latter it begins usually in the superjacent mucous membrane. These growths may be:

Sarcoma. Periosteal sarcoma of the maxilla is usually of the round or spindle-celled type and of rapid growth.

Carcinoma. The upper jaw may be involved by a squamous-celled carcinoma originating in the mucous membrane covering the hard palate or by a similar growth commencing in the gum, though here it is less frequently met with than in the lower jaw.

Another variety of epithelial malignant tumour involving the maxilla is a columnar-celled carcinoma, arising probably from the glands of the antral mucous membrane (Bolam, *Newcastle-upon-Tyne Journal of Path. and Bact.*, 1898, v, p. 65): owing to its destructive nature it has been called boring epithelioma (*épithélioma térébrant* of Réclus).

(ii) **Cancer of the naso-pharynx.** Excision of the upper jaw may be required for the removal of malignant tumours of the naso-pharynx. (See also Osteoplastic resection of the upper jaw, p. 314.)

(iii) **Odontomes and necrosis of the maxilla.** Complete removal of the upper jaw for either of these conditions is rarely called for.

Though no attempt has been made in this article to detail the points, consideration of which determines the presence of a malignant growth in the upper jaw, it cannot be superfluous to insist that even in the hands of the most experienced surgeon considerable difficulty may be met with in definitely diagnosing the presence of a malignant growth and in excluding the possibility that the antrum is distended with pus and granulation tissue.

In all cases where the slightest doubt exists as to the nature of the lesion, before an operation for removal of the maxilla is commenced an exploratory puncture should be made through the canine fossa into

the antrum with a trocar, and should this not supply sufficient information to determine the point, the opening should be enlarged with a
gouge.   When the material evacuated cannot be definitely stated to be
either inflammatory tissue or growth, it must be subjected to a microscopical examination before the patient is exposed to the risk of a possibly unnecessary removal of the maxilla.   Cases scattered through surgical literature impress upon us the importance of this preliminary
investigation, and show that mistakes have been made by surgeons of
repute even where the diagnosis has been apparently of no difficulty.

The selection of cases favourable for operation.   Before
undertaking so severe an operation it is necessary not only to inquire
into the history, but also to determine, by the presence or absence of
proptosis and by the freedom or limitation of movement of the eyeball,
whether the orbital plate has become involved or not; to examine the
palatal surface of the maxilla, and by anterior and posterior rhinoscopy
(or if the latter be impossible, by examination of the post-nasal space
with the finger) to determine as far as possible whether the growth has
extended beyond the limits of the maxilla.   Palpation of the hollows
above and below the zygoma will detect or exclude gross involvement of
the zygomatic and temporal fossæ, but it is well to remember that when
exposed in the course of an operation, such growths are often found to
extend further upwards or backwards than had been previously suspected.

Malignant tumours, commencing at the back of the jaw or in the
spheno-maxillary or pterygo-maxillary fossa, and secondarily affecting
the maxilla, usually give rise to protrusion of the eyeball at an early stage
and are clearly unsuitable for surgical interference.   Again, tumours of
rapid growth intensify the gravity of the prognosis, and as the malignant
infiltration in these cases readily extends upwards into the ethmoidal
cells, the walls of which are so thin as to offer but feeble resistance to its
extension, displacement outwards of the eyeball or swelling in the region
of the inner canthus, both suggestive of this complication, must be regarded as of grave significance.   However, it is well to bear in mind, as
Cheyne and Burghard (*Manual of Surgical Treatment*, Part V, p. 215)
point out, that, provided the tumour is of slow growth, the fact that the
eyeball is thus displaced does not render the case inoperable, because
the growth may fill up the ethmoidal cells without involving the bones,
and can therefore be eradicated without grave risk of recurrence.

Similar considerations apply to cases in which a mass of growth is
found on posterior rhinoscopy to fungate into the naso-pharynx.

Involvement of the skin of the face, while not in itself an absolute
contra-indication to operation, necessitates free removal of the soft parts
over the jaw if recurrence is to be avoided, and so usually results in

considerable deformity, which further plastic operations will probably only remedy incompletely. Consideration of each individual case will alone determine whether, under these circumstances, operation is justifiable, and before negativing operation the surgeon must make certain that the soft tissues are actually involved and not merely thinned and stretched over the growth while still movable upon it.

Secondary deposits in the submaxillary or cervical glands, resulting in so much enlargement that these are recognizable on digital examination before operation, may generally be taken as contra-indicating operation.

The cases which are most suitable for operation are those of some months' duration, arising either in the antrum or involving only one surface of the bone, and which, as far as physical examination can determine, have not extended into the adjacent cavities.

Besides the immediate and remote risks dealt with below, which are inseparable from such an operation usually undertaken in a patient beyond middle life, complete removal of the upper jaw possesses several disadvantages.

Of these the chief is the tendency of the eyeball to drop after losing the support of the orbital plate of the maxilla. This may be so marked that the affected eye may look downwards, and may not only become useless to the patient, but may cause considerable annoyance owing to the diplopia which results. When it is clear that the growth does not involve the orbital plate, this may be left, the operation being modified in the manner detailed below (see p. 310). When, however, removal of the orbital plate is essential in order to avoid the risk of recurrence, which is the chief consideration in all these operations, the ingenious plastic operation of König (see p. 309) may be employed. At the same time it is true that, provided the internal and external tarsal ligament—by which the suspensory ligament of Lockwood is supported—are not interfered with by too free removal of the nasal and malar processes respectively, sinking down of the eyeball is unlikely to be a serious complication.

A second disadvantage is that by removal of the hard palate the mouth is left in free communication with the nasal cavity. This may be overcome in a small proportion of cases by leaving the palatal process of the upper jaw when this is clearly not involved by the growth. In a greater number of cases even when it is deemed advisable to remove the bone in this situation, the muco-periosteum covering the hard palate may be peeled off, so that the above-mentioned disadvantage is eliminated.

While cases undoubtedly occur for which these modifications of the complete operation may be adopted, it is essential that the first consideration in the operator's mind must always be as free a removal of the malignant tumour as possible, which must never be departed from one iota for mere cosmetic considerations.

Operation. As before any other operation within the mouth all carious teeth must be removed and an antiseptic mouth-wash, such as hydrogen peroxide or chinosol (1 in 500), must be employed for several days in order to diminish the risk of oral sepsis as far as possible.

The patient is either placed in the supine position, with the head, unsupported by pillows, turned towards the affected side, or advantage will be gained by the adoption of the Trendelenburg position. Opinions are widely divided as to the advisability of performing a preliminary laryngotomy. Jacobson (*Operations of Surgery*, fifth edition, p. 483), who is in favour of this, points out that it is a much less severe operation than tracheotomy, and considers that the success of laryngotomy is due to its being performed through a fixed part of the air-passages and to the fact that the tube is removed as soon as the operation is finished. The writer's experience confirms the value of preliminary laryngotomy in eliminating the risk of inhalation pneumonia. Further, as the anæsthetic throughout the operation can be given from a Junker's apparatus through a rubber tube introduced into the laryngotomy tube, this procedure gives considerable freedom to the operator, who can carry out the operation without any fear of interfering with the anæsthetist. When preliminary laryngotomy is employed a large sponge is introduced into the pharynx, so as to block the upper laryngeal orifice completely, and this in itself considerably lessens the danger of pulmonary complications resulting from the inhalation of blood during the operation. When laryngotomy is not employed, these risks may be partially, but not so completely, overcome by plugging the naso-pharynx with a sponge. This, if large enough and firmly packed in position, will not tend to be dislodged, so as to cause any danger by being drawn into the air-passages. Some operators, however, advise that the sponge introduced into the naso-pharynx should be fastened to a long piece of silk or wire, the other end of which is secured externally.

Kocher (*Operative Surgery*, English translation, p. 102) recommends a preliminary ligature of the external carotid, pointing out that the high mortality, even in the present day, of excision of the upper jaw is largely due to hæmorrhage in patients whose vitality is insufficient, or to aspiration pneumonia, and that both of these dangers are diminished by this preliminary procedure. Jacobson (*loc. supra cit.*) quotes Dr. J. D. Bryant of New York as being in favour of it, especially in patients exhausted by hæmorrhage and cachexia, and himself recommends that it should be a routine part of the operation. The time taken up by this preliminary is more than repaid by relieving the assistants of much sponging, and by saving time in securing vessels; further, it enables the operator to see exactly what he is doing at every stage of the operation, so that he incurs less risk of leaving fragments of growth behind.

It is usually desirable to remove the glands, both at the angle of the jaw and those deeply situated in front of the sterno-mastoid on the same side. For this Kocher advises a curved incision running from the apex of the mastoid process downwards behind and below the angle of

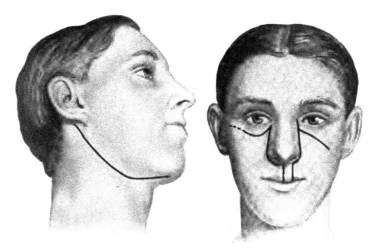

FIG. 139. INCISION FOR EXPOSING THE CONTENTS OF THE SUBMAXILLARY AND UPPER CERVICAL TRIANGLES.

FIG. 140. INCISIONS FOR REMOVAL OF THE UPPER JAW. Right side, Fergusson's; left side, Kocher's incision.

the jaw to the middle of the hyoid bone (see Fig. 139). He points out that in the course of removal of the submaxillary and deep cervical set of glands there is an excellent opportunity for ligature of the external carotid. This is carried out before the operation of laryngotomy, which necessitates some risk of infection of the hands and instruments.

For the removal of the upper jaw itself the classical incision of Fergusson is most suitable in the majority of cases (see Fig. 140).

In carrying this out the upper lip is divided in the middle line as far as the columella nasi. The incision is then carried downwards below the nostril, and passing in the sulcus between the ala of the nose and the cheek is carried upwards to a point just below the inner canthus, so as to avoid opening the lachrymal sac. It is then continued outwards along the infra-orbital ridge to a point below the outer canthus. This incision is carried down to the bone throughout its extent, and the flap formed by raising the soft parts from the surface of the maxilla is turned outwards. While this is being done free hæmorrhage from the superior coronary (labial), lateral nasal, and angular branches of the facial will ensue unless preliminary ligature of the external carotid has been undertaken. This hæmorrhage may be controlled by digital compression of the facial trunk as it crosses the lower jaw, and by grasping the two halves of the upper lip between the fingers as it is divided. In turning this large flap outwards care must be taken both to avoid the growth, should it have fungated through the facial aspect of the maxilla, and yet to cut the skin flap thick enough to avoid any risk of subsequent sloughing. The mucous membrane is divided horizontally along its reflection from the upper lip on to the alveolus to a point behind the last molar tooth, and the flap formed by the soft tissues is reflected backwards as far as the anterior border of the masseter.

Attention must now be paid to all bleeding points, which are secured by Spencer Wells's forceps. The orbital periosteum, when not involved, is now raised throughout the whole extent of the floor of the orbit, and in doing this the origin of the inferior oblique will be detached and carried upwards with the other orbital contents. On the inner side the incision should have passed into the nose by dividing the fibrous tissue and mucous membrane along the concave margin of the bony anterior nasal orifice. The nasal (frontal) process of the superior maxilla and the adjacent portion of the nasal bone should now be divided with bone-forceps, so placed that the cut will extend backwards towards the inferior border of the sphenoidal (superior orbital) fissure (see Fig. 141, A). The junction of the maxilla with the malar bone must now be severed, and this is best carried out by free separation of the soft parts to expose the anterior extremity of the spheno-maxillary fissure, through which a Gigli's saw may be passed from above downwards, and the bone divided from behind forwards. The line of this bone incision must necessarily vary according to the extent of the disease, but when there is no reason to fear that the growth has extended into the temporal and zygomatic fossa, it should lie only just outside the malo-maxillary suture, and should avoid the anterior fibres of origin of the masseter muscle, as when the malar prominence can be left behind less deformity will result from sinking in of the normal prominence of the cheek (see Fig. 141, B).

The mouth is now opened in order to free the palatal attachments of the upper jaw, and if necessary the central incisor is drawn. The hard palate is divided in the middle line from before backwards by an incision dividing the muco-periosteum of the gum over the alveolus, and extending backwards down to the bone to the posterior margin of the hard palate. From this point it is continued transversely outwards to the tuberosity of the upper jaw. When the soft palate has been detached with a rugine, the hard palate is sawn through along a line corresponding to the division of the mucous membrane in an antero-posterior direction with a saw introduced through the nose (see Fig. 141, c). Where it is possible to leave the muco-periosteum of the hard palate the division of the palatal surface may be more easily carried out with a Gigli's saw or bone-forceps. Free sepa-

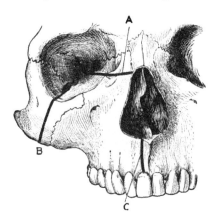

ration of the cut surfaces along all the bone incisions may now be completed with forceps, and when the bone has been sufficiently loosened it may be freed with lion forceps and forcibly withdrawn, bone-forceps inserted at the inner and outer limits of the jaw being used as a lever to assist this process. If the upper jaw be still held at any point it will probably be owing to its attachment behind to the pterygoid process: this may be severed by passing

FIG. 141. LINES OF BONE SECTION IN REMOVAL OF THE UPPER JAW.

the bone-forceps transversely inwards from behind the tuberosity of the jaw. As the maxilla is removed, all connecting soft parts, especially the superior maxillary nerve, are cleanly divided with scissors.

It is not unusual, when the bone has been considerably softened by infiltration with new growth, to find that it can only be extracted piecemeal, and when this is done, careful inspection, aided if necessary by artificial light, will alone ensure that all doubtful tissues are freely cut away.

At this stage of the operation free hæmorrhage is frequently met with, and this is temporarily controlled by packing the cavity with a large sterilized sponge, by which means capillary hæmorrhage is arrested. When this is withdrawn all the bleeding vessels are secured with Spencer Wells's forceps and ligatured with catgut.

When all severe bleeding has been controlled it is well to inspect the whole cavity carefully in order to ensure that no growth remains behind, and in doing this comparison of the mass just removed with the cavity remaining will direct the operator's attention to the points at which this is most likely, for if the upper jaw has been broken in removal, and a portion of the capsule of the growth is adherent at any point, it is probably there that remains of the growth have been left behind. All irregular rough fragments of bone must be carefully removed with bone-cutting forceps : such trimming of the bony cavity will probably be called for at the upper and back part of the wound, where fracture of the maxilla rather than separation of the whole bone from the palate and ethmoid is likely to take place.

When it is quite certain that the whole growth has been removed, and when all hæmorrhage has been arrested, the cavity is firmly packed with one long strip of iodoform gauze wrung out in weak carbolic lotion. Before this is done Cheyne and Burghard recommend that the raw surface should be mopped over with a solution of zinc chloride (40 grains to the ounce), and Jacobson (*loc. supra cit.*) is in favour of using a similar application, or Whitehead's varnish (containing benzoin, ethereal solution of iodoform, and turpentine), but when possible he is in favour of omitting to plug the cavity. Other surgeons soak the gauze packing with an emulsion of sulphur in glycerine.

In the writer's experience careful search for detached particles of growth, aided if necessary by an electric forehead-light, and their free removal with scissors or bone-forceps, is better than to trust to the action of any caustic applications, and in his experience the subsequent bleeding has been so slight as not to call for the use of local styptics.

The opening between the nose and the mouth is now narrowed as much as possible by sewing the detached half of the soft palate to the cut margin of the mucous membrane of the cheek and to the other half of the palate.

The edges of the skin wound may now be brought together with superficial catgut sutures. Jacobson advises that especial care should be paid to the insertion of these sutures at two points : one the angle of the flap near the inner canthus, where, if sloughing of the skin takes place, ectropion will follow ; the other at the lower margin, where care must be taken that the red line of the upper lip is accurately sutured. Further, it is important to carefully suture the mucous aspect of the lip, in order to avoid the possibility of the lip becoming adherent to the cut edge of the alveolus, when imperfect movement will result.

Modifications of and additions to the above operation. Numerous modifications of Fergusson's incision have been employed, of which the following are the most important.

Kocher recommends the adoption of *Nélaton's incision* in cases where free access to the regions of the orbit and malar bone is not required. This is similar to Fergusson's, but stops short at the inner canthus of the orbit. When, however, more room is required above, Kocher carries the incision downwards and outwards at a lower level than Fergusson's incision, along the lower edge of the orbicularis palpebrarum (oculi), but above the origins of the levator labii superioris (caput infraorbitale) and zygomatic muscles. This is so placed that it falls between the upper and lower areas of the distribution of the facial nerve (see Fig. 140).

Kocher employs, for extensive growths, a modified *Dieffenbach's incision* (see Fig. 142, A), which is carried perpendicularly through the upper lip, and then upwards along the nose, just external to the middle line. The inner canthus is then divided, and the incision runs along the inferior conjunctival fornix to the outer canthus, beyond which it is continued horizontally as far as may be necessary. In such operations Kocher recommends that the eyeball should be removed, for by this means free access is obtained for the removal of growth in the region of the ethmoid, where he says recurrence is specially apt to occur after operation for tumours in advanced stages. As it is impossible to be sure before the commencement of such an operation to what limits the growth may have extended, it is always well to obtain the patient's consent to removal of the eyeball before operating. This will, however, only be called for when the soft tissues of the orbit are actually involved, or the growth has fungated to such an extent into the ethmoidal cells that free access is impossible while the eye remains in position.

Modifications of the original incision will be required when the growth has fungated, and is involving the soft parts covering the facial aspect of the maxilla. In this case the incision must be planned so as to give the invaded tissues a wide berth, the only point to be considered being that the growth shall be freely got rid of. After this a plastic operation on the face will be necessary, skin flaps being obtained from the cheek, frontal or cervical regions.

König's operation. As is pointed out above, removal of the orbital plate of the maxilla may result in serious disfigurement from falling downwards of the eyeball and from associated œdema of the lower lid. König has introduced a plastic operation to prevent this deformity (Schlatter, *v. Bergmann's Surgery*, vol. i, p. 731). He tries to prevent dislocation downwards of the eyeball and sinking down of the lower lid by supporting the eyeball with a flap taken from the temporal muscle.

From the insertion of the temporal muscle to the lower jaw he takes a strip of muscle of half a finger's breadth attached to a piece of the anterior border of the coronoid process of the inferior maxilla, which he chisels away as far as the horizontal ramus. He then carries this transversely inwards below the eyeball, where it is attached to the remains of the frontal process of the maxilla, so as to support the eyeball.

In order to overcome the disadvantage of the free communication between the nasal cavity and the mouth, Bardenheuer (Schlatter, v. Bergmann's Surgery, vol. i, p. 731) uses the nasal septum to fill up the defect in the hard palate. The septum is detached from the anterior portion of the frame of the nose and the base of the skull, and is turned outwards upon its inferior attachments until it assumes a horizontal position. It is then sutured to the soft palate behind and to the edge of the mucous membrane of the buccal flap externally.

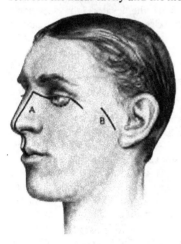

FIG. 142. INCISIONS FOR OPERATIONS UPON THE JAWS. A, Dieffenbach's incision for removal of the upper jaw; B, Incision for operations upon the inter-articular fibro-cartilage, or for excision of the condyle of the mandible.

This deformity may be overcome when the parts are soundly healed by the fitting of an obturator carrying a denture.

It has been pointed out above (see p. 302) that, when the growth is limited to the upper part of the jaw, the palate may be left entire, or when it is considered unsafe to leave the bony palate the muco-periosteum of the roof of the mouth may be saved. The first-named modification is very rarely safe, but when possible it may be carried out, after reflection of the facial flap and free exposure of the maxilla, by sawing horizontally outwards with a fine saw introduced into the nose immediately above the level of the hard palate. This procedure will be rarely available, as it interferes considerably with later inspection of the highest and deepest part of the cavity, and it must be borne in mind that it is here that it is most difficult to deal radically with the growth. When the operator intends to save the muco-periosteal covering of the palate, this may be divided along the mid-line and raised outwards as far as or beyond the alveolus after it has been cut through transversely behind at its junction with the soft palate : or, as advised by Cheyne and Burghard (*loc. supra cit.*), the muco-periosteum may be reflected inwards after an incision has been made on the side affected within the alveolus, extending from the mid-line in front to the hamular process behind; in either case the soft palate should be detached behind. After the jaw has been removed, the palatal flap is replaced and sutured to the cut margins of the buccal mucous membrane and to the soft palate behind with interrupted catgut sutures.

Similarly, when the lower part of the upper jaw is alone involved, and the parts have been exposed by Nélaton's incision described above, the orbital plate of the maxilla may be left intact. When this is possible it should always be done, as it obviates some of the gravest objections to removal of the upper jaw. In order to carry this out, the maxilla is divided horizontally below the infra-orbital ridge, partly with a saw, partly with a chisel and mallet,[1] the lower part of the maxilla being removed by the method previously described.

After-treatment. The patient is returned to bed, and is well propped up on a bed-rest or pillows, in order to hamper the movements of the chest as little as possible. Feeding for the first few days is to be carried out with nutrient enemata, but water *ad libitum* should be given through a drinking-cup, in order to quench thirst and to wash away unpleasant discharge. The mouth should be frequently mopped out or sprayed with sanitas, and the patient allowed to gargle with potassium permanganate or resorcin lotion. After two or three days fluids may be given by the mouth through a long india-rubber tube attached to a feeding-cup. The gauze packing is removed after twenty-four hours, and the cavity is lightly repacked. This is repeated until granulation commences.

Owing to the frequency of pulmonary complications it is well to allow the patient to sit up in bed on the third or fourth day, and to leave his bed for an arm-chair or wheeled couch within a week of the operation.

Dangers and difficulties. The chief risks of this operation are due to hæmorrhage, which is best overcome prophylactically either by preliminary ligature of the external carotid or by compression of the arteries likely to be divided, as mentioned in the account of the operation. Bleeding is also dangerous from the possibility of blood entering the larynx, resulting in coughing and dyspnœa, and inspiration of blood-stained saliva which is likely to give rise to a dangerous or fatal bronchopneumonia. These complications are best avoided by preliminary

---

[1] Or a Gigli's saw may be passed from without inwards through the pterygo-maxillary (pterygo-palatine) fissure into the nose (Schlatter), when the maxilla may be cut through at whatever level is desired.

laryngotomy and plugging of the pharynx, though Cheyne and Burghard state that they have not met with a case in which they have thought this necessary.

Shock. In the aged, those suffering from advanced arterial degeneration or defective nutrition due to inability to take food readily before the operation, or in those suffering from malignant cachexia, this is likely to be marked. In Eve's opinion (*Brit. Med. Journ.*, 1907, vol. i. p. 1525) the preliminary operations of laryngotomy and ligature of the external carotid tend to decrease shock and do not prolong the operation, as much time is saved in sponging and securing vessels. Rapid operation, great care in limiting the amount of hæmorrhage, and hypodermic injections of adrenalin are the most important antidotes for this condition.

Recurrent or secondary hæmorrhage may be dealt with by the application of an ice-bag to the face or by douching with cold water. The gauze packing may be soaked in a solution of adrenalin chloride (1 in 1,000). Should these fail, ligature of the external carotid may be called for if this has not been done as a preliminary measure.

Inhalation pneumonia is a considerable risk during the first few days, when the patient's power of expectorating discharges is reduced. Infection of the wound, followed by cellulitis or erysipelas, is likely to occur in feeble patients, the subjects of advanced disease, where the growth has already undergone necrosis, and must be dealt with as in other parts of the body by free incisions, and fomentations of boric or mercuric perchloride lotion, frequently applied.

Results. Krönlein (*Arch. f. Klin. Chir.*, 1901, vol. lxiv, p. 265) states that in 1872 Dangenbeck, owing to the great diversity of opinion as to the immediate danger in this operation, expressed the wish that statistics might be collected as to the mortality, but the repeated attempts which have been made to do so by the *Deutsche Gesellschaft für Chirurgie* have not met with much success. Langenbeck considered that the risk was undoubtedly very great, especially in individuals of sixty and upwards, whilst Volkmann believed that death very rarely resulted from resection of the upper jaw. Baum puts the mortality at a little over 10%.

In 1847 Dieffenbach performed more or less extensive resections in 32 cases, none of these patients dying from the operation and its immediate results; it is not, however, stated how many were total resections. Before the antiseptic period (1844 to 1870), out of 115 total resections found in the literature there were 37 deaths, that is to say, a mortality of 32.1%, whilst during the antiseptic period (1871 to 1897) out of 158 cases there were 33 deaths, or 21.5%. Krönlein points out that this decrease of mortality is by no means general. For example, in the cases reported by Küster and König the mortality was 29.1%, whilst in those reported by Heyfelder, Reid, Esmarch, and Baum there were 19 deaths out of 55 operations, or 16.3%. König (1898) states that the immediate mortality is especially high after total resection for malignant growths, and puts it at about 30%. Butlin (*Operative Surgery of Malignant Disease*, p. 136) is of opinion that the mortality after removal of the upper jaw is still very high. Eve (*loc. supra cit.*) records a mortality of 16.6% in 12 operations undertaken in the last six years. Before the antiseptic period pyæmia, septicæmia, erysipelas, and meningitis were the most common causes of death, whilst during the last decades disorders of the air-passages predominate, death resulting from septic bronchitis, broncho-pneumonia, and suffocation, owing to flooding of the air-passages with blood during the operation.

The late results of these operations are even more disappointing. Schlatter (*loc. supra cit.*) records recurrence in an average of 3.9 months in all his cases where the whole maxilla was involved. Küster obtained no permanent good results: in the statistics of the Erlangen Clinic there was one permanent cure in 17 cases, in those of the Greifswald Clinic no cure in 17 cases; Estlander had 10 recurrences in 12 cases. Martens reports 72 total resections in the Göttingen Clinic, resulting in 23 deaths and 16 permanent cures, the disease recurring in all the other cases. In 13 cases of complete resection for carcinoma of the upper jaw reported by Stein in von Bergmann's Clinic (1890 to 1900) there was recurrence in every instance in an average of 3.6 months, death usually resulting in about thirteen months. In 11 cases in which total resection was performed for sarcoma death occurred in 3, recurrence in 2, whilst 6 remained well up to the time when the cases were reported. Stein reports 47 cases in which total resection was carried out in the Berlin Clinic, with 12.6% cures. In the cases of partial resection reported, permanent cure for at least three years occurred in 50%.

PARTIAL REMOVAL OF THE UPPER JAW

Indications. (i) For the removal of malignant growth not involving the whole maxilla: modifications of Fergusson's operation required in such cases have been described above.

(ii) For epulis. This is a term applied clinically to tumours arising from the gum close to the teeth and includes growths of widely varying characters. While all arise in the alveolar periosteum or in the periodontal membrane, they may be benign fibrous growths or fibro-sarcomata of slight but definite malignancy. Eve (*loc. supra cit.*) states that among 30 cases removed at the London Hospital recurrence took place in 18.2%.

Operation. Under a general anæsthetic a tooth on either side of the epulis is extracted. A vertical cut is then made upwards, lateral to the sockets of the extracted teeth, through the alveolus with an Adams's saw. The muco-periosteum of the gum is divided within the limits of that part of the alveolus isolated by the saw-cuts, and this portion of the alveolus is detached with a Gigli's saw, chisel and mallet, or bone-forceps. Bleeding is now controlled by pressure, and a small gauze dressing is packed into the gap. The mouth is frequently rinsed out with a non-irritating antiseptic lotion. The mucous membrane is allowed to re-form so as to cover the gap in the alveolus, which at the same time undergoes considerable atrophy. After a period of six months the resulting deformity may be reduced to a minimum by the provision of a well-fitting plate carrying teeth to replace those removed at the operation.

OSTEOPLASTIC RESECTION OF THE UPPER JAW

Indications. (i) For the removal of naso-pharyngeal benign growths, such as fibromata. This will rarely be called for, as they can usually be removed without danger of recurrence by a snare introduced through the nose, or by Moure's operation (see Vol. IV).

(ii) For the removal of malignant growths growing from the base of the skull and projecting into the naso-pharynx, or extending into it from the spheno-maxillary fossa or nose. Here osteoplastic resection of the jaw is only called for when it is thought that sufficient space will not be obtained by Gussenbauer's method (Schlatter, *v. Bergmann's Operative Surgery*, vol. i, p. 733). In this operation the muco-periosteal covering of the hard palate is divided in the median line, and reflected with an elevator to either side as far as the alveolar processes. The palatal processes of the maxillæ and palate bones are then resected, and the mucosa covering the floor of the nose and the lower part of the septum is removed. After extirpation of the tumour the two lateral flaps of the palatal muco-periosteum are sutured.

The advantages of the above operation, which is very similar to that described by Nélaton, and to which his name is given by some, are firstly that no deformity of the face from scarring results, and secondly that it is followed by less hæmorrhage than results from Langenbeck's operation. But its great disadvantage is that, owing to the limited space available, considerable risk is run of leaving behind portions of the growth, so that recurrence is more probable than after the more extensive operation of Langenbeck.

Dr. Robin Massé collected 26 cases dealt with by Nélaton's operation, of which 13 were successful. Walsham (*Med. Soc. Trans.*, vol. xix, 1896, p. 394) found that by this means he had succeeded on several occasions in obtaining adequate space for the removal of naso-pharyngeal growths. He advocated the operation because, though such growths may extend into the nose and even cause the eyeball to protrude, only rarely do they invade the upper jaw or turbinates, and consequently he thinks that as a rule osteoplastic resection of the jaw is unnecessary. Further, in his opinion osteoplastic resection entails the following disadvantages:

some scarring of the face, interference with the lachrymal duct, and sometimes œdema of the lower eyelid, which is prone to persist. He adds that reflection of the maxilla is attended with considerable shock and often severe hæmorrhage.

Operation. *Langenbeck's method.* A skin incision is made from the inner canthus of the eye along the infra-orbital ridge, extending to the middle of the zygomatic arch: from this point it curves downwards, and turns inwards to the lower border of the ala of the nose (see Fig. 143). The soft tissues are not reflected, but are turned inwards, together with the bone, at a later stage in the operation. After detaching the origin of the masseter from the lower border of the zygoma, an

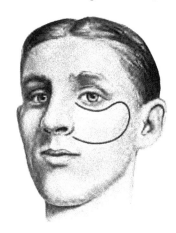

FIG. 143. INCISION FOR LANGEN-BECK'S OSTEOPLASTIC RESECTION OF THE UPPER JAW.

elevator is passed through the pterygo-maxillary (pterygo-palatine) fissure into the spheno-maxillary (pterygo-palatine) fossa, and guided by this an Adams's or a keyhole saw is introduced towards the naso-pharynx, where its extremity is caught by the index-finger of the left hand, which has been inserted into the naso-pharynx through the mouth. The upper jaw is now sawn through horizontally above the level of the hard palate, as far as the anterior nasal orifice, thus freeing it from below (see Fig. 144, C). It is detached externally by dividing the zygoma with a saw or bone-forceps and by freeing the malar bone from the soft parts (see Fig. 144, A). The superior attachments of the jaw are severed by dividing the frontal process of the malar bone as far as the spheno-maxillary fissure, and by cutting through the orbital plate of the maxilla with bone-forceps, carefully avoiding the lachrymal sac (see Fig. 144,

B and D). By means of an elevator inserted under the malar bone the portion of the upper jaw outlined by the saw-cuts can now be levered inwards towards the median line, in doing which the deep connexions of the maxilla with other bones will be fractured. The tumour can then be lifted from the naso-pharynx or adjacent fossæ, and its pedicle detached from the base of the skull by means of a knife, scissors, or thermo-cautery. Finally the jaw is replaced and secured in position by skin sutures.

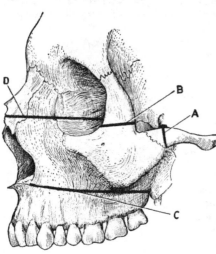

Dangers and difficulties. Unless the posterior connexions of the jaw have been thinned by the naso-pharyngeal growth, and the fossæ at the back of the jaw have been enlarged from the same cause, there will be great difficulty in separating this portion of the upper jaw, which has so many articulations with the other bones of the face; and even when this has been done this method will often provide insufficient access if the growth be of large size. Undue force again is likely to crush the part of the upper jaw removed, or to break through adjacent delicate bones, so

FIG. 144. LINES OF BONE SECTION IN LANGENBECK'S OSTEOPLASTIC RESECTION OF THE UPPER JAW.

that necrosis may result. If the portion of bone to be resected be clear on one side, but remains attached and fixed at another, severe hæmorrhage, which cannot be located so as to be controlled, is likely to ensue. The risk of any blood entering the air-passages should be eliminated in the same way as was recommended in removal of the upper jaw (see p. 304), namely, by conducting the operation in the Trendelenburg position and by performing a preliminary laryngotomy, after the pharynx is firmly packed with sponges. Lastly, difficulty is often met with in replacing the bone accurately, and fitting it in place.

Owing to the above serious dangers and disadvantages it is scarcely surprising that many surgeons advocate, for cases requiring more extensive operation than can be ensured by the intranasal or by Moure's method, that the upper jaw should be partly or completely removed.

In favour of partial or complete removal of the jaw for naso-pharyngeal growths is the fact that much freer access to the roof of the nasopharynx, from which growths usually spring, is obtained by an operation such as Fergusson's.

The operation of osteoplastic resection of the jaw entails a similar disfiguring scar upon the face, and preliminary laryngotomy is, as pointed out above, equally desirable here as it is as a preliminary to complete removal of the jaw. Cheyne and Burghard (*Manual of Surgical Treatment,* Part V, p. 230), in advocating partial removal of the jaw rather than osteoplastic resection, point out that it is unnecessary to remove the orbital plate, and that the periosteum of the hard palate can be retained. For details of this operation the reader is referred to p. 304.

CHAPTER V

OPERATIONS UPON THE LOWER JAW AND THE TEMPORO-MAXILLARY JOINT

OPERATIONS UPON THE TEMPORO-MAXILLARY JOINT

OPERATION FOR SUBLUXATION OF THE INTERARTICULAR FIBRO-CARTILAGE

Indications. When local medication has failed to relieve the symptoms operation may be undertaken as follows :—

Operation. An incision one inch long is made obliquely from before backwards and downwards over the joint, and is carried down to the capsule (see Fig. 142, B). In making this incision the chief structures to be avoided are branches of the facial nerve. This may be done by planning the incision so that it shall run forwards and upwards in the same direction as the temporal branches, and by taking care that any filaments exposed are carefully drawn aside. The superficial temporal artery and vein, with the auriculo-temporal nerve, lie more deeply between the condyle and the tragus, and should be in no danger of injury.

Attention must now be paid to bleeding points, and the outlying lobules of the parotid gland, which often overlap the condyle, must be turned backwards; the masseter is defined in front of the joint, so that the latter may be freely exposed. When this has been done the capsule is opened by a vertical incision, and the fibro-cartilage is seized with forceps and dragged back into its natural position, where it is sutured by stout catgut sutures at the temporo-maxillary capsule as near as possible to its attachment to the margins of the glenoid fossa. When the interarticular fibro-cartilage cannot be replaced by this method, or when it is fenestrated or torn considerably, relief may be obtained by its complete removal.

The capsule is now re-sutured and the wound closed. Active movements are controlled as far as possible for a week, during which time the patient is fed by fluids through a tube. Annandale (*Lancet*, 1887, vol. i. p. 411) records the results of operation upon two women, aged respectively 38 and 18. The movements of the joint became natural and the jaws could be opened and closed perfectly.

OPERATION FOR AN UNREDUCED DISLOCATION

When dislocation of the lower jaw resists replacement by manipulation, even under an anæsthetic, open operation must be resorted to. The joint is exposed in exactly a similar method to that which has just been described (see p. 318), when the condyle is levered into position with an elevator.

Open operation facilitates reduction by enabling the surgeon to remove part or the whole of the interarticular fibro-cartilage, which is one of the possible obstacles to reduction by manipulation. Kocher (*Operative Surgery,* 4th edit., p. 106) states that he has reduced by open operation a dislocation of the jaw of four months' duration, and obtained an excellent result.

Should reduction, even after free division of the capsule, with or without removal of the meniscus, be impossible, excision of the condyle should be undertaken in order to restore movement.

EXCISION OF THE CONDYLE OF THE LOWER JAW

This operation, sometimes termed excision of the temporo-maxillary articulation, only deals with that portion of the articulation formed by the condyle of the mandible, and therefore the heading used above more correctly defines its nature. It is required when a patient is unable to open his mouth sufficiently to take food, or when the inability to open the mouth results in fœtor of the breath and difficulty of speech, which condition is frequently increased by the presence of septic roots. This operation will only avail when the fixation of the lower jaw is due to pre-existing disease of the temporo-maxillary joint or to an unreduced dislocation.

Bony or fibrous ankylosis may result from pyæmic arthritis, suppurative arthritis following a punctured wound, gonorrhœal and rheumatoid arthritis, or from a fracture of the condyle involving the joint. Unreduced or recurrent dislocation may also call for a similar operation, which may be required on one or both sides.

Operation. An incision is made from in front of the lower end of the tragus upwards and forwards for 1½ to 2 inches. This is carried through the skin and the deep fascia. As in the preceding operation, care must be exercised to avoid the branches of the facial nerve and the superficial temporal vessels. A vertical incision is now made, so as to open the capsule freely and to expose the neck of the lower jaw. The capsule is divided sufficiently to allow the condyle to be levered out of the glenoid fossa with an elevator, and after those fibres of the external pterygoid attached to the neck of the jaw have been freely

detached with scissors the neck of the bone is divided with bone-forceps
or with a Gigli's saw (see Fig. 145, c). If diseased, the interarticular
fibro-cartilage is excised, and, when the operation is undertaken for
recent suppurative arthritis or for tuberculous disease, the glenoid fossa
is carefully scraped with a Volkmann's spoon. The mouth should be
opened to its full extent with a Mason's gag or a wooden wedge, and,
if this cannot be done, it may be necessary to remove an additional piece
of bone below the condyle. The wound is now sutured without drainage.

Arbuthnot Lane (*Clin. Soc. Trans.*, vol. xxix, p. 1), in recording
four cases of excision of the temporo-maxillary
joint for bony ankylosis in children, draws attention to the difficulty experienced in removing enough of the bone, which in cases of
ankylosis developing early in life and remaining fixed for a long period is always abnormally
broad and thick. He says that the part of the
jaw which 'is con-
tinuous with the
squamous portion of
the temporal bone
must be freely re-
moved,' and that its
excision was in some
of his cases a matter
of much difficulty.
He recommends that
the surgeon should
remove very much
more bone than

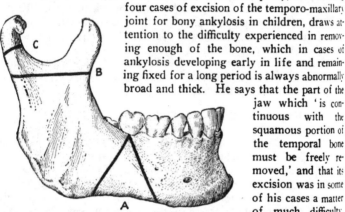

FIG. 145. OPERATIONS UPON THE LOWER JAW. Lines
of bone section for: A, Esmarch's operation; B, Excision of both processes of lower jaw; C, Excision of
condyle of lower jaw.

would at first sight seem necessary if he wishes to secure a good joint.
He also is of opinion that the formation of a new articulation after
such an operation is more successful in childhood than in adult life.

Mears (*Amer. Journ. of Med. Sci.*, 1883, p. 459) quotes the case of
a girl in whom excision of the condyle was undertaken for unilateral
bony ankylosis of seventeen years' duration, due to a gunshot wound.
This did not allow separation of the jaws, which could, however, be
forced apart to the extent of one inch after the coronoid process and
a bridge of new bone which had formed near it had been freely resected.
Jacobson (*loc. supra cit.*) obtained a favourable result by this method
in another case.

After-treatment. Care must be taken to avoid any relapse, and
in order to do this, passive movements must be employed on the second

day, and forcible opening of the mouth must be frequently carried out, if necessary under a general anæsthetic.

Kocher (*loc. supra cit.*) remarks that mobility readily returns after unilateral excision, and even after a bilateral operation a satisfactory result may be ensured if active movements are at once carried out. To prevent the recurrence of bony ankylosis Helferich places part of the temporal muscle between the glenoid fossa and the mandible, while Kusnagow uses a slip cut from the masseter for the same purpose.

OPERATIONS UPON THE LOWER JAW

PARTIAL REMOVAL OF THE LOWER JAW

Indications. Partial removal of the mandible may be required:

(i) *For epulis.* The observations made upon epulides and the operation for their removal when arising in the upper jaw equally apply here; the operation is carried out in exactly the same way as described on p. 314.

(ii) *For the removal of an epitheliomatous growth arising in the floor of the mouth or upon the lip, and extending on to the gum.* Under these circumstances removal of a portion of the lower jaw may be necessary, as it must be borne in mind that it is impossible to remove the mucous membrane of the gum so freely as to eliminate the possibility of recurrence without detaching the nutritive periosteum from the bone, when necrosis is likely to ensue. Again, when an epitheliomatous growth arising in the gum has been stripped off the lower jaw it is not uncommon to find that the growth recurs upon the bone, so that when there is any suspicion that the periosteal surface of the gum is involved it is wiser to resect the affected portion of the jaw with the muco-periosteum covering it, in one piece and at one operation, rather than to wait until recurrence occurs which will necessitate a more extensive removal of the bone. At the same time it is well to bear in mind that at first epithelioma will only involve the alveolus, so that it may be possible to remove the affected part widely without destroying the continuity of the lower jaw. Cheyne and Burghard (*loc. supra cit.*) point out that this is of extreme importance, owing to the difficulties in mastication which are likely to ensue after resection of a portion of the whole thickness of the mandible, from alteration in the line of the teeth.

(iii) *For the removal of myeloid sarcomata of the mandible.*

(iv) *For extensive necrosis of the lower jaw,* the result of periostitis following dental caries, fracture, or phosphorus poisoning. The last-named affection is now of extreme rarity in this country, and, as it is

mainly due to tuberculous disease, it is dealt with separately by Mr.
Stiles (see p. 156).

Operation. When the lower jaw is involved by the extension
of an epitheliomatous growth, it is usually the body which is affected,
and therefore it is this portion of the jaw which most commonly requires
removal. A vertical incision is made through the lip to below the chin,
from which a curved incision, convex downwards, is carried on one or
both sides to the hyoid bone, then backwards and upwards to the top of
the mastoid process (see Fig. 146) ; the greater part of the above incision
is required for the removal of the growth from the floor of the mouth

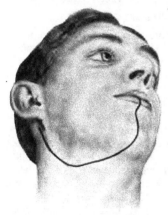

FIG. 146. INCISION FOR EXCISION OF
THE LOWER JAW. (*After Kocher.*)

and of the submaxillary and upper
cervical lymphatic glands rather
than for the resection of the bone,
though its removal is somewhat
simplified by carrying out the full
incision at an early stage of the
operation. The inferior coronary
and other divided arteries having
been secured, the soft parts are detached and reflected laterally as far
as may be necessary. The level of
bone sections being decided upon,
one or more teeth are extracted on
either side of these lines. The bone
may now be divided with an Adams's
saw working from the external surface ; or the soft parts may be detached on the inner surface of the
jaw, sufficiently to allow of the pas-
sage of a Gigli's saw, with which the bone is more easily divided from
within outwards. It is easier to saw the bone three-quarters through, and
then, after making the second section, to complete the first with bone-
forceps, rather than to divide it completely at one spot before beginning
the second cut. Care should be taken that the affected bone and soft
parts are removed in one piece, and that the tongue, which must necessarily be deprived of its muscular attachments if the section involves
the symphysis, does not fall back and produce serious dyspnœa.

Removal of part or of the whole of the horizontal ramus is called for
in dealing with a myeloid sarcoma, or in cases of extensive necrosis.
The details of the operation have been mentioned above ; in the case
of removal of bone for necrosis it is usually possible to preserve the
periosteum, so that new bone will be formed within it.

When, however, a complete section of the lower jaw and its periosteum has been removed, it is important to overcome the tendency which the remaining portions manifest of being drawn together towards the middle line by the unopposed external pterygoid muscles: unless this is done the lower jaw becomes contracted, and its teeth cannot be apposed to those of the upper jaw. The ideal method here is the employment of immediate prosthesis, using a perforated metal plate secured at either end to the separated parts of the mandible, so that the remaining teeth in the lower jaw are maintained in accurate alinement with those of the upper. Of the numerous mechanical appliances which have been devised on this plan, Claude. Martin's apparatus (Schlatter, *v. Bergmann's Operative Surgery*, vol. i, p. *722*), or one of its various modifications, is the most suitable, but as these entail the fixation of the jaw by a metal bar held in position by screws or pegs, the risk of oral sepsis and possibly of necrosis is considerable. In many cases a metal interdental splint made from plaster casts taken before operation and fitted while the patient is under the anæsthetic fulfils all requirements and can be more easily kept clean: occasionally it is better to rely upon secondary prosthesis when a metal interdental splint to bridge over the gap resulting from the operation and to restore the normal outline of the remaining teeth is fitted as soon as the wound in the floor of the mouth is covered with healthy granulations. Whatever method of prosthesis is employed, it is necessary to place the patient in the hands of a dentist for the application later on of a permanent denture to replace the teeth which have been lost. In every instance septic roots must be extracted and carious teeth stopped before such an operation is undertaken.

Schlatter (*loc. supra cit.*) speaks favourably of the use of a metal plate, which is fastened to the stump of the lower jaw on the outer side of the teeth, to which it is connected by wires: the metal plate is directed upwards and outwards, and when the mouth is open projects beyond the upper teeth. In mastication the teeth of the upper jaw impinge upon this inclined plane, and thus tend to push outward that fragment of the lower jaw to which it is attached.

In some cases the deficiency can be supplied by a plastic operation, using material from the remaining portion of the jaw, or from the femur, clavicle, or frontal bones.

Krause (*Centralb. f. Chir.*, 1904, No. xxv, p. *767*) describes a method which he has adopted. Four to seventeen days after resection of the lower jaw, he fills up the defect from the neighbouring intact portions of the jaw; from these he forms a flap of skin, muscle, periosteum, and bone, 5 to 7 centimetres in length and more than a centimetre in height, which remains connected along its lower border with the neighbouring soft tissues. This flap is inserted into the defect, and the extremities of the bone graft are fixed to the free ends of the lower jaw by two silver wire sutures, the soft parts being sutured together. The resulting defect in the neck is diminished by means of sutures, so arranged that they do not involve the flap. There is no danger of necrosis of the bony portion of the flap, and the actions of swallowing and opening the mouth are accomplished without difficulty .

Pichler and Ranzi (*Arch. f. klin. Chir.*, 1907, vol. lxxxiv, p. 198), in an article on prosthesis of the lower jaw, state that Claude Martin's method of immediate prothesis did not meet with the favourable reception which might have been anticipated, owing to the apparent danger of the entrance of septic foreign bodies into the wound, though good results have been obtained from it. Attempts have been made to replace the defect by a simple sterilizable apparatus, such as Sauer's bandages, Bönnecken's metal splint, &c. The more recent prostheses have been constructed upon Martin's original idea, namely, replacement by an intact portion of the lower jaw under strict asepsis. The apparatus employed by Stoppany-Schröder and Fritzsche consists of a massive central piece of tin, fitted with a perforated strip of metal on either side, the latter being attached by means of metal wire to the stump of the jaw. The splint is not firmly attached to the metal strips, but can be removed by taking out the pegs (or rods), rendering inspection of the wound possible. After resection of one half of the lower jaw the apparatus usually has a metal strip at one end for attachment to the intact half of the jaw, whilst the other extremity is inserted into the glenoid cavity as an artificial condyloid process. In one case, in which this method was employed after resection of the lower jaw for carcinoma involving the floor of the mouth and the lower jaw, the temporary apparatus was replaced five weeks later by a permanent one, furnished with artificial teeth. There was no recurrence six months after the operation, and the cosmetic and functional results were good.

Pichler and Ranzi state that in some cases the weight of the tin appliance is unpleasant to the patients, and that it may, partially at least, be replaced by rubber. Prosthesis must of course in all instances be preceded by dental treatment, which is essential both for the maintenance of asepsis, and for the establishment and firmness of the apparatus; the process is also facilitated if models of both jaws are taken before operation.

Sébileau (*Bull. et Mém. Soc. de Chir. de Paris*, 1906, vol. xxxii, p. 1174) recommends a permanent apparatus only after complete cicatrization of the wound, though from the time of the operation the portions of the lower jaw should be kept apart by a temporary wire splint.

REMOVAL OF ONE HALF OF THE LOWER JAW

The usual indication for this operation is the presence of a periosteal
.rcoma. Here, no less than in the upper jaw, exploration of a doubt-
illy malignant tumour is always indicated in order to avoid unneces-
.ry resection of bone.

Operations. The patient is placed in the Trendelenburg position,
· in the horizontal position with a firm pillow under the cervical spine,
ı that the head will fall backwards. Preliminary laryngotomy will
;ually be unnecessary when the operation is being carried out for
:moval of a tumour confined to the bone itself; but when adjacent soft
ırts are implicated, or when it is necessary to remove affected sub-
axillary glands, laryngotomy is a wise precaution. Similarly, when
ıe operation involves a free dissection of the tissues in the submaxillary
iangle, hæmorrhage may be avoided, time saved, and shock obvi-
:ed by a preliminary ligature of the external carotid artery, which
ıould be carried out below the origin of the lingual and facial
ranches.

The actual incision will vary with the above-mentioned conditions.
:ocher advises the employment of a median incision dividing the lower
p and extending down to the hyoid bone, which will give free access
·hen only the symphysis and the horizontal ramus are involved. He
oes not recommend the employment of a lateral incision, as he considers
ıat it impairs the mechanism of swallowing by division of muscles and
erves, and so the risk of aspiration pneumonia is increased. When,
owever, access to the angle and ascending ramus of the jaw is required,
r when (as is usually the case in the writer's opinion) it is necessary
ɔ remove the submaxillary and other cervical lymphatic glands, Kocher
Operative Surgery, translation of 4th edit., p. 105) continues his
ıcision on the side affected ' from the hyoid bone along the submaxillo-
ɛrvical crease to a point a finger's breadth behind and below the angle
f the jaw, and from thence up to the apex of the mastoid process '
see Fig. 146, p. 322). The level of this incision is insisted upon in
rder to spare the branches of the facial nerve supplying the muscles
ı this region.

The flap outlined by this incision is now turned upwards, care being
ıken to include the muscular structures of the lower lip and chin by
eeping as close to the bone as possible. Near the posterior margin of
ıe wound the facial artery and vein must be isolated and divided be-
ween ligatures. The glandular contents of the submaxillary triangle
re exposed and dissected upwards, so that they may be removed in one
iece with the lower jaw. The lower jaw is now divided at or near the

middle line: though it is usually necessary to cut the bone in the mid-line, yet when practicable and without risk of recurrence advantage is gained by making the bone section lateral to the origin of the genial muscles on the side affected; by doing this the movements of the tongue in swallowing and speaking are less likely to be interfered with. Removal of one of the incisors may be necessary, when the jaw may be divided with an Adams's saw; or detachment of the muco-periosteum on the inner surface will allow of the introduction of a Gigli's saw, by which the jaw may be quickly divided from behind forwards.

The affected half of the mandible is now drawn strongly outwards, and the mucous membrane of the floor of the mouth and the attachments of the muscles to its inner surface, namely, the digastric, mylo-hyoid, genio-hyoid, and genio-hyoglossus, are quickly divided. The external surface of the vertical ramus is laid bare by the detachment of the masseter, and by careful separation with a blunt dissector of the soft parts along its posterior margin. The incision in the mucous membrane of the mouth is carried up along the anterior border of the vertical ramus, when the internal pterygoid is detached from its insertion with a knife, and the soft parts are separated backwards with a blunt dissector. Where the superior constrictor has been divided at its attachment to the posterior end of the mylo-hyoid ridge care must be taken to avoid the lingual nerve, which curves forwards at this point. The inferior dental nerve is divided as it enters the inferior dental foramen, and the inferior dental artery lying behind the nerve is divided after ligature at the same spot, the jaw being strongly pulled outwards while this is being done. The bone is now firmly depressed, when a few touches with a knife will expose the attachment of the temporal muscle to the coronoid process; this is carefully divided, and the jaw is pulled down to expose the anterior surface of its neck. Here the external pterygoid will require division, and troublesome hæmorrhage is likely to arise from the masse-teric and temporal branches of the internal maxillary artery. The capsule of the temporo-maxillary joint is now more freely exposed with a blunt dissector and its fibres are gradually divided. This, with the detachment of any remaining fibres of the external pterygoid, may be most safely accomplished with a pair of blunt-pointed scissors or by a scalpel kept close to the bone and used in a saw-like manner. In freeing the condyle care must be taken to avoid the internal maxillary artery as it passes between the neck of the jaw and the internal lateral ligament. Pre-liminary ligature of the external carotid will have eliminated the possi-bility of troublesome hæmorrhage at this stage of the operation.

As in the case of removal of the upper jaw, so here, fracture is likely to occur when the bone is extensively implicated by the growth, and this will add to the difficulty of removal of the coronoid process and condyle.

When all hæmorrhage has been arrested, the wound is sponged over with hot saline solution, and the whole raw surface is carefully inspected for remaining fragments of growth. The margins of the wound in the mouth may now be, at least partially, brought together by interrupted catgut sutures, connecting the mucous membrane of the floor of the mouth with the mucous membrane of the cheek. The external skin wound is accurately sutured with interrupted sutures of salmon gut or catgut. When the submaxillary triangle has been freely opened up by the removal of the salivary and lymphatic glands it is wise to insert a drainage tube in the posterior angle of the wound, which may be removed after forty-eight hours.

After-treatment. For the first three or four days the patient must be fed by rectal enemata or by a nasal tube, but during this period a free supply·of cold water may be given by the mouth, and the patient may be allowed to suck ice to check capillary oozing. From the first the mouth must be frequently washed out with a weak antiseptic, such as chinosol (1 in 500), and at a later period after each feed given by the mouth the nurse should be instructed carefully to mop or spray the whole region of the wound with the same solution.

Difficulties and dangers. Shock and hæmorrhage, unless the soft parts are extensively involved, are not so severe as after removal of the upper jaw, and for this reason aspiration pneumonia is not likely to occur. The importance of disturbing the muscular attachments as little as possible, so as not to interfere with the patient's power of swallowing, has been previously referred to.

COMPLETE REMOVAL OF THE LOWER JAW

This may be required when both halves of the bone are symmetrically involved by a periosteal sarcoma. The operation is carried out in the same way as that for removal of half the lower jaw by dividing it in the middle line, and removing each half in turn.

OSTEOPLASTIC RESECTION OF THE LOWER JAW

This is a valuable procedure preliminary to the removal of growths, usually malignant, from the floor of the mouth, tongue, tonsil, fauces, and pharynx. .

Mesial division of the jaw. When employed as an aid to obtaining better exposure of an epithelioma of the floor of the mouth or

tongue, resection of the lower jaw forms a part of the classical operation of Syme and of Kocher's newer operation, as described in the fourth
edition of his *Operative Surgery,* p. 109. By division of the lower jaw
in the middle line, followed by separation of the mucous membrane
muscles along that side of the floor of the mouth which may in each
individual case seem most convenient, free access can be obtained to
all the structures between the lips and the posterior pillar of the
fauces.

Details of the different operations above indicated will be found
elsewhere; here reference will only be made to that part of these operations which is concerned with the lower jaw itself.

With the patient under an anæsthetic and placed in the Trendelenburg position, a median incision is made through the lower lip to a point
below the chin. Hæmorrhage from the inferior coronary arteries having
been controlled by Spencer Wells's forceps, the soft parts are reflected
from the body of the lower jaw for a distance of half an inch on either
side of the middle line. The line of the vertical saw-cut to be made
through the bone is now outlined by a few movements of the saw, after
which a hole is drilled on either side of this notch through the whole
substance of the bone, and division of the jaw is then completed with a
Gigli's or Adams's saw, when the position of the drill-holes on the inner
surface of the bone may be defined by slight detachment of the soft parts
laterally. Before proceeding with the operation it is well to locate the
two drill-holes for further recognition by passing a short piece of silver
wire through each; the two ends of each of these pieces may now be
twisted together so as to form a loop on either side, which will form a
very useful retractor for the separation of the two halves of the jaw during the later stages of the operation.

When the removal of the growth for which the operation has been
undertaken has been completed the two halves of the lower jaw are accurately brought together by a piece of silver wire passed through the drill-
holes on both sides. These are now twisted as tightly as possible and
cut short, after which the lower lip is sutured.

Lateral division of the jaw. When the tonsil, the pillars of
the fauces, and the pharyngeal wall behind these are the seat of new
growth, easier access may be obtained by division of the lower jaw at the
junction of the body and ascending ramus than by division in the middle
line. A similar procedure has been employed by Mikulicz as a step in
the operation for neurectomy of the third division of the fifth nerve.
The site of bone section may be exposed by Langenbeck's perpendicular
incision, which passes vertically downwards from the angle of the mouth,
but König prefers to expose the bone by turning a flap of the soft parts

upwards after making a curved incision in the neck, carried from the apex of the mastoid process downwards and forwards to the hyoid bone, and curving upwards towards the chin (see Fig. 147). When the soft parts have been reflected upwards as a flap, the facial artery and vein are ligatured as they cross the inferior border of the mandible. The soft tissues are now raised from the external surface of the mandible, and the mucous membrane of the mouth is divided on its inner aspect, after which the bone is drilled and divided in a similar manner to that described in connexion with the mesial operation. Kocher advises that the line of section should be carried from the lower border upwards and backwards, as, after the parts are replaced, the sawn extremity of the posterior fragment has a tendency to be drawn inwards and upwards by the muscles attached to it.

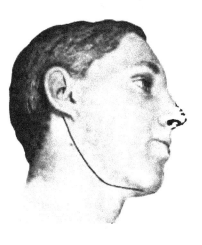

FIG. 147. INCISION FOR LATERAL DIVISION OF THE LOWER JAW IN OSTEOPLASTIC RESECTION. (*After König.*)

OPERATIONS FOR CLOSURE OF THE JAWS

Various operations upon the mandible have been introduced in order to overcome closure of the jaws, due either to cicatrization of the soft parts or to ankylosis of the temporo-maxillary joint. For the latter condition osteotomy of the neck of the mandible may be undertaken as an alternative to excision of the condyle (see p. 319), and Rochet (Schlatter, *Von Bergmann's Surgery,* vol. i, p. 717) resects a portion of the ascending ramus of the lower jaw, and interposes a flap from the masseter to prevent bony union recurring. Grieg, in order to avoid the branches of the facial nerve, makes an incision at the level of the supraorbital ridge, running backwards above the malar bone nearly to the external auditory meatus and continued downwards just in front of the tragus to the level of the lobule. This flap is turned downwards and forwards, and the superficial temporal artery divided and ligatured if necessary; the fascia over the masseter is divided, and turned down with the parotid. The jaw can then be freed, from the condyle downwards, when the neck is divided transversely.

Küster for the same purpose makes an incision upon the posterior border of the ascending ramus, to avoid the internal maxillary artery and facial nerve. The soft parts are dissected away from the internal and external surface of the jaw. Access, however, is not so free by this method as by Grieg's incision. Von Bergmann succeeded in improving the deformity of the receding chin by extensive resection of all the processes and subsequent displacement forwards of the entire jaw by a dental apparatus.

Another method applicable to this class of case is a cuneiform osteotomy, so devised that the base of the wedge is at the angle of the jaw. Mr. Swain's case, referred to below, will serve as a good example of the indications for and results of this method. When the closure of the jaw is due to cicatrization within the mouth, osteotomy of the horizontal ramus is required, which is best carried out after the manner devised by Esmarch.

Esmarch's operation. Indications. For the relief of inability to separate the teeth, due to cicatrization within the mouth or to ankylosis of the temporo-maxillary joint, which cannot be dealt with by excision of the condyle. It is clear that the operation is only applicable to cases where the cicatrices are behind the teeth, as osteotomy can only be successful if carried out in front of the restricting bands.

The beneficial effect of Esmarch's operation is greater when it is only necessary to perform it on one side, and it is held by some that loss of power over the central fragment will usually result from the employment of Esmarch's operation on both sides. Jacobson (*loc. supra cit.*) quotes, as showing that this contention is certainly not universally true, a case operated on by Mr. Swain of Plymouth (*Lancet*, 1894. vol. ii, p. 189), in which, by a modification of Esmarch's operation, a wedge-shaped portion of the lower jaw at its angle was removed on both sides for closure of the mouth after scarlet fever. In this case relapse did not occur and excellent power of control of the body of the lower jaw was retained.

Operation. An incision two and a half inches long is made under the lower border of the mandible, and is placed so that its posterior extremity is in front of the cicatrices which are limiting the movements. When the incision has been carried through the skin the soft parts are raised with the fingers of the left hand, so that the skin wound is drawn up to the bone. The incision is then carried down to the bone, and in doing it the facial artery and vein will usually be exposed, and must either be drawn aside or divided between ligatures. With an elevator the overlying soft parts are carefully and freely raised from the periosteum on both the inner and outer surface of the mandible. The periosteum is now divided on either side of the wedge of bone to be removed. With a keyhole or Gigli's saw a triangular wedge of bone, having its apex at the alveolus, is now freed: the base of the wedge which is formed by the lower border of the mandible measuring at least one and a quarter inches in an adult, and in a child about three-quarters of an inch. Manipulation of the chin will not indicate whether sufficient bone has been removed, and whenever there is any doubt on this question it is better to remove an additional piece owing to the risk of relapse. In the section of the bone the inferior dental artery and nerve are of course divided: hæmorrhage from the former is usually not serious, but if necessary it may be controlled by crushing inwards the cancellous bone upon the cut surface of the jaw.

In order to prevent bony union between the two cut surfaces Helferich detached a portion of the masseter, and sutured it between the apposed surfaces. The wound is now sutured, with or without drainage, after which any teeth loosened during the course of the operation may be removed.

After-treatment. Active and passive movements should be begun on the third day, if necessary under an anæsthetic, and continued daily. The mouth must be frequently washed out with an antiseptic solution, such as resorcin (10 grains to the ounce) or chinosol (1 in 500).

Results. The great tendency after this operation is for relapse to occur. This may be obviated partly by ensuring that a sufficiently large wedge of bone has been removed, and partly by persistence in active and passive movements after the operation. Swain (*loc. supra cit.*) considers that by this modification of Esmarch's operation, if a sufficiently large wedge is removed, the danger of relapse is very remote, but the experience of other surgeons of this operation for cicatrization, such as results from cancrum oris in children, is on the whole discouraging.

TEMPORO-MAXILLARY ANKYLOSIS (MURPHY)

Murphy has studied this question of proper operative procedure in cases of ankylosis of the jaw. He has operated upon 23 cases and the experience gained by him makes his opinion worthy of serious consideration.

The work of Murphy has been summarized by Kreuscher in the *Interstate Medical Journal.* The following description of his work is given:

(a) The intra-articular bony ankylosis (true ankylosis); (b) the intra-articular fibrous ankylosis; (c) sub-zygomatic cicatricial fixations: (d) inter-alveolar buccal fixations.

Under c belongs the fixation in the sub-zygomatic area, resulting in scar tissue, which binds the coronoid process to the cranium. Under d belong the cicatricial fixations due to the sloughing of muscle and mucosa in the mouth or cheek.

Routes of Invasion. Murphy described four routes of infection invasion into or surrounding the temporo-mandibular articulation, namely:

First and most frequent, an extension of the suppuration from the middle ear.

Second, an osteitis or osteomyelitis of the mandible extending into the glenoid cavity.

Third, the metastases from foci of infection within the mouth or elsewhere in the body, or part of general metastatic arthritis.

Fourth, ankylosis may result from a transmitted trauma from the tip of the chin to the articulation, giving a traumatic osseous fibrous arthritis.

The glenoid cavity alone may be involved in the ankylosis, or the bony bridge may extend forward to include the zygomatic and coronoid processes.

Diagnosis. In the osseous type or firm fibrous type the diagnosis as to which side is involved is often extremely difficult. However, in nearly all the cases one is able to detect the ankylosed side from a close study of the physical findings, which were described by Murphy as follows:

1. There is a flattening of the jaw on the unaffected side, most pronounced near the tip of the chin. The side which appears normal is the one which is involved in the ankylosis and the flattened side is the one in which the joint is not fixed.

2. When the patient attempts to open his mouth, the teeth move from 1 60 to 1 100 of an inch downward and deviate a little in the direction of the ankylosed side. This is due to a sliding forward of the mandibular articulation on the unaffected side, as the muscles of the neck are put on tension in the effort made to open the mouth.

3. A sliding motion on the unaffected side can be felt by the palpating finger, and the muscular activity on that side is very much greater on attempted opening and closing of the mouth than on the ankylosed side.

4. The muscles on the ankylosed side are more atrophied than those on the unaffected side.

5. The distance by measurement from the lower edge of the zygomatic arch to the lowest point on the ramus of the jaw is less on the affected side than on the well one. This is true especially when there has been some destruction of the upper end of the mandibular articulation or when the ankylosis occurs in infants or children. As a general rule, the earlier the ankylosis has occurred in life the greater the deformity of the face, due to the fact that the epiphysis of the condyle is the means through which the ramus grows in length. The growth is arrested by the ossification across the epiphyseal line before the normal time for ossification at this point, which is in the fifteenth year.

Details of the operation. The technique of the operation as originally described by Dr. Murphy and later improved by him is as follows: In all the cases of ankylosis of the jaw of the intra-articular type the operation has been a typical and uniform arthroplasty, employing the pedicled flap, consisting of the aponeurosis of the temporal muscle and fat. In the earlier operations the flap was fixed by suture to the connective-tissue and internal portion of the capsule. Now the flap is fixed at the basal angles only, thus avoiding the danger of injuring the internal maxillary artery, an accident which was encountered in one of the early cases. The joint is exposed by a perpendicular incision just in front of the ear, extending from 1½ inches above the zygoma in the hair-line downward to the lower border of the zygomatic (Fig. 148). This incision then curves forward on the superior margin of the zygoma for a distance of about ¾ of an inch and then curves upward slightly so as to avoid injuring the temporal and orbicular branches of the facial nerve. This leaves a very slight scar, most of it being hidden in the hair-line. It gives better access to the joint than does the perpendicular incision and is an improvement on the incision which was made several years ago.

Various means have been devised for dividing the head and neck of the mandible at the line of bony ankylosis, including chisels, Gigli saws, and olive-tipped dental burrs driven by electric motors. The last are much more rapid, but on the whole not so satisfactory as the chisel. It is needless to point out that the greatest caution is necessary in the use of the chisel and burr because of the close proximity of the internal maxillary artery and also the brain, which is separated from the head of the mandible by a very thin transparent plate of bone only. To avoid the injury mentioned, Murphy had devised special periosteotomes, the tip of which passed directly beneath the neck of the mandible and lay between that and the internal maxillary artery. One periosteotome is placed in position from each side, and all the bone lying anterior to them may be cut without any danger (Fig. 150). Bone-cutting forceps or nippers may also be used and are more convenient than the chisel for smoothing off the surface of the bone (Figs. 149, C and D). The Gigli saw may be used in dividing the mandible (Fig. 151).

After the incision has been made as described above, the edges of the wound are drawn downward, the lower lip being displaced below

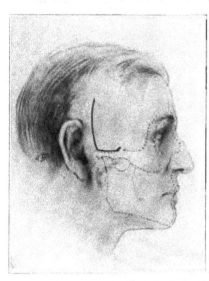

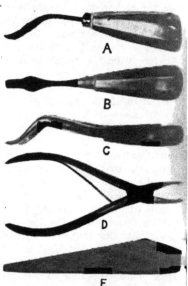

FIG. 148. THE LINE OF INCISION AND THE BONY OUTLINES AT THE POINT OF ANKYLOSIS. (*Murphy*.)

FIG. 149. A, B, DR. MURPHY'S PERIOSTEOTOME, SIDE AND BACK VIEW (somewhat reduced); C, D, bone-cutting forceps or nippers, side and front view (somewhat reduced); E, the interdental block designed by Dr. Murphy to maintain the desired separation of the jaws. It is made of wood, and since it is wedge-shaped, the degree of opening can easily be regulated by withdrawing or pushing in the block. (*Murphy*.)

the lower border of the zygoma. This gives a good exposure of the joint. The tissues are then pushed away with the special curved periosteotome all around the anterior surface of the line of union, and further separated with a similar instrument around the posterior surface. When the bone is laid bare, the two instruments are passed behind the neck of the bone, one on each side, so that when they are in place

ey completely encircle the neck of the mandible behind, hugging close
the head, holding the soft parts retracted during the excision of the
ıne (Fig. 150). The insertion of these instruments and their retention
position during the excision of the bone formed the key to the success
ıd safety of the operation. Injury to the internal maxillary artery,
hich closely hugs the neck of the mandible, is thus avoided. The

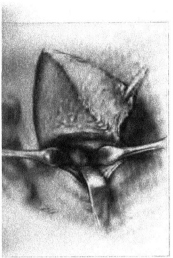 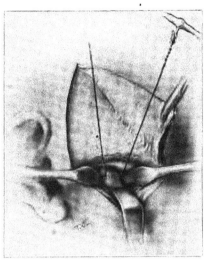

50. Special Periosteotomes in Po-   Fig. 151. The Gigli Saw used to divide
        sition. (*Murphy*.)   the Mandible. (*Murphy*.)

:traction of the soft tissues brought about by these instruments keeps
ıe field wide open during all the work. The chisel or burr then re-
ıoves a section of bone ½ inch wide clear across the neck of the
ıandible (Fig. 152). This must be done carefully and ample bone
ıust be removed so as to admit of the free insertion of the interposing
ıp of fat and fascia (Figs. 153 and 154). The periosteum should be
ıcised with the bone. The deeper fragments of bone can be taken out
ith a small rongeur. If one desires to use the Gigli saw for dividing
ıe neck of the mandible, a small full-curved aneurysm needle carrying
silk thread may be passed around the neck between it and the
ıriosteotome. This thread acts as a carrier for the Gigli saw. The
ifficulty of inserting the saw is slight, but the acute angulation of the
ire which necessarily occurs, occasionally causes it to break, putting

one to the inconvenience of replacing
that it is handled quite as easily as
completely divided, the mouth can b
The interposing fat and fascia flap
sary, the perpendicular incision is ex
1½ to 2 inches. Then a U-shaped

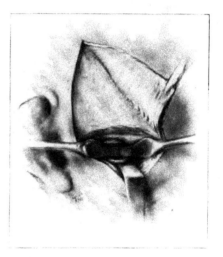

FIG. 152. THE GAP LEFT AFTER THE
EXSECTION, WITH THE CURVED PERIOSTEO-
TOMES STILL IN POSITION. (*Murphy*.)

over the temporal muscle. This fla
long and has its base at the upper
from above downward, folded dow
into the bony gap previously describ
few catgut sutures at its anterior an
The skin wound is accurately closed
subiodide, and sealed with collodion
ing needs to be applied.

No special effort should be mad
it is important that the lower jaw sh
in order that the wooden block inse
tain the wide separation of the me

has healed in. This block also prevents the muscular contraction from compressing and necrotizing the flap.

After much experience with arthroplasties, it has been learned that a hæmatoma very often forms about the field of operation, and if permitted to remain, will be disastrous to the result, the same as it would be in the knee or in the hip-joint. A hæmatoma following an arthro-

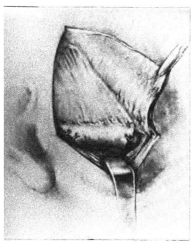

FIG. 154. THE FLAP IS NOW IN PLACE D THE WOUND READY FOR CLOSURE. 'urphy.)

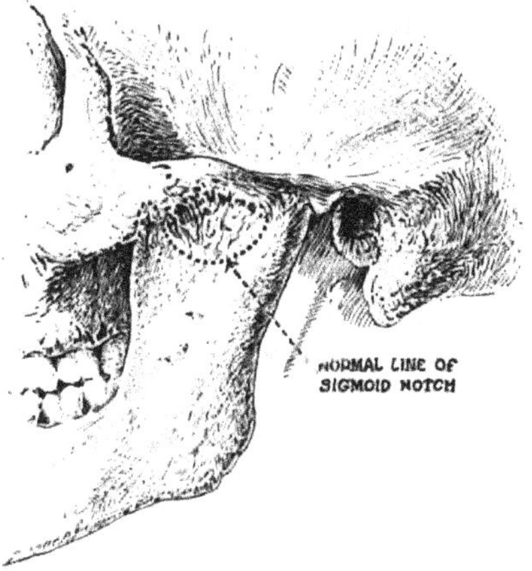

FIG. 155. SHOWING HOW THE SIGMOID NOTCH IS ENTIRELY FILLED WITH NEW-FORMED BONE. (*Murphy.*)

plasty is a disadvantage in three ways: First, it may necrotize a portion or all of the interposing flap; second, it may necrotize the skin overlying the operative field; third, and most important, it acts as a splendid culture medium in which organisms may grow and thence become destructive. To avoid such sequelæ it is important that the condition of the wound should be watched very carefully after the operation. If there is the slightest evidence of a hæmatoma, a small hypodermic or aspirating needle is inserted and the blood is drawn off. This may be repeated on the second day, and again on the third and fourth days or even more often, if necessary.

We have found that the position in which this wooden plug is held is of considerable importance. If the wedge is placed between the upper and lower incisors the jaws are kept apart, but the pressure which is necessarily exerted upon the flap by the neck of the mandible, with the masseter muscles acting as a fulcrum, must eventually destroy at least a portion of the flap which has been interposed. If, on the other hand, the wedge is passed backward between the upper and lower molars, the jaws are kept apart, with the additional advantage of keeping the freshly made bony surfaces from lying in apposition. In other words, the wedge serves the same purpose in husbanding the flap as the Buck extension does in arthroplasties of the knee, hip, and shoulder.

In the 3 cases of extra-articular fibrous fixation Dr. Murphy employed the method which we believe is original with him. It consisted in the utilization of mucous membrane pedicled flaps taken from the hard and soft palates and the tongue margin of the buccal mucosa, as an interposing medium between the divided cicatricial connective-tissue masses, for the purpose of preventing a recurrence of the fixation.

Operative complications. The location of the artery must always be borne in mind in the removal of the head and neck of the mandible, as it hugs the neck on the inner side very closely, and can easily be injured. If it is injured, the external carotid artery should be ligated opposite the cornu of the hyoid bone, where it is most accessible and readily reached. In one case it was necessary to resort to this procedure. In another case the external carotid was ligated as a pre-operative precautionary measure.

The second element of danger is realized on consideration of the facial nerve. This nerve leaves the skull through the stylo-mastoid foramen, passes forward across the lower portion of the parotid, where it is distributed to all the muscles of expression of the face. If this nerve is injured there is danger of inducing permanent paralysis, particularly of those fibres that pass to the temporal and supra-orbital zones. These can all be avoided by the L-shaped incision made just above the zygomatic level. The third element of danger lies in the fact that one is almost certain to penetrate the base of the skull if he endeavours to divide the ankylosis in the line of the original articulation. Therefore the condyle of the inferior maxilla is removed, but there is no attempt to clean out the glenoid fossa.

Post-operative treatment. The after-treatment is very important. Mastication should be started at the end of two weeks to avoid the formation of too much fibrous tissue between the ends of the divided bone. The wooden wedge should be placed between the molars on the operated side and kept there day and night for at least two weeks to prevent a possible compression necrosis of the interposing flap. If a hæmatoma forms under the flap, this must be aspirated repeatedly until all oozing has ceased.

CHAPTER VI

CORRECTION OF DEVELOPMENTAL OR ACQUIRED DEFORMITIES OF THE LOWER JAW

By Major Vilray P. Blair, M.D., F.A.C.S.

THE lower jaw is a long bone which lends itself readily to all of the ations that come within the scope of good surgery of long bones ther parts of the body. For both cosmetic and functional reasons, rmities of this bone are of more consequence in proportion to their nt than of any other long bone. It carries the inferior dental nerve, ch must be divided in most resections of this bone, but apparently nerve usually regenerates. The complicated shape of the bone and powerful muscles attached render the fragments difficult of control external splints, but the teeth give more exact anchorage than can obtained on any other bone. Contamination which might lead to mity or may be mortality in a resection of another long bone is an ost negligible incident in resection or fracture of the jaw-bone, and : ununited fractures are extremely rare. The most common de-nities of the lower jaw are: Forward protrusion, absolute, relative, oth; backward recession, which may also be either absolute, relative, oth; open bite, in which either or both jaws may participate; de-nities of the alveolar process. These deformities may be unilateral bilateral or there may occur as combinations of the above types. se deformities may be dependent upon mal-union or loss of bone, -occlusion or abnormalities of growth, and possibly atavism.

In the early formative age, these deformities may be completely or ially corrected by orthodontic procedures, which are more effective halting their further development than correcting them when fully blished.

Forward protrusion of the lower jaw. This is due most com-ily to an increase in the length of the body of the jaw, evidenced by rdental spaces in the molar regions, or to an increase of the angle i possibly increased length of the ramus, or to a combination of the ve conditions. Regardless of the cause, if sufficiently pronounced equire correction, we believe that removal of a properly shaped sec-

339

tion from the body of the bone on one or both sides is a better operati?
than attacking the angle, ramus, or neck of the condyle. The simplest
operation is an open section of the bone on one or both sides.

Transmucoperiosteal operation for protrusion of the lower jaw.
The mouth having been properly prepared, the shoulders are raised, an
the head drawn back.

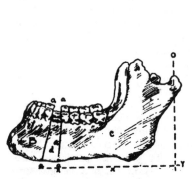

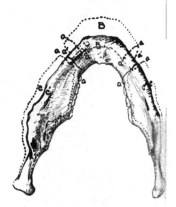

FIG. 156. ABNORMALLY LONG JAW
WITH INTERDENTAL SPACES IN THE BI-
CUSPID REGION. Showing position of
cuts for correction. (Blair, *Oral Surgery*.)

FIG. 157. RECONSTRUCTED JAW
SHOWING HOW BOTH FORWARD AND
LATERAL PROTRUSIONS ARE CORRECTED
BY REMOVING BONE SECTIONS. The dotted lines indicate the jaw-bone shown in
the preceding figure. (Blair, *Oral Surgery*.)

Fixing the jaw. In order to render the jaw rigid, a pine block is
inserted between the molar teeth, on one side, behind the site of the
proposed bone section. The jaws are closed firmly on the block, and
held there by wires passing between the molars. This will fix the lower
jaw securely; this fixation cannot be as completely obtained by means
of a mouth gag.

Cutting the bone. Corresponding to the site of the bone which is
to be removed, the skin lying under the border of the jaw is drawn
upward, and a cut 2 or 2½ centimetres is made parallel with this border. This will render the scar inconspicuous when the operation is
complete. The incision extends through the skin, fascia, and platysma.
The tissues are dissected from the outer surface of the jaw-bone, but
without on any account injuring or even exposing the periosteum. The
dissection is continued upward until the mouth is opened through the

co-alveolar cul-de-sac, the mucous covering of the gum being left
ct.

Before inserting the saw-blade, the exact position of the first saw-
is determined, and a flat piece of metal may be inserted into the

ind and turned on edge so as to rest
inst the bone just to the outside of
l parallel with the first cut. This will
ve as both a guide to the saw and a
tection from the soft tissues which
uld deflect the blade from its proposed
irse. The handle of a knife or the
de of another saw can be used. No
tter what kind of a saw is used, for
ious reasons the bone should not be
entirely through in any place until the
ation holes are drilled near the lower
der and all of the other saw-cuts are
least three-fourths of the way through.
e have a mechanical saw, very narrow
l probe-pointed (a nasal saw modi-
l), run by an engine and cable, that
is very rapidly; but a sharp, narrow-
ded metacarpal saw will suffice, and
probably safer. We use also an ad-
stable probe-pointed double-bladed saw,
lich is ideal for making parallel cuts.

**Submucoperiosteal operation for
otrusion of the lower jaw.** If the
erdental spaces are not sufficiently
ge, the teeth from the sites of the pro-
sed bone sections must be removed at
ist one month before the operation so
it the gum tissues will be entirely
aled. It is even better to wait until

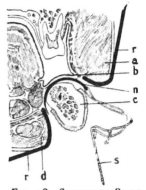

FIG. 158. SUBMUCOUS RESEC-
TION OF THE LOWER JAW. Coronal section through the body
of the jaw and the surrounding
tissues. a, Tissues of the cheek;
b, mucoperiosteum of the gum
raised from the body of the
jaw; c, body of the jaw, covered with periosteum on its
lower part; d, submaxillary tissues; n, curved needle passed
over the body of the jaw; r, retractors holding back the cheek
and submaxillary tissues; s,
wire saw, with ring replaced by
a sharp bend, attached to the
needle by a silk carrier. (Blair,
Oral Surgery.)

nsiderable absorption of the alveolar process has taken place.

The mouth is prepared for operation as usual. The exact site of
e piece of bone to be removed should be marked on the skin with a
ncil or a knife scratch. This will correspond to the centre of the
in incision. After the skin of the face and neck is prepared a sterile
ith or towel is sewed across the face from ear to ear on a line running
tween the mouth and the chin. This towel is turned upward over the
ier mask and prevents contamination from coughing or vomiting.

It is not necessary to fix the jaw, as it can be held up with the finger of an assistant.

Cutting of the bone. An incision 3 or 4 centimetres long is made along the under border of the jaw down to the periosteum. The soft tissues are dissected from the periosteum half-way up the inner an outer surfaces of the body of the jaw; from here up to within a short distance of the necks of the teeth, the dissection is subperiosteal. If th

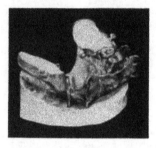

FIG. 159. LATERAL VIEW OF ANGLE SPLINT, SHOWING FLANGES DRILLED FOR BOLTS, AND ALSO BICUSPID TEETH THAT WERE REMOVED AT OPERATION. (Blair, *Oral Surgery*.)

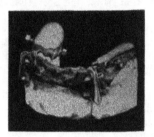

FIG. 160. ANGLE SPLINT AFTER OPERATION, LATERAL VIEW. To allow for inaccuracies, the distance between the flanges was made larger than the section of bone to be removed. After operation the space between the plates was filled with a piece of lead plate, beaten and cut to the proper shape. (Blair, *Oral Surgery*.)

necks of the teeth should be exposed, there would be a communicatic between the wound and mouth. It is easier to make the whole dissectio subperiosteally, but the vitality of the bone is better assured when t exposed ends are not entirely deprived of this source of nutrition. A the site of the interdental spaces a curved, blunt needle is passed ove the alveolar border of the jaw, hugging the bone closely; on no accou must this be allowed to penetrate into the mouth. It is followed by silk or linen carrier which in turn draws a Gigli saw into place (Fi 158).

The ring on one end of the Gigli saw is to be cut off, and the e bent into a sharp hook; this takes less room than the ring and is l liable to injure the mucoperiosteum of the gum. The eye of the opera is his only guide in making the cuts. Before making the cuts, the bone should be drilled for wires, and no saw-cut should be completed until all of the others in both sides are almost entirely through; otherwise one will be dealing with fragments that are difficult to control. For this reason it is better to use four saws. It is better to remove too little than too much bone; for, though the jaw-bone is extremely hard, it can be rongeured away with a good instrument or a coarse bone bur. While doing this, each fragment can be held with a pair of sharp-toothed lion forceps that will grasp the bone but will not tear its coverings.

Adjusting the bone. The bone sections having been removed, the new arch is formed by wiring the remaining fragments with silver wire, which was put through the holes drilled before the saw-cuts were made. The final twisting of these wires is not done until the intraoral fixation is made.

Fixation is accomplished chiefly by dental anchorage, either with a splint of the Angle type (Figs. 159 and 160) or by bands (Fig. 161). These are fixed in the mouth before the operation is done. In undertaking operations for forward protrusion of the lower jaw one must remember that much of the protrusion may be relative, and that in making a prominent lower jaw correspond accurately to the receding upper jaw, one may destroy the one strong feature in an otherwise weak face.

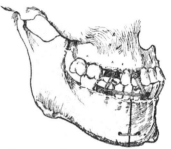

FIG. 161. FIXATION OF THE JAW BY WIRES AND BANDS, AFTER REMOVING A SECTION FROM THE BODY. The lower wire should show, bent downward. (Blair, *Oral Surgery*.)

Backward recession. If there is a full quota of teeth present, the recession is due to a change in the angle or to a lack of length in the ramus. Lack of teeth in the developing period will cause a lack of development of the body in that area. When possible the correction is most satisfactorily made by resection of the ramus on one or both sides and dragging forward of the body. If the recession follows an early ankylosis, the condyle on the ankylosed side may be removed and the ramus sectioned on the other.

Operation for retraction of the lower jaw.—Cutting the bone. The operation is done in this manner: An incision 2 centimetres long is made through the skin over the posterior border of the mandible. The skin is drawn forward and the parotid sheath is opened at the anterior border of the gland, which latter is drawn backward until the posterior border of the ramus can be felt. A large, strong, curved needle on a handle, threaded with a heavy silk carrier, is now passed between the parotid gland and the masseter muscle behind the ramus, hugging the bone closely. It passes forward between the ramus and the internal pterygoid muscle and emerges through the cheek without penetrating the mucous lining of the mouth. The diameter of the curved part of the needle should be a little greater than the width of the ramus.

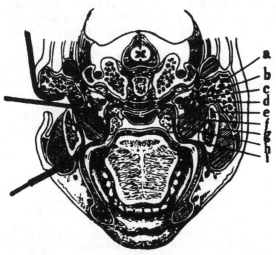

Fig. 162. Transverse Section of the Face at the Level of the Occlusal Surfaces of the Molars. On the left is shown the wound through the skin and fascia. The parotid gland is drawn back with a retractor and the wire saw is seen passing around the ramus and out through the cheek. Where it emerges, the skin of the cheek is protected by passing the saw through a thin metal tube. On the right side are indicated; a, parotid gland; b, temporo-maxillary vein; c, internal carotid artery; d, external carotid artery; e, ramus of the jaw containing the inferior dental nerve and vessels; f, internal pterygoid muscle; g, masseter muscle, h, tonsil; i, wall of the pharynx. (Blair, *Oral Surgery*.)

It is followed by a Gigli wire saw with which the bone is cut through (Fig. 163).

Hæmorrhage is controlled by packing the space with sterile or mildly antiseptic tape, which is left in place for one day. In this operation the parotid gland is pushed out of the way, as is also the cervico-facial division of the facial nerve, which lies at the posterior border of the jaw. The temporo-maxillary vein is also avoided, and the external carotid lies well out of the way. These anatomical points were verified by thirty special dissections (Figs. 162 and 163).

The needle used is full-curved. The curved portion, being almost one-half of a circle of 4 centimetres in diameter, must extend to the point in order to round the anterior border of the ramus without penetrating the mucosa. The point is so formed that it will dissect the soft structures from the inner surface of the bone rather than penetrate them (Fig. 164). In this way bleeding is avoided, and there will ordinarily be no danger of penetrating the mouth. To prevent damage of the skin, after the saw is in place, a short, small steel tube is passed over the anterior end of the saw, through the skin, and down to the bone. Posteriorly, the parotid gland is held back with a small retractor. In cutting the bone, the saw is held as straight as possible, and the operator should be familiar with the peculiarities of the Gigli saw (Figs. 162, 163).

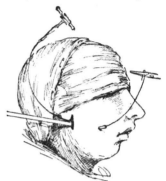

Fig. 163. Subcutaneous Section of the Ramus. Showing points of entrance and exit of the wire saw. (Blair, *Oral Surgery*.)

This operation presents three distinct problems: (1) the cutting of the bone, which is the easiest of the three; (2) the placing of the jaw in its new position; and (3) holding it there.

Adjusting the bone. The posterior part of the occlusal plane of the molars inclines upward and backward. On account of this obliquity

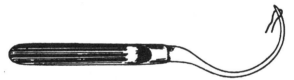

Fig. 164. Needle used for passing a Carrier around the Ramus of the Jaw. It is important that the curve of the needle extends up to the point. If the point end of the needle is somewhat straight, the needle is very apt to pierce the buccal mucosa and enter the mouth. (Blair, *Oral Surgery*.)

the body of the lower jaw can be brought forward only by lengthening the ramus; theoretically, the line of tthe saw-cut should be slightly down-

ward and forward about 5 millimetr
to allow the body to be moved dov
completely separating the several fra
ever, X-rays show that the fragmei
at the posterior border in the opera
difficult to exactly gauge the positioi

It is only the posterior part of t

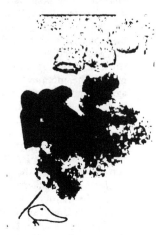

Fɪɢ. 165. X-ʀᴀʏ sʜᴏᴡɪɴɢ Cᴏɴᴅɪᴛɪoɪ
ᴛɪᴏɴ. Notice the obliquity with which tl
meets the lower portion. In this case tl
ankylosed joint, and on that side there is
ends of the ramus. Later this union b
excise the ankylosed joint. The nail an
piece of costal cartilage in place. (Blai

the rotation thus produced lessens tl
which is a very distinct advantage.

In order to lengthen the ramus i
and internal pterygoid muscles. P
done carefully as they are easily l
toothed lion forceps, the jaw may l
body, the teeth of the forceps penetr
osteum.

Fixation is immediately applied
Obliquity of the chin. If, as w

dontic or a bone-cutting operation for a receding jaw, the obliquity of the chin is so pronounced as to detract materially from the result, it may be improved by either injecting paraffin into the chin or inserting a piece of cartilage or rib.

Transplantation of bone or cartilage. To fill out the chin with bone or cartilage, an incision is made under the chin, and all of the tissues excluding the periosteum are reflected from the mental portion

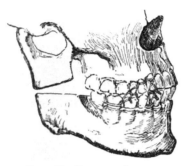 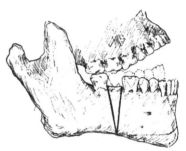

Fig. 166. Showing Jaw wired in its new Position after Section of the Ramus. (Blair, *Oral Surgery*.)

Fig. 167. Open Bite of an Extreme Type in a Young Man, showing how Correction might be made by a V-shaped Excision. This would have the disadvantage of shortening the jaw considerably, as shown in the reconstructed jaw indicated by dotted lines. The operation shown in Fig. 168 was done in this case. (Blair, *Oral Surgery*.)

of the mandible. Bleeding should be controlled by pressure. Next, the seventh or eighth costal cartilage is exposed, and a section removed, including its perichondrium. This should be done without wounding the pleura or the intercostal vessels, though we have several times wounded the pleura in a dog without any apparent evil consequences. The cartilage is picked up with toothed forceps and trimmed with a bone-cutting forceps; the finger with or without gloves should not be put into either wound. As soon as each skin wound is made, the knife that cuts through the skin should be discarded, and the skin excluded from the operating field by attaching sterile cloths to the cut edges with tenaculum forceps or safety pins. The cartilage can be fastened to the bone with one or two wires or nails. The bone and cartilage having been drilled, the wound is closed without drainage by deep through and through silkworm-gut sutures. If suppuration should oc_cur, neither the sutures nor the cartilage are to be removed unless the infection be of a virulent character. We have had two pieces of cartilage and one piece of the tibia stay in place and unite to the soft tissues by its perichondrial or periosteal surface when there was suppuration

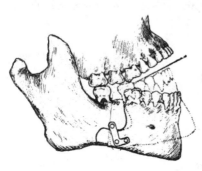

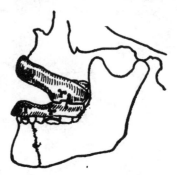

FIG. 168. SHOWING OPERATION BY S-SHAPED BONE-CUT, THAT LENGTHENS THE JAW-BONE AND GIVES A BETTER CLOSURE OF THE MOUTH. The silver splints at the site of the bone-cut are absolutely necessary and increase the risk of sepsis. The bone spaces will fill in satisfactorily, but the transverse part of the 'S' cut must be in hard bone. (Blair, *Oral Surgery*.)

FIG. 169. SHOWING A MODIFICATION OF THE GUNNING SPLINT THAT MAY BE USED FOR ANY CASE IN WHICH THE JAWS ARE TO BE HELD APART. This is made in two pieces, which are fastened together after each half has been fixed in place. Its application is very much simpler than is that of the original Gunning splint. (Blair, *Oral Surgery*.)

occurring in its deep surface. In one of the cartilage cases, an injection of Beck's bismuth paste stopped the suppuration.

Open bite. This deformity has been corrected by bone cuts shown in Figs. 167 and 168 or division of the bone at the angle. Considerable difficulty has been encountered in holding up the mental fragment in its new position owing to the pull of the suprahyoid muscles. This is best overcome by dressing the mouth wide open (Fig. 169). If the open bite is due to a mal-union at the angle, then this latter plan cannot be followed, but the body of the jaw must be placed and maintained in its proper position at once.

Deformities of the alveolar process. These are to be treated according to the type encountered. One of the first recorded cases of resection of the jaw for correction of pure deformity was by Hullihan of West Virginia in 1848, who made a deep resection of the alveolar process without disturbing its contained teeth for a deformity caused by scar contraction. It was held in its new place by a swaged splint.

The correction of these deformities should not be undertaken by the general surgeon without the aid of a competent dental oral surgeon. He should be called in before and not after the operation is done.

SECTION IV

PLASTIC SURGERY AND BURNS AND SCALDS

PLASTIC SURGERY

BY

T. P. LEGG, M.S. (Lond.), F.R.C.S. (Eng.),
Lieutenant-Colonel, R.A.M.C.(T.)
Surgeon to the Royal Free Hospital

BURNS AND SCALDS

BY

J. M. MacLEOD, M.A., M.D., F.R.C.P. (Lond.)
Physician for Diseases of the Skin, Victoria Hospital for Children.
Physician for Diseases of the Skin, Charing Cross Hospital

PRINCIPLES OF PLASTIC SURGERY

BY

H. D. GILLIES, F.R.C.S. (Eng.), B.A. (Cantab.),
Major, R.A.M.C.(T.)
Surgeon to Throat and Ear Department, Prince of Wales Hospital, N.

CHAPTER I

GENERAL PRINCIPLES: SKIN-GRAFTING

PLASTIC SURGERY is the method by which a surgeon attempts to remedy some deformity or to restore, as far as possible, a lost portion of the body. It is also the means by which a surgeon attempts to repair an organ, or some part of it essential to the carrying on of its proper function, which may have been accidentally damaged or injured as the result of some operative procedure. For centuries, plastic operations on the face have been performed. The operation of rhinoplasty appears to have been known to and practised by the ancient Egyptians. The Indian method dates from very early times, and the Italian (Tagliacotian) method from the year 1597, but it is only since the early part of the last century that the development of plastic surgery may be said to have taken place. In 1869 Reverdin published his method of skin-grafting; afterwards, Thiersch, using large grafts, obtained more satisfactory results and further added to the advancement of this branch of surgery, which until quite recent years was concerned with the restoration of a defect which was on the surface of the body. At the present time the internal organs have plastic operations performed on them, and even the blood-vessels have been successfully sutured after having been partially divided.

GENERAL PRINCIPLES

Sound and rapid healing is essential for the successful performance of plastic operations. The patient must be in the best possible state of health, and the neighbouring tissues free from disease. These operations must be deferred, therefore, till such conditions are present. Failure to obtain the desired effect by the first operation makes subsequent attempts less likely to succeed, as such failures always leave behind scar tissue. The best results are obtained with fresh, healthy structures, and though it is possible to succeed even when a certain amount of scar tissue is present, the ultimate result is never so satisfactory as when working with the normal tissues. In some cases scar tissue may have to be utilized, but it can never be relied upon; in other cases, the local conditions may render a repetition of the operation impossible; moreover, it is possible that an unsuccessful plastic operation may leave the patient in a worse condition than that before it was attempted.

An attempt to do too much at one operation is another source of failure. It is better to avoid trying to attain the total restoration of a defect when the tissues are scanty and to proceed by stages rather than to risk a complete failure as the result of one operation. By a series of operations, and by allowing a sufficiently long interval to elapse

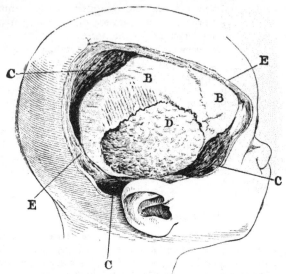

FIG. 170. CLOSURE OF A LARGE DEFECT BY MEANS OF FLAPS. The patient was a boy aged two years, who had a large part of his scalp torn off as a result of a street accident. B, B are the cranial bones. D is the dura mater exposed by the removal of a large part of the squamous portion of the temporal bone, which was extensively fractured and depressed, and ingrained with dirt. The dura is shown covered with granulations. C, C, C are the deeper tissues of the scalp and pericranium; E, E, the edges of wound in the scalp. (*From a photograph.*) See also Fig. 171.

between them, it is sometimes possible to make use of the same tissues over again. It is courting failure to attempt plastic surgery on the aged or very feeble, or in the neighbourhood of active disease, *e.g.* syphilis or tubercle, but provided these diseases are cured or quiescent, excellent results may be obtained.

Septic infection is another potent cause of failure, and therefore special attention must be paid to the details of asepsis in these operations.

Methods of cutting and using flaps. Each particular case has to be treated on its merits, success often depending on the ingenuity of the operator. Flaps must be thick and include the subcutaneous tissue, but not as a rule the deep fascia, so that their vitality is not impaired. Besides the skin, flaps containing other structures, such as bone or

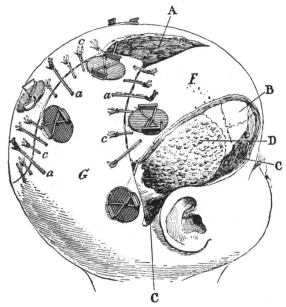

Fig. 171. Method of closing a Large Defect by means of Flaps. *Author's case.*) The incisions marking out the flaps are parallel to the lines of he vessels. The flap F was taken from the fronto-parietal region, and the flap from the occipital region, each being glided into its new position. They con-ined all the layers of the scalp except the pericranium, A, which is exposed. *a, a* are silver wire sutures; *c, c, c,* silkworm-gut sutures. The method of ing silver wire and lead buttons is also shown. By subsequent operations the fect was closed more completely. (*From a photograph.*)

riosteum, are occasionally employed, as in some of the operations r restoration of the nose. In cutting a flap, it is better, whenever ssible, to use curved rather than straight incisions; more tissue is this way obtained, and there is consequently much less tension when it fixed in position. The incisions marking out the flap should be made rallel to the line of the blood-vessels, or placed so as to interfere with the vascular supply as little as possible (Fig. 171). The knife must be directed towards the deep fascia so that the blood-supply to the skin. which is derived from the subcutaneous tissues, is not cut off, and care should be taken that the flap is neither button-holed nor scored on its deep aspect. Its length is proportional to the width of the pedicle, which should be as broad as is consistent with the flap being accurately and readily applied in its new position; in doing so the pedicle must not be twisted or stretched to such an extent as to occlude the blood-vessels.

The raw area from which the flap has been taken is closed by undermining the adjacent skin and subcutaneous tissues, or by skin-grafting.

The method most frequently employed is to simply *glide* the flap obtained from the neighbourhood of the defect into its new position, where it is fixed by sutures (Fig. 171); extensive wounds, such as those left by the removal of the breast for carcinoma, malignant disease of the cheek, &c., are frequently closed in this manner. Sometimes the flap is *transplanted* from another part of the body; the extent and completeness of the union with the surrounding tissues, especially at the distal end of the flap, determines the time when it is safe to sever the pedicle; on an average this is in ten or fourteen days. The flap gradually adjusts itself to its new surroundings, and there is ultimately no difference in the sensibility of it and that of the adjacent parts, but secondary operations are frequently necessary to correct various irregularities in the flap.

Flaps may also be employed in three other ways. *The reversed flap,* in which the cuticle is directed inwards and the deep surface outwards, the latter being covered by skin grafts. *Superimposed or double flaps* (Fig. 214, p. 413); the outer or raw surface of a reversed flap is covered by a second flap with its cuticle directed outwards, the two flaps having their raw surfaces in apposition. Instead of a superimposed flap. the first one may be folded on itself after the pedicle has been divided (Fig. 213, p. 411). *Granulating flaps;* the flap is dissected up, but is left attached by both its extremities for some ten to fourteen days, or longer if necessary. During this time, *i.e.* whilst it is granulating, the deep surface of the flap is prevented from uniting to the adjacent tissues, by the insertion of a sterilized piece of protective. The vitality of the flap in its new position is more likely to be assured after the pedicle is divided if its deeper parts are granulating. This method of using a flap has some advantages. In the first place, it may be cut much longer in proportion to its width, without fear of sloughing; as a rule the length should not exceed three times its width, these dimensions being marked out according to the size of the area to be covered, due allowance being made for shrinkage. The limits of the flap having been determined.

it is dissected up freely, carefully, and completely throughout its whole extent down to the deep fascia or aponeurosis. At the end of ten to fourteen days the flap will have become thick and vascular; one pedicle may then be divided and the flap turned into the place prepared for its reception. Secondly, such a flap will adhere in a short time if care is taken to excise and divide every portion of cicatricial tissue and to have a freshly made raw surface; two weeks is an average time for adequate vascular union to occur in its new position, but the final severance of the flap is a matter of some importance and must depend on the amount and soundness of the union which has taken place. The disadvantage of this method of 'granulating flaps' is that it is very complicated and cannot often be employed.

In the *Indian and French methods* the flap is taken from the parts adjacent to the area to be occupied by it. In the *Italian* (*Tagliacotian*) *method* the flap is derived from a distal part, such as one of the arms.

Whenever a flap is being used to close a cicatrizing area, the scar tissue must be removed and the edges carefully refreshed so that everywhere there is a fresh raw surface on which to place it. At the same time care must be taken not to remove too much of the scar tissue without some good reason. Immediate and secure union of the refreshed surfaces with the flap is most essential, and therefore they must be carefully fixed in position by sutures with a minimum amount of tension. If the edges are not in perfect apposition at all points a good result may still be obtained, and attempts to obtain a complete apposition should not be made at the expense of undue tension or dragging on the flap. The position of the flap is maintained by sutures, with or without some form of retentive apparatus (as in the Tagliacotian operations).

Methods of suturing. The suturing is most important, and a good deal of the success or want of success of a plastic operation depends on this factor. Of the many materials used for sutures, silkworm-gut and silver wire are the best. Catgut may be used for buried sutures and for uniting mucous membranes. The great advantage of silkworm-gut is that it does not absorb moisture, and is only slightly irritating unless tied tightly. Fine horsehair, sterilized by boiling, may be used for delicate tissues, whenever it is important to avoid stitch marks and when the parts can be readily brought into apposition, but fine silkworm-gut is equally efficient. Whatever material is chosen, all sutures should be just tight enough to hold the parts in apposition, and there must be no tension or dragging after they are tied.

As soon as the knot is tied the effect on the flap and skin should be noticed. Any suture which is causing tension produces an area of whiteness, which persists in the parts adjacent to it. If a suture is not tied too tightly the blanching which follows its insertion passes away in a few minutes, and is followed by a red blush. After the operation there is always some swelling of the flap and tissues around it; a stitch, therefore, which appears to be slack, will become tighter, and if any

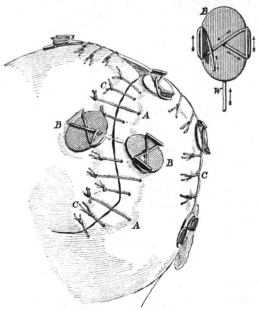

FIG. 172. DIFFERENT METHODS OF USING SUTURES. A, A are silver wires used as deep sutures, and passed some distance from the edges. The ends of the wire are twisted round one another. B, B are ' relief of tension,' or ' relaxation' sutures, fastened to leaden buttons. The smaller figure shows more clearly how the wire, w, is fastened to the button. C, C, C are the superficial, or ' stitches of apposition ', passed not far from the edges. Instead of being interrupted, it is often preferable to put them in as a continuous stitch. There should be no tension at all on these stitches.

are tied too tightly, a zone of inflammation with a greater degree of swelling will follow. The pressure of the stitch may lead to a local sloughing, and therefore prevent primary union, and should this happen around several of them, a considerable area of the flap may be destroyed. Under these circumstances, the advent of sepsis is not infrequent and further sloughing takes place, resulting in complete or partial failure of the operation.

It is often necessary to use *deep* or *'relief of tension'* stitches in addition to those uniting the edges. They should be passed at some distance from the margins (Figs. 171 and 172) and tied only just tight enough to bring the deep parts into apposition. Silver wire may be employed for these stitches. The ends of the wire may be passed through a leaden button and fixed by fastening them to the button in 'a figure-of-eight,' or they may be loosely twisted round one another (see Figs. 171 and 172). Under each button a pad of gauze must be placed to prevent local sloughing from its pressure. In the absence of the silver wire and buttons, stout silkworm-gut, fastened to small pieces of india-rubber

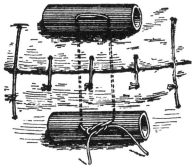

Fig. 173. The Method of using India-rubber Tubing and Silkworm-gut as 'Relief of Tension' Sutures. The gut is first passed through one piece of the tubing, then through the tissues, and finally through the other piece of tubing. As it is tightened, the edges of the raw area will be approximated, and they are then united by the superficial sutures.

tubing, does excellently (Fig. 173). When these sutures are applied it is generally possible to bring the edges together without tension by the *superficial stitches* or *stitches of apposition*. If they cannot be completely united, as much as possible should be sutured, and the unclosed portions will heal by granulating, or if an area of some size remains, it may be skin-grafted. In passing the sutures, those should be inserted first which bring the important points opposite to one another and all the deep before the superficial ones.

The deep and 'relief of tension' stitches may be removed about the fourth or fifth day; as a rule they should not be left longer than a week. A little local ulceration may follow from the pressure of the button, if one is used. The remaining stitches are removed when the edges appear to be firmly united, or at such times as may appear to be advisable.

When the flap is taken from a distal portion of the body, such as a limb, it is necessary to fix the limb to the part being restored. A special apparatus may be required, or a casing of plaster of Paris may be employed. Trials should be made before the operation is performed in order to find the most comfortable and tolerable position of the limb, and the pedicle in these cases should be wide, so that the flap may be as long as possible and capable of being adjusted without tension.

THE CLOSURE OF TRIANGULAR GAPS

1. If the gap is small and forms an equilateral triangle, the edges may be brought into apposition simply by undercutting them.

2. If the gap is large, one of the following methods may be used:—

(*a*) An incision, B D, continues the side A B.   The triangular flap

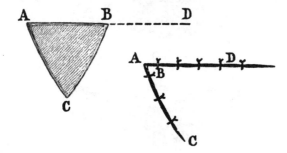

FIG. 174. METHOD OF CLOSING A TRIANGULAR GAP OF SMALL SIZE. By making an incision, B D, the flap C B D can be raised so as to allow B C and A C to be united by sutures, as in the figure.   More accurate apposition may be obtained by the use of a continuous suture.

C B D, consisting of skin and subcutaneous tissue, is then dissected up to allow B C to be sutured to A C (Fig. 174).

(*b*) If one flap is not sufficient, another similar flap, E A C, may be raised from the opposite side of the triangle and the edges A C and B C brought together in the middle of the gap. If there is much tension on the flaps, parallel incisions may be made beyond the points D and E. When the flaps are in position, oval-shaped gaps are left which will heal by granulation, or these may be closed by further undercutting the tissues around them (Fig. 175).

(*c*) Instead of a straight incision, a curved incision, as in Fig. 176, p. 362, is often preferable for marking out the flaps when the defect is large, and when it is desirable to have a scar as little evident as possible.

THE CLOSURE OF QUADRILATERAL GAPS

A gap, A B C D, may be closed by making the incisions B E and D F dissecting up the flap E B D F so that B D and A C can be united by hes (Fig. 178, p. 363). If one flap is insufficient, a second flap,

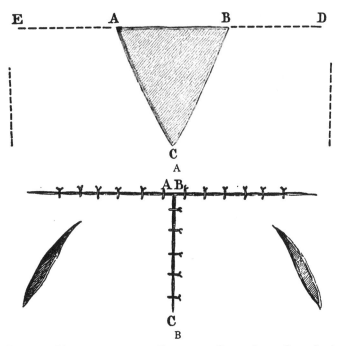

FIG. 175. METHOD OF CLOSING A TRIANGULAR GAP OF LARGE SIZE. In A the es E A and B D represent the incisions made to allow of the flaps E A C and ʒ C being raised, so that A C and B C may be united by sutures as in B. If ːre is much tension on the flaps, incisions, in A represented by the vertical tted lines, may be made to allow the edges to be readily approximated, and the al-shaped gaps left by making these incisions are shown in B.

A C H, may be obtained from the opposite side of the gap by making e incisions G A and H C and sliding the two flaps inwards over the p, so that A C and B D meet, and are united by sutures. These inci-ɔns must be sufficiently long to allow the flaps to meet without tension ʔig. 179, p. 364).

THE CLOSURE OF ELLIPTICAL GAPS

This may often be effected by simply undermining the skin around t
edges of the gap (Fig. 180, p. 365), or by means of a curved incisi
E D F, parallel to one of its margins.   An incision, C D, divides the a

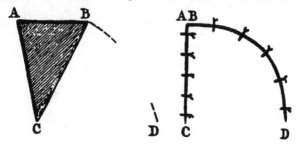

FIG. 176. METHOD OF CLOSING A TRIANGULAR GAP BY USING A CURVED
INCISION. The flap C B D is dissected up and B C united to A C.

E A B F into two flaps, E D C A and F D C B, which are glided over the n
area so that A C and B C are united to the edge A G B (Fig. 181, p. 36

In the closure of any defect, attention must be paid to the followi
points: (1) As far as possible the incisions should be made parallel to t
lines of the vessels, and the division of important nutrient arteries m

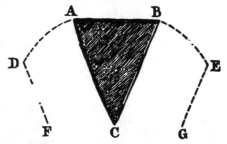

FIG. 177.   METHOD OF CLOSING A LARGE TRIANGULAR DEFECT BY MEANS
FLAPS. A quadrilateral flap, F D A C and G E B C, is raised on each side of t
defect and then glided inwards, so that A C and B C are in contact and united
sutures.

be avoided; (2) the incisions should be made in the natural lines
cleavage of the skin; the scars will then be least visible; (3) free und
cutting of the adjacent subcutaneous tissue, provided the whole or great
part of it is taken up and the skin is not scored on its deep aspect.

SKIN GRAFTING

Skin-grafting is one of the most important and widely applicable rms of plastic surgery. It may be used when other methods are not itable or available, or in conjunction with them, and is most valuable obtaining rapid and sound healing, not only of granulating wounds it also of large freshly-made wounds, which cannot otherwise be

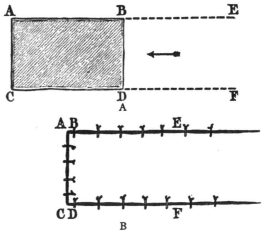

FIG. 178. METHOD OF CLOSING A SMALL QUADRILATERAL DEFECT. A. The icisions B E and D F are made, continuing the sides A B and C D of the gap utwards into the surrounding tissues. A flap, E B D F, is raised sufficiently freely o allow B D to be sutured to A C without tension. This is accomplished by iaking B E and D F longer than they are here represented.

B. The flap is in position, and its edges are sutured to those of the defect.

losed. It is often required when large raw surfaces are left, such as ollow burns, sloughing of the skin after cellulitis and injuries, ulcers, xtensive lupus, and the large wounds remaining after removal of a odent ulcer or a cancer of the breast, &c. In such cases, a sound supple car is desirable, and whenever it is important to avoid contraction, ine of the methods of skin-grafting may be employed. To obtain these esults it is essential to carry out the operation with great attention to the irinciples which underlie its successful performance. Moreover the zeneral state of health of the patient plays an important part, and unless ill these details are attended to, the result will be a failure.

The first point is that the raw surface to be grafted must be healthy, or if it be an ulcer, it must have commenced to heal, as shown by the presence of a thin bluish-red epithelial line at its edges. When these conditions are present, the sooner the raw area is grafted the better will be the ultimate result, because the amount of contraction will be the least possible. A large raw surface left by the removal of a tumour may be grafted at once. It is useless to attempt to graft a septic ulcer or wound.

Secondly, the tissues in the neighbourhood of the area to be grafted must be in a healthy condition. If they are congested or in-

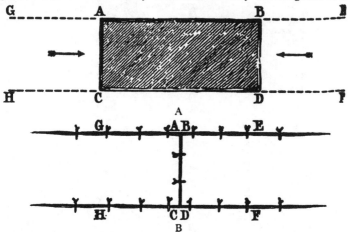

FIG. 179. METHOD OF CLOSING A LARGE QUADRILATERAL DEFECT. A. Two flaps (one from each side of the defect) are dissected up, in a manner similar to that shown in Fig. 178. B. They are then pulled towards the centre of the defect and the apposing edges sutured.

flamed, or otherwise diseased, the grafts are certain not to take, and therefore, before the operation is undertaken, every means must be employed to get the parts into a healthy condition. It is well recognized that many ulcers show no signs of healing so long as the surrounding tissues are diseased. This may be due to local and general causes, and before undertaking skin-grafting any such influences must be remedied; thus, in the case of a chronic ulcer of the leg, varicose veins may require removal, or if the ulcer is due to tertiary syphilis the patient must be given anti-syphilitic remedies. Tertiary syphilis in itself is not necessarily a contra-indication to skin-grafting, and very successful results may be obtained in such patients provided the general health of the patient and local conditions are satisfactory. In fact, it may be said that if the ulcer shows signs of healing as evidenced by the

ate of the edges, the patient's general health is such that the grafting
ill probably be successful. In old and feeble patients with a poor
rculation, or in diabetics or those with extensive disease of the lungs,
‹in-grafting will not succeed.

Thirdly, the situation of the raw surface to be grafted has an impor-
int bearing on the result. Absolute rest and firm pressure are essential
‚ success, and therefore in parts of the body, such as the limbs, a
uccessful result is more frequent than where immobility is less easy

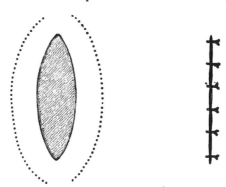

Fig. 180. The Closure of an Elliptical Area by undermining the
Skin and Subcutaneous Tissues around it. The dotted lines indicate the
extent to which this should be done. The edges are then united by a continuous
or interrupted suture.

to secure, *e.g.* the neck and back. In the neighbourhood of joints,
excellent and permanent results may be obtained provided that care
is taken to prevent movements being carried out too soon after the
raw surface has been grafted and healed. Lastly, the after-treatment
is most important.

The principles of the operation itself may be considered under the
following heads :—

1. The preparation of the raw area to be grafted, and of the area
from which the grafts are to be taken.

2. The method of grafting.

3. The after-treatment.

The preparation of the raw area to be grafted. It has been
pointed out that the raw area must be as aseptic as possible and therefore means must be taken to obtain this condition. The surrounding
skin must be shaved and thoroughly washed with ether soap and water, or

ordinary soap and turpentine may be used, the parts being thoroughly scrubbed with a nail-brush. The skin is then washed with 1 in 500 biniodide of mercury in spirit and afterwards with 1 in 2,000 perchloride of mercury lotion. If an ulcer, hot fomentations are applied and changed every three or four hours. The fomentations may be made with boro-glyceride, sanitas and water, or chlorinated soda if the ulcer is very foul.

The use of strong germicides may be discussed here. There is no doubt that these are very efficacious in destroying septic granulations,

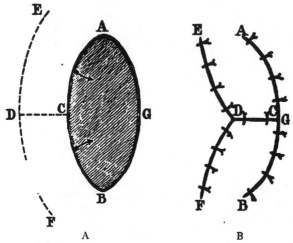

A   B

Fig. 181. Closure of a Large Elliptical Area by means of Flaps. In A the curved incision E D F is made parallel to the edge A C B, and the intervening portion of skin and subcutaneous tissue is divided by the incision D C into two flaps, which are glided over the raw area, and sutured as in B. The tissues on the outer side of E D F and A G B may require to be undermined, so that the edges may be sutured without tension.

but they also impair the vitality of the underlying healthy tissues, and should therefore be only used sparingly and at the commencement of the preparatory treatment. It is unnecessary to use any such agents when the ulcer is not very foul; they lower the vitality of the young growing cells and render them more susceptible to any micro-organisms which may gain access to the wound. Of these powerful germicides, undiluted carbolic acid is the best: it is applied by dipping a small piece of sponge or wool into the acid, thoroughly rubbing the surface of the granulations and edges of the ulcer, and allowing it to act for some minutes. A good deal

)ain is temporarily produced, but it passes off in a short time. An-
:r efficacious way of getting rid of the foul granulations is to scrape
n with a sharp spoon, whilst the patient is under a general anæsthetic:
Whilst the preparatory treatment is being carried out, every
ins should be taken to improve the local conditions, the skin
·ounding the ulcer being regularly washed and disinfected. Eighteen
twenty-four hours previous to the operation, the whole region is
in purified and enveloped in a dressing of sterilized gauze, wrung
of 1 in 2,000 perchloride of mercury, covered with protective and
daged.

**The preparation of the area from which the grafts are to
taken.** The area from which the grafts are taken should be as
: from hairs as possible. The front of the thigh, the flexor aspect
the arm or forearm, will therefore usually be the sites selected.
: skin must be thoroughly disinfected by scrubbing with ether soap,
·it and biniodide lotion (1 in 500), followed by 1 in 2,000 perchloride,
I then a dressing wrung out of the latter lotion and covered with
ta-percha tissue is put on. It is advisable to do this preparation
ty-eight hours before the operation, and to repeat it in twenty-four
irs' time.

The method of grafting. Under this heading the following
nts have to be considered :—

1. The final preparation of the ulcer.
2. The cutting of the grafts.
3. The dressing and after-treatment.

1. **The final preparation of the ulcer.** The patient having
·n anæsthetized, the ulcer is first scraped with a sharp spoon, to remove
soft granulations and to leave a smooth, raw, even bed of new-formed
·ous tissue. The edges of the ulcer must be removed at the same time,
ier by scraping or cutting them away. The raw surface bleeds freely,
I it is essential to arrest the hæmorrhage, after having first washed
ay the separated granulation tissue by douching with 1 in 2,000 per-
oride of mercury lotion, followed by sterilized normal saline solution.
essure is the most efficient means of arresting the bleeding. A
ficiently large piece of dextrinized protective or gutta-percha tissue,
ich has previously been sterilized by keeping it for a prolonged time
1 in 20 carbolic acid lotion, is laid flat on the raw surface and covered
layers of gauze. A sterilized bandage is then firmly applied out-
e the gauze, or, if the area is small, an assistant can make the desired
:ssure manually. It is well to make some small holes in the protective,
iich must be rinsed in sterilized salt solution or boracic acid lotion
fore it is used. The protective or gutta-percha tissue is applied to the

raw surface in preference to making direct pressure by gauze, because the latter adheres to the raw surfaces; and when removed fresh bleeding occurs. One of the most essential points to be attended to is that there should be no oozing going on when the grafts are placed in position. Whilst the hæmorrhage is being arrested, the grafts are prepared, but before doing this it is advisable for the operator to thoroughly disinfect his hands or to put on sterilized gloves and during the remainder

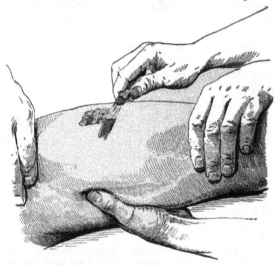

FIG. 182. THIERSCH'S METHOD OF SKIN-GRAFTING. To show how the knife should be held, and the position of the hands to steady and make tense the skin. On the right leg it is convenient to cut the grafts from below upwards and in the reverse direction on the left leg.

of the operation to use sterilized salt solution or dilute boracic acid lotion.

2. **The cutting of the grafts.** There are three methods of cutting the grafts: (1) *Thiersch's*, (2) *Reverdin's*, (3) *Wolfe's*. Thiersch's is the best and most widely applicable method, but there are occasions when it may be desirable to use one of the other methods. Whichever is employed the utmost delicacy and care in handling the grafts must be exercised.

1. *Thiersch's method* (Figs. 182 and 183). The grafts consist of the whole thickness of the epidermis together with the superficial portion of the cutis vera, so that the tips of the papillæ are just severed. If the

;rafts are cut too thick they curl up and become very difficult to manipu-
ate. The proper thickness of the grafts is obtained when the raw sur-
ace left by their removal shows numerous minute punctiform hæmor-
hages. If this thickness of skin only is removed no scarring follows.
n the course of time it becomes almost impossible to distinguish the
)lace from which the grafts were taken, though a certain amount of
ight brown pigmentation may be left; in fact the same site can be used,
f necessary, for providing a second series of grafts.

Very few simple instruments are required; these are a knife, a
)air of scissors, dissecting forceps, a couple of fine probes, and possibly

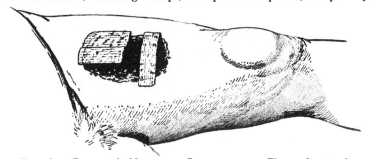

FIG. 183. THIERSCH'S METHOD OF SKIN-GRAFTING. The grafts are shown
in position on the area to be covered. The overlapping of the grafts, and of the
latter over the edges of the raw area, is shown.

a broad smooth metallic spatula (Fig. 184) for transferring the grafts.
Thiersch's razor, which has a broad flat surface (Fig. 185), is used by
many surgeons, but an amputating knife with a blade four or five inches
long is the best kind of knife to use. Whatever kind of cutting instrument is employed, it must be extremely sharp in order to work easily;
therefore in sterilizing it some means must be taken to protect the edge.
Whilst the grafts are being cut the blade should be kept moistened with
normal saline solution or boracic acid lotion; unless this is done the
grafts adhere to the blade and curl up.

The skin is kept as tightly stretched as possible in the long axis of
the limb, the assistant placing his hands one above and the other below
the selected area (Fig. 182). The operator grasps the limb from behind
forwards with his left hand and keeps it on the stretch in a lateral direction, at the same time pushing the muscles forwards so as to have a flat
surface. The blade of the knife is placed at such an angle, that when it
penetrates the skin, the graft shall be of the requisite thickness. The
graft is cut by a rapid, even, lateral sawing movement and should be as

large as possible. With practice, grafts four or five inches or more in length and two inches wide may be easily cut. The final severance of the graft is often best accomplished by cutting with scissors. The number required will depend on the size of the raw area to be covered and the size

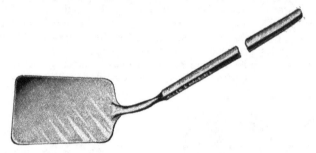

FIG. 184. A BROAD SMOOTH METALLIC SPATULA FOR TRANSFERRING THE SKIN GRAFTS.

of the individual grafts. If many are needed, each one as it is cut may be left lying on the bleeding surface or may be transferred to normal saline solution at a temperature of 100° F. Either of these methods is preferable to the immediate transference of each graft to the area to be covered.

The dressing is cautiously removed from the raw area and any blood is carefully wiped away from its surface. The graft is gently lifted by

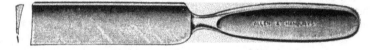

FIG. 185. THIERSCH'S KNIFE FOR CUTTING SKIN GRAFTS.

the forceps, or if it is large, placed on the spatula with the raw surface downwards, and transferred to the wound, where, by means of the probe, it is uniformly and evenly spread out. Each graft must be placed in close contact with its neighbour or their edges be allowed to overlap; if this is not done any uncovered area would become covered with skin, but the scar at such places is likely to be thin and to break down. The margins of the ulcer or wound should likewise be overlapped by the grafts for about one-eighth or a quarter of an inch (Fig. 183). No air or fluid must be allowed to remain between the under surface of a graft and the raw area. Any such accumulation may be got rid of, by making firm pressure on the grafts by means of long broad pieces of sterilized protective grasped at each end and stretched tightly across the grafts. Once the grafts are in position, every care must be taken not to displace them.

2. *Reverdin's method.* This method consists of snipping off small pieces of the superficial layers of the epidermis and placing them on the surface of the ulcer at short distances (half an inch) from each other. These pieces form foci from which the epithelium spreads over the ulcer and if the grafts be placed close enough together the ulcer is soon cicatrized. If the separate growths of epithelium do not coalesce, the intervening granulation tissue becomes converted into bands of scar tissue, which is very likely to be the starting-point of fresh ulceration.

This method is inferior to Thiersch's, but it is useful in some cases of burns on the face and in large burns on the trunk when the whole area cannot be covered in by the Thiersch grafts. It hastens the healing process and to some extent diminishes the amount of subsequent contraction.

3. *Wolfe's method.* The whole thickness of the skin without any of the subcutaneous fat is employed to form the graft. The size of the graft must be larger than the area to be covered to allow for the contraction of the skin, and it must be taken from some part (usually the thigh) where the cicatrization of the wound left by its removal will produce the least amount of inconvenience.

The graft must be taken from a part of the body which is free from hair, as the normal structures in the skin are neither absorbed nor destroyed. The whole of the fat is removed, and the graft is well stretched before placing it in position. It may be fixed by means of a few stitches. When successful this method provides a thick and complete covering for the part. The amount of scar tissue is greatly diminished, and thereby the tendency to reproduction of the deformity. It is therefore especially useful for cases of burns of the hands and fingers.

Instead of a portion of skin, the healthy prepuce removed by circumcision may be employed; but it is not easy to sterilize, and there is a great tendency for it to curl up. It should be divided into small portions, which are placed close to one another.

The objection to the method is that it is not so successful as Thiersch's: part or even the entire central portion of the graft may slough; in any case the superficial epithelium is shed in the course of a few days, but provided the deeper part remains, the wound is speedily covered in.

3. **The Dressing and After-treatment.** As soon as all the grafts are in position, they are covered by a sterilized layer of protective or a perforated piece of thin silver foil, outside which a thick layer of sterilized gauze is applied, and the whole is firmly and uniformly band-

aged. If necessary some sort of splint may be used. Complete and absolute rest must be secured, in order that the grafts may adhere to the raw surface. The place from which the grafts were obtained is dressed in a similar manner, this dressing being left undisturbed for a week or ten days, by which time the surface will usually be healed.

The dressing on the grafted surface will require changing about the fourth or fifth day. In those cases where the asepticity of the wound is certain, it is possible to defer the first dressing for a week. Especial care must be taken not to disturb the grafts during the removal of the protective, and if on removal of the gauze there is no pus or discharge the protective need not be disturbed. To detach the protective, plenty of normal saline, or 1 in 4,000 perchloride of mercury lotion, must be used. If the grafts are of a pink or reddish colour they are living; if whitish or greyish, they no longer live. The protective is reapplied with fresh outside dressings and bandages as before, and the wound is dressed subsequently as often as seems necessary.

In the after-treatment it is important to protect the newly grafted area, both from injuries, and from being detached by movement of the adjacent structures; therefore a period of prolonged rest is necessary to get a permanently sound scar; this is especially indicated in the case of chronic ulcers of the leg. At the same time appropriate means to improve the nutrition of the surrounding skin must be adopted. A dilute, bland, unirritating ointment or oily preparation should be kept constantly applied when there is any tendency to thickness or cracking of the epidermis of the grafts.

CHAPTER II

RHINOPLASTY

GENERAL PRINCIPLES

PLASTIC operations on the nose are performed for congenital and acquired defects. In this chapter only the external defects or abnormalities will be considered. True congenital defects are very rare and in the vast majority of the cases which require rhinoplasty, the deformity is due to injury, an operation, or disease. These defects or deformities may be divided into three classes: (1) The nose may be totally destroyed, usually by syphilis, and be represented by one or two openings on the face and some cicatricial tissue. Occasionally such a condition is due to injury. (2) Partial destruction, usually of the cartilaginous portions—the alæ, the tip, and septum—the bony portions remaining intact. Such defects may be the result of syphilis, lupus, injury, frost-bite, or an operation for the removal of tumours. (3) Deformity from sinking in of the bridge, secondary to an injury or syphilis. As a result of syphilitic necrosis, or defective development due to congenital syphilis, the bony bridge may be almost absent, and the nostrils are directed forwards instead of downwards.

Rhinoplastic operations are divided into (1) **complete,** in which the whole nose has to be re-formed, and (2) **partial,** in which the restoration of some part, such as the tip, the alæ, the septum, or the bridge, is required. In any case, a flap operation is almost invariably employed, the flap being taken from the forehead or face, or from more distal parts, such as the arm.

When a complete rhinoplastic operation is required one of the following methods may be used:—

(a) *In the Indian method* the flap is obtained from the forehead and twisted into position. An obvious objection is the large scar which is left on the forehead; and, of course, the method is inapplicable when the forehead is the seat of cicatrices. (b) *In the French method* the flaps are obtained from the adjacent portions of the cheek. It is most suitable for those cases in which the upper part of the nose is intact. (c) *In the Italian or Tagliacotian method* the flap is taken from the arm. It has not been widely adopted, and is only to be used when other methods are inapplicable or unavailable. The chief objections to this method are

373

the constrained position of the arm and the cumbersome apparatus required to keep the parts in apposition. Moreover, the flap is not so well adapted for the purpose as one obtained from the forehead. Which-ever of these three methods is employed the final results are never very satisfactory when the whole nose has to be restored. The chief draw-backs are (1) the difficulty of forming a columella, and (2) the tendency to continued contraction of the anterior nares of the new nose, a tendency which persists for many months. The new-formed nose at first may appear to be very good, but it shrinks, in such a way that sooner or later a shapeless mass of skin is left on the face. In addition the scarring causes marked disfigurement when the flaps are taken from the adjacent portions of the face or from the forehead. These operations are rarely practised at the present day, and before performing them the surgeon should see whether a better cosmetic effect cannot be obtained by the use of a carefully moulded and coloured artificial nose.

Partial rhinoplastic operations are much more satisfactory and are frequently practised. For the restoration of the bridge, bone has been successfully transplanted, in some cases, from an animal such as the rabbit; and during recent years the subcutaneous injection of paraffin has been largely and very successfully employed to restore the shape of the bridge.

It is, perhaps, hardly necessary to reiterate the caution already given, that all signs of active local disease, syphilis, tubercle, or other inflam-matory conditions, must be absent before undertaking any of these operations.

COMPLETE RHINOPLASTIC OPERATIONS

THE INDIAN METHOD

A piece of gutta-percha tissue to indicate the size and shape of the flap is laid flat on the forehead in the position from which it is proposed to take the flap, which is then marked out fully one quarter or a third of an inch larger in all its dimensions, in order to allow for shrinkage. The edges of the defect are refreshed and freed from the underlying parts, so that the attachment of the frontal flap may be made more secure with the borders of the skin around the defect. If there is any healthy skin left at the root of the nose it should be detached from above downwards, as a quadrilateral flap, its attached margin being at the lower end (see Fig. 186, c). The raw surface of this flap will then be directed out-wards; it serves to support the frontal flap, and at the same time dimin-ishes the amount of subsequent shrinkage. The forehead flap should be more or less pyriform in shape (Fig. 186, A) or cut after Langenbeck's method (Fig. 186, B), and should be placed obliquely on the forehead, especially when the latter is a low one and the line of the hair comes far down, but care must be exercised not to place it transversely, as the con-

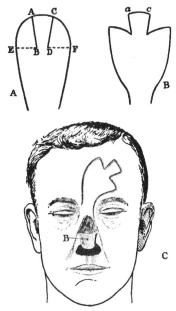

FIG. 186. THE INDIAN METHOD OF RHINOPLASTY. A is the outline of a pyriform-shaped flap. A B and C D represent the lines for marking out the columella. The dotted lines B E and D F indicate the lines along which the flaps A B E and C D F are folded to form the alæ of the nostrils. A C is sutured to a prepared raw area on the upper lip.

B represents Langenbeck's method of cutting the flap. The prominent part forms the columella, a c being sutured to the upper lip.

C. The flap is shown in position on the forehead: one margin of the pedicle ceases at the inner limit of the eyebrow and the other reaches to the raw area on the nose. B is a quadrilateral flap, turned downwards from the outer surface of the nose: its point of attachment is at the lower extremity of the nasal bones: its raw surface is directed forwards, and is covered by the forehead flap which it serves to support.

traction of the scar may then draw up the corresponding eyebrow. The obliquity of the flap serves to minimize the risk of the vessels being unduly compressed in the pedicle when it is twisted into position. One limb of the incision is carried down into the refreshed area, the other one ceases about the level of the inner end of the eyebrow (see Fig. 186, c); the latter incision may be continued horizontally outward, if necessary, to make the turning of the flap easier. The pedicle is thus placed at the root of the nose and is made as broad as possible and contains one nutrient artery, viz. the frontal. The incisions are carried down to the bone; the whole flap, including the periosteum, is then dissected up. (There are two possible objections to dissecting up the periosteum: (a) the frontal bone may superficially necrose, (b) the periosteum has no bone-forming function and therefore is useless from this point of view. Most surgeons, however, include the periosteum in the flap.) It is also recommended to remove by a chisel a thin layer of bone and transplant it together with the flap in order to better retain the shape of the nose. All hæmorrhage being arrested, the flap is rotated into position, taking care not to twist the pedicle more than necessary. If a pyriform flap has been made, the two longitudinal cuts, A B, C D (see Fig. 186, A), are made, dividing it into three parts; the middle part forms the columella, and the two lateral parts, after being bent back along the lines B E, D F, form the alæ nasi.

The septum is formed from the middle portion of the flap by folding it longitudinally and securing this longitudinal fold by means of catgut sutures. The two lateral portions are also doubled on themselves (Fig. 186, A) for the formation of the alæ nasi, and secured in the same way by catgut sutures. If by the doubling of the lateral portions the alæ are made too thick and the nostrils too small, the excision of a small wedge-shaped portion or the removal of the subcutaneous tissue may be employed to overcome the difficulty.

The flap is sutured to the defect with fine silkworm-gut or horse-hair sutures, the edges being carefully brought into apposition without tension. If a columella has been formed, it is sutured to a groove or bed made for it in the mid-line of the lip, but in many cases, when the forehead is a low one, it is advisable to form the columella from the upper lip, either at once, or at a later period. The lower aperture of the nose must be supported by gauze plugs, or if the nostrils have been formed, a small drainage tube is inserted into each. The defect in the forehead is closed as completely as possible by sutures, any remaining portion being grafted by Thiersch's method.

The new-formed nose may be left without a dressing or else a simple collodion dressing may be applied. The sutures remain untouched for four or five days, and their removal is then gradually accomplished. The gauze in the lower opening will require to be changed twice or thrice daily; the drainage tubes should be changed frequently, but not finally removed for some weeks. The pedicle of the forehead flap is divided at the end of four to six weeks, the redundant portion being removed or replaced in the lower portion of the forehead wound. Secondary operations will probably be required to improve the alæ, but these should never be undertaken till the nose has ceased to shrink.

THE ITALIAN METHOD

In this method the flap is taken from the anterior surface of the upper arm and sutured to the defect. The arm is fixed to the forehead, and kept in this position for three or four weeks, when the pedicle is severed and the operation completed. A full account of the method may be found in a paper by the late Sir William MacCormac in the *Clinical Society's Transactions*, vol. x, p. 181.

PARTIAL RHINOPLASTIC OPERATIONS

OPERATIONS FOR DEFECTS OF THE BRIDGE

Saddle-back nose. In a typical case, the bridge is completely depressed and on a level with the cheeks, the cartilaginous portion being tilted upwards so that the nostrils look forwards instead of downwards. The deformity may be due to a depressed fracture, or to necrosis after injury, or may have followed congenital or acquired syphilis. In the latter cases there is likely to be a considerable amount of scar tissue, and the results are not so good as in the former cases.

The objects of the operation are: (1) to restore the shape of the bridge by some means which will be permanent; (2) to correct the position of the nostrils. Very many operations have been devised, including the use of frameworks made of gold, amber, aluminium, &c., but at the present day these latter are not employed.

Sir Watson Cheyne's method [1] (Fig. 187, ᴀ). A median vertical incision is made from the root of the nose downwards on to the cartilaginous portion, extending on the latter for a quarter of an inch. Transverse incisions are then made at the upper and lower ends of this incision, thus forming two lateral flaps, which are dissected up, taking if possible any periosteum and fragment of the nasal bones which may be present. The cartilaginous portion of the nose is then separated from the remains of the bony portion, the nasal cavity being opened and the cartilaginous septum divided sufficiently to enable the tip of the nose to be readily pulled into its normal position. Two vertical and parallel incisions, each about an eighth of an inch on either side of the median line and beginning half an inch above the root of the nose, are carried upwards on the forehead to the margin of the hair, and their upper ends are

[1] Cheyne and Burghard, *Manual of Surgical Treatment*, Part V, p. 154.

united by a transverse cut. These incisions divide all the structures down to the bone. A narrow chisel being introduced along each lateral incision and into the upper transverse incision, a portion of the external table of the frontal bone is separated together with the soft parts. The flap is then turned downwards, and when the lower end is reached the bone is broken across. The flap is rotated so that when in position it will have on its outer surface a thin layer of bone and on its deep surface the soft parts of the forehead, *i.e.* the skin is directed towards the nasal cavity. The flap must be long enough for

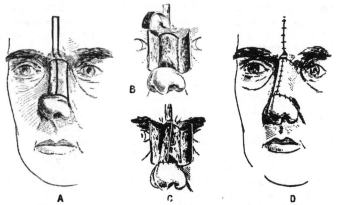

A **B** **C** **D**

Fig. 187. Sir Watson Cheyne's Method of restoring the Bridge of the Nose. A shows the lines of incision for the various flaps. In B the flaps have been reflected and the tip of the nose freed and brought into position. In C the reflected flap from the forehead is sutured in position, while in D the lateral flaps have been brought together over the reflected forehead flap. The small triangular gap left at the root of the nose is afterwards filled by the divided pedicle of the forehead flap, which is trimmed into shape and turned up again. (Cheyne and Burghard's *Manual of Surgical Treatment*.)

its free end to be attached to the cartilaginous portion when this is pushed into its proper position, and to enable this to be done without tension it may be necessary to prolong the lateral incisions a little downwards on each side of the root of the nose; but a sufficiently broad pedicle must be left for the proper nutrition of the flap. The flap is stitched to the freshened end of the cartilaginous portion of the gap, so that its cutaneous surface covers the aperture between the bony and cartilaginous portions of the nose. Above this gap the skin on the deeper surface of the flap is carefully shaved off, in order to make it readily adhere to the remaining refreshed surfaces of the bridge. At the root of the nose there is a certain redundance of the skin from the folding of the pedicle, which will be divided subsequently and the excess turned upwards. The lateral flaps are finally replaced and united over the raw surface of the reflected forehead flap. The upper transverse incisions should be curved downwards and outwards; this allows a certain amount of sliding of the flaps downwards so that they can cover the opening between the tip of the nose and the new bridge. The incision in the forehead is readily stitched up and leaves a hardly perceptible scar. At the end of three weeks the base of the reflected flap is divided and the little portion remaining is trimmed into a triangular shape and fitted in at the lower part of the vertical incision.

The new bony bridge tends to sink downwards as healing occurs and will as a rule not be high enough.

Bone transplant in nasal depressions. When there is a marked depression of the bridge of the nose, which often follows marked injury or destruction of the tissues due to syphilis or other diseases, the ordinary plastic operation employing soft tissues would be of no avail. In this type of case the bone transplant offers by far the better solution.

Technique. A curved incision with the convexity downward is made at the root of the nose. The incision is carried through the subcutaneous tissues to the bone. A blunt-pointed dissector is inserted at this point, carefully separating the skin and subcutaneous tissues over the bridge of the nose from the underlying bone structure. The cutaneous flap should be made thick enough to avoid danger of subsequent necrosis and great care should be used that the instrument does not perforate the mucous membrane of the nose. The dissection is carried well down to the tip of the nose and laterally to the junction of the nose with the cheek. A small bone graft is taken from a rib and is cut and trimmed to a suitable size to fit the individual case. This graft is inserted into the furrow prepared. The tip of the graft should come well down toward the point of the nose, the upper edge being securely fastened under a little ledge prepared in the periosteum of the frontal bone. The skin incision is closed by fine horsehair suture without drainage and a dressing applied. Care should be used that the graft is not misplaced until fixation occurs.

Beckmann advises the use of a cartilage splint in place of the bone splint. When cartilage is used it can be taken from the costal cartilage and it is comparatively simple to trim this graft with an ordinary scalpel to the exact form and size desired to reconstruct the nose. It is placed in position in the same manner as in the previously described operation.

The success of either operation depends upon absolute asepsis and careful technique to avoid injury of the underlying structures in the nose, thereby lessening the possibility of infection travelling through the mucous membrane about the place of the graft.

The Subcutaneous Injection of Paraffin for the Restoration of the Bridge. This method was first introduced by Gersuny in 1900, and has been extensively employed in the correction of saddle-back noses. The most suitable cases are those in which the deformity is secondary to a depressed fracture of the nasal bones, and those in which there is defective development of the bridge due to congenital syphilis. The skin over the bridge should be supple, thick, and freely movable: if it is thin, cicatricial, or closely adherent to the periosteum, the case is not so suitable, and the results are not so good; when these adhesions are present they may be divided by introducing a tenotome, and cutting them with the blade parallel to the skin.

The best kind of paraffin to use is one which has a melting-point of 110° to 115° F. A special syringe with screw pressure is desirable. The skin of the nose must be efficiently disinfected. The paraffin, syringe, and needle are first sterilized and then placed in a water bath at a temperature of 6° or 7° above the melting-point of the paraffin, which is allowed to become semi-solid or opaque in the syringe before it is injected. The injection must be given slowly and gradually. The skin having been pinched up, the needle with its point directed upwards and passed well under the skin, is entered on one side of the mid-line and some distance below the place where the bridge ought to be.

The quantity to be injected varies, and should be rather less than that required to entirely remove the deformity. The needle should not be withdrawn until the required amount is injected, and it may be necessary to repeat the operation to improve still more the appearance of the patient. After the withdrawal of the needle, the puncture is sealed with a collodion dressing. The skin at first becomes white and tense, the degree depending on the quantity of paraffin employed; some inflammatory reaction may follow in a few hours, the redness slowly subsiding, or perhaps persisting for many days. Pain is not usually complained of, but there may be some tenderness. The results obtained by this method in suitable cases are excellent and permanent, but it is important to recognize that it has its limitations. Many accidents have occurred from the use of hot paraffin, which are avoided by the use of cold paraffin. This method is superior to that in which melted paraffin is employed. In the latter the operation has to be done very quickly, and diffusion of the paraffin into the eyelids is not uncommon. Moreover, in the former method an assistant is not necessary. There is no fear of poisoning and very little of sloughing or suppuration if the

kin is healthy. Failure is usually due to insufficient antiseptic precau-
ions or because too much paraffin has been used.

Paraffin has also been successfully employed for elevating depressed
cars, especially those on the face, for filling large bony cavities and the
epressions remaining after removal of the upper jaw. It has also been
ised with success in the treatment of prolapse of the rectum and of the
agina.

OPERATIONS FOR RESTORATION OF THE SOFT PARTS

Syme's operation. When the end of the nose only has been de-
troyed this operation (Fig. 188) may be employed. Two flaps are
narked out, one on each cheek, having a median conjoint pedicle at the

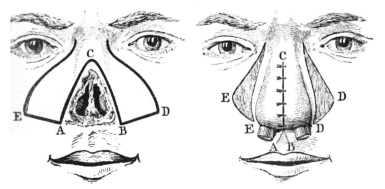

FIG. 188. SYME'S OPERATION FOR THE RESTORATION OF THE SOFT PARTS OF
·HE NOSE. In the left-hand figure the incisions marking out the flaps are shown,
ind the raw area on the nose, the edges of which are refreshed. In the right-
iand figure the flaps are in position, and the edges A C, B C sutured. A small
iiece of drainage tube has been placed in each nostril. The areas from which
he flaps are raised are closed, partly by undermining the adjacent cheek and
iartly by skin-grafting.

·oot of the nose between the inner canthi. The size of the flaps is regu-
ated by the size of the nose which it is required to restore according to
neasurements previously made. The area to be closed having been care-
:ully refreshed, the flaps are dissected up and united in the middle line
ifter all bleeding has been arrested. The outer edges of the flaps are
iutured to the raw area at a proper distance to form the nasal orifice. It
s advisable, if possible, to fold over the free inferior margin of the flaps
ind unite the apposed raw surfaces in order to have a cutaneous surface
it the margin of the new nostrils which are supported by drainage tubes.

The septum may be formed at a later date from the upper lip. The edges of the wounds left in the cheeks are brought together as closely as possible, any unclosed area being left to granulate, or it may be skin-grafted. By this method a conspicuous frontal scar is avoided, but the nose is apt to be very flat, as there is a good deal of shrinkage.

Keegan's method. This method was introduced to restore noses which had been mutilated by injury, and is only applicable, in its fullest extent, to those cases in which the skin and tissues over the nasal bones have been undamaged. Superimposed flaps are employed; one flap is taken from the forehead, the size of it being proportioned to the face of the patient. This flap is placed obliquely on the forehead, with the pedicle at the internal angle of the orbit, and it must contain the angular artery. The other flaps are taken from the skin of the bridge. The method is thus described in the *Lancet*, vol. i, Feb. 21, 1891: 'The cavities on both sides of the septum are plugged with pledgets of wool, to which sutures are attached. The operation is begun by carrying two converging incisions from two points slightly external to the roots of the alæ nasi to two points about three-quarters of an inch apart on the bridge of the nose where a pair of spectacles would rest. These two points on the bridge of the nose are now joined by a horizontal incision. A F (Fig. 189). This horizontal incision is bisected and a perpendicular incision, B D, E G, is drawn downwards from the point of bisection nearly as far as where the nasal bones join on to the cartilage of the nose. In other words, this perpendicular incision follows the course of junction of the nasal bones, but is not carried down as far as their inferior borders. The skin and tissues are now dissected from off the nasal bones from above downwards in two flaps, A B C D and E F G H (Fig. 189). The two inferior borders of the flap, C D and G H, are not interfered with and constitute the attachment of the flaps to the structures and tissues which clothe the inferior borders of the nasal bones where they join the cartilage of the nose. If these two flaps are reflected downwards so that their raw surfaces look forwards and their cutaneous surfaces look backwards, it will be found that they overlap in the centre. The surgeon has, therefore, a redundancy which he can utilize a little later on, when he has raised the flap from the forehead. He now proceeds to do this.' The flap has the shape shown in Fig. 189, its size being marked out according to that of the nose to be restored. ' This flap should embrace all the tissues down to the pericranium, and should be handled as little as possible. The sides of the gap in the forehead are approximated as quickly as possible with horsehair sutures, and it is surprising how small a raw area is left behind on the forehead if the approximation of the sides of the gap be carefully and rapidly carried out. Attention is now directed to preparing a bed for the reception of the columella, and this does not require any description. The two flaps, A B C D and E F G H, which have already been raised from off the nasal bones, are now reflected downwards, and as they overlap in the centre, two triangular pieces are cut away and placed in the middle of the gap left in the forehead, in order to expedite the healing of the frontal scar. The forehead flap is now

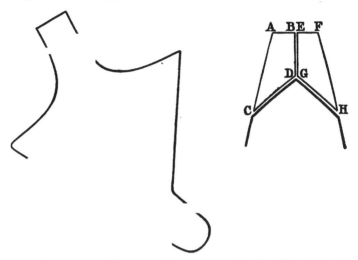

FIG. 189. KEEGAN's METHOD OF RHINOPLASTY. On the left hand the shape of the forehead flap is shown; on the right hand, the incisions marking out the nasal flaps. (*Lancet*, February 21, 1891.)

brought down over the nasal bones and rests inferiorly on the two re-flected flaps, A B C D and E F G H, which have already been raised from the nasal bones. The raw surface of the frontal flap inferiorly lies on the raw surfaces of the two reflected nasal flaps, and the nostrils of the newly formed nose are therefore lined inside with the skin of the reflected nasal flaps. The free inferior margins of the forehead flap and the nasal flaps are now brought together by horsehair sutures. The columellar portion of the forehead flap is now fixed in the bed prepared for it by sutures, and the two original incisions drawn from the root of the alæ nasi on either side to the bridge of the nose are deepened and bevelled off for the reception of the sides or lateral margins of the forehead flap. The lateral margins of the forehead flap are most accurately stitched by horsehair sutures to the bed prepared for them. Two pieces of drain-

age tube are inserted into the newly formed nostrils. If the root or
pedicle of the newly formed nose is broad enough and is not dragged
upon, and the angular artery has not been wounded, there need be no fear
of sloughing, and the new nose will largely adhere by first intention.'
The pedicle is divided at the end of a fortnight and a wedge-shaped slice
is cut out of the root, so that the new nose may not be parrot-shaped.
As the inside of each nostril is lined by skin, the drainage tubes can be
discarded at the end of ten days.

OPERATIONS FOR RESTORATION OF THE ALÆ NASI AND SIDE OF THE NOSE

It is impossible to give a detailed account of the actual operation
which may be required in any given case. A flap will be required in all
cases, and this may be obtained (1) from the opposite side of the nose:
(2) from the same side of the nose above the defect; (3) from the
adjacent portion of the cheek. The first and second methods can be employed only when the skin of the nose is sound.

By a flap taken from the sound side of the nose. *Langenbeck's method.* The base of the flap is placed near the inner angle of
the orbit of the affected side. The edges of the defect are refreshed and
sutured to those of the flap. The raw area left by elevation of the flap
is covered by skin-grafts, or by undercutting the skin of the cheek and
gliding it over the raw area. The flap should be long enough to allow
the lower border to be folded on itself to form a more natural margin for
the nostril. and a small drainage tube is placed in the newly formed
nostril to support it (Fig. 190).

By a flap taken from the same side of the nose.[1] A straight
incision, A B D (Fig. 191), is made down to the periosteum along the
anterior edge of the defect up to a point a short distance below and
internal to the inner canthus of the eye. A second curved incision.
B E C, of about the same length is made downwards and outwards along
the upper border of the naso-labial fold to a point about one inch external
to the outer margin of the gap. The flap, thus obtained, is then dissected downwards and includes everything down to, but not including
the facial artery and vein. The neighbouring parts of the cheek and
upper lip are freely raised by undercutting them.

The tissues on either side of A D are dissected up to form a deep
groove for the reception of the edge of the transplanted flap. The latter
is folded on itself and then twisted inwards and downwards. so that
the upper angle, B, is brought down to the tip of the nose at A. The
upper half, B E, of the outer edge of the flap is then sutured to the lower

[1] Berry, *Clinical Society's Transactions,* vol. xxxviii, p. 174.

half, A D, of the first incision along the side of the nose. The raw inner edge, D B, of the flap is thus left free to form part of the anterior edge of the restored nostril; this granulation edge curls inwards and disappears behind the new ala. The lower part, C E, of the outer edge of the flap is acutely doubled upon itself, and this portion of the flap is thus made to present a prominent angle in imitation of the prominent

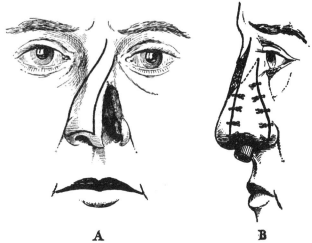

A   **B**

FIG. 190. LANGENBECK'S METHOD OF RHINOPLASTY. In A the flap is shown marked out on the sound side of the nose. In B it is stitched in position and the nostril is supported by a drainage tube. The stitches holding the folded lower margin of the flap in position are shown.

part of a normal ala. The triangular raw area, D B E, can be closed by undercutting, chiefly on the side of the cheek. Deep tension sutures will be probably required, or the gap may be closed by skin-grafting if its edges cannot be brought together.

In the patient illustrated in Fig. 192 the lower part of the septum and the whole of the left ala of the nose had been destroyed by gangrene following a specific fever. An incision, A D B, was made, the point A being just below the level of the lower limit of the nostril of the opposite side, and the point B just above the inferior margin of the nasal bone. The incision completely separated the remains of the ala along B D. On each side of A D the scar tissue was freely removed, so as to form a broad raw surface. An oblique incision, B C, then separated the whole thickness of the soft parts below C B D as a thick flap, which was detached from the nasal bone. The whole flap, c b d, was rotated downwards so that d was opposite a and the part of the incision b d opposite d a. A

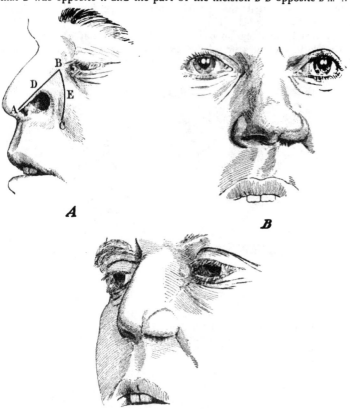

A

B

C

FIG. 191. RESTORATION OF THE ALA NASI BY A FLAP TAKEN FROM THE SAME SIDE OF THE NOSE. In a the defect and the lines marking the incisions are shown. In b the front view, and in c the lateral view, of the restored nostril is shown. The figures are drawn from photographs. Three and a half years after the operation there had been no shrinkage, and the result was excellent. (*Mr. J. Berry's case.*)

gap was thus left on the side of the nose above the displaced flap. By freely undercutting the skin of the adjacent part of the cheek and pulling it inwards, this gap was easily closed. The margin, b d, was united

y silkworm-gut sutures to the raw surface along D A. The effect and the
:sulting scar are shown in Fig. 192, B and C.

FORMATION OF A NEW COLUMELLA ·

A new columella may be formed from either the upper lip or the
orsum of the nose.

From the lip (Fig. 194, p. 389). Two parallel incisions, separated
:om one another about a quarter of an inch, are made through the whole

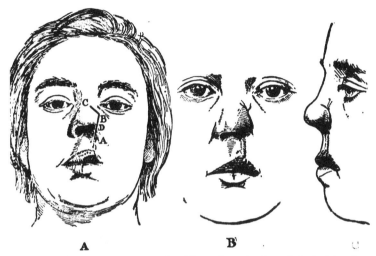

A   **B**   C

FIG. 192. RESTORATION OF THE ALA NASI. In A the line of the incision for
marking out the flap is shown. In B the front view, and in C the side view, of the
restored nostril is shown. The scars in the lip are the results of an operation to
restore it (see Fig. 203, p. 401). Taken from photographs. (*Author's case.*)

hickness of the central portion of the upper lip. The pedicle of the
lap is at its upper end and the lower end is formed by the free border
)f the lip. The flap is twisted upwards after the frænum has been
livided, so that the mucous membrane looks forwards, and the skin
surface towards the nasal cavity. The free end of the flap, after its
mucous membrane has been removed, is sutured to the prepared raw
surface on the tip of the nose. In time the exposed mucous membrane
)ecomes thickened and resembles the skin. In males it is advisable to
lissect off the skin and hair follicles from the flap before placing it in
position. The upper lip is restored by separating it on each side of the

gap from the underlying bone and uniting the raw edges together (Fig. 143, B), especial care being taken to preserve the line of continuity of the skin and mucous membrane and in the formation of the free border of the lip, that a V-shaped depression is not left.

From the dorsum of the nose (Fig. 195 A, p. 389). A long flap, including the periosteum, is dissected up, having the pedicle near the tip of the nose. The flap is then twisted into position and its lower margin

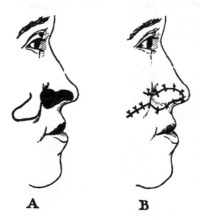

A   **B**

FIG. 193. RESTORATION OF THE ALA NASI BY A FLAP TAKEN FROM THE CHEEK. The flap may be placed in the defect with its cutaneous aspect directed outwards, or it may be so placed that its raw (deep) surface is directed outwards and its cutaneous surface towards the nasal cavity. The former is then skingrafted.

is sutured to a raw area prepared for it in the mid-line of the lip at its upper border. The raw area of the nose is closed by suturing its edges (Fig. 195. B), or by skin-grafting.

PLASTIC OPERATIONS ON THE AURICLE

The deformities of the external ear which require a plastic operation are (1) undue prominence, (2) excessive size. Other malformations are occasionally seen, but these are often associated with defects of the auditory apparatus, which preclude the necessity of performing any operation.

To reduce undue prominence, an incision is made immediately behind the attachment of the auricle, from the adjacent posterior surface

f which a triangular or elliptical portion of the skin is removed. It
sometimes necessary to excise a portion of the cartilage, and the

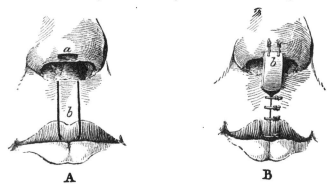

A   **B**

FIG. 194. FORMATION OF THE COLUMELLA FROM THE UPPER LIP. In A the
ap *b* in the upper lip is marked out, and the raw area, *a*, on the tip of the
ose, to which the free end of *b* is attached, is shown. In B the operation is
ompleted.

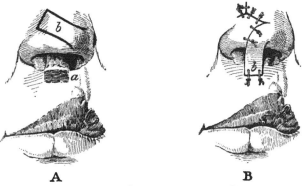

A   **B**

FIG. 195. FORMATION OF THE COLUMELLA FROM THE DORSUM OF THE NOSE.
n A the raw area, *a*, on the upper lip, to which the extremity of the flap *b* is
titched, is shown. In B the operation is completed. The upper lip had also
een restored.

imount of skin and cartilage removed depends on the degree of the
leformity. When the margins of the defect are sutured together,
:he ear should be in its normal position and it is well to unite the cut
:dges of the cartilage by separate sutures. The operation is not called

CHAPTER III

PLASTIC OPERATIONS ON THE LIPS, MOUTH, AND FACE

GENERAL PRINCIPLES

THESE operations are frequently required to remedy defects which follow operations, and the deformities which are the result of injuries or the effects of cicatrization following ulceration. The earlier operations for the restoration of the lips were designed at a time when it was the custom to remove epitheliomata with a minimum amount of surrounding tissues. At the present day a much greater amount of these tissues is removed; thus most of the earlier plastic operations are inapplicable and need not be described. The whole thickness of the lip or cheek is not infrequently removed by an operation, and if the defect is not closed, great deformity will follow. The defects left by these extensive operations are very varied in shape and size; each case has to be considered on its merits, and the operations described are only those which have been actually used and found to be satisfactory. To obtain the best result a combination of methods may have to be employed; thus skin-grafting and the use of flaps are often necessary. In some cases, especially when the superficial portions of the cheek only have been removed or destroyed, skin-grafting alone is sufficient. In other cases, when the whole thickness of the cheek is deficient, flaps may be the only possible means of remedying the defect or deformity, and they may be obtained from the structures adjacent to the defect, or from distal parts, such as the neck or one of the upper limbs. Whatever method is employed, it is very probable that a certain amount of subsequent contraction will occur, and this is especially the case when the operation has been undertaken for the repair of a cicatricial deformity.

Curved incisions are especially useful in marking out the flaps, and they should be so placed that the resulting scars are as little visible as possible.

More than one operation is frequently necessary; it is also better to do what is required in separate stages rather than to endanger the whole effect by attempting too much at one operation. Secondary operations are often needed to correct some of the results of the primary operation and these should be delayed rather than done too soon.

When the whole of the lower lip has required restoration, although the external appearance may be very good, the muscular tone may be deficient, and the saliva is liable to dribble away from the mouth for some time, if not even permanently. There may be also some difficulty in preventing the escape of food during the process of mastication.

The proximity of the mouth and teeth introduces a septic element to all these operations; therefore before doing them all stumps should be removed, decayed teeth stopped, and the mouth rendered as aseptic as possible and kept so during the process of healing.

Transplantation of fat. In the correction of deformities, especially the depressions due to scar tissue, free transplants of fat may be used. These transplants may vary in size from an almond to several inches in width. Kanavel has discussed this subject in several contributions. The fat is generally obtained from the abdominal wall, although if the patient is excessively obese or if the fascia lata is transplanted at the same time, transplants from the leg may be found satisfactory. Where possible sutures are not used to retain the flap in position, and if they are used the finest of silk is preferred. Care should be taken to prevent the development of a hæmatoma in the field.

Fat may be used to soften cicatrices and to restore mobility or to repair deformity. In the first instance through incisions small pads of fat $\frac{1}{4}$ of an inch in thickness and about $\frac{1}{2}$ inch in width are inserted into various areas, care being taken not to undercut too large an area if the scar be extensive, because of the danger of sloughing from poor blood-supply. In the latter instance the fat is inserted underneath the scar so that the entire depressed area is elevated. Nicety of plastic surgery suggests that where possible the incision made in the skin for the insertion of the fat should be at a distance from the scar and if possible at a concealed site, such for instance, as under the jaw or in the hair area. In the latter instance the undermining may be carried for some inches.

The illustration shows a patient who had an extensive burn of the lower lip and neck, which was corrected by a plastic procedure so that the ectropion of the lip, which had been present, was repaired and at subsequent periods deposits of fat were placed in the scar tissue rounding out the face and restoring its mobility.

Transplants may also be made about vessels which have been exposed and where it is feared that the contracting scar tissue may cause œdema of an extremity, as for instance after a dissection of an inguinal region. It may also be used to surround nerves which are repaired or are exposed in the scar tissue. Kanavel has also used it extensively in free flaps of fat about tendons which were exposed in scar tissue or after suture, and the results were very satisfactory. Here a small section of fat about ¼ of an inch in thickness, 1 or 2 inches in length, and 1 inch in width is wrapped about the tendon. Fat has also been used as a transplant in brain defects. Its use around artificial tendons made from silk is also discussed in the section upon that subject.

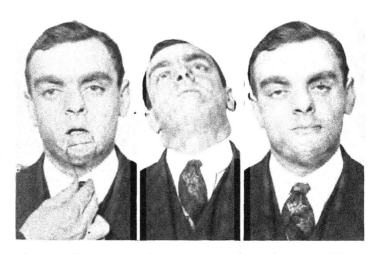

Fig. 196. Photograph of Patient in whom Lower Lip was restored by Plastic Operation with Subsequent Transplantation of Fat to ensure its Mobility and soften the Area. Photograph on left shows attempt to represent defect before operation, since unfortunately no photograph had been taken to represent this. (*Kanavel.*)

The transplantation of large pads of fat in potentially infected areas should always be approached with conservatism because of the possibility of infection. Transplantation into joints to restore their mobility, and into bones in cases of old osteomyelitic cavities, has not been followed with brilliant results.

The use of fat as a transplant after excision of the sternocleidomastoid muscle in wry neck is presented in another section. Its use in the restoration of the contour of the breast after excision will be presented in that chapter.

OPERATIONS ON THE LIPS: CHEILOPLASTY

For ectropion.   Ectropion or eversion of the lip is generally the result of extensive cicatrization following burns or ulcerations due to syphilis or lupus.   In the worst cases the teeth and gums are exposed and when the lower lip is affected the saliva constantly dribbles away.

The operation may be either easy or difficult according to the amount and depth of the scar tissue and the extent of the involvement of the muscles.

1. *For slight cases.*   (*a*) A curved transverse incision is made at the junction of the mucous membrane and skin.   The mucous membrane

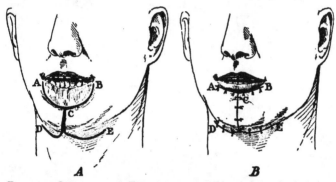

A   *B*

FIG. 197. OPERATION FOR ECTROPION OF THE LOWER LIP. In A the everted mucous membrane is separated as a thick flap by the incision A C B, and is then placed in its proper position. The curved incisions C D and C E mark out the flaps, A C D and B C E, which keep the lip in position. In B the method of suturing is shown. (*After Cheyne and Burghard.*)

is separated sufficiently to form a flap to over-correct the deformity, and this flap must be as thick as possible.   The raw area on the outer surface is then skin-grafted by Thiersch's method.   It is difficult to maintain the grafts in position and to keep the wound from becoming infected from the mouth.   In order to keep the flap in position it has been suggested that a sharp-pointed stiff probe should be passed through the flap, entering it a quarter of an inch outside the angle of the mouth on one side and bringing it out at a corresponding place on the opposite side.   The probe traverses the flap of mucous membrane and is left in position till the grafts have taken.

(*b*) An incision (A B, Fig. 197) is made along the edge of the everted mucous membrane from one side to the other.   A vertical incision is then made from the mid-point of this transverse incision to the chin, and it is then carried in a curved direction in the submaxillary region of each side for a sufficient distance. The mucous membrane of the lip is dissected up as a thick flap and restored to its natural position. The two flaps, A C D and B C E, containing the subcutaneous tissue are freed by undercutting and then united as in Fig. 197. The stitches may be removed on the fifth day.

2. *For severe cases where there is much scar tissue* (Fig. 198). An incision, *c d*, is made along the muco-cutaneous border of the lip, which

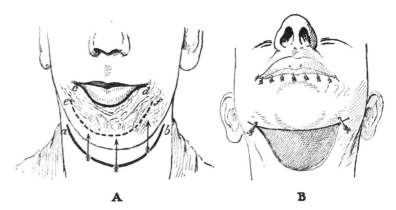

A   **B**

FIG. 198. OPERATION FOR SEVERE ECTROPION OF THE LOWER LIP, WITH MUCH SCAR TISSUE. The flap is taken from the submental region. In A, *a b* is the line of incision marking out the lower limit of the flap; *c d*, the incision for raising the mucous membrane to its proper position; *e f*, the line along which the scar tissue may be excised; the arrows indicate the direction in which the flap is displaced upwards. In B the flap is in position and sutured to the mucous membrane of the lip. The shaded area is the gap left by the displacement of the flap.

is elevated to its proper position by free dissection through the scar tissue. If there is much scar tissue, portions of it may be excised. A transverse incision (*a b*, Fig. 198, A) four or five inches long is made in the neck about the level of the hyoid bone. This incision should be slightly convex downwards. The bridge of tissue between the two incisions is completely raised from the underlying deep fascia, and then glided upwards over the chin. The flap is stitched by its upper margin to the edge of the mucous membrane of the lip (Fig. 198), and to prevent it slipping downwards, two or three buried sutures attach its deep surface to the periosteum of the jaw and muscles of the chin. The gap left in the submental region is closed, partly by undercutting the adjacent skin and partly by skin-grafting.

3. *In the worst cases* the scarring or destruction is so extensive that there is no possibility of obtaining flaps locally, and skin-grafting would not correct the deformity. In such a case, the flaps must be taken from a distal part, such as the upper arm; Mr. Brown [1] of Leeds obtained an excellent result by means of this method. The child was aged 11, and

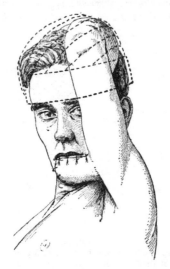

FIG. 199. RESTORATION OF THE LOWER LIP BY MEANS OF A FLAP TAKEN FROM THE UPPER ARM. The method of fixing the limb to the head is shown.

some years previously had been severely burnt about the head and neck. Salivation was profuse; the head was drawn downwards, and to remedy this, a cut was made across the neck from angle to angle of the jaw; all the scar tissue was divided, the head was pushed into its proper position and the wide gaping wound which resulted was closed by flaps of skin taken from the shoulders. When this wound had completely healed the lip was restored by making a transverse incision at the junction of the mucous membrane and skin; the lip was elevated into its natural position and kept there by means of a stitch. The large raw area was then closed by suturing a flap taken from the bicipital surface of the arm to the margins of the gap, the arm being brought across the face and fixed

[1] *Brit. Med. Journ.*, Jan. 7, 1905.

there by an apparatus. The pedicle was divided at the end of fourteen days, the flap being living and healthy. The patient was kept quiet by small doses of opium, and the necessary dressings were done under an anæsthetic. Berger also speaks highly of restoring the lip by taking a flap from the arm in these severe cases. He divides the pedicle on the tenth or fourteenth day. Secondary operations are usually required

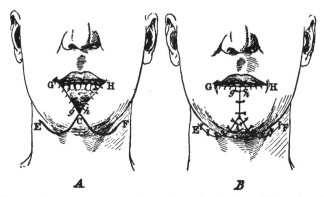

A   B

Fig. 200. Restoration of the Lower Lip. In A a large V-shaped portion, g c h, of the lip has been removed. The mucous membrane is sutured to the skin along the lines g *g* and h *h*, to form the margin of the new lip. From the apex of the V (the point c), curved incisions, c e and c f, are made on each side into the submaxillary region. In B the operation is shown completed. It may be necessary to undermine the skin to bring the edges together. (*After Cheyne and Burghard.*)

to complete the adjustment of the flap and to restore the angles of the mouth.

Feeding is often a difficult problem in these cases and may be accomplished by means of a tube and funnel. The dressings should be kept as dry as possible and will require to be frequently changed.

For restoration of the lips. This operation is required after the removal of a carcinoma involving the whole of the lip. Either a V-shaped portion with the apex at the margin of the jaw or a quadrilateral portion of the lip and chin will have been removed.

First method (Fig. 200, a and b). From the apex of the V a curved incision is made on each side down to the level of the hyoid and is then continued backwards and upwards towards the angle of the jaw. The whole thickness of the tissues of the lip and chin is dissected off the jaw and deep fascia, care being taken that the facial artery of each side is not divided. The edges of the original V are then brought together in the horizontal line to form the lip; the mucous membrane on the deep surface of each flap is elevated as far as may be necessary, so that it can be sutured without tension to the skin to form the red margin of the new lip. The edges of the flaps are then united vertically in the median line.

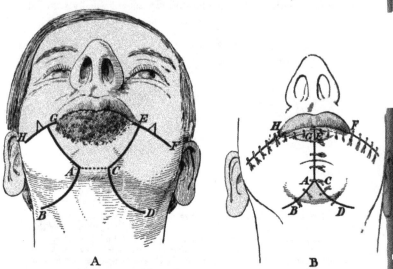

A   B

FIG. 201. RESTORATION OF THE LOWER LIP. In A the lines G A, C E show the incisions for the removal of an epithelioma. The dotted line A C completes the incision for the portion, G A C E, to be removed; this should be more quadrilateral in shape. A B and C D are curved incisions in the submaxillary region; they extend down to the deep fascia. H G and E F are horizontal incisions carried outwards from the angles of the mouth; they divide the whole thickness of the tissues of the cheek, but the mucous membrane should be divided at a higher level, in order to allow of it being sutured to the skin to form the new lip. The flaps H G A B and F E C D are raised from the lower jaw and sutured as in B. The small triangular areas above H G and E F may be excised, if necessary, to make the flaps come together more easily. (*Dowd.*)

The skin beyond the lower edges of the incisions in the neck will probably require to be undermined in order to close this portion of the wound.

Second method (Fig. 201, A and B). From the apex of the V or the lower angles of the quadrilateral space, curved incisions, A B and C D, are carried backwards on each side into the submaxillary region nearly as far as the angles of the jaw. From the corners of the mouth horizontal incisions, E F and G H, are made outwards through the substance of the cheek for a sufficient distance to allow the flaps H G A B and F E C D to be approximated. These latter incisions are carried down to the mucous membrane, which is then divided one-third of an inch higher to allow of its being stitched to the skin without tension in order to form the new lip. The flaps are then glided inwards and united in the median vertical line. Any excess of tissue in the cheeks above the horizontal incisions may be removed by the excision of small wedge-shaped portions (Dowd).

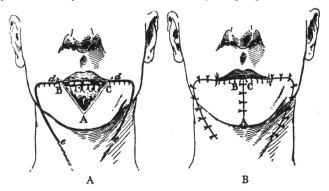

A   B

FIG. 202. RESTORATION OF THE LOWER LIP. In A the thick black line *d e* represents the incision on each side for raising the flaps: the new lip is formed by stitching the mucous membrane to the skin along the horizontal portion, *d*, of the incision. In B, B A and B C are shown united by sutures in the middle line, the flaps being displaced inwards to allow of this being done. (*After Cheyne and Burghard.*)

The facial arteries must not be damaged in dissecting up the flaps, which contain the whole thickness of the tissues down to the periosteum.

By these two methods the nerve-supply to the muscles in the flaps is preserved, and they are well nourished.

Third method (Fig. 202, A and B). In this method the flaps are obtained wholly from the cheek. A horizontal incision is made from the angle of the mouth on each side to the edge of the masseter, dividing the whole thickness of the cheek. The incision then curves downwards over the mandible and then forwards in the submaxillary region nearly as far as the hyoid. The mucous membrane is divided vertically at the anterior border of the masseter and horizontally where it is attached to the jaw. When the flaps have been raised sufficiently they are glided inwards to meet in the middle line, where they are united by their edges. Before uniting the mucous membrane to the skin to form the lip, it must be separated so that there is no tension on it; with this object in view it is well to divide the mucous membrane in the horizontal part of the incision at a higher level than the skin and muscles. This method produces much more scarring on the face; the nerve-supply to the muscles is more interfered with and the vascular supply is inferior to that in either of the other two methods, and in marking out the flaps the pedicle must be made sufficiently wide. Free undercutting of the skin on the outer sides of the incisions will be necessary to close the gap left by sliding the flaps into their new position.

RESTORATION AFTER INJURIES AND SLOUGHING OR LOCAL ULCERATION

The operation required to restore the lips in these cases depends on the extent of the injury and the amount of destruction of the adjoining parts of the chin and cheek.

Fig. 203 is taken from a patient whose upper lip on the left side had been almost completely destroyed. A wide gap extended from the left angle of the mouth to the right of the mid-line. There was a large amount of scar tissue, and ectropion of the mucous membrane of the right half of the lip. The scar tissue was excised and the lip freely separated from the alveolus on the right side; in order to allow this portion of the lip to be glided over the defect, a horizontal incision was made at its junction with the right nostril and then curved round the margin of the latter (see Fig. 203, *d e*). The margins of the gap on each side were completely refreshed, the mucous membrane of the lip being separated and preserved along the free border. The left cheek was widely detached from the upper jaw, the line of reflection of the mucous membrane from the cheek on to the jaw being divided as far as was found to be necessary. It was then possible to unite the refreshed surfaces: a broad lip was made, but with some eversion of the mucous membrane and leaving a notch in the free margin, which was corrected by a subsequent operation (Figs. 192 and 195).

This method of gliding the margins of the gap towards each other can be usually employed, if the cheek and lip be freely separated from the jaw. Their whole thickness must be elevated and the elasticity of the tissues is sufficient to allow of them being united without undue tension. Another great advantage of this method is that there is a minimum amount of visible scar tissue.

When the defect is so extensive that the whole length of the lip has been destroyed, Dieffenbach's operation (Fig. 204) may be employed A quadrilateral flap is marked out on each side of the defect. The base of the flap is at its lower end and thus a good blood-supply is ensured

The flaps which contain the whole thickness of the cheek are turned inwards, so that A B is sutured to C D, and the gap left by the displacement is closed by undercutting and uniting its edges.

In some cases not only is the lip destroyed, but there is also extensive loss of the adjacent tissues, such as the chin, and a very wide gap is left. If it is impossible to close such a gap by one of the methods above

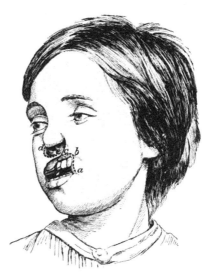

FIG. 203. RESTORATION OF THE UPPER LIP, FOLLOWING AN INJURY. The dotted line *a b c* represents the incision to free the left half of the lip and excise the scar tissue; *d e*, an incision to allow the right half of the lip to be separated from the nose. The dark line at the junction of the mucous membrane and skin represents the incision to allow the former to be separated from the latter. By freely separating the cheeks from the maxillæ the margins of the defect were sutured, and the resulting lip is shown in Figs. 192 and 195. (*Author's case.*)

described it is necessary to take a flap from some distal part, such as the arm (Fig. 199, p. 396). A very successful case in which this method was employed is reported by Watts in the *Annals of Surgery* for January, 1905. Another method is illustrated in Fig. 205. On each side of the defect two rectangular flaps, A B C D and D E F G, comprising the whole thickness of the cheek, are marked out. The mucous membrane at the upper margins, B C and E F, of each is stitched to the skin to form the new lip. The flaps are then displaced towards the mid-line, and their adjacent edges, C D and D E, are sutured together. By freely raising the cheek from the bone, the gaps left by the displacement of the flaps may be closed (Fig. 205, B).

When the upper lip has to be restored, the proximity of the nose and the small amount of space render necessary some slight modifications of these operations. When only a part has to be restored, it is possible by freely separating the remainder of the lip from the jaws to bring the edges of the defect together (Fig. 203). In order to prevent the nostrils being unduly compressed, an incision should be made round the ala on each side (Figs. 203 and 206), removing, if necessary, an elliptical portion of the skin (Fig. 206). When the whole lip is removed or has

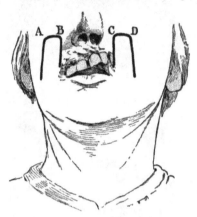

FIG. 204. DIEFFENBACH'S OPERATION. The flaps on each side of the gap contain the whole thickness of the tissues of the cheek and are rotated inwards so that A B and C D are sutured. The scar tissue must be sufficiently removed A similar operation may be employed to restore the lower lip.

been destroyed, the incisions round each ala should meet in the mid-line below the septum. If scar tissue is present, it must be excised. The flaps on each side are freely raised and the mucous membrane is stitched to the skin along the margins of the raw surface to form the new lip which is then brought down to its proper position. The portions of the incision below the nostrils are stitched together to make a median vertical line, on either side of which the tissues will form the lip proper (Fig. 207).

Operations for microstoma (Fig. 208, p. 406). This condition is often the result of extensive ulceration, not infrequently syphilitic in origin; sometimes it is due to an injury or an operation.

To restore the mouth to its proper size, an incision (*a b*, Fig. 208, B) is made outwards on each side of the contracted orifice through the whole thickness of the cheek and sufficiently long to make the new mouth large enough. The mucous membrane is carefully freed as much as possible from the tissues of the neck and stitched to the skin to form the red margin of the lips (Fig. 208, c). If the mucous membrane is deficient the skin must be turned inwards and stitched to it. Especial care must be taken in the formation of the angles of the mouth, that the skin

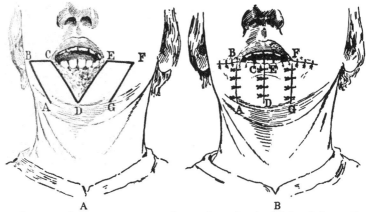

Fig. 205. Restoration of the Lower Lip. In the left-hand figure the quadrilateral flaps, A B C D and D E F G, are marked out. They contain the whole thickness of the cheek, and the mucous membrane is stitched to the skin along B C and E F to form the new lip. In the right-hand figure the method of suturing the flap is shown.

and mucous membrane in these places are very accurately united, in order to prevent recurrence of the contraction. In some cases it is better to dissect up at the new angle a thick triangular flap of skin with its base directed outwards. The mucous membrane is then divided as far as the new angle and the flap of skin turned inwards and sutured to the mucous membrane to form the angle of the mouth (Fig. 209, p. 407).

In all these operations the dressings should be of the simplest nature, and changed frequently. It is often best, *e.g.* in cases of restoration of the lips and for microstoma, not to apply any dressings at all. The vascular supply is so abundant and union occurs so rapidly that they are unnecessary. It is also most important to keep the parts as dry as possible, and this cannot be done if an elaborate dressing is used. Of course, if extensive incisions in the submaxillary region have been made, a dressing

should be put on, but at the same time the mouth and lip should not
be kept covered up.

It is perhaps hardly necessary to point out that before undertaking
these plastic operations on the lips and mouth, all signs of active disease
and ulceration must be absent, or to emphasize the importance of curing
any constitutional disease, such as syphilis.

PLASTIC OPERATIONS ON THE CHEEK

These are required to close recent defects remaining after surgical
operations, or those which follow extensive destruction from ulceration,

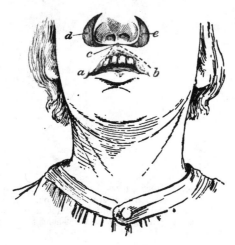

Fig. 206. Restoration of the Upper Lip. The dotted lines indicate the line
of incision for removal of the scar tissue. *d* and *c* represent elliptical portions of
skin removed from each cheek in order to prevent compression of the nostrils
when the lip is completed. It may not be necessary to remove these. The mucous
membrane is stitched to the skin along *a c* and *b c* in order to form the free
margin of the lip; *c* is then drawn downwards and the operation completed as in
Fig. 207.

cancrum oris, &c. In the latter group of cases there is often closure
of the jaws, either from cicatricial contraction in the structures attached
to them, or the cheek is firmly adherent to the jaw, and if it is separated
by division of the adhesions, it is exceedingly likely to become again
adherent. If the defect which is left by the removal of the whole thickness of the cheek is not closed by an immediate plastic operation, ex-

tensive contraction and adhesions to the jaw may also occur. There are, therefore, a number of factors to be considered which materially influence the result of these operations.

All active ulceration must be at an end and the condition of the teeth must be investigated, and when necessary, stumps must be removed and the mouth rendered as aseptic as possible.

Attempts must be made to remedy the cause of the closure of the jaws before undertaking the operation to close the defect. It may be possible to overcome the closure by stretching the cicatricial tissue by

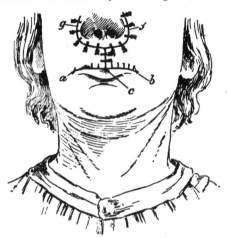

Fig. 207. Restoration of the Upper Lip. Completion of the Operation shown in the previous Figure. It is important to make the depth of the lip as great as possible.

various kinds of gags. If the scar tissue is divided, some means must be employed to prevent its reproducing the closure, and this can often only be done by means of a flap. In very bad cases, the adhesions are so dense and firm that it is almost impossible to divide them completely and to prevent them reforming, so that an operation to make a false joint becomes necessary; or excision of the temporo-maxillary joint may be undertaken, but the latter operation is not often beneficial in these cases.

When flaps are employed to close the defect, they may be obtained from the adjacent parts of the cheeks, (a) the masseteric area, (b) from above or below the defect; or (c) from more distal parts, viz. the forehead or temporal regions, and from the neck or from the arm.

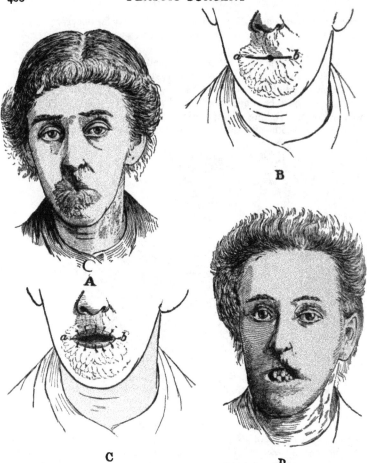

FIG. 208. OPERATION FOR MICROSTOMA. A shows the condition before the operation. In B the line of the incision *a b* for dividing the scar tissue, and in C the method of stitching the mucous membrane to the skin, is shown. Especial care must be taken in stitching the mucous membrane to the skin at the angles of the mouth. D shows the result some months after the operation. (*Mr. Burghard's case.*)

When the flap is taken from the masseteric region, it is usually twisted on its pedicle so that its cutaneous surface is directed inwards. The continual growth of hair into the mouth is a serious drawback to the patient's comfort, and therefore in males, whenever possible, some other flap should be used. It may, however, be possible to dissect out the layer containing the hair bulbs; it is probably useless to attempt to destroy the hair follicles by X-rays. The outer surface of the flap is covered by a superimposed flap taken either from some convenient

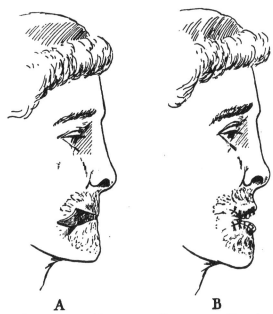

A   **B**

Fig. 209. Operation for Microstoma. Formation of New Angle of the Mouth. In A a triangular flap of skin is turned back and the dotted line shows the place of division of the mucous membrane. In B the flap is turned in around the new angle and sutured in position.

part of the neck or from the tissues over the inferior maxilla (Fig. 215, c), or it may be skin-grafted. When the flap is taken from above or below the defect it is not necessary to reverse it—it can be glided into position with its raw surface inwards (Figs. 211 and 212); this will cicatrize and remain non-adherent to the mucous membrane of the jaw, and thus the mouth can be satisfactorily opened. If a flap is taken only from the cheek above the defect, considerable distortion of the eyelids and mouth may follow, and therefore this method is rarely available.

In cutting the flaps from the cheek, the direction and position of the parotid duct must be remembered and care taken not to injure it. After the flap has become united in its new position, subsequent operations will be required to form the angles of the mouth, &c.

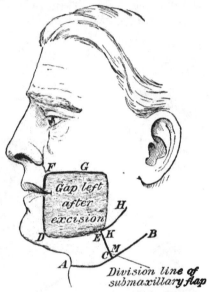

FIG. 210. METHOD OF CLOSURE OF A LARGE GAP IN THE CHEEK BY TRANS-PLANTATION OF A FLAP FROM THE SUBMAXILLARY REGION. The patient had an epithelioma of the cheek and angle of the mouth, and its wide removal left the large gap shown in the figure. The incision A C B was made low down in the sub-maxillary region and a large flap of skin and subcutaneous tissue was raised; part of the upper border of the flap was formed by the lower margin of the gap. The incision E C divided the flap into two portions, A C E D and B M K H, which were placed in the gap as in Fig. 211. The glands were removed from the submaxillary region after the flap had been raised. It will be noticed that the raw deep surfaces of the flaps are directed towards the mouth, which could be opened widely after union had occurred. (*Mr. Cunning's case.*)

A flap from the forehead and neck has the great advantage of being hairless. The former leaves a very obvious scar, but has a plentiful vascular supply. The raw area left on the forehead may be considerably diminished in size by undercutting the adjacent scalp and at once uniting the apposed edges, but in doing this the hair must not be brought too low down, or the effect may be more conspicuous than a scar. Any uncovered area may be skin-grafted. The skin of the neck is said to shrink a great deal, but excellent results may be obtained by its use, provided the flap is made long enough.

Whatever method is used, the flap must be large enough to allow

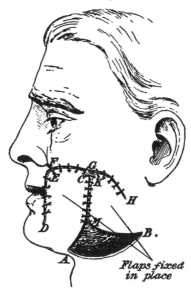

FIG. 211. RESTORATION OF A LARGE DEFECT IN THE CHEEK. COMPLETION OF THE OPERATION SHOWN IN FIG. 210. The margins of the flaps and defect are united by sutures. The raw area, A M B, was closed by undermining the skin below A B. Drainage tubes should be placed on the deep aspect of the flaps. (*Mr. Cunning's case.*)

for its contraction, and thereby to reduce the subsequent distortion to the smallest amount.

Closure of a large defect (Figs. 210 and 211). A large defect, such as one left after the removal of an epithelioma, may be closed in the following manner:—A curved incision, A C B, is made low down in the submaxillary region, and a flap of skin and the whole of the sub-cutaneous tissue is dissected up. The upper margin of this flap is formed by the lower edge of the defect, and from the point K the incision K H is carried backwards. Care must be taken not to divide the facial artery. The flap has therefore two pedicles, and is divided by the incision E C into two parts. The anterior portion, A C E D, is twisted

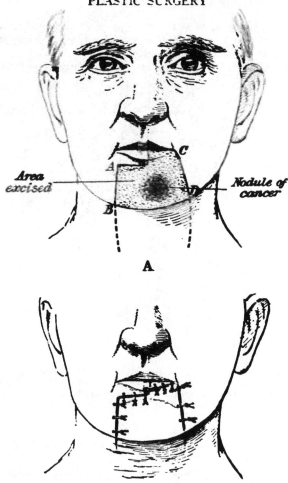

A

B

Fig. 212. Closure of a Defect in the Cheek by gliding a Flap from the Submaxillary Region. In A the lines of incision for the removal of a nodule of cancer and the surrounding portion of the skin are shown. The dotted lines indicate the prolongation of these lines into the submaxillary region in order to form a flap which was displaced upwards into the gap, B, and sutured to its margins. (*Mr. Cunning's case.*)

into the gap so that E C and F G are united by sutures; the posterior
portion, B M K, is then placed in the remainder of the gap, and the apposed edges are sutured to one another. A large raw area is left in the
submaxillary region, and this is closed by freely undercutting the surrounding skin. A drainage tube is placed on the deep aspect of the
flaps and brought to the surface at the lowest point of the operation area.

Another method of closing a large gap by means of a submaxillary
flap glided upwards into the defect is shown in Fig. 212, A and B. The

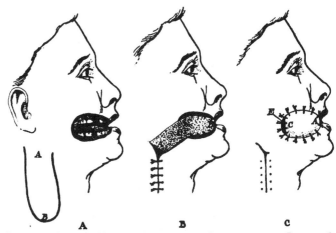

| A | B | C |

FIG. 213. ISRAEL'S METHOD OF CLOSING A DEFECT IN THE CHEEK. In A
the flap A B is marked out, having its pedicle near the angle of the jaw and its
lower end reaching nearly to the clavicle. In B the flap is stitched to the refreshed margins of the gap; the part A C bridges over the skin behind the defect.
The raw area in the neck is closed by sutures. In C the part of the flap A C is
shown folded over B C, so that the raw surfaces are in contact and the edges are
united to those of the defect. A hole, E, is left communicating with the mouth.
This is subsequently closed by the sutures (shown dotted) after refreshing the
apposing edges. A secondary operation will be required to form the angle of the
mouth.

patient had a recurrent nodule of cancer in the position shown in the
figure. It was excised with a wide margin of skin and deep tissues
from all sides of it. The incisions A B and C D were prolonged downwards and a large rectangular flap was dissected up, having its broad
pedicle at the lower end. The flap with its deep surface directed inwards
was placed in the gap, and the apposed edges sutured to one another
as in Fig. 212, B. A small amount of sloughing took place at the junction

of the mucous membrane of the lip and flap. A drainage tube .hould be placed beneath the lower end of the flap. This method may also be usefully employed to close the gap left after the removal of a cancer situated at the angle of the mouth.

Israel closed a large gap by taking a long **flap from the neck** (see Fig. 213). The pedicle, placed near the angle of the jaw, is made broad whilst the lower end of the flap reaches nearly to the clavicle The flap, consisting of skin and subcutaneous tissue, is placed in the defect, so that its distal extremity, B, is at the situation of the angle of the mouth, and the upper portion of the flap A C ' bridges over' the skin behind the defect. The edges of the flap and those of the defect are then united by sutures. The pedicle is severed in about seventeen days. The posterior part, A C, of the flap (Fig. 213, B) is then folded over and placed on the raw outer surface of the anterior portion, A being placed at the angle of the mouth. The borders of the flap are united to the upper and lower edges of the margins of the defect. After union has taken place between the edges of the flap and those of the defect, it is necessary to close the opening, E. into the mouth, which exists at the place where the flap was reduplicated on itself (Fig. 213, C). This is accomplished by refreshing the raw edges of the gap and excising the posterior end of the flap. The two raw surfaces are then accurately united by sutures. A further operation will be necessary to make an angle for the mouth by dissecting up the mucous membrane of the lips and uniting it to the anterior edge of the flap. The wound in the neck is closed by sutures, after undermining the surrounding subcutaneous tissue.

Flap from forehead. This method may be employed as an alternative to taking the flap from the neck, or it may be used in conjunction with a neck flap, the latter being superimposed on the former (Fig. 214). The flap, consisting of skin and subcutaneous tissue. is made sufficiently large to enable it to be turned downwards, and fixed without tension to the margins of the defect, which are pared, except the upper which is not touched at this stage. As a rule the pedicle will be in the region of the zygoma, and must be made broad; the upper end of the flap may reach as high as the hair and anteriorly the edge will skirt the outer margin of the orbit (Fig. 214). It may be necessary to make a backward prolongation of the flap in order to provide a covering for any raw surface on the inner aspect of the ascending ramus of the jaw remaining after adhesions have been freely divided in this region, and to enable the mouth to be opened. When the flap is in position, its cutaneous surface will be directed inwards. The raw surface of the backward prolongation is sutured to the raw surface of the inner aspect of the jaw, by means of stitches which pass from the flap through the whole thickness of the cheek; the knots being tied on the cheek, the stitches can be easily removed.

The second flap for superimposing on to the raw surface of the deep or forehead flap is obtained from the skin and subcutaneous tissue of the neck (Fig. 214). This superficial flap has, of course, its cutaneous surface directed outwards, the two raw surfaces of the flaps being

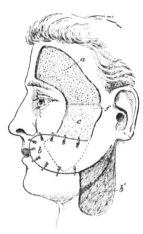

Fig. 214. Method of closing a Defect in the Cheek by Superimposed Flaps. A large forehead flap, *c*, is being used to close a defect in the lower part of the cheek, and has superimposed on it the flap *b* taken from the neck. This flap is also sutured to the margins of the gap. After the division of the pedicle of the forehead flap the upper edge of the defect is refreshed and united to the edge of this flap. *f* is the redundant portion of the forehead flap, and is replaced in the raw area *a*; *b'* is the raw area in the neck, which is closed by undermining its edges. Drainage must be provided at the lower borders of the flaps. Any uncovered area on the flap *c* may be skin-grafted.

apposed to one another. It is sutured to the deep flap and to the margins of the gap, and is also used to close any portion of the defect not covered in by the forehead flap. It is well to provide for drainage, the tube being placed between the flaps and brought to the surface at the lower margin of the superficial flap. The raw area left by transplanting the neck flap is closed by undercutting the edges and bringing them together by sutures in the usual way.

The pedicle of the forehead flap is divided in about a fortnight or three weeks. The upper margin of the gap is now refreshed and united to the upper edge of the deep flap by silkworm-gut sutures. Any redundant portion of the pedicle is replaced in the raw area on the forehead, the remainder of this area being skin-grafted.

Further operations will be required to make an angle for the mouth, and to correct any displacement of the eyebrow or eyelids. These operations are employed to close large defects, when there is no sound skin or the latter has been removed, as in some cases of excision of the upper jaw or of a rodent ulcer.

Closure of a small defect. (a) When the defect is small and the mouth can be freely opened, it may be possible to close it by dis-

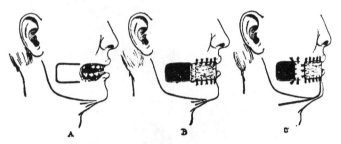

A   B   C

FIG. 215. To illustrate the Closure of a Small Defect by a Flap taken from the Skin over the Masseter. In A the flap is marked out, having its pedicle a short distance behind the gap. In B the flap is shown sutured to the refreshed margins of the gap; the cutaneous surface is directed towards the buccal cavity. In C the pedicle is divided after union of the flap and the edges of the gap has taken place; the redundant portion of the pedicle is also shown replaced in the raw area, the remainder of which is closed by skin-grafting or by a flap raised from over the lower jaw. The thick black line indicates the line of incision for raising this flap, which also covers the outer surface of the flap in the defect. Another operation will be required to form the angle of the mouth. (*After Cheyne and Burghard.*)

secting up the cheek freely on each side of the gap; the cheek below the gap should be the more widely displaced in order that the eyelids may not be distorted. The edges of the gap are then accurately united by sutures. Or a single flap may be taken from the cheek behind the gap (Fig. 215. A). The flap is turned forwards on its pedicle so that the cutaneous surface looks inwards. The pedicle should be attached a little distance behind the posterior margin of the defect and may be severed at the end of a fortnight; any redundant portion is replaced in the area from which it was taken. The outer surface of the flap is covered by skin-grafting or by a superimposed flap taken from the tissues over the lower jaw (Fig. 215, c).

(b) When the defect is small and there is inability to open the mouth on account of cicatricial contraction, **Gussenbauer's operation** (Fig. 216), performed in two stages, is most useful, provided the skin is abundant. A flap of skin and subcutaneous tissue, somewhat broader at its posterior end than at its anterior end, is dissected up, the pedicle being placed about the anterior border of the masseter. The cicatricial tissue is divided from before backwards and the mouth widely opened. The skin flap is turned into the defect so that its anterior free border is inside the mouth; its edges are stitched to those of the defect, the raw (deep) surface of the flap being sutured to the inner aspect of the internal pterygoid muscle. At the end of four weeks the pedicle *b b* is divided and the

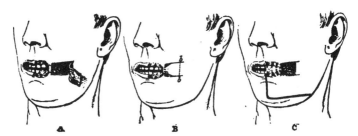

FIG. 216. GUSSENBAUER'S OPERATION. In A the flap is dissected backwards: the dotted lines indicate the incisions for dividing the mucous membrane. In B the anterior end of the flap is shown carried round into the mouth, preparatory to being stitched in position. *b b* is the line along which the flap is subsequently divided and turned forward into the gap, to the margins of which it is sutured in C. The thick black line in C indicates the incision for marking out the flap which is placed on the outer surface of the one filling the gap. The raw surface left where this flap is taken from may be skin-grafted or closed by undermining the adjacent skin. (*After Cheyne and Burghard.*)

posterior part of the flap is brought into the anterior part of the defect and sutured to its refreshed margins. The cutaneous surface of the flap is thus directed towards the mouth and the exposed raw surface is covered by a superimposed flap taken from over the lower jaw (Fig. 216, c).

Flaps from the arm have been used to close very large defects when other methods have been unavailable or inapplicable. The method of employing them is similar to that described under restoration of the lips (Fig. 199).

Defects in the mucous membrane of the cheek remaining after the removal of large portions, have been closed by transplanting a flap from the neck to the inside of the mouth through an incision made in the cheek in front of the masseter. The pedicle of the flap must be broad and the flap must be long. The raw surface of the flap is applied to the raw surface in the mouth and united to it by sutures, the pedicle being divided after the lapse of ten days to a fortnight. The excess of flap is replaced in the gap left by its removal, the remaining portion being closed by undermining its edges. This may be done either at the first operation or when the pedicle is divided. Finally, the incision in the cheek is closed by silkworm-gut sutures.[1]

PLASTIC OPERATIONS FOR SYPHILITIC AFFECTIONS OF THE PALATE

As a result of syphilitic ulceration, the hard or soft palate may be more or less completely destroyed. In the hard palate a round or oval hole is usually produced by necrosis of the palatal processes of the superior maxillæ; when the soft palate is affected, the loss of tissue is often extreme and the most striking feature is the formation of adhesions between the remains of the palate and the pharyngeal wall. These may be so abundant as to completely shut off the naso-pharynx from the oro-pharynx, or the communication may be so small that only a probe or small-sized bougie can be passed through it. Nasal respiration may be rendered difficult: much mucus may collect in the nose and only be got rid of with difficulty, and progressive deafness, accompanied by attacks of earache, may follow. The voice becomes nasal and indistinct, and this is the usual symptom which the patient wishes to have remedied.

If the perforation is in the hard palate, an obturator made by a dentist is generally the best method of treatment. It should never fit into the hole tightly, but always take the form of a plate, which can be readily removed for cleansing purposes and easily replaced. Such an appliance will restore the natural character of the voice and prevent food and liquids passing into the nose. If it is desirable to operate, the hole may be closed by means of flaps of the muco-periosteum, raised on each side of it, as in the ordinary operation for cleft palate, the raw edges being united by silkworm-gut sutures. A better method is to raise the flaps as in Davies-Colley's operation for cleft palate, making the flaps as large as possible in order to allow for their subsequent contraction.

When the soft palate is adherent to the pharyngeal wall, the operation is performed in the following manner :—A Smith's gag is introduced into the mouth, which is opened as widely as possible compatible with free respiration. The adhesions are divided by means of an angular cleft-palate knife or by curved scissors; a cleft-palate raspatory is also sometimes useful in separating them. There may be a good deal of hæmorrhage, but by keeping the head low, and using sponge-pressure, it is

[1] See Keetley, *Lancet*, March 4, 1905.

controlled without much difficulty. The soft palate is drawn forwards as much as possible, and fixed by silkworm sutures either to the muco-periosteum of the hard palate, or by sutures, one on either side, passed through the whole thickness of the palate, the free ends being brought forwards and fixed round the front teeth. Instead of silkworm-gut sutures, silver wire may be employed. The sutures are left to cut their way out, which they will do in the course of one or two weeks. During this time, healing of the raw surfaces will have taken place to a considerable degree, but it will be necessary to keep the opening into the naso-pharynx patent by the regular passage of bougies, and from time to time by stretching the soft palate with a blunt hook or the finger passed behind it from the mouth. During the stage of healing after division of the adhesions, union of the raw surfaces may be prevented by using a piece of lead plate cut to the full breadth of the naso-pharynx and so bent that one arm of it rests on the upper surface and the other on the lower surface of the palate, the separated margin being received between the two portions of the plate and apposed to the bend in it. Silk threads being fixed to the four corners of the piece of lead, the two from the upper corners are passed, one through each nostril, and the two lower ones are brought forward across the hard palate to the interval between the lateral and central incisor teeth of each side. The upper and lower threads of each side are then tied together in front, over the upper lip, after being passed through a piece of rubber tubing, in order to prevent them cutting. The plate is left in position for a fortnight.[1]

In all these cases the chief difficulty is to prevent recurrence of the adhesions. The immediate results of the operation are often good, but in the course of time contraction frequently occurs again. As an almost complete occlusion of the passage from the naso-pharynx to the oro-pharynx may exist without causing any evidences of discomfort, these operations should not be undertaken in the absence of some definite symptoms such as those already enumerated, nor should they be performed so long as ulceration is present, or shortly after the ulcer has healed, and bearing in mind that the patient is syphilitic, iodides and mercury should be given in full doses.

[1] Robinson, *Trans. Laryngol. Soc.*, vol. xiv, p. 106.

CHAPTER IV

OPERATIONS FOR CONGENITAL AND ACQUIRED DEFORMITIES

OPERATIONS FOR WEBBED FINGERS

GENERAL PRINCIPLES

WEBBED fingers present varying degrees of deformity.

1. The web may be only slightly longer than normal.

2. The fingers may be united by a band of tissue extending their whole length. This band may either be thick and loose, or thin and binding the fingers closely together.

3. The fingers may be united by bone, the phalanges of the individual fingers being more or less completely fused.

The operative measures to be adopted depend on the variety and degree of the union, and it not infrequently happens that different operations have to be used in conjunction; if several fingers are affected one method may be suitable for some, and another for the other fingers. A great variety of operations have been practised, but none of them are completely satisfactory except in the cases where the web is broad and thick and there is plenty of tissue. The web has a great tendency to reform, and when the union is close and thin, there is a great likelihood of subsequent contraction of the fingers taking place. If the separation of the fingers leaves a scar on the palmar aspect, flexion is very likely to follow from its contraction. Unless it is quite certain from the mobility of the fingers on one another that there is no bony union, an X-ray photograph should be obtained before an operation is undertaken; the extent of the union and the possibility of improving the state of affairs can then be more accurately estimated. If several fingers are fused together and a shapeless digit is present, it is generally best not to attempt any operation at all; though unsightly, such a hand is often very useful and may be made much worse by an unsuccessful operation. If two fingers are united by bone and their usefulness is thereby considerably impaired, some improvement may be obtained by the removal of the bones belonging to one finger. In these cases it is not possible to give the patient two separate fingers as the covering of skin is insufficient.

The hand in cases of webbed fingers is smaller and does not develop to the same extent as the normal hand. Therefore, to improve the usefulness of the hand, to encourage its development and to remove if possible an unsightly deformity, it may be necessary to operate, but this should not be done before the third or fourth year. It is not advisable to operate in early infancy, for the parts are so small and the tissues so delicate that a good result cannot be expected, and if the operation is a failure, the prospects of success from later operations is much diminished. It is advisable also not to attempt to correct the deformity of all the fingers by one operation, but to take them in pairs. The effect can then be observed, and the succeeding operations modified, or if necessary entirely changed. Some weeks or months may elapse between the dates of the operations; this applies especially to cases in which flaps have been taken from the dorsum˙of the hand—the succeeding operations should not be undertaken until the scar and the flap are soundly healed.

Whatever method is adopted, the dressings must be applied to each finger in such a way that they are kept separate during the healing process.

The after-treatment is most important. To prevent subsequent contraction it is necessary that the patient should wear a splint, at first both by day and night, subsequently at night only. The exact time the splint should be worn varies, but in any case it will be for months. When the splint is being worn constantly, it should be removed daily in order that passive movements may be carried out. Some form of moulded splint is the best; it should be applied on the dorsum of the hand and fingers, and should be long enough to reach from just above the wrist to the ends of the fingers. It must be well and carefully padded, so as not to exert pressure on the parts.

The available methods of operating are:—

1. Simple division of the web and union of the raw surfaces.

2. Division of the web combined with the formation of a triangular flap at its base.

3. The formation of a dorsal and palmar flap from the conjoined fingers (Didot's operation).

4. A combination of one of these methods with skin-grafting, where there is not enough tissue to cover all the raw surfaces.

5. Removal of the bones of one finger when there is osseous union.

SIMPLE DIVISION OF THE WEB AND UNION OF THE RAW SURFACES

This method may be used when the web is large and thick, and may be combined with perforation of the apex of the web by means of a stout silver wire which is kept *in situ* till the perforation is healed and a round hole remains (Fig. 217). The web is then divided throughout the rest of its extent; any excess of tissue is removed and the raw surfaces

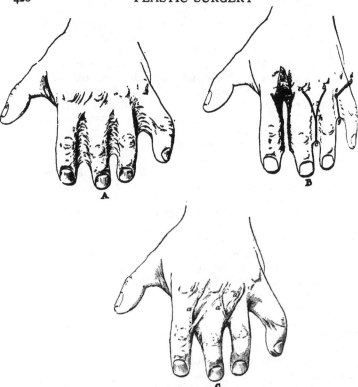

FIG. 217. OPERATIONS FOR WEBBED FINGERS. In A a well-marked web is shown between each of the fingers. In B two methods of operating are shown. The web between the third and fourth fingers has been perforated at *e*, and a stout silver wire, *e d*, has been inserted. This is left *in situ* till the perforation is cicatrized. The remainder of the web is then divided along the line *e g*. any redundant portion is removed, and the raw edges are sutured to one another on the sides of each finger.

    A better method of operating is shown on the webs between the other fingers. *a h* and *b h* show the incisions marking out a dorsal V-shaped flap; *h c* is the incision for splitting the remainder of the web; *f* is the flap dissected up: this is sutured to the palmar surface between the fingers to form the new web. The raw area on the sides of each finger is closed by stitching the margins together after any redundant portion has been removed. In c the result of operating by this method on the hand A is shown. The webs between the first and second and the second and third fingers have re-formed to some extent; *a, a', a"* are the scars. The operation on the web between the third and fourth fingers was quite successful. (*Author's case.*)

of the two flaps on each finger are united by sutures. It is a tedious and not very satisfactory method.

TRIANGULAR FLAP AT THE BASE OF THE WEB

This method should be employed when the web is a broad one, whether it is partial or complete. A triangular flap having its apex at the centre of the web and its base opposite the metacarpo-phalangeal joint of the finger is marked out on the dorsal aspect. The flap must be long

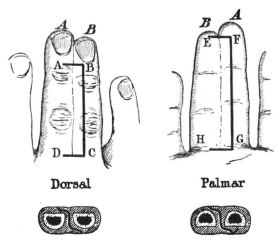

Dorsal   Palmar

FIG. 218. DIDOT'S METHOD OF OPERATING FOR WEBBED FINGERS. The lines of the incision for the dorsal and palmar flaps are indicated. The smaller figures represent a transverse section of the fingers, and show the direction of the line of separation. The dorsal flap should be sufficiently broad to be united to the incision on the palmar aspect of the finger.

enough to be turned into the palm and stitched in position without tension, and it must also be as thick as possible. The remainder of the web is divided along its median line (Fig. 217, B). The flap is then passed between the fingers and its apex stitched to the palmar edge of the cleft, the margins being united to the skin of the edges of the wound at the sides of the fingers. Any excess of tissue left after splitting the web, or any protruding fat, is removed and the raw surfaces on each side of the fingers are then united.

Instead of a long dorsal flap, two smaller flaps, one from the dorsum and one from the palmar aspect of the web, may be employed. These flaps having been dissected up, and the remainder of the web divided, are then united together and form the new web. The raw edges of the web attached to each finger are then sutured together as accurately as possible, any excess of subcutaneous tissue being removed.

DORSAL AND PALMAR FLAPS. DIDOT'S OPERATION
(Figs. 218 and 219)

This method is employed when the web is narrow and thin. An incision, B C, is made along the dorsal aspect of one finger, and at each end

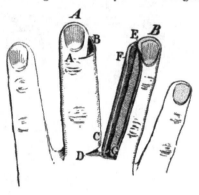

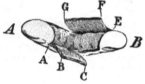

FIG. 219. DIDOT'S METHOD OF OPERATING FOR WEBBED FINGERS. This figure shows the flaps dissected up and being applied to the raw area on each finger. The lower figure is another view of the same stage.

of this incision, short incisions, A B and D C, are made. On the palmar aspect of the other finger an incision, F G, is made, and transverse cuts, E F, H G, are made at the ends of the longitudinal incision. These flaps, which should be as thick as possible, are carefully dissected up, the rest of the tissues between the fingers being divided and their separation completed. One finger (A) thus has a dorsal flap, and the other (B) has a palmar flap, attached to it. Each flap is carried round the side of its own finger and stitched in position to the edges of the raw surface. It rarely happens that both flaps are sufficiently large to cover the whole of the raw surfaces; one finger may be well covered and the other incompletely. Skin-grafting will be necessary to cover any raw area, and should be carried out at the same operation.

There is also a difficulty in making a satisfactory web unless it is possible to make a triangular flap from the dorsum of the hand between the bases of the fingers. Again, the finger which has the scar on its palmar aspect is more likely to become flexed, and therefore, in planning the flaps, an endeavour should be always made to give this finger the better flap to cover it, that is, the dorsal flap should be the larger. Lastly from the thinness of the tissues used to form these flaps, the operation should not be done before the patient is four or five years old.

REMOVAL OF THE BONES OF ONE FINGER WHEN THERE IS OSSEOUS UNION

If it is necessary to perform an operation when osseous union is present, a rectangular flap is dissected up from one side of the conjoint finger, and the bones of one finger removed after the tendons, &c., have been separated. The flap should be taken from the palmar aspect, and after removal of the bones, it is applied to the raw surface and sutured with silkworm-gut. A dorsal scar is thus made. The majority of these cases are, however, often best left without an operation.

OPERATIONS FOR SUPERNUMERARY DIGITS

These are a not infrequent congenital deformity; they are often symmetrical, either the fingers or the toes being affected. From an operative point of view, the most important point is the method of union of the digit. This may be simply by a band of fibrous tissue, or the extra digit may be attached, with or without an articular surface, to the side of the metacarpal or metatarsal bone. Much more rarely the extra digit has also a metacarpal or metatarsal bone, and then there is an articulation with the carpus or tarsus. Sometimes the terminal phalanx alone is affected and is more or less completely divided, so that a bifid digit results.

If the union is fibrous, all that is necessary is to cut through the bond of union after making an elliptical incision in the skin round its attached base so as to form a flap and then unite the edges by sutures. When there is an articular surface or projecting piece of bone on the side of the metacarpal, this must be removed after the amputation, so as to leave a smooth level surface on the bone; otherwise, as growth continues, a very obvious projection will be formed. Flaps consisting of the whole thickness of the tissues down to the bone are dissected up, care being taken in shaping them that they do not contain any excess of tissue. If the supernumerary digit has an extra metacarpal bone, this must be removed together with the digit; any projecting articular facet left after the removal of the extra bones must be smoothed down with a chisel, and, as some part of the carpal joints may be opened strict precautions against sepsis will be necessary. The operation is performed in the manner described in Vol. I, p. 229.

When the terminal phalanx is bifid, it is necessary to remove one portion, and that part which is the more deviated from the line of the digit should be excised. If the phalanx is only partially divided, it must be completely split down to its base and one part removed. It may be necessary to divide the ligaments of the joint, in order to put the remaining part of the phalanx in a straight line with the rest of the finger. By means of a splint fixed round the wrist and applied to the finger, the latter must be kept as straight as possible during the healing process and for some time after. Massage or passive movements are required to restore the mobility of the joints, but the splint will have to be worn for some weeks.

When the toes are affected similar methods of treatment should be employed, if it is thought desirable to do any operation, but very often the presence of the additional toe causes no inconvenience.

OPERATIONS FOR ACQUIRED CONTRACTIONS OF THE FINGERS

General principles. Acquired contractions and adhesions of the fingers are often due to burns and scalds. These cases are most difficult to treat, (1) because of the extensive cicatrization and adhesions between the various structures; (2) the great liability to reproduction of the deformity, as healing and contraction occur after the parts have been freely separated; (3) the skin is usually destroyed and replaced by thin scar tissue which is almost useless for any plastic operation; and (4) the small size of the parts and the difficulty in getting healing to take place by first intention.

Where such scar tissue causes contracture it is absolutely essential that it should be excised thoroughly. The slightest amount left will impair the result. If the area is small, by under-cutting the edges of the healthy skin it may be sutured over the area, but where the defect is of any size or is subject to tension or trauma, transplantation of pedicled flaps of skin is the only satisfactory method. For the back of the hand these may be taken from the abdomen, but for the palmar

surface they should be taken from the buttock, care being exercised to
choose an area free from hair and to raise the skin with a minimum
amount of fat. This latter is emphasized since an excess of fat absorbs
only after years of use. The whole hand may be inserted under the flap

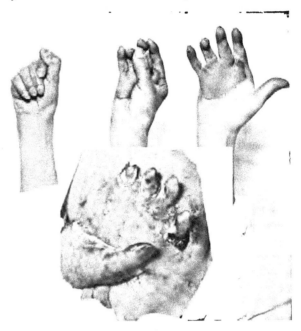

FIG. 220. PHOTOGRAPH OF HAND INSERTED IN POCKET ON BUTTOCK AND
FINAL RESULT ONE YEAR AFTERWARDS IN THIS CASE, WHICH WAS SO CONTRACTED
THAT HAND COULD NOT BE OPENED AT ALL. (*Kanavel.*)

and if the fingers are also involved, these may be included, each finger
being made to make its exit through small puncture holes in the skin.
In such cases care must be taken to make the web out of skin also and
not have the suture line along the free edge of the web, since in such
cases the contraction of the scar as the time passes ends in a webbing
of the proximal phalanges. This can be avoided partially at least by
making a flap of skin to pass between the fingers with its line of sutures
on the dorsum of the hand. This web should be as short as possible.
One begins to cut the pedicle about the eighth day and it is completely
detached by the tenth to fourteenth day, varying with its size and

condition. Such pedicled flaps have been used by one of the editors (Kanavel) in a considerable number of cases with complete satisfaction. The arm and hand are held immobile in a plaster cast before the pedicle

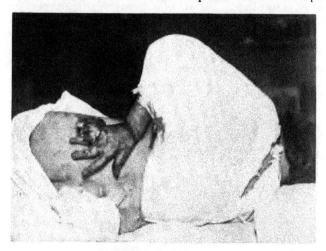

FIG. 221. ILLUSTRATION DEMONSTRATES THE METHOD OF TAKING LARGE FLAP AND GRADUALLY CUTTING V-SHAPED SECTION, SO THAT FLAP OF SKIN MAY ULTI- MATELY BE CARRIED BETWEEN BASES OF FINGERS SO AS TO PREVENT CONTRACTION INCIDENT TO TIME IN SCAR TISSUE. (*Kanavel.*)

is cut. Passive and active movements should be begun at once on de- tachment of the hand.

Where tendons or nerves are exposed they may be wrapped in pedicles of fat cut from the surrounding tissue.

OPERATIONS FOR DUPUYTREN'S CONTRACTION

Operations for this deformity very often end in disappointment owing to several factors. Among these may be mentioned the recur- rence of the scar tissue and the sloughing of the skin. Operations may be done either by the subcutaneous or open method. The latter is to be preferred, but requires a high degree of surgical judgment and technique.

Subcutaneous division of the fascia through multiple incisions (Adams's operation) is performed as follows: The skin is thoroughly cleansed and a small sharp-pointed tenotomy knife is introduced parallel to the skin. The cutting edge is then turned toward the contracted fascia and the bands divided, being careful not to cut the vessels and nerves, also not to attempt too much in any puncture. This puncture is repeated at various sites until as much is done as is thought advisable. The operation is repeated at later periods. Meanwhile the hand is kept extended—under moderate tension only. The splints must be worn at

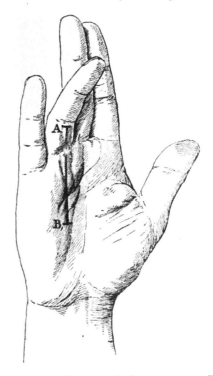

Fig. 222. Operation for Dupuytren's Contraction by Excision of the Contracted Fascia. a b is the line of incision for exposing the fascia; the short transverse lines at each end of it enable the skin to be reflected in the form of two flaps.

night for months, meanwhile active and passive motion continued. Others have cut the bands under open incision

The treatment is so prolonged and the outcome so problematical that a majority of surgeons do not favour the method.

Division of skin and fascia by V-shaped incision. By this method the skin and fascia are incised by the V-shaped incision (see Fig. 223) and the finger straightened. The incision is then sutured, resulting in a Y-shaped line. This method gives temporary relief, but suffers from

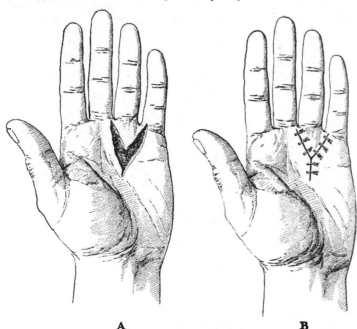

A   **B**

FIG. 223. OPERATION FOR DUPUYTREN'S CONTRACTION BY A V-SHAPED INCISION. In A the raw area left after the skin and fascia have been divided and the finger has been straightened is shown. In B the method of uniting the edges of the raw area is indicated. Any unclosed part should be covered with a skingraft.

the probability of a return of the contracture. The adjacent scar tissue may be excised but seldom adds much to the result.

Excision of the contracted tissue. This procedure alone offers assurance of definite results but often ends in disappointment due to sloughing of the palmar skin in some instances, and return of the contracture in others, if the surgeon has been too timid. The surgeon is between the horns of the dilemma. It is manifest, as Kanavel has emphasized. that if the surgeon wishes for definite results, he must take the responsibility and excise completely all contracted tissue and then cover the area by the palmar skin if possible, but if not possible, or if sloughing occurs, by a transplant of skin.   In his judgment the result is improved if a transplant of fat is used to replace the contracted tissue.   His procedure as described comprises also the excision of the entire palmar fascia if the deformity is at all marked.   Excision may be

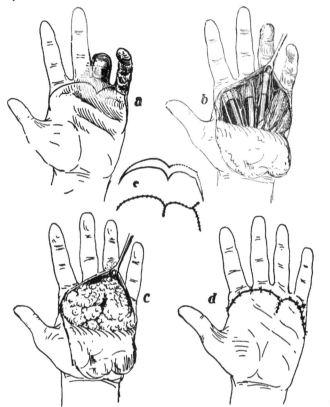

Fig. 224. Dupuytren's Contracture-Technique of Operation for Excision of Palmar Fascia and Transplantation of Fat. (*Kanavel.*)

made through a Y-shaped incision or through a longitudinal incision with transverse incisions at the ends to permit rolling back the skin.   In the latter incision sloughing is a possibility.   Kanavel has described the following technique in severe cases:

A longitudinal incision is made just to the inside of the hypothenar eminence, extending down to within a thumb's breadth of the base of the ring finger. Two wings then descend, forming a V. The ulnar wing goes down to the base of the little finger and over the ulnar side of the hand nearly to the dorsum. The radial wing extends down to the base of the middle finger. This permits one to excise the entire palmar fascia over to the thenar and hypothenar spaces. The skin over the finger is raised and the contracted bands along the fingers excised.

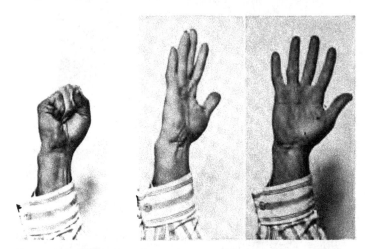

FIG. 225. PHOTOGRAPH OF PATIENT SHOWING RESULT AFTER OPERATION FOR DUPUYTREN'S CONTRACTURE, WITH REMOVAL OF PALMAR FASCIA AND TRANSPLANTATION OF FAT. Photograph taken one and one-half years after operation. (*Kanavel.*)

The palmar skin being mobilized to the thenar and over the hypothenar areas may now be brought together. After the fingers are straightened the palmar V is changed into a Y. Before final closure of the skin a free transplant of fat taken from the abdominal wall is inserted into the palm and prolongations carried up under the skin of the fingers. The fat transplant is $\frac{1}{4}$ inch in thickness and covers the entire palm. Before proceeding to this stage, however, the surgeon must convince himself that the skin can be closed and that it is viable. This is generally so if the operation has been done properly. If the skin cannot be closed or if the surgeon believes the skin is not viable, it is better for the patient if the issue is met squarely and the hand placed in a skin pocket on the buttock as described above. These skin transplants, if properly done, are almost certainly successful and end in complete function of the hand. The operation is not difficult and the disability not much longer than by the other methods. The patient, however, is confined to bed for a couple of weeks, but the certainty of success more than compensates for this in doubtful cases.

If the first procedure is tried and sloughing of any size occurs, the surgeon should not depend on Thiersch grafts or splints or manipulation to secure a result, but resort at once to pedicle flaps as the quickest and most satisfactory method of securing function.

OPERATIONS FOR CICATRICIAL DEFORMITIES AFTER INJURIES

The deformities which follow cicatrization are so various that it is impossible to describe any operation which will meet an individual case. Thus one patient will have an arm closely bound to the side of the chest; another will have a large mass of scar tissue preventing movements in a joint; and a third will have a cicatrix binding the chin down to the neck.

The general principles to be followed in these cases are :—

(1) Division of the scar tissue till healthy tissues are reached. Tight bands and large masses of cicatricial tissues will need to be excised, but care must be exercised not to remove unnecessary portions; at the same time, the whole area and its edges must be completely refreshed. As a result there will probably be a good deal of bleeding, which must be arrested by pressure before proceeding further with the operation.

(2) The means by which the deformity may be prevented from recurring: these are (a) skin-grafting, (b) the use of flaps. (a) As regards skin-grafting, Thiersch's method does not permanently prevent the recurrence of the contraction, especially when the area to be grafted is large, and it is essential in these cases to have a thick sound covering of skin. Moreover, when a very large area requires to be covered, it may be almost impossible to get enough skin. Wolfe's method is not so suitable for these cases and is also inferior to the use of flaps. Therefore skin-grafting should be used for small areas and when other methods are not available, or in conjunction with these methods.

(b) Flaps are the best means of treating these cases; these may be obtained either from adjacent parts, or from a distal part of the body, such as a limb. The flap may be raised and immediately transplanted to its new position, or it may be glided into position or may ' bridge over ' an intervening portion of the skin. For example, if the arm is firmly bound down to the chest (following a severe burn or similai injury) a flap may be raised from the chest (Fig. 226) or back of the shoulder. The distal end of the flap is sutured to the raw area on the scar tissue prepared to receive it. When union has taken place, the

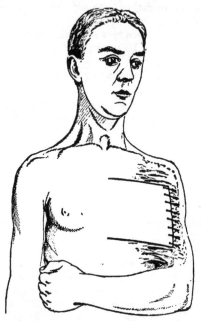

FIG. 226. TO SHOW HOW A FLAP MAY BE USED TO CORRECT CICATRICIAL CONTRACTION. The arm is bound to the side of the chest by adhesions; a large flap has been raised from the thorax and stitched at its distal end to a prepared raw area on the arm. When union has taken place, the pedicle of the flap is divided, and the arm is freed by dividing the cicatricial bands. A raw area is thus made on the inner side of the arm, to which the flap is sutured.

pedicle is divided and at the same time the remaining adhesions uniting the arm to the side of the thorax are cut through, thus freeing the limb and leaving a large raw area on the inner side of the arm. The proximal portion of the flap is then applied to this area and sutured to its edges. The flap must be made broad in proportion to its length and does not always correspond exactly in size and shape to the raw area, but care should be taken to make their relative sizes equal as far as possible, and especially to obtain primary union between the raw area and the distal end of the flap, because this portion is the most likely to slough. The pedicle may be usually divided in ten days or a fortnight, the exact time depending on the amount of union between the flap and raw area and the condition of the flap.

Instead of transplanting the flap at once, it may be raised, left attached by both ends, and allowed to granulate. Such a flap may be taken from an adjacent portion of the body; thus, in the case of a large contracted area on the inner side of the arm or forearm, it may be obtained from the outer surface of the limb. The incisions must be made parallel to the line of the blood-vessels and so arranged as to allow the flap to be readily twisted into its new position. The flap must be thick, and the raw area left by its elevation should be closed as much as possible in order to diminish the amount of contraction which follows the healing of the wound. A piece of sterilized gutta-percha or oiled silk is placed beneath it, especial care being taken to prevent union occurring in the angles between the pedicles and the raw surface. In about two or three weeks' time, the flap is transplanted by division of one of the pedicles and sutured to the edges and surface of the raw area prepared for it. When union has taken place, the other pedicle is severed and the remaining portion is then sutured in position. At first the flap is very bulky and unsightly, but in the course of time it shrinks and flattens out.

Another method of using a double-pedicled flap is shown in Figs. 227 and 228. This method is particularly useful in the case of the forearm and hand, and especially for the palmar surface of the latter, where elasticity and resistance are required. Instead of taking the flap from the buttock or thigh, it may be taken from the abdomen. The flap has two pedicles and should not be cut too thick; it must contain a part of the subcutaneous tissue and must be long enough to be free from tension. The edges of the raw area are dissected up, to make their union with those of the flap more easy of accomplishment. The pedicles of the flap are divided at different times, the first in ten to fourteen days, and then the other after a further lapse of some days, viz. about the third week. If the fingers have to be covered they should be first separated as widely as possible and the flap marked out with them in this position, so as to ensure a sufficient amount of covering. It may be possible to make separate pockets for each finger, the attached portions of the flap between the fingers being subsequently divided. This also should be done in stages, one finger at a time, and each portion sutured to its proper finger. When this method is used, the nails must be cut quite short and thoroughly cleaned, every care being taken to minimize septic influences. A large raw area will be left on the buttock

or from wherever the flap is taken; this is closed as far as possible
by undercutting the adjacent skin and stitching together apposed surfaces, Thiersch's grafts being used to cover any remaining uncovered
parts.

(3) During the various stages the parts must be kept absolutely at
rest and it is therefore often necessary to employ some form of fixation

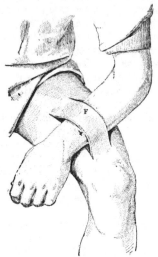

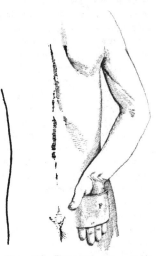

FIG. 227. TO ILLUSTRATE THE USE OF
A FLAP, F, WITH TWO PEDICLES.

FIG. 228. TO SHOW HOW THE PALM
OF THE HAND MAY BE COVERED WITH
A FLAP, F, TAKEN FROM THE BUTTOCK.

apparatus. Plaster of Paris is one of the most useful and easily applied:
a window may be left so that the wound can be dressed without disturbing the flap, or the whole case may be put on in such a way as to be
easily removable.

(4) Many operations will probably be required to obtain a good result, and no attempt should be made, except in the least serious cases, to
effect a complete cure by one operation.

Here it may be helpful to give some indications as to the positions
from which these flaps may be obtained.

1. For the upper arm and axilla, the flap may be taken from the
chest (Fig. 226).

2. For the forearm and dorsum of the hand, from the abdomen
(Fig. 229) or thigh (Fig. 227). For the dorsum and palm of the hand,

and the fingers, the buttock may be used to supply the flap (see Fig. 228).

3. For the lower limbs, the opposite limb may be used (Fig. 230).

4. For the neck, the back of the shoulder or upper part of the chest may be employed to supply the flap.

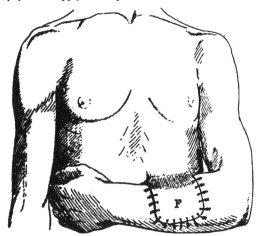

Fig. 229. To show how a Flap, f, may be taken from the Skin of the Abdomen and applied to the Forearm.

OPERATIONS FOR HAMMER-TOE

This deformity is characterized by dorsal flexion of the first phalanx at the metatarso-phalangeal joint and plantar flexion of the second phalanx on the first. The terminal phalanx may be in its normal position or in the same straight line as the second phalanx. The condition is primarily due to a shortening of the lateral ligaments of the first inter-phalangeal joints, and complicated in bad cases by contraction of the glenoid ligament, of the flexor tendons, and of the skin on the plantar aspect of the toe. Hallux valgus frequently accompanies this deformity, and in cases requiring operative treatment there is usually a corn on the dorsal aspect of the first inter-phalangeal joint or at the extremity of the toe. The patient usually seeks advice on account of this painful corn or because he wishes to enter one of the public services. The pressure of the boot on the displaced toe interfering with walking is another indication for operation.

The operative measures available are: (1) division of the contracted structures around the joint; (2) excision of the head of the first phalanx;

(3) amputation of the toe. The first method is suitable only for slight cases; in the majority of cases the choice lies between excision and amputation and generally excision is to be preferred. Amputation is certainly an effective means of relieving the deformity, but it is an unnecessarily severe remedy, which increases the amount of hallux valgus,

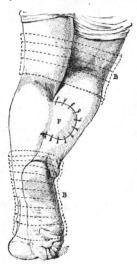

FIG. 230. TO SHOW HOW A FLAP, F, TAKEN FROM ONE LEG, MAY BE APPLIED TO THE OTHER. B is the appliance (a plaster of Paris casing is very convenient) for fixing the limbs immovably together.

if this is present, and favours its occurrence in every case. Moreover, the loss of the toe may prevent the patient from entering one of the public services. If a marked degree of hallux valgus is present, this should be rectified at the same time that the hammer-toe is operated on.

Division of the contracted structures around the joint. The foot having been thoroughly cleansed and sterilized, a small sharp-pointed tenotome is entered on one side of the toe, opposite the first interphalangeal joint, at the junction of the dorsal and lateral aspects. The lateral ligament is made tense and divided, and the knife is carried across the plantar aspect of the joint, dividing the glenoid ligament, the long flexor tendon, and opposite lateral ligament. If the flexor tendon and plantar ligament are not contracted, the knife may be withdrawn and a fresh puncture made on the other side of the joint in order to divide the plantar ligament of that side. The toe is then straightened, and in doing so the skin may be lacerated, or may require to be divided if it is tense. An antiseptic dressing is applied to the toe, and a well-padded splint is placed on its plantar surface. The splint should be made of thin metal and be T-shaped; it should extend far back on the sole, the transverse limb being fixed to the foot by an elastic band passing round the instep, and the longitudinal limb fastened to the toe by another band. Instead of these elastic bands, it is sometimes more convenient to use a bandage.

Excision of the head of the phalanx. A longitudinal incision is made on one side of the extensor tendon down to the bone. The soft structures are separated from the bones and the tendon displaced to one side. The ligaments of the joint being divided, the head of the phalanx is made to project out of the wound and is then divided above the articular cartilage by means of sharp bone forceps. Enough bone must be removed to allow the toe to be easily and completely straightened. The corn which will usually be present must be excised before the wound is closed by two or three sutures. An antiseptic dressing is applied, and the toe is placed on a well-padded splint with an extra amount of padding beneath the terminal phalanx, to keep it in a straight line. After the wound is healed, the toe should be kept on a splint, or put in a silicate bandage for three or four weeks.

Amputation. The method of amputating the toe is described in Vol. I, p. 275.

CHAPTER V

BURNS AND SCALDS

By J. M. H. MacLeod, M.A., M.D., F.R.C.P. (Lond.)

BURNS are due to dry heat and scalds to moist heat. Scalds are usually less severe than burns, but the area involved is generally more extensive. Burns vary in severity according to the degree of heat and the length of time the skin has been exposed to it.

Symptoms. It is customary to describe the local effects of excessive heat as being of six degrees, and this division, though purely arbitrary, is useful in emphasizing the points in which burns differ according to the degree of heat.

1. Burns of the first degree are caused by a temperature of about 60° C. and consist of erythema, which may be accompanied by swelling from a transudation of fluid into the tissues, and is associated with a burning sensation and tenderness. This subsides quickly, generally leaving slight scaliness.

2. Burns of the second degree are the result of a temperature of about 100° C. In them the inflammation and burning pain are more severe and the transudation of fluid into the tissues leads, either at once or in a few hours, to the formation of vesicles and bullæ. The bullæ are rapidly ruptured by injury or by increased exudation, and dry up to form a scab which may separate without leaving a scar. Occasionally the fluid in the bleb becomes absorbed and the bleb collapses without breaking. On the other hand, the bleb may become infected with septic micro-organisms and suppuration and ulceration supervene, followed by scarring.

3. Burns of the third degree are caused by a temperature greater than 100° C. and are intensely painful. In them not only the epidermis but the deeper layer of the skin is destroyed, forming an 'eschar' which is firmly adherent to the underlying tissue, is ashen-grey or black in colour and leathery in consistence. It soon becomes surrounded by an inflammatory halo, in a few days pus appears at the edges, and in course of time it sloughs off, leaving a granulating surface which, on healing, is followed by a scar.

4. In burns of the fourth degree the skin is involved in its whole

depth, and when the eschar separates irregular scars and unsightly contractures are produced.

5. In burns of the fifth degree not only the skin but the underlying tissue and muscles are affected.

6. In burns of the sixth degree the charring involves the whole of the tissues, including the bone, and loss of parts and deformity occur.

One of the most serious complications of burns is secondary infection with septic micro-organisms, which not only causes ulceration followed by unsightly hypertrophic scars, but may lead to a severe cellulitis or, from absorption, to septicæmia.

Constitutional effects of burns. The constitutional effects of burns vary with the situation and extent of the skin involved and are far more severe than those which occur after other injuries involving an equal destruction of tissue. Burns involving about one-half of the skin surface are usually fatal, death resulting from shock a few hours after the burn, the patient dying in a state of profound collapse. Sometimes the patient may remain comparatively well during the first twenty-four hours, except for the local pain, and then gradually succumb, with symptoms of prostration preceded by spasms, restlessness, and distress over the region of the heart. In the majority of the fatal cases death from shock supervenes within forty-eight hours. Should prostration be delayed for forty-eight hours or longer the prognosis becomes more favourable. On the other hand, the state of collapse may be safely passed through, and yet the patient be in danger from acute inflammatory symptoms supervening from septic absorption.

A curious complication of severe burns is ulceration of the duodenum, indicated by epigastric pain after food and, possibly, hæmatemesis or melæna; this may lead to a fatal issue from perforation into the peritoneum or bleeding from an eroded artery.

Histo-pathology. The initial action of heat is to cause dilatation of the blood-vessels throughout the corium, clinically evident in erythema, an exudation of serum, and an infiltration of leucocytes. The serous fluid passes up between the cells of the epidermis, causing them to be œdematous, interfering with the process of cornification, and giving rise to scaliness. When the heat has been more severe the exudation is greater, takes place more rapidly, and collects in the epidermis forming vesicles or bullæ. The bulla is the result of the fluid stretching, weakening, and breaking the inter-epithelial fibres and accumulating in the space so formed. This process is facilitated, partly by the softening of the epidermal cells by the heat and the transformation of any moisture into steam, which, forcing its way between the prickle-cells, separates them and prepares a passage for the fluid; and partly by the toxic action of the softened or dead epidermal cells causing a positive chemotaxis and attracting more serum.

In more severe degrees of burn the epidermal cells are destroyed and charred and separate as an eschar, leaving a more or less deeply ulcerated surface. When the ulcer heals there is an organization of the small round cells of the cellular infiltration into new fibrous tissue which may be so abundant as to result in a keloidal scar.

Diagnosis. The diagnosis of slight burns from other localized patches of erythema is rendered easy by the destruction of the hair and the associated burning sensation. Nor need any difficulty be experienced in distinguishing the bullous state from other bullous conditions like pemphigus or erythema bullosum, for in the case of burns there are marked subjective symptoms, a definite history, and a localization of the lesions to the burnt area instead of an irregular distribution over the cutaneous surface.

Prognosis. The prognosis in burns of a minor degree is excellent, and even in cases where bullæ have formed, provided the burnt surface is not too extensive and suppuration has not occurred, healing may take place without scarring. The time occupied in recovery depends on the extent of the area involved and the general condition of the patient. In children and old people shock is apt to supervene unless the burn is very limited, and this delays healing. Where the burn is deep and the corium implicated, more or less severe scarring and contracture result. The danger from burns is dependent on the extent of the area rather than on the depth of the injury, and even in milder degrees of burn a fatal issue is almost inevitable if the area affected be more than one-third of the body.

Treatment. In mild degrees of burn the pain may be relieved by a suitable occlusive dressing or by immersion of the affected part, or of the whole body if necessary, in warm water at 100° F. The skin should then be mopped dry and covered with cottonwool. Where the pain is excessive it may be necessary to resort to injections of morphine.

Should shock supervene the patient should be stimulated by the administration of hot drinks or, better, by an injection of normal saline solution, either subcutaneously or per rectum.

As soon as the recovery from shock takes place, completely charred parts should be amputated, sloughs removed, and suitable dressings applied.

Where the burn consists simply of erythema the lesions should be powdered thickly with talc or zinc oxide and covered with cottonwool under a bandage. This dressing should be kept on for a few days until the inflammation subsides.

Where the area involved is considerable and the skin unbroken, but the burning sensation intense, relief is obtained by applying compresses of sodium bicarbonate lotion 10 grs. to the oz., lead lotion, or, best of all, by a 2 to 5% aqueous solution of ichthyol. The time-honoured Carron oil, or Linimentum calcis, which was once so popular, should not be employed, as its greasiness is apt to conserve the heat and may increase the discomfort, while if any abrasion of the skin be present it is liable to lead to sepsis. A substitute for it which is soothing and may be used with safety is equal parts of almond oil and lime water, with the addition of 10% of zinc oxide and ½% of carbolic acid; this cream should be applied gently over the burnt area, the superfluity wiped off, and the part then dusted over with zinc oxide or talc powder and covered with cottonwool kept in place by a loose bandage. On no account should waterproof tissue be used, as, like Carron oil, it is apt to induce heat.

When bullæ are present the clothes should not be dragged off but should be carefully cut away and the skin cleaned with 1 in 4,000 biniodide of mercury, each bulla should be slit in the dependent part and drained, the cuticle being left as a protective covering. The area should then be dressed with lint soaked in the following solution of picric acid 1½ drs., absolute alcohol 3 ozs., and distilled water 40 ozs., or in a 10% watery solution of aluminium acetate, covered with a layer of wool and retained in position by a bandage. When the burn is re-dressed, any wool adhering to raw surfaces should be soaked off by warm boric lotion and the dressing re-applied.

Where suppuration has supervened it must be treated on antiseptic principles and the burn thoroughly cleansed and dressed with boric ointment or with a salve containing eucalyptol and vaseline.

A new method of treatment of burns by paraffin has come into vogue during the present war and has been found to be very successful in the treatment of extensive burns due to liquid fire, etc. It was introduced by de Sandfort who employed a patent French preparation of paraffin called ' ambrine '; Lieut.-Colonel Hull, R.A.M.C., has advocated a substitute for this which has also given satisfactory results and which consists of :—

Beta naphthol	.	.	.	.	.	0.25 per cent.
Eucalyptus	.	.	.	.	.	2.0 "
Olive oil	.	.	.	.	.	5.0 "
Paraffin molle	.	.	.	.	.	25.0
Paraffin durum		.	.	.	.	67.75

The method of employment is as follows :—The burn is first washed with sterile water and dried by pressing a dry piece of gauze over it.

It is next painted over, or sprayed, with a layer of paraffin at a temperature of 50° C., then a layer of cottonwool is placed over the paraffin and covered with a second layer of paraffin, and the dressing is completed by a pad of cottonwool and a bandage. The burns are dressed daily at first, and later on, every second day, and any dead skin or sloughs removed. In this way it is claimed that healing rapidly takes place with the minimum of scarring and pain, and the need for grafting in large burns is to some extent avoided.

The hypertrophic scarring which results from burns may be reduced by applications of radium or the X-rays. The hypertrophy is usually most marked immediately after healing has taken place, tends to diminish after six or seven months, and then to remain permanent. It is in the early stages that most benefit can be derived from the treatment.

In extensive burns scarring can be prevented to some extent by Thiersch grafting of the granulating surfaces and severe deformities mitigated by suitable plastic operations.

CHAPTER VI

PRINCIPLES OF PLASTIC SURGERY

By H. D. Gillies, F.R.C.S., M.R.C.S., L.R.C.P.,
Major, R.A.M.C., Surgeon-in-Charge
The Queen's Hospital for Sailors and Soldiers suffering from Facial
Injuries, Frognal, Sidcup, Kent

FACE INJURIES

THIS little practiced branch of surgery, owing to the ravages of shell and bullet, has come so insistently to the fore that future work on surgery will embody many present-day developments of this art.

On the whole, its problems and their solutions are similar to those encountered in other branches of surgery; function and form are so dependent on each other that the restoration of one is usually correlated with the restoration of the other. All the principles of surgery in relation to asepsis, to immobilization of the parts by suture and splint, and to the general conservation of the tissues find their full scope in this work.

In addition, considerable boldness in action and opportunism in design are desirable qualities in the plastic surgeon. As in other branches of medicine, sometimes it is the waiting policy that pays, and oftentimes inaction means the loss of a golden opportunity. On the whole, however, after the earliest stage of the injury, the safest policy is to wait patiently until the individual, both in his local and general condition, is fit for operation. This delay is necessary not only between wound and first operation, but also between the operations of the various stages. So much is this necessary that the War Office authorities have sanctioned and recommended the sending home of these men between stages.

The early stages of an injury to the face, though not strictly pertaining to plastic surgery, are so important that a brief reference to them should be made here. There are in this connection three main classes of cases :—

(1) Without loss of tissue, mostly civilian type of injuries.
(2) With loss of tissue, mostly gunshot wounds.
(3) The separate class of burns.

The early treatment of burns is so well known that the very remarkable results by the 'Ambrine' wax method (W. O. Paraffin No. 7) needs no further mention.

For the other two classes of facial injuries, with or without loss of tissue, the following guiding principle is, I think, a sound one :—

That what is left of the tissues should be replaced into and retained in its normal position at the earliest possible moment by the best available means. A corollary of this might be expressed thus :—

That no attempt should be made in the early stage to bridge over gaps due to loss of tissue by over-stretching and stitching the normal tissues across the gap. More harm than good is done thereby, as the reactionary swelling and the usual suppuration cause more scar tissue than would otherwise have to be dealt with, and the stitches nearly always give way.

In addition to this undue stretching of the damaged tissues, the early cutting of flaps is, in my opinion, to be condemned; for even when this procedure is successful no obvious gain in time or appearance is obtained, while considerable risk of suppuration has been run. It evolves, practically, that split lips, lacerated noses, and gashed cheeks, where the loss of tissue is negligible, should be accurately and carefully sewn up as soon as possible, but that where the detached portions do not easily fill the gap caused by the injury the uncovered portion is best left to granulate, to be closed later by properly designed flaps. Every effort, therefore, should be made to replace tissues into normal position by stitches, strapping, head-gear apparatus, nasal supports and splints,[1] but not into abnormal positions. There is one exception to this which deserves mention, that tags of mucous membrane and of lip should, faute de mieux, be roughly attached to any neighbouring raw surface to preserve their shape and vitality.[2]

The use of strong, deep, approximating sutures is advocated wherever possible to take the tension off the uniting edges of the skin.

The displaced and fractured bones should likewise be replaced to their normal position at the earliest date possible and retained there by all possible means. In the case of mandible and maxilla, the closest co-operation between the surgeon and dental-surgeon should be the rule. Early wiring of the mandible has had, in my experience, very few successes, many failures, and a few disasters. It is comparatively easy for a dental surgeon of experience to control the fragments in the early

[1] Much developed by Hon. Major V. Kazanjian.
[2] This is rightly advocated at the front, notably by Hon. Major Valadier, C.M.G.

stages by some temporary buccal apparatus whereas if the bones are allowed to remain displaced ' until the patient is better ' the difficulties of both surgeon and dentist are greatly multiplied.

Only those teeth which are in danger of falling down the throat should be removed in the early stages, as valuable supports for the dental-surgeon to control the fragments may thereby be lost. Similarly, only completely detached pieces of bone should be removed.

When all suppuration has been controlled and the scars defined, the problem of the restoration must be considered from two points of view, of which the one—function—is considerably more important than the other—appearance. For instance, it is obvious that it is useless to build a man a new nose without the restoration of the air passages, and, similarly, it is bad practice to make new lips without giving due regard to the prevention of cicatricial bands which will interfere with the function of the mouth and jaws. As a rule, however, the complete restoration of form is usually accompanied by an adequate return of function, with the exception of cases when the facial nerve is paralyzed, or when there are no muscles of expression in the restored part.

The details of the restoration may conveniently be discussed under the following headings :—

(a) The general shape of the part to be remade.

(b) The skin covering.

(c) Incisions, sutures, dressings.

(d) The after-treatment.

THE CONTOUR

The general shape plays the most important rôle in the majority of severe facial injuries and presents the greatest difficulty to be encountered in this fascinating work. As in any branch of medicine, when one finds a long list of drugs to choose from or a considerable variety of recommended surgical procedures the cure of the condition is sure to be elusive; so here when the formidable array of possible methods of restoring the shape of the face is set forth one is inclined to surmise that none of them is of much value. However, owing to the immense opportunity of the present time, the methods so long advocated, but hitherto inadequately tested, have been well sifted by practical experience. For instance, in this matter of the general form of the part all sorts of artificial implantations have been tried. Metallic plates and filigrees, celluloid plates and injections of liquid celluloid, solid slabs of wax and injections of molten wax have all been used to build up the missing contour. Speaking very generally, these foreign bodies are to be condemned whenever it is possible to substitute a graft from the patient himself. The former all tend to give trouble either immediate or late, whereas the latter, if successful in the early stages, continue satisfactory. One celluloid plate which I used to replace a zygomatic prominence developed over it a sort of cold abscess five months after its implantation. The healing had been primary, and when the abscess burst the skin again healed over the plate. But by far the greater number of celluloid plates had to come out within two months of their insertion. Very satisfactory results appear to be attained by very cautious and repeated injections of paraffin wax in small quantities, but this is not suitable for the larger restorations, and imbedded solid blocks of paraffin have not been tolerated in my experience.

The little experience I have had with buried metallic or vulcanite plates does not encourage me to experiment any further with them. There is no panacea for the plastic surgeon with these artificial means of building up the skeleton of the face, and he must return to the harder road of pure surgery. Of the various autogenous grafts available, I have had enough experience to form some conclusions. Cartilage for large cosmetic purposes stands unrivalled. It is available in sufficient quantity, is easily fashioned to the desired shape, and, what is most important, remains permanently in the shape and size in which it is imbedded. This statement requires modification only in cases where there is suppuration following the operation, when part of the cartilage may necrose and a corresponding secondary deformity may arise. This is also the case when a part of the cartilage is left exposed in a mucous cavity. The clinical evidence of the permanence of cartilage is borne out by the experimental work of Staige Davis (*Annals of Surgery*, Feb., 1917).

When a softer contour is desired than would be provided by cartilage, local fat and muscle flaps are used to fill the smaller hollows. This method is most satisfactory and should be employed for all depressed scars. For larger hollows free fat and muscle grafts are used; these are naturally more uncertain of result. All I feel it possible to say of fat grafts is that when successful the result is very satisfactory, and diminution of the size of the graft from absorption has not occurred in any appreciable extent while the case has been under observation. (It is not yet established how they will be affected in conditions of war time, or yet in old age.) The fat graft often, however, undergoes a partial absorption from fat necrosis, which is carried to a greater extent if the products of this disintegration become infected; but even in this latter unfortunate occurrence not all the fat (or muscle) comes away, and eventually there is left sufficient substance to very materially aid any future work on the part. Fat is frequently recommended as a preliminary to bone graft, and in my opinion rightly so.

The bone graft proper is almost entirely confined, when speaking of facial injuries, to those of the mandible. An ever-growing percentage of these are entirely successful, and when suitable cases are chosen and immobility of the graft in its bed is attained the percentage is a remarkably high one. The attainment of immobility is enormously aided by the presence of sound teeth on the fragments, and, failing these, it must be sought in careful wedging of the graft into the mandible, or vice versa.

When the fragments can be controlled with the aid of the teeth the use of osteoperiosteal grafts has given great satisfaction, and when the case is suitable for wiring the superimposition of this method of graft gives a most rapid and solid union. In connection with wiring bone fragments, soft iron wire is a long way better than silver wire, but there is little tendency to callus formation, and the addition of the osteoperiosteal graft from the tibia seems to result in a much quicker union.

Of other ways of building up the facial scaffold I should like to draw attention to the following, which are available only in certain localities: The malar prominence may satisfactorily be simulated by advancing the flap of the adjacent temporal muscle, as described by me in the *St. Bartholomew's Hospital Journal* of May, 1917, and the muscular action of this flap will give a certain amount of expression to the face which the usually accompanying upper facial paralysis has left expressionless.

Similarly in rhinoplasty, partial or complete, considerable help is obtained by turbinate grafts and mucocartilaginous flaps of the septum in building up the sides or bridge of the nose before the skin covering is brought into place. These intranasal transplantations are of considerable use in the closure of palatal perforations.

There remains the question of using a graft from another patient. The only experience in this respect I have had is with cartilage (six cases). Five behaved similarly to an autogenous, but the sixth, after apparent success, was completely absorbed. It is possible that animal cartilage might succeed.

THE SKIN COVERING

When one comes to the question of the skin covering the method of flaps is, by far, the most satisfactory. Skin grafting does not come up to the required standard when dealing with the face. Thiersch grafts give such a thin epithelium that they are not suitable, while whole thickness grafts are, in my small experience, not very certain, and at the same time appear to be subject to a good deal of contraction later. Their site of election appears to be in the eyelids. Hairy transplantations in the upper lips might also prove satisfactory, but when there is a strong beard a pedicled bridge flap from the chin will give an excellent moustache. Free grafts are, naturally, of more value in burnt faces, where the finding of flaps is sometimes impossible.

There is hardly any new skin flap of the face that can be thought of. They have nearly all been enunciated long ago in the books on Plastic Surgery, and the following flap methods are also old methods that have been proved sound by practical experience. Many of them have been developed greatly beyond their original design. The simplest flap is an advancement, and the most typical place in which I have used this method is in providing the skin covering to the upper part of the nose. It always has the disadvantages of tension at the point of union and of difficulty of sewing neatly a long loose edge to a tight one. Relaxation sutures are here indicated, as in every case where there is likely to be tension.

Another simple flap method is the swinging flap. For the larger gaps transposed flaps are mostly used and, providing they are well planned, give excellent results. There are, however, in war surgery so many scars which interfere with the taking of flaps that all points of the case must be considered. For instance, scar tissue across the line of a flap will often cause a sloughing of part of the flap, but when either the flap is very thick or the scar superficial, this risk is considerably lessened.

In one of a long series of similar procedures the guiding principle is to take the flap from the opposite, or sound, side of the orifice which it is proposed to restore. Similarly this principle is used in correcting the level of the corners of the mouth or of the ocular angles.

The place from which this transposed flap is taken must be carefully considered. Thus, when scar conditions allow, it should be taken as far away from its new home as its blood supply will allow, as under those conditions the secondary closure of the place whence it comes has no influence on the flap in its new position; whereas if this flap is transposed from a position only separated by a small amount of tissue the net gain is considerably lessened by the secondary closure.

Roughly, a sound flap may be swung 90° without fear of local gangrene; but they have often been turned through a much bigger angle, especially when the base of the flap lies in the course of an artery. A good example of this lies in the turning down of a frontal flap in Rhinoplasty. I have seen very few flaps that have lost a portion through gangrene. Apart from those examples which had scar tissue in them or around their base the other cases occurred when there was so much tension or torsion that white bloodless streaks were noticeable across the flap at the time of operation.

The double pedicled flap is also a transposed flap, and in relation to the eyelids (operation of Tripier) gives excellent results. Its development in other regions of the face, and on a much larger scale, is in process and presents considerable possibilities.

Another flap which gives excellent results and is more particularly indicated in those cases where a successful free graft would meet the difficulty, is the bridge flap. Here the end portion of the flap is sewn into the new position, while the basal portion lies free over an untouched skin surface. At the end of ten days the unattached portion is divided from the attached and the former refitted into its original position, which is particularly adapted for transposing hair-bearing skin to the upper lip or eyebrows.

The double pedicled bridge flap is a still larger development and combination of methods which I have employed with success. A large strip of scalp, extending from ear to ear, was swung over the face and sutured in its middle portion to a position below and round a new cartilaginous chin in a case in which the whole of the lower lip and body of the mandible had been shot away. On the tenth day both pedicles were divided and replaced in the scalp, leaving a large hair-bearing island of skin over and beneath the chin.

Conversely I have designed and carried out with satisfactory results a new method of covering hopelessly scarred and burnt faces by means of an extensive double pedicled bridge-flap taken from the neck and chest.

In cutting transposed flaps it is of considerable importance to run them to a point, thereby greatly facilitating the secondary closure. Additional advantage is gained in adjusting these pointed flaps in position, as they may be dovetailed to give greater or less depth, and, when sutured, they give a larger surface of union than do square-ended flaps.

Esser, in the *Annals of Surgery*, March, 1917, greatly favours this method of forming the lower lip from the lateral nasolabial region, and my own experience corroborates his opinion as to the good results obtained from this design. These overlapping flaps are, however, available in other parts of the face, and since early in 1916 I have used them to advantage not only for the lower lip but also in restorations of the upper lip, chin, and eyelids. Double epithelial flaps are particularly indicated in forming the new nose, and wherever a piece of epithelialized scar tissue, or small flap, can be turned skin-surface downward to the cavity of the nose to line that organ it is attended with good results. But it is astonishing how little contraction occurs in a rhinoplasty when its raw surface is left exposed to the nasal cavity, and in restorations of the buccal cavity it is possible in the large majority of cases to obtain a mucous membrane covering by suitable flaps without sacrificing the function of the parts to their appearance.

Occasionally the procedure of turning a second flap inward is indicated, and in certain regions can be carried out without much additional scarring.

In the freeing of adherent lips, in shrunken eye sockets, and in many mucous membrane contractures, the method of epithelial inlay, as advocated by Esser in the same article, is full of possibilities, and so far has given me excellent results.

Relaxation cuts are occasionally useful, and when used should be sewn up styptically.

There are many points in connection with the incision and suture of the skin in plastic operations of the face that require consideration. The very essence of the work lies in obtaining the minimal scar; to ensure absence of scar, or the unnoticeable one, is a problem of great interest, and, to my mind, as yet unsolved. I believe there is some special quality in the individual skin which determines the character of the scar, quite apart from the surgical treatment of the incision and suture, and this individual quality prevents one from pronouncing that it is *usual* to produce an invisible scar on the face. The usual result, as seen from three to six months after operation, is a visible but practically unnoticeable scar, and one giving a pleasing appearance. In certain cases scars are quite indistinguishable at an early date; others, on the other hand, show stitch marks and are noticeable and unpleasant after three months, and a few are keloidal in type. In long operation scars of the cheek it is often observed that part of this becomes invisible, while the rest remains visible, the whole having received, apparently, the same treatment; but the good parts are those which have the least tension. Simple incision of linear scars or ragged wounds without loss of tissue are examples where there is no tension and a perfect result is to be expected. Suppuration will, of course, always mar the effect, but the absence of tension plus the accurate adaptation of the extreme edges are, in my opinion, the most important factors in obtaining the desired result. I am still open-minded as to the best suture material, as good results have followed the use of fine silkworm-gut, silk, thread, or horsehair; but the latter is preferred.

There are only two outstanding principles—one that the tension of the retracting skin must be taken up by sutures other than those making the ultimate union, and the second that a really accurate application of edge to edge be achieved by as many carefully placed fine sutures as are necessary. The needle should be inserted very near the free margin. A continuous close blanket suture is indicated in simple linear scars, but in the majority of plastic operations one edge has more tension than the other and frequent interrupted stitches are necessary. When required, mattress sutures are useful in everting the edges and in taking up the tension. These mattress sutures may be placed with advantage at intervals along the line and may be placed a quarter of an inch from the edge for horsehair, or half an inch from it for silkworm-gut when it is desired to overcome a slightly greater tension. For the more important tension sutures buried catgut or thread sutures should be used whenever possible, either with or without threads of stout silkworm-gut or wire sutures tied over a vulcanite plate. They can usually be left in ten days without causing any serious pressure mark on the skin, but this point naturally requires watching.

Another procedure which is very commonly practiced, and which I strongly believe in, is the incision of the skin on the slant, so as to produce a bevel edge. This latter was described in the *Lancet* of September 1, 1917, and the reason that I use it is because there appears to me that a larger area of epithelial surface is available for union, while the thin edge, having the character of an epithelial graft, tends to fuse with the opposite skin and to produce an indefinite and rapidly fading scar. This incision is not indicated in complicated flap operations, for the ultimate vis-à-vis bed of these flaps cannot be determined at the time of their delineation. When employing it I frequently use a semi-subcutaneous mattress suture which must usually be supplemented with a few interrupted edge-to-edge stitches. The four or five single knot lies well for this purpose. The subcuticular catgut or other stitch does not appear to be so well adapted for the face as the neck, but on this point I plead insufficient experience.

In regard to dressings there can be no hard-and-fast rule; but in order to protect the wound from flies, from the patient's fingers, and from the bedclothes, some covering is indicated. Plain gauze is the best, but when discharges from the nose, eyes, or mouth are likely to flow over the wound a collodion or mastisol dressing is advisable, and when it is desired to have a covering which will not stick, paraffin wax (No. 7) is an excellent application. If kept on for more than three days, however, it tends to produce a softened moist condition, and a dry dressing should then be substituted. An excellent dressing for Thiersch graft areas, both at site of origin and of implantation, is to be found in the combined use of paraffin wax (No. 7) and collodion. A piece of gauze the exact size of the raw or grafted area is impregnated with wax and laid in position; over it, covering a large area of healthy skin, is laid a single layer of gauze which, by means of collodion, firmly holds the wax pad in position. This dressing may be removed without it adhering to the graft or wound and yet maintain its position.

After-treatment. When an operation wound suppurates, Biers cupping is, next to establishing drainage, the soundest procedure.

Electro-therapeutics, as represented by X-rays, galvanism, high-frequency current, and ionization have their sphere of usefulness.

The 1,000 C.P. light also has been used, somewhat empirically, in a large number of cases, and I believe in the efficacy of its rays, the increased blood supply to the part being obvious. At the same time it is impossible to be honestly convinced that cases do better with light treatment than they would without. I have often exposed wounds to the effect of the rays while the sewing up is in progress, in the faint belief that introduced infection is eliminated, and although these cases have done well, the belief is not deep-rooted.

Carefully regulated massage is a necessary procedure for the scars and flaps both before and after the operation, and I attach a good deal of importance to this auxiliary treatment. Frequently when the nutrition of a flap is in doubt judicious early massage, combined with one of the electro-therapeutical methods of producing increased blood supply will turn a probable failure into a success; whilst the discreet pricking of the surface of a flap in which venous and lymphatic stasis is apparent, allows for the necessary drainage until the new circulation is established.

With these few principles from actual experience, I hope to have indicated what a vast amount of care and thought must be given to the study of this art, of which no man can be master.

SECTION V

OPERATIONS UPON THE TONGUE, TONSILS, · PHARYNX, AND ŒSOPHAGUS

PART I

OPERATIONS UPON THE TONGUE

BY

H. J. WARING, M.S. (Lond.), F.R.C.S. (Eng.),
Brevet Colonel R.A.M.C.
Surgeon to and Joint Lecturer in Surgery, St. Bartholomew's Hospital;

OPERATIONS UPON THE TONSILS

BY

GEORGE E. WAUGH, M.D., F.R.C.S. (Eng.)
Surgeon to the Hospital for Sick Children, Great Ormond Street;

OPERATIONS UPON THE PHARYNX

BY

WILFRED TROTTER, M.S. (Lond.), F.R.C.S. (Eng.)
Captain R.A.M.C. (T.)
Assistant Surgeon, University College Hospital.

CHAPTER I

OPERATIONS FOR NON-MALIGNANT AFFECTIONS OF THE TONGUE

By H. J. WARING, M.S. (Lond.), F.R.C.S. (Eng.)

OPERATIONS FOR ACUTE ABSCESS AND CELLULITIS OF THE TONGUE

THE operation which is of most value for these conditions is free longitudinal incision or incisions deeply into the substance of the tongue on the dorsal aspect and as near the median line as possible.

Before making incisions of this kind into the tongue, it is advisable for the patient to be anæsthetized and to have the jaws held apart by a strong gag. In addition, a pair of tongue forceps will also be of value for pulling the tongue forward, and often it will be found convenient to pass a strong suture through the substance of the tongue and leave it tied in a loop. Both these precautions aid the operator in preventing the tongue falling backwards into the oral part of the pharynx, and so seriously interfering with respiration.

Local abscesses of the tongue are very uncommon. They are treated by free incision into the abscess cavity, if possible, from the dorsal aspect, care being taken that the cut is made in the long axis of the tongue.

After-treatment. The cavity of the mouth and the surface of the tongue should be frequently and regularly washed out with a solution of peroxide of hydrogen, or some other dilute antiseptic.

OPERATIONS FOR CHRONIC ULCERS OF THE TONGUE AND LEUKOPLAKIAL PATCHES

The forms of chronic ulcer which most frequently require surgical treatment are those due to tertiary syphilis and tubercle. Patches of leukoplakia—local manifestations of chronic superficial glossitis—and the condition to which the term 'pre-cancerous' is applied, also often require local excision. Before carrying out any operation for the excision of any form of localized ulcer of the tongue in chronic glossitis, it is necessary that all septic stumps be removed and carious teeth either treated or extracted.

The chief precautions to be observed when removing local ulcers of

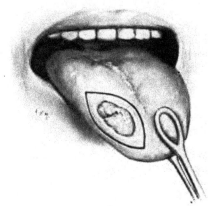

FIG. 231. CHRONIC ULCER OF THE TONGUE. Position of the incision.

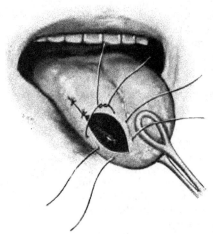

FIG. 232. CHRONIC ULCER OF THE TONGUE. Ulcer removed and sutures
inserted, but not tied.

the tongue are to ensure free and complete exposure of that portion of
the tongue which is to be operated upon and to use a strong gag for
keeping the jaws apart. When the ulcer is situated far back, the sound

side of the tongue should either be transfixed with a needle carrying a strong ligature or held by a special pair of tongue forceps.

When the ulcerated area is small and situated anteriorly, excision may be carried out under local anæsthesia. When, however, the area

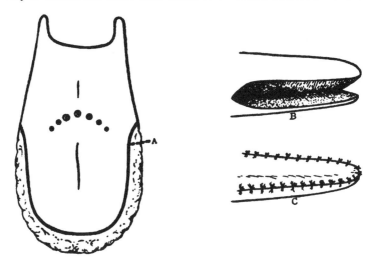

Fig. 233. Excision of Chronic Disease limited to the Border of the Tongue. A the dorsal incision; B shows the gap left after excision of the area, and c the method of closing it. (*Butlin.*)

to be excised is comparatively large, or is situated posteriorly, then general anæsthesia is preferable.

Operation. The tongue having been pulled forward and the ulcerated area fully exposed, an oval-shaped excision is made around the ulcer in the manner depicted in Fig. 231. In making the incision into the tongue a space of about 1 to 1½ centimetres from the margin of the ulcer should be allowed. The cut into the substance of the tongue is made in a wedge-shaped manner, the apex of the wedge being opposite the central line of the ulcer. By these means the affected portion of the tongue is freed and removed. All bleeding points are picked up with fine pressure forceps and ligatured with catgut. The entire field of operation is sponged dry and a series of sutures introduced after the manner shown in Fig. 232. It is advisable to introduce all these sutures before any are tied. The sutures are then knotted and the ends cut short.

After-treatment. Frequent washing out of the mouth with peroxide of hydrogen or dilute antiseptic solution should be practised, and in a week or ten days the sutures are removed.

The marginal portion of the anterior half of the tongue is frequently the site of superficial glossitis with, in places, small areas of leukoplakia or even induration.   Occasionally, also, small chronic ulcers are found along the margins.   The late Sir Henry Butlin devised an operation for the removal of the diseased tissues under these conditions.   The stages of the operation which he practised are shown in the diagram, Fig. 233.

OPERATIONS FOR NON-MALIGNANT TUMOURS OF THE TONGUE

The most common local tumours of the tongue are papillomata or warty growths, localized areas of lymphangioma, venous nævi, and solid tumours such as lipomata, fibromata, and adenomata.   The basal portion of the tongue in addition may be the seat of a cyst derived from the remains of the thyreo-glossal duct, whilst occasionally the dorsum of the tongue posteriorly may be the site of a considerable tumour—a so-called lingual thyreoid gland.

REMOVAL OF PAPILLOMATA AND LOCALIZED LYMPHANGIOMATA

The operations for the removal of these conditions are essentially similar.   Small warts and papillomata can be removed quite easily under local anæsthesia by seizing the affected portion of the tongue with serrated forceps and excising the wart and adjacent mucous membrane by one cut with a strong sharp pair of scissors.   The margins of the wound thus made can then be approximated by the insertion of one or two sutures of fine catgut, in a manner similar to that shown in Fig. 234.

Removal of larger papillomata and lymphangiomata. The affected portion of the tongue having been exposed in the manner described in connexion with chronic ulcers, an oval-shaped incision is made into the substance of the tongue and surrounding the tumour as shown in Fig. 234.   The mucous membrane within the margins of the incision and the underlying superficial tissues of the tongue are cut away with a pair of scissors.   By these means a localized growth is removed; hæmorrhage is then arrested and the margins of the wound are brought together by the insertion of a series of sutures similar to those recommended after removal of a chronic ulcer.

REMOVAL OF A VENOUS NÆVUS

Venous nævi of the tongue most commonly involve the anterior part, and often the margin not far from the tip.   The operation which offers the best prospect of a cure is excision of a wedge-shaped portion of the tongue, the wedge removed containing the diseased area. In determining the position of the wedge-shaped incision, attention must be paid so to locate the limbs of the incision that when the margins of the wound are brought together the tongue shall not be too pointed.

Operation. The tongue is drawn forward as in the previous operation and a strong suture passed through its substance posterior to the affected area and also on the opposite side. A strong pair of sharp scissors is used and a wedge-shaped portion of the tongue enclosing the affected area cut out. Hæmorrhage may be somewhat severe, but usually can readily be arrested by picking up the bleeding points with pressure forceps. Considerable assistance may be obtained in temporary control

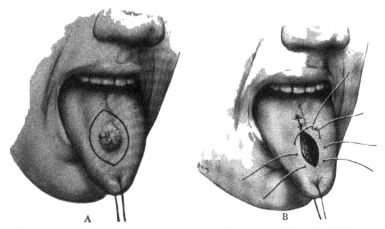

Fig. 234. REMOVAL OF A PAPILLOMA FROM THE TONGUE. A shows the incision, B, the insertion of the sutures.

of the bleeding by pulling forward the tongue with the two sutures, or with the forefinger hooked round the dorsum. When the hæmorrhage has been arrested the two raw surfaces are approximated by the insertion of a series of interrupted sutures of catgut.

REMOVAL OF A LIPOMA, FIBROMA, OR ADENOMA

Localized tumours of the tongue of this kind are usually small and removal can readily be effected.

Operation. The mouth being held open by a gag and the anterior part of the tongue seized with a pair of tongue forceps, the organ is so manipulated that the portion of the tongue in which the tumour is situated is fully exposed; with a scalpel an incision is made through the mucous membrane overlying the tumour and in the long axis of the tongue. An enucleator is then taken and the small tumour separated and dislodged from its bed of fibrous tissue. The walls of the cavity from which the tumour has been taken are approximated by several points of interrupted sutures. If there is too much redundant mucous membrane the margins of the wound can be pared before suture.

OPERATIONS FOR GENERAL LYMPHANGIOMA OF THE TONGUE OR MACROGLOSSIA

Certain cases of macroglossia due to a general condition of lymphangioma of the tongue can be very much improved by excision of the anterior half of the affected organ.

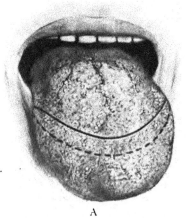
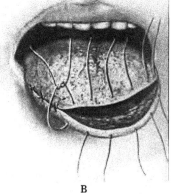

A   B

FIG. 235. OPERATION FOR MACROGLOSSIA. A shows the incisions for removal of the anterior half of an enlarged tongue, B, the method of inserting the sutures after its removal.

Operation. The patient having been anæsthetized and the mouth widely opened, two incisions are made in the tongue almost transversely and in the position shown in Fig. 235, A. These incisions are deepened in a wedge-shaped manner until they meet posteriorly, when the anterior protuberant half is set free. Next, all bleeding points are picked up and ligatured, special care being taken to apply ligatures to the main branches of the lingual artery, as they lie in the lower part of the incision.

The wound surfaces are sponged thoroughly dry, approximated, and fixed in close apposition by a series of interrupted sutures of No. 1 chromicized catgut, after the manner shown in Fig. 235, B.

After-treatment. This is similar to that already described in connexion with the removal of small tumours.

REMOVAL OF A CYST OF THE TONGUE DUE TO A PERSISTENT THYREO-GLOSSAL DUCT

The tumours of the tongue which are caused by the presence of a thyreo-glossal cyst usually occupy the basal portion and protrude as a swelling in the neck, immediately above the body of the hyoid bone and below and behind the posterior aspect of the symphysis menti. Consequently the best route of surgical approach for the removal of cysts of this kind is from the neck.

Operation. The patient having been anæsthetized, a large sandbag is placed underneath the neck and the head thrown back. This manœuvre fully exposes the supra-hyoid and submental regions. The exact position of the cyst is determined by palpation, and then an incision of sufficient length is made over it either in a line extending from the centre of the body of the hyoid bone to the mandible or transversely across the neck immediately above the superior margin of the hyoid bone. The skin and fascial tissues are cut through and the external surface of the cyst exposed as it lies between the muscles and in the mid-line of the base of the tongue. By careful dissection or separation with a blunt dissector, the cyst is separated from its surroundings. Usually it will be found that a band of fibrous tissue passes upwards and backwards towards the region of the site of the foramen cæcum. This fibrous band should be cut through above, and any other prolongations of the capsule of the tumour downwards towards the body of the hyoid bone are similarly treated. By these means, the cyst can usually be removed entire. The walls of the cavity from which the cyst has been taken should now be approximated by the insertion of a few points of buried catgut suture, any bleeding vessels being first ligatured. The external wound is then closed.

OPERATION FOR LINGUAL THYREOIDS

The dorsum of the tongue in the region of or immediately behind the foramen cæcum is occasionally occupied by a firm, solid tumour which histologically has the structure of the thyreoid gland. Often tumours of this kind occur in patients in whom the thyreoid gland is congenitally absent. Consequently, operations should not be recommended for the removal of such tumours unless it is clear that the patient has a thyreoid gland in the normal position. Sometimes, however, these tumours increase in size and interfere with swallowing; then it may be necessary partially to remove them. This can be effected either by shaving off the protuberant portion of the tumour, or better, perhaps, by excision of a wedge of tissue from the more prominent portion.

Cases have been reported in which, after operations of this kind, in which the entire lingual swelling has been removed, the patients have developed symptoms of myxœdema.

CHAPTER II

OPERATIONS FOR MALIGNANT DISEASE OF THE TONGUE AND FLOOR OF THE MOUTH

By H. J. Waring, M.S. (Lond.), F.R.C.S. (Eng.)

Malignant disease of the tongue and floor of the mouth in nearly all cases is histologically a squamous-celled carcinoma (epithelioma). The varieties of carcinoma of the tongue which are the most favourable for operative procedures and are followed by the best results are the hypertrophic and the localized and indurated forms. The ulcerative and the diffuse infiltrating varieties are less suitable for operation and give the worst results, especially the last. It cannot be too strongly pointed out that carcinoma of the tongue and floor of the mouth in the early stages is a localized disease, and does not extend beyond the tissues in the immediate neighbourhood and the primary groups of lymph glands which receive lymph vessels from the infected area. Also when deep infiltration has taken place even extensive operations do not offer good prospects of a permanent cure.

When infiltration of the tissues in the base of a carcinoma occurs it is especially liable to travel along and within the sheaths of the intrinsic and extrinsic muscles of the tongue. The muscles which are mostly involved are the genioglossus, the styloglossus, the hyoglossus, and the inferior lingualis. Clinically, infiltration of muscles or extension along the fascial muscular sheaths must be suspected when, on examination, a definite outline of the tumour cannot be distinguished by careful digital palpation.

The lymph vessels from the tongue in the main empty themselves into the submental, submaxillary, or deep cervical groups of lymph glands along the course of the upper portion of the jugular vein. The submental lymph glands receive the lymph vessels from the tip and the anterior part of the tongue, the submaxillary group those from the middle portion, whilst the lymph vessels on the posterior part pass into the deep cervical glands which lie in close relation to the jugular vein. There is one important lymph gland located close to the bifurcation of the carotid artery which receives lymph vessels directly from the median and lateral portions of the tongue. In the main, the lymph vessels from one lateral half of the tongue pass to the lymph glands on the same side of the neck, but it must be borne in mind that, in the region of the tip and of the posterior part, and also in the region of the median fibrous tissue septum, there are communications between the lymph vessels of the two sides; consequently, when carcinomata are situated in one or other of these regions, the lymph glands on both sides of the neck are very prone to be simultaneously involved. Fig. 236 shows the general distribution of the lymph vessels of the tongue and the groups of lymph glands into which they

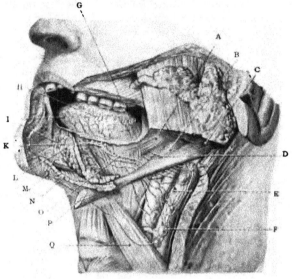

FIG. 236. DISSECTION OF THE SUBMENTAL, SUBMAXILLARY. SUBLINGUAL, AND DEEP CERVICAL REGIONS. The drawing shows the arrangement of the lymph vessels and the lymph glands in connexion with the tongue and floor of the mouth. A, Styloglossus; B, Stylohyoid; C, Digastric; D, Afferent vessels to deep cervical glands from posterior third of tongue; E, Common facial vein; F, Upper deep cervical lymph glands; G, Vallate papillæ; H, Superficial lymph vessels of side and dorsum of tongue; I, Lymph vessels of apex of tongue; K, Afferent vessels to mandibular glands; L, Sublingual gland; M, Submental gland; N, Mylohyoid (cut); O, Afferent vessels to deep cervical glands; P, Anterior belly of digastric (cut); Q, Omohyoid. (*Robinson.*)

open. In addition, it must be borne in mind that the lymph glands in close proximity to the parotid and submaxillary salivary glands are liable to escape notice in the early stages of enlargement, on account of the dense fibrous tissues which surround them.

The object of the surgeon when treating by operation a carcinoma of the tongue or floor of the mouth must be to remove the neoplasm, the affected portion of the tongue comprising the overlying mucous membrane and underlying muscular and fascial tissues, together with all the lymph glands which receive lymph vessels directly from the affected area. When the disease has made considerable progress, it is necessary to remove, in addition to the primary lymph glands, the lymph vessels and the lymph glands of the next series. This in all cases necessitates a deep dissection of the neck on one or both sides and complete removal from below of these secondary lymph glands, together with the lymph vessels and lymph glands above them. In a dissection of the neck for the removal of the primary lymph glands, it is necessary in all cases to excise the submaxillary salivary gland of the affected side; otherwise small, submaxillary lymph glands are certain to escape detection and removal.

When a patient suffering from carcinoma of the tongue comes under observation at an early stage, the operation to be recommended is removal of the diseased portion of the tongue, together with a marginal area of two-thirds or three-quarters of an inch all round the growth, and at the same time to remove the lymph glands on the same side of the neck. Usually, it will be found advisable and convenient first to perform the operation on the lymph structures in the neck and at the same time ligature the lingual artery. The wound in the neck is then completely closed and the affected portion of the tongue removed on the lines already mentioned.

Excision of the tongue, either partial or complete, may be effected by operation carried out through the mouth, through the mouth after division of the lower lip and the mandible in the median line, or through an incision commencing at the angle of the mouth on the affected side and extending outwards and downwards into the neck, with simultaneous division or removal of the portion of the horizontal ramus of the mandible opposite the diseased area.

CHOICE OF OPERATION FOR THE REMOVAL OF MALIGNANT DISEASE OF THE TONGUE

The important factors which govern the determination of the variety of operation for removal of the cancer of the tongue are in the main the following:—

The position and extent of the primary growth. When the carcinoma is limited to the tongue and has not infiltrated deeply or spread to the mucous membrane of the floor of the mouth or become attached to the periosteum of the mandible, excision of the growth is best carried out through the mouth; favourable cases are those in which the affection is limited to the anterior two-thirds of the tongue and especially when the lateral half only is involved. In these cases good results can usually be obtained by cutting away the affected half of the tongue with scissors. When, however, the disease is located in or extends to the posterior third of the tongue, and especially when it has spread to the adjacent portion of the fauces, it is necessary, in order to effect complete removal, to enlarge the field of operation by dividing the lower lip, the lower jaw, and the tissues in the submental region. When the carcinoma chiefly involves one lateral margin of the tongue and spreads towards the inferior aspect and the adjacent mucous membrane of the floor of the mouth, it is usually necessary to remove several teeth opposite the growth and a segment of the alveolar portion of the horizontal ramus of the mandible. This procedure very greatly facilitates complete exposure of the diseased area and enables the operator to ensure, as far as possible, complete local excision of the diseased tissues. In those cases in which the disease is situated far back and extends outwards to the fossa between the base of the tongue and the inner aspect of the mandible, and is attached to the latter, the most complete exposure is obtained by making a curved incision commencing at the angle of the mouth on the affected side and running downwards and outwards to the horizontal ramus of the mandible, a little in front of the angle, and then downwards and forwards in the neck as far as the hyoid bone. When the soft tissues of the cheek and neck have been cut through and turned aside, the mandible should be divided in such a manner that the portion to which the growth has extended is included within the lines of section.

The duration of the disease and involvement of the lymph glands. Carcinomatous growths of the tongue or floor of the mouth offer the best chances of successful operative removal and least liability to non-recurrence when they come under observation at a comparatively early stage and before extensive infiltration of adjacent tissues has occurred. The definite palpable enlargement of the primary lymph glands which receive lymph vessels from the diseased area cannot generally be detected in these early stages. It must not be assumed, however, that because enlargement of these lymph glands is not obvious that they are not already the site of deposits of carcinoma cells which will ultimately cause the development of secondary growths. Unfortunately, as regards hospital patients, too frequently they fail to come under surgical observation before the disease has made considerable progress. Patients of the educated classes generally discover carcinomatous disease of the tongue at an early stage and seek advice. The rate of growth of carcinoma of the tongue varies considerably in different individuals. Patients who are confirmed alcoholics and are the subjects of tertiary syphilis generally present the most quickly growing varieties of this disease. Consequently, in patients of this kind, the outlook as regards the permanent relief from operative interference is not good. As far as the author's observation goes, in young patients who suffer from carcinoma of the tongue, growth is usually rapid and the prognosis is not so good. Therefore, in young patients, wide excision of the diseased tissues is very important. If the carcinomatous growth has extended to and involved the periosteum covering of the mandible, extensive operation is necessary and the outlook is not so good.

When in a patient suffering from carcinoma of the tongue it is found that the disease has infiltrated deeply and the tongue has become fixed to the jaw, it is not usually advisable to recommend any operation, since it is not possible to take away the entire disease. The position of a patient who has been submitted to an incomplete operation for the removal of a cancerous growth, either of the tongue or the floor of the mouth, is far worse than if no attempt had been made to free him from his disease. When the dorsum of the tongue is also the seat of a carcinomatous growth, and this extends backwards and affects the superior orifice of the larynx, especially the arytæno-epiglottic folds, then in the great majority of instances even extensive operation does not offer any prospect of success.

In cases of cancer of the tongue which cannot readily be dealt with through the mouth alone—that is to say, when the disease is placed far back and involves the dorsum of the tongue, the posterior part of the root, and the folds of the fauces and the tonsil—the operation of choice ought to be median division of the lower lip followed by division of the mandible in the region of the symphysis. This method of surgical approach will, in practically all cases which are amenable to operative interference, enable the surgeon satisfactorily to remove the disease. When both sides of the dorsum of the tongue are involved it will be necessary to remove the entire organ down to the root, on account of the serious interference with the blood-supply of the anterior portion.

There is one further class of case which requires to be treated somewhat differently. I refer to those cases in which the disease involves the anterior part of the posterior half of the tongue and has spread and become fixed to the horizontal ramus of the mandible. These cases are best treated by dividing the cheek laterally and cutting through the horizontal ramus of the mandible in front of and behind the disease.

Some surgeons have recommended, in those cases of carcinoma of the tongue which spread towards the upper aperture of the larynx, that the route of surgical approach should be through the neck, immediately below the body of the hyoid bone. I do not think, however, that this method of subhyoid pharyngotomy offers any advantage over the operations already recommended.

PRELIMINARY PREPARATIONS

Before commencing an operation for the removal of the tongue, partial or complete, the cavity of the mouth should be rendered as clean as possible. This can best be effected by removal of all carious teeth and decayed stumps, complete removal of all tartar from the bases of the remaining teeth, and the regular use of an antiseptic mouth-wash. The daily use of a dilute solution of peroxide of hydrogen for a few days before operation gives considerable assistance. It is not possible, of course, to render the buccal cavity and the tongue entirely aseptic.

CHOICE OF ANÆSTHETIC

As a general rule, removal of the tongue can best be effected under general anæsthesia. Localized growths, however, when situated in the

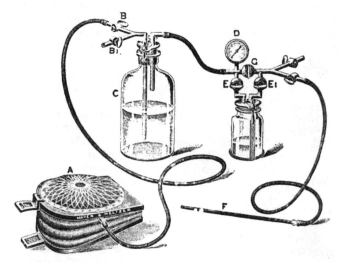

Fig. 237. Apparatus for Anæsthetization by the Intra-tracheal Method. A, bellows driving air through tap B into wash bottle C. Through the tube B 1 oxygen can be also passed if desired. Attached to the ether bottle is the gauge D and the regulating taps E, E 1, and G. F is the tracheal tube. (*Boyle & Gask.*)

anterior part of the tongue, can easily be removed with infiltration anæsthesia. The advantages, however, of local anæsthesia are very small, since it can only be employed satisfactorily in the case of small growths and it does not allow of simultaneous removal of the affected cervical lymph glands. Ordinary anæsthesia with ether or chloroform is available in most cases in which the disease is situated in the anterior or middle portion of the tongue. When, however, the base of the tongue is the seat of disease, or it is necessary to perform an extensive operation with resection of a segment of the mandible, it is necessary either to administer the anæsthetic by the intra-tracheal method, with a tube passed down through the pharynx and larynx into the trachea (Fig. 237), or to perform preliminary laryngotomy. After the introduction of the laryngotomy tube, the cavity of the lower portion of the pharynx is packed with a sponge, in order to prevent the passage of blood or other fluids downwards into the chest. From many points of view anæsthetization in these cases is best effected by the intra-tracheal method. This, however, requires the services of an anæsthetist skilled in the use of the intra-tracheal tube. Preliminary laryngotomy has many advantages, it is easier of application and does not of necessity require the services of such a skilled anæsthetist. The chief advantage of the intra-tracheal method of anæsthetizing a patient is that the larynx is not opened by a wound from the outside.

SIMULTANEOUS REMOVAL OF PRIMARY GROWTHS IN THE TONGUE AND OF LYMPH GLANDS ON THE AFFECTED SIDE OF THE NECK

As a general rule it is advisable, when operating upon a patient with carcinoma of the tongue, to remove both the primary growth and the lymph glands at the same sitting. The best method of effecting this is to perform the cervical portion of the operation first and, when the neck has been opened up, to ligature the lingual artery. After closure of the wound in the cervical region and careful protection by dressings, the intra-buccal removal of the affected portion of the tongue is carried out. Occasionally, however, it will be found, especially in hospital cases, owing to the extent of the primary disease and the septic condition of the oral cavity, it is safer to perform the operation at two sittings. In these cases, it is usually preferable to perform the cervical operation first and at the expiration of ten to fourteen days to remove the disease from within the mouth. It will often happen if the diseased portion of the tongue is removed first, that the patient will decline to have the second operation for the removal of the affected lymph glands.

EXCISION OF ONE HALF OF THE TONGUE THROUGH THE MOUTH

This operation is often referred to as 'Whitehead's operation,' and consists in cutting away the greater part of one half of the tongue with scissors.

Operation. The patient is placed in the dorsal posture with the head somewhat raised. This position helps in preventing blood being drawn into the respiratory passages and also facilitates the administration of the anæsthetic. The mouth is fixed widely open with a strong gag. The operator stands on the affected side of the patient and his assistant directly opposite to him. The tongue is drawn forward and a piece of thick salmon-gut or silk passed through each lateral half about 1 inch from the tip. Care should be taken in passing the salmon-gut through the diseased half to avoid the region of the growth. Each piece of gut is knotted in a loop and serves to draw the tongue forwards and helps in preventing the dorsum falling backwards and so impeding respiration. The loop on the sound side is given to the assistant whilst the operator draws the tongue forwards with the other. An incision is now made with a knife through the mucous membrane on the superior and inferior aspects of the tongue in the median line, as far backwards as an inch beyond the limit of the growth. Scissors are next taken and traction exerted laterally by means of the loop ligatures. The median fibrous tissue septum of the tongue is defined by a few snips of the scissors; when this has been done, the tongue is separated into two halves by cutting backwards with the scissors until the limits of the growth have been passed. The two halves are then pulled upwards and towards the sound side, and the diseased half cut through transversely at the base from below and on the lateral side upwards and inwards. The lingual artery, which lies quite close to the mucous membrane on the inferior aspect and a short distance from the median septum, should be picked up with pressure forceps when it has been recognized. If a ligature has not already been applied to it during an operation for the removal of the lymph glands after the lingual artery has been dealt with, the remaining substance of the tongue is cut through by a series of further cuts with the scissors. The affected portion of the tongue including the growth is thus removed. After the portion of tongue containing the carcinomatous growth has been removed, it should be carefully examined in order to determine the extent of the disease and whether sufficient surrounding tissue has been taken away, since it sometimes happens that the disease has extended further than was originally recognized. When there is doubt as to the complete removal of the diseased tissues, a further portion must be cut away before suturing the margins of the divided mucous membrane on the superior and inferior aspects of the tongue. All bleeding points are picked up with pressure forceps and the cut margins of the mucous membrane on the under aspect joined to those on the dorsum by a series of interrupted sutures of catgut. The stump of the tongue is

FIG. 238. EXCISION OF ONE HALF OF THE TONGUE FOR LOCALIZED CARCINOMA BY THE INTRA-BUCCAL METHOD. Two stages of the operation are shown. 1, Carcinoma; 2, median septum of the tongue; 3, Palato-glossal fold; 4, division of the mucous membrane; 5, lingual nerve; 6, sub-lingual salivary gland; 7, proximal end of the lingual artery; 8, proximal end of the lingual nerve; 9, divided muscles of the tongue.

allowed to fall back into the mouth, and the salmon-gut suture which had been passed through the sound half of the tongue may be fixed to the external aspect of the cheek with a small piece of strapping. This suture readily enables the tongue to be drawn forward if hæmorrhage should occur due to non-ligature of a blood-vessel or slipping of a ligature.

After-treatment. The field of operation and also the entire buccal cavity should be regularly washed out at short intervals either with a solution of peroxide of hydrogen or a dilute antiseptic. The patient should be kept in bed as little as possible and encouraged to remain in the sitting posture. When asleep, he should lie on the affected side with the head turned towards that side, whilst frequent sponging or washing out of the mouth should be practised; the object of these precautions is to avoid the secretion from the floor of the mouth and the field of operation being drawn into the bronchi and lungs during inspiration, since, when this happens, ' inhalation pneumonia ' is liable to be set up.

EXCISION OF THE TONGUE AFTER MEDIAN INCISION OF THE LOWER LIP AND THE SUBMENTAL TISSUES AND DIVISION OF THE MANDIBLE

Operation. The patient is placed in the dorsal posture with the head and shoulders raised. In these cases it will usually be found advisable to anæsthetize the patient by the intra-tracheal method. In other cases, a preliminary laryngotomy may be first performed and the pharynx packed with a sponge. The operator stands on the right side of the patient and his assistant directly opposite to him. A vertical incision is first made through the lower lip and the submental and suprahyoid regions, commencing above the central point of the lower lip and extending downwards to just above the upper border of the body of the hyoid (Fig. 239). The soft tissues of the lip, including the mucous membrane on its buccal aspect and the periosteum on the outer aspect of the mandible, are incised together with the skin and fascial tissues in the submental and sub-hyoid regions. The flaps thus formed are held aside after the coronary arteries have been seized with pressure forceps, whilst the lower jaw is supported by the assistant. Next, the mandible is pierced with a bone-drill about one-third of an inch on each side of the median line. The two apertures thus made are for the introduction of a wire suture when the operation is being completed. If necessary the central incisor tooth on the affected side is extracted, and the bone just to one side of the symphysis menti is sawn through. This division of the jaw can be effected either with a strong saw or a wire saw passed behind the symphysis. The mandible having been thus divided, the two halves are pulled apart and the genioglossi muscles separated. This will expose the inferior aspect of the tongue and the floor of the mouth. A loop of strong salmon-gut is passed through the anterior portion of the tongue, and with this the organ is pulled forward towards the sound or the less affected side. Strong scissors are now taken and the mucous membrane of the floor of the mouth on both sides is divided from before backwards, the division being made as wide as possible of the tissues involved in the disease. When the mucous membrane has been thus divided, the lingual vein will be exposed as it lies upon the hyoglossus muscle and the lingual nerve on the inferior aspect of the tongue near the lateral margin and close underneath the mucous membrane. The hypoglossal nerve will be found somewhat deeper upon the external surface of the hyoglossus and sending forward branches to supply the genioglossus.

These branches should not be divided if they can be safely preserved so as to leave the floor of the mouth and base of the tongue in as satisfactory a functional condition as possible. If, however, the margins of the neoplasm render this impossible, the surgeon should not hesitate to divide them, otherwise local recurrence will be probable. The lingual artery will be readily recognized passing upwards between the hyoglossus and genioglossus, and should be picked up and ligatured. The hyoglossus is next cut through, the tongue pulled further forwards, and the mucous membrane on its

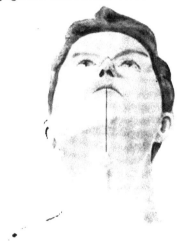

Fig. 239. Excision of the Tongue with Median Division of the Lower Lip. Position of the incision.

dorsal aspect divided. In those cases in which the disease extends far backwards it may be necessary, in order to ensure the incision being made well beyond the margins of the disease, to cut through the adjacent portions of the soft palate, the tonsil, and the lateral wall of the pharynx. Similar incisions are next made on the other side and then the base of the tongue is cut through with scissors and the organ containing the new growth removed. Some prefer to make the section of the tongue with the knife or a thermo-cautery on account of the small amount of hæmorrhage which results from this form of division and the lessened probability of recurrence. Hæmorrhage, however, is not usually severe, since, as the tongue is being pulled forward, each bleeding-point can be readily picked up and ligatured and, as regards recurrence in the stump of the tongue which is left, it is not my experience that it is more frequent after removal with scissors than after removal with the thermo-cautery.

All divided blood-vessels are now ligatured, the stump of the tongue is drawn forward, and the margin of the divided mucous membrane on the dorsal and lateral aspects fixed by sutures as accurately as possible to the margin of the divided mucous membrane on the anterior part of the floor of the mouth. In effecting this fixation, several of the sutures should be passed deeply through the tissues in the floor of the wound. This method of fixation of the stump of the tongue helps to avoid falling backwards of the organ. It also hastens union and enables the patient to swallow more readily. The field of operation is now sponged dry and the two sawn surfaces of the mandible are brought together and fixed in exact apposition by a silver wire introduced through the holes already made.

When the carcinomatous growth involves both halves of the tongue no attempt should be made to split the organ along the median raphé. The entire tongue with the contained growth should be removed in one piece.

A rubber drainage tube is passed through the lower portion of the wound from the neck and the parts around are packed with strips of gauze. Finally, the margins of the divided lip and the wound in the neck are approximated by salmon-gut sutures. The lower portion of the cervical part of the wound is left open for the exit of the drainage tube. The dressing is then applied.

After-treatment. The after-treatment is similar to that already mentioned on p. 472. The main points to be borne in mind are that free drainage should be established, discharges should not be allowed to collect in the mouth, and frequent irrigation should be practised after the operation; the patient should be allowed to sit up as much as possible, and encouraged to sleep in this position.

EXCISION OF A CARCINOMA OF THE TONGUE AND THE FLOOR OF THE MOUTH AFTER LATERAL SPLITTING OF THE CHEEK AND DIVISION OR RESECTION OF A PART OF THE HORIZONTAL RAMUS OF THE MANDIBLE

This operation is of the greatest value in those cases of carcinoma of the tongue and the floor of the mouth in which the disease extends

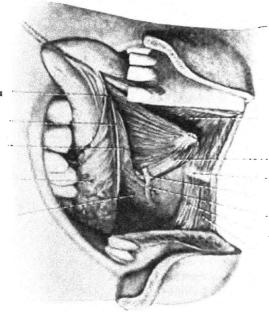

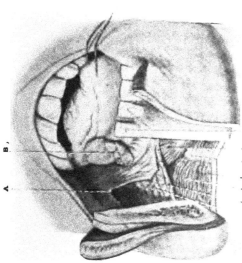

FIG. 240. EXCISION OF THE TONGUE AFTER DIVISION OF THE LOWER LIP AND THE MANDIBLE. Two stages of the operation are shown. I—A, Buccal mucous membrane; B, New growth; C, Sublingual duct; D, Sublingual gland; E, Mylohyoid; F, Digastric; G, Median raphé; H, Mylohyoid; I, Incisor teeth. II—A, Hyoglossus; B, Sublingual gland; C, D, Sublingual duct; E, Mucous membrane; F, G, Mylohyoid; H, Lingual vein; I, Lingual artery; K, Median raphé; L, Right genioglossus (cut); M, Left genioglossus.

backwards to the region of the fauces, the anterior part of the tonsil, and the adjacent part of the lower jaw. The best results can be obtained when only the alveolar process of the lower jaw is involved.

Operation. It is necessary in practically all cases where this operation is necessary to administer the anæsthetic by the intra-tracheal method or to perform a preliminary laryngotomy. In the latter case the lower portion of the pharynx is plugged with a sponge.

The patient is placed in the dorsal posture with a firm pillow or sandbag underneath the head and shoulders and the head turned towards the unaffected side. The surgeon stands on the affected side and the assistant opposite to him.

The assistant first grasps the cheek on the affected side in order to control the circulation, and then the surgeon makes an incision somewhat semilunar in shape commencing at the angle of the mouth and extending backwards and downwards to the anterior margin of the masseter muscle; then downwards over the anterior margin of this muscle as far as the inferior margin of the horizontal ramus of the mandible and thence onwards to the anterior margin of the sterno-mastoid muscle in the submaxillary region whence it is curved inwards and forwards towards the outer part of the body of the hyoid bone. This incision divides all the tissues of the cheek and exposes the lateral surface of the mandible and the anterior margin of the sterno-mastoid muscle. On the outer part of the incision, near the anterior margin of the masseter, the external maxillary artery will be divided and require ligature. The other vessels which require ligature are the coronary arteries at the angle of the mouth. The flap thus formed, consisting of the tissues of the cheek and neck, is dissected downwards and forwards so as

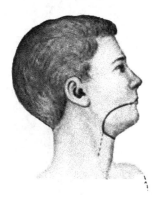

FIG. 241. POSITION OF IN-CISION FOR REMOVAL OF THE TONGUE, AFTER SPLITTING THE CHEEK AND DIVIDING THE MAN-DIBLE.

fully to expose the external aspect of the horizontal ramus of the mandible and the structures in the submaxillary triangle of the neck. When the disease involves the periosteum covering the posterior portion of the horizontal and the lower portion of the vertical ramus of the mandible, the posterior margins of the incision, including the insertion of the masseter, should be separated from the underlying bone and strongly

ding to whether
l aspect or not.
e latter is sawn
nterior segment
ie opposite side,

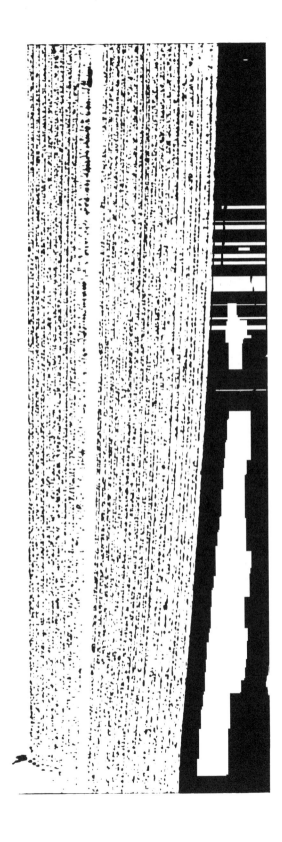

HE FLOOR OF THE
OR RESECTION OF
has been divided
ect of the tongue
ius membrane; D,
land; G, Sterno-
ssels.

and backwards.
d to the alveolar
ould be effected
s of the disease,
eans the lateral

aspect of the tongue and floor of the affected side of the mouth and the regions of the tonsil and fauces are fully exposed.

The mucous membrane of the floor of the mouth is next cut through with scissors, some distance beyond the margins of the diseased area. The glosso-palatine fold is divided if necessary, and the tongue cut through some distance behind the infiltrated or ulcerated area. When only one-half of the tongue is involved in the disease the mucous membrane covering it should be divided along the middle line on both dorsal and ventral aspects, and the organ split backwards into two lateral halves. These cutting operations can be most easily carried out with scissors. When cutting through the substance of the tongue, particular care should be taken when dealing with the ventral aspect to locate the position of the lingual artery, and when seen this should be grasped with pressure forceps before division. The sublingual salivary gland can generally be removed at the same time as the tongue.

When the diseased portion of the tongue and the adjacent structures have been thus removed, the submaxillary triangle should be dealt with and the submaxillary salivary and lymph glands excised. It is desirable also in all cases of this kind to remove the vertical chain of lymph glands which lie deep to the anterior border of the sterno-mastoid and in close relation with the jugular vein. Occasionally it will be found that these lymph glands are so closely connected to the jugular vein and its fascial sheath that it may be necessary, in order to effect complete removal of all diseased tissues, to excise a segment of the jugular vein. When doing this great care must be taken in order to avoid injury to the vagus nerve and sympathetic chain, both of these structures lying in connexion with the posterior aspect of the carotid sheath. When the disease is found to spread beyond the middle line of the tongue, it is necessary, in addition, to remove the entire organ by the method described in the previous operation.

All the diseased tissues having been excised, the field of operation is well investigated for bleeding points, all of which are ligatured with catgut. Next, the margin of the mucous membrane on the dorsal aspect of the stump of the tongue is approximated to the margin of the mucous membrane of the floor of the mouth by a number of interrupted catgut sutures. In addition, it is advisable to pass a few deep sutures through the soft tissues in the base of the wound in order to obliterate as far as possible any 'dead space.' This method of suturing tends to prevent the falling back of the stump of the tongue upon the superior aperture of the larynx and also facilitates healing in the deep portions of the wound. In those cases in which the lower jaw has been divided and it has not been found necessary to take away any part of the bone, the two frag-

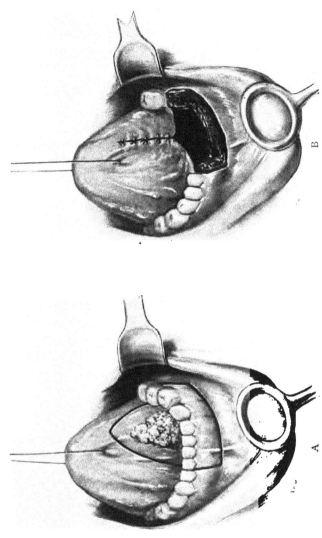

FIG. 243. EXCISION OF A CARCINOMA OF THE FLOOR OF THE MOUTH, OR OF ONE SITUATED ON THE LATERAL AND VENTRAL ASPECTS OF THE TONGUE, EXTENDING TO AND INVOLVING THE MUCOUS MEMBRANE OF THE FLOOR OF THE MOUTH. A, Position of the incisions through the mucous membrane and the mandible. B, Suture of the mucous membrane after removal of the bone.

ments are brought into apposition, drilled with a bone-drill, and fixed by a silver wire suture. When, however, it is necessary to remove the section of the horizontal ramus, the cavity of the wound is packed with strips of gauze after all hæmorrhage has been arrested. Finally, the margins of the wound in the cheek and neck are united by interrupted sutures of salmon-gut with the exception of the most dependent portion which should be left open for the exit of a strip of gauze and a rubber drainage tube. During the suturing particular attention should be directed to securing exact coaptation in the region of the angle of the mouth.

After-treatment. The rubber tube and strips of gauze should be removed at the end of twenty-four or thirty-six hours. The entire wound should be frequently irrigated and great care taken to ensure free exit and early removal of all discharges which may collect.

EXCISION OF A CARCINOMA OF THE FLOOR OF THE MOUTH, OR ONE SITUATED ON THE LATERAL AND VENTRAL ASPECTS OF THE TONGUE EXTENDING TO AND INVOLVING THE MUCOUS MEMBRANE OF THE FLOOR OF THE MOUTH

The majority of cases of carcinoma of the floor of the mouth begin either at the frænum or in the mucous membrane immediately adjacent to it on one or other side. Occasionally I have seen a carcinoma of this kind begin in the mucous membrane which covers the anterior part of the sublingual salivary gland. When the mucous membrane of the posterior part of the floor of the mouth is the seat of the carcinoma, it has usually arisen by direct extension from a primary focus on the lateral margin of the posterior portion of the tongue. Carcinoma of the floor of the mouth, commencing at or in the region of the frænum, at first forms either a small warty prominence or an ulcer with a hard indurated base. By many surgeons carcinoma commencing in this region has been regarded as a very fatal form of the disease, and as one offering small prospect of a permanent cure by operation. In my experience, however, I have found that this disease is not so fatal as has often been thought. When the disease is recognized comparatively early and is subjected to free local removal, together with excision of the lymph glands in the submental and submaxillary regions, good results can be obtained. The hypertrophic or warty form of carcinoma appears to give a much better prognosis than those cases in which ulceration is a marked feature. Carcinomata of this latter kind appear to have a considerable tendency to extend forwards and involve the periosteum upon the posterior aspect of the adjacent alveolar process of the mandible. On this account, I have found it advantageous when treating these cases to remove the teeth from the portion of jaw opposite the growth and also to excise the under-

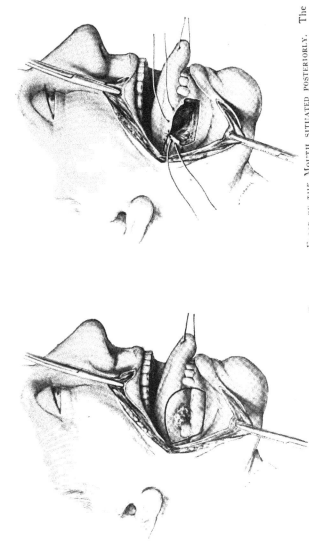

FIG. 244. EXCISION OF A CARCINOMA OF THE TONGUE AND FLOOR OF THE MOUTH SITUATED POSTERIORLY. The two stages of the operation showing the cheek split, the incision for removal of the growth and portion of the mandible, and the method of inserting the sutures.

lying segment of the alveolar process. I have seen cases in which this has not been done quickly recur in the mucous membrane attached to the alveolar process. The ulcerative form of carcinoma in this position is very liable to escape notice since the ulcerated area appears to contract and so render the site of disease difficult to see. Its presence, however, can often be suspected when protrusion of the tongue is limited and the patient complains of soreness in the region of the frænum. Digital exploration of the floor of the mouth will readily enable one to discover the indurated area. Another point of importance in connexion with this disease is the fact that the submental lymph glands on both sides are very prone to become the site of secondary growths at an early stage; consequently, at every operation, these glands must be freely removed on both sides.

Operation. The patient is placed in a semi-sitting posture with the head slightly depressed. The mouth is held open by a strong gag, and a strong salmon-gut suture is passed through the substance of the tongue and made to serve as a tractor. The lower lip is retracted and the exact site, extent, and connexion of the growth determined. Next, a tooth beyond each limit of the growth is removed from the lower jaw and then the remaining teeth, if any, opposite the growth. Next, the mucous membrane and periosteum covering the external aspect of the mandible are cut through along the lines shown in Fig. 243, A. The alveolar process is sawn through on each side at each extremity of the area from which the teeth have been removed. Next, the alveolar process within the two saw-cuts is cut through with a chisel and mallet along the horizontal portion of the line shown in Fig. 243' A. The region of the growth is now sponged dry, the mucous membrane of the floor of the mouth cut through all round the growth and about half an inch to two-thirds of an inch from its margin. The separated segment of the alveolar process is lifted up and the soft tissues of the floor of the mouth underlying the site of the disease and the adjacent portions of the ventral aspect of the tongue are cut through with scissors. During this process of separation the lingual artery may be exposed; if so, it is seized with pressure forceps before division and then ligatured. The carcinomatous growth, together with all adjacent tissues, can now be removed. Next, the field of operation is sponged dry, all bleeding points are picked up and ligatured with catgut, and then the margins of the divided mucous membrane in the lingual portion of the incision are approximated by the sutures. The remaining portion of the incision is packed with strips of gauze.

After-treatment. This is similar to that recommended in removal of the tongue and the floor of the mouth.

In all cases of carcinoma of the floor of the mouth the submental lymph glands of both sides, when the disease is in the region of the frenum, and the submaxillary lymph and salivary glands on the affected side must be removed through an incision in the neck. Details of this operation are given later. (See p. 484.)

REMOVAL OF A CARCINOMA OF THE FLOOR OF THE MOUTH (POSTERIOR PORTION) IN WHICH THE DISEASE HAS EXTENDED TO THE ALVEOLAR PROCESS OF THE MANDIBLE

As already mentioned, carcinoma involving the mucous membrane of the posterior part of the floor of the mouth usually spreads to it by extension from the adjacent portion of the tongue. Occasionally, however, cases are met with in which the disease appears to be primary in the mucous membrane. The operation which is most suitable for disease in this region is a modification of that described in connexion with excision of the tongue after lateral division of the lower jaw.

Operation. The patient is placed in the dorsal posture, with the head and shoulders well raised and the head turned towards the sound side. the lips being grasped by the fingers of an assistant so as to control hæmorrhage, an incision is made commencing at the angle of the mouth and extending backwards and outwards to the anterior margin of the masseter muscle. A controlling ligature of salmon-gut is passed through the anterior portion of the tongue and this organ is drawn towards the sound side. The site of the carcinomatous growth is carefully examined, and the extent and connexion of the disease made out. The flaps formed by the tissues of the cheek are well retracted, the jaws separated by the gag and the teeth of the lower jaw opposite the growth extracted. The muco-periosteum on the external aspect to the jaw is incised, and the alveolar process divided with a saw and chisel in the manner already described. Next, the mucous membrane of the floor of the mouth in front of the growth, on the lateral aspect of the posterior part of the tongue and in the region of the glosso-palatine fold of the fauces, is cut through. The divided portion of the alveolar process is then lifted up and the tissues underlying the carcinomatous growth cut through wide of the diseased area. By these means the growth is set free and is removed. Next. the field of operation is sponged dry, all bleeding vessels are picked up and ligatured, and then the divided margins of mucous membrane approximated as far as possible by catgut sutures (Fig. 244). The space from which bone has been removed and any non-approximated part of the wound in the floor of the mouth are packed with strips of gauze. Finally, the mouth is sponged clean, and the cheek sutured, special care being taken to ensure exact coaptation at the angle of the mouth.

After-treatment. This is similar to that described in the previous operation.

The lymph glands in the submaxillary region and in the deep cervical region along the jugular vein, together with the submaxillary salivary gland, must be removed through a separate incision in the neck.

EXCISION OF THE CERVICAL LYMPH GLANDS, SUBMAXILLARY SALIVARY GLAND, AND FASCIAL STRUCTURES OF THE NECK FOR CARCINOMA OF THE TONGUE AND FLOOR OF THE MOUTH

Operation. The patient is placed in the dorsal position, the head turned towards the opposite side, the shoulders slightly raised in order to throw the head backwards and so give better exposure of the submaxillary, submental, and deep cervical regions.

An incision, semilunar in shape and so planned as to lie as far as possible in the natural fold or crease of the upper part of the neck, is made, commencing behind over the anterior border of the sterno-mastoid muscle and a little below the lower level of the mastoid process, and carried downwards and forwards to the middle line of the neck at a point midway between the prominence of the chin and the body of the hyoid bone. From the convexity of this incision and a short distance in front of the anterior margin of the sterno-mastoid a second incision is made, which extends downwards to the level of the cricoid cartilage or lower according to the extent to which the cervical lymph glands are involved. Some recommend that the lower limb of this incision should be carried to the upper border of the sterno-clavicular articulation. This, in my opinion, is not generally necessary.

When these incisions have been made, three flaps, each consisting of skin and subcutaneous tissues, are dissected free: one upwards, one downwards and outwards, and one downwards and inwards, as shown in Fig. 245, A.

The deep cervical fascia is next divided along the internal and external boundaries of the triangular-shaped space thus laid bare; the dotted lines in Fig. 245, B show the position of these incisions in the deep fascia. Commencing with the inferior angle, a triangular-shaped flap of deep cervical fascia and underlying and attached lymph glands is dissected upwards until the horizontal ramus of the lower jaw is reached. Great care must be taken in making this dissection to separate all the cervical lymph glands and fascial tissues and to avoid causing injury to the carotid sheath and its contents. The external maxillary artery should be sought for in the upper part of the dissection and can readily be recognized where it enters the groove in the submaxillary salivary gland. This

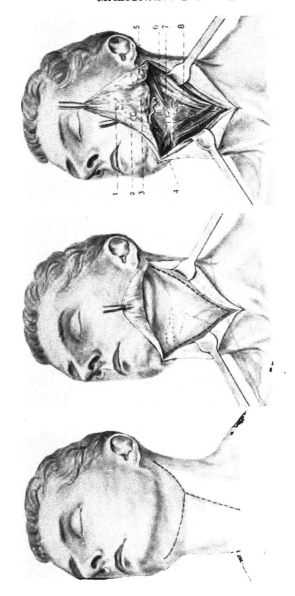

FIG. 245. REMOVAL OF THE CERVICAL LYMPH GLANDS. A shows the skin incisions, B the dissection of the skin and platysma from the deep fascia, and C the deep dissection of the region. 1, Platysma; 2, superficial lymph glands; 3, Submaxillary salivary gland; 4, Mylohyoid; 5, Parotid lymph glands; 6, Internal carotid artery; 7, External carotid artery; 8, Jugular vein.

vessel should be seized in two places with pressure forceps and divided. Next, the submaxillary salivary gland together with the attached submaxillary lymph glands is isolated from its deep connexions and the duct ligatured close to the floor of the mouth. The entire mass of cervical lymph glands, submaxillary salivary glands, submental lymph glands, and fascial tissues can be removed by cutting through the upper attachment along the horizontal ramus of the mandible. During this division the distal portion of the external maxillary artery will be again cut as it lies upon the ramus of the mandible in the region of the anterior margin of the masseter muscle. A number of facial veins will also be cut and require ligature. When effecting the separation near the prominence of the chin, great care must be taken to ensure that all the submental lymph glands and adjacent connective tissues are removed. The submental, submaxillary, and deep cervical regions are carefully sponged and all hæmorrhage arrested. The margins of the flaps, consisting of skin and subcutaneous tissue, are brought into exact apposition by interrupted sutures of fine salmon-gut. A small portion of the wound should be left unsutured and through this a drainage tube is inserted into the deep part of the wound in the submaxillary region. If this is not done an accumulation of blood and serum is liable to occur in the deep parts of the wound, which may become a source of septic trouble. The drainage tube can usually be removed at the end of twenty-four or thirty-six hours.

CRILE'S BLOCK DISSECTION

Crile has advocated in such cases as this a block dissection of the regional lymphatic system, as well as the removal of the primary focus, on exactly the same lines as Halstead has suggested for cancer of the breast. Such a dissection is suggested whether the glands are or are not palpable. He lays great stress on the avoidance of all handling of the carcinomatous tissue so long as the lymphatic channel remains intact. His dissection is begun at the lower end of the neck and includes excision of the veins as well as of the lymphatics. He describes the technique of his operation as follows:

Assuming all preliminary preparations to have been made, the patient is given an injection of $\frac{1}{4}$ morphin and 1-100 atropin half an hour before beginning anæsthesia. After completion of anæsthesia the pharynx is cocainized to prevent reflex inhibition from manipulation: two rubber tubes closely filling the nares and having perforations at the distal end are pushed down to the level of the epiglottis, the tongue is then drawn well forward, a large piece of gauze packed firmly into the pharynx, completely filling it, the brunt of the packing being made at the sides of the tubes, preventing their compression; the patency of the tubes and easy respiration is readily verified; a T-tube is then connected up with an inhaler and the anæsthetizer takes his place a foot or more from the field of operation, giving him the opportunity of continuing an even, uninterrupted anæsthesia, allowing the surgeon full control of the operative field, absolutely preventing the entrance of any blood into the pulmonary tract and permitting the operator to place the patient in any position he wishes.

The patient is then placed in the inclined posture, head up, and the skin incision over the common carotid artery just above the clavicle is made. The artery is exposed by an intermuscular separation of the sterno-mastoid, its outer sheath nicked, the vessel exposed and temporary closure made. The complete skin incisions are then made, the skin reflected back over the entire area of the field. The sterno-mastoid is divided, the internal and external jugulars are secured, tied double and divided at the base of the neck. The dissection is then carried from below upward into the deep plane of the neck behind the lymphatic glands, working first at the sides, then posteriorly, carrying upward all the fascia, muscles, veins, fat, and connective tissue until the floor of the mouth is reached. The lower jaw is then divided at a safe distance on each side of the growth. The floor of the mouth and the border of the tongue are then similarly divided, completing the block.

The following paragraphs, which deal with special points and statistics of operations, are taken from the article by the late Sir Henry Butlin in the previous edition of this work.

Special considerations connected with the removal of the diseased portion of the tongue. *How much of the tongue is it necessary to remove?* On this question there always has been considerable difference of opinion. Nothing less than ' removal of the entire tongue ' satisfied certain operators thirty years ago, and it appears to be still the practice of a few surgeons. The entire tongue is not usually removed by those who profess to perform the operation, for large portions of the muscles attaching the tongue to the jaw or hyoid bone are habitually left behind. Removal of the entire tongue does not guarantee the patient from recurrence in the floor of the mouth or in the tonsillar region, which areas are much more likely to be attacked than the other half of the tongue. In addition, a large number of the patients would be deterred from submitting to operation if they expected to lose the ' entire tongue ' for cancers of small or moderate size. It has been my own practice to remove the disease with, if possible, about $\frac{3}{4}$ inch of adjacent non-infected tissues. In relation to this point the statistics of the late Sir Henry Butlin ' show the following results:—

Out of the 197 cases operated upon by him there were 99 in which there was no recurrence in the tongue. They are classified as follows:—

Died of affection of the glands	39
Died of affection of the glands on the other side of the neck . .	2
Died of cancer of the lungs	1
Died of cancer of the other border of the tongue	2
Successful	55
Total	99

Professor Kocher,[1] in support of limited excision for limited cancer as against removal of the 'entire tongue,' states that he had only nine local recurrences in thirty-eight cases of recurrence of cancer of the tongue.

Special considerations connected with removal of the lymph glands. *Has the removal of the contents of the anterior triangle thus far justified the practice as a routine operation?*
The following table of Sir Henry Butlin of 114 cases in which he removed the contents of the anterior triangle in 70, and did not remove them in 44 cases, clearly shows the advantage of removing the contents of the anterior triangle as a routine operation.

ANALYSIS OF FORTY-FOUR CASES IN WHICH THE CONTENTS OF THE ANTERIOR TRIANGLE WERE NOT REMOVED

To these should be added 8 cases in which the patients returned at a later period for removal of enlarged glands, which were not intended to be removed when the tongue was treated, making a total of 52 cases.

Died of operation	6
Died of recurrence in the mouth (in 3 of these the operation was abandoned)	7
Died of affection of glands (in 5 of these the glands were enlarged at the time of operation on the tongue, but were not removed for various reasons)	15
Died of cancer of opposite border of tongue	1
Cases not countable	3
Successful cases	12
Total	44

In 52 cases there were 23 (15 + 8) in which the glands either were affected at the time of the operation (5) or became affected later (18). The successful cases were 12 in number, and there are 3 cases still not countable. Eight of the cases in which the glands became affected afterwards are included in the following table:—

[1] *Chirurg. Operationslehre*, 5th ed., 1907, p. 605.

ANALYSIS OF SEVENTY CASES IN WHICH THE CONTENTS OF THE ANTERIOR
TRIANGLE WERE REMOVED

Died of the operation 6
Lost sight of after operation 1
Died of recurrence in the mouth 9
Died of recurrence, uncertain where (in one of these the glands
could not be entirely removed; operation abandoned) . . . 7
Died of recurrence in the glands (in one of these the submaxillary
salivary gland was left and the disease recurred beneath it; in the
other seven cases the glands were enlarged at the time of their
removal, and in five of these they were demonstrably cancerous) 8
Died of cancer on the opposite side of the tongue 1
Died of affection of glands on opposite side of neck . . . 2
Died of other diseases within three years 1
Cases not countable 11
Successful cases 24
                                                                   —
        Total 70

The number of patients who died of recurrence in the glands on the same side
is only eight, but it is probable that several of those who died of recurrence, 'uncertain where,' should be added to the eight. The successful cases number
twenty-four, and there are several others out of the eleven 'not countable' cases
which may possibly at a later date be added to them.

Should the operation be performed in every case of cancer of the tongue?
May not the very early cases be allowed to pass, and is not cancer of some parts
of the tongue less dangerous in this respect than cancer of some other parts?
Very small, and, presumably, recent cancers were removed in eighteen of Sir
Henry Butlin's cases, and from different parts of the tongue. No fewer than six
of the patients died of affection of the glands without recurrence in the mouth.
One of the smallest cancers [1] was successfully removed by a local operation, but
proved fatal more than three years later by involving the corresponding lymph
glands.

In order to discover the influence of the seat of the primary disease, Sir Henry
Butlin made the following analysis of his cases. In 23 cases out of his entire
series of 197, only the primary disease was removed, but the patients remained
free from recurrence *in situ* and from affection of the glands (successful cases).
The seat of the disease, roughly noted, was as follows:—

Dorsum:
    Anterior 8
    Further back 2
Border:
    Near the tip 1
    At various points 4
    Beneath the border 7
Tip:
    Under surface 1
                                      —
        Total 23

[1] Figured in the Second Scientific Report of the Imperial Cancer Research,
p. 45, Fig. 35, 1905.

For comparison with these cases, he gives 23 cases (between the 87th and the 197th) in which the glands were not removed, but became affected at a later period:—

Dorsum:
    Anterior 4
Border:
    Near the tip 5
    At various points 9
    Beneath the border 2
    Frænum 2
Extensive disease 1

        Total 23

This points strongly to the belief that, although the anterior portion of the dorsum of the tongue may perhaps be less dangerous to the lymph glands than any other part, it is not wise to act as if it were so. The proper course is to remove the lymph glands in every case of cancer of the tongue in which there is reason to believe the patient will recover from the operation.

Is there any advantage in postponing the removal of the glands until they are enlarged? The great hope of success lies in early removal of the glands. The operation is easier and the results are better.

In support of this Sir Henry Butlin quotes 56 cases, in which the results are known:—

Glands enlarged at the time of operation, 34:
    Died of recurrence in the neck . . . 7
    Successful 11
Glands not enlarged at the time of operation, 22:
    Died of recurrence in the neck . . . 1
    Successful 13

It will be seen that the evidence is largely in favour of not deferring the operation until the glands are enlarged.

In the single case of recurrence in the neck in the second series, the submaxillary salivary gland was not removed, but was raised up for the removal of the glands beneath it. Recurrence took place in the lower part of the salivary gland, presumably due to affection of a lymph gland which had been overlooked.

When should the operation on the lymph glands be performed? In the absence of a decided indication to the contrary, the tongue and the neck should *not* be operated on at the same time. There are cases, however, of small cancers and strong patients, in whom it would be almost absurd to operate at two sittings. But, in most cases, the double operation is a great strain upon the patient, the neck wound is liable to be infected and suppurate, and the risk to life is much greater than when the operation is performed at two sittings. As a rule, the operation on the tongue should take place first and the operation on the neck as soon as the wound in the mouth is free from sepsis and the patient can take food easily. But there are cases in which the lymph glands may be advantageously treated first; when the external carotid artery or some of its branches can be tied, and the second operation thus made much more easy and less dangerous.

Is the removal of the contents of the anterior triangle of the affected side as a routine operation sufficient? Removal of the submaxillary salivary gland should be practised in every case; the dissection carried well up into the parotid region, with removal of the lower portion of the parotid salivary gland in most cases; and the lymph glands beneath and behind the sterno-mastoid muscle should certainly be removed in those cases in which the lymph glands in the parotid region are affected.

Some surgeons remove the contents of both anterior triangles in all cases in which the patient will submit to the operation. This, in my opinion, is not necessary. The following conditions appear to indicate the performance of the operation on both sides:—

(i) Those cases in which the lymph glands on both sides of the neck are enlarged.

(ii) Those cases in which the lymph glands are affected only on the side of the neck opposite to the disease.

(iii) Those cases in which the disease is seated on both sides of the tongue, or in which it reaches to the middle line of the tongue.

(iv) Perhaps it ought to be done in those cases in which microscopical examination gives reason to believe that, although the primary disease is apparently only of small extent and depth, it is much more malignant than usual—when, for instance, columns of cancer-cells are found running deeply down between the muscular fibres.

Removal of the tissues between the primary disease in the tongue and the lymph glands. It may be said that the aim of the modern surgery of cancer is to remove the primary disease and the lymph glands, together with the intervening tissues, whenever this is possible. It is quite feasible in most cases of cancer of the tongue, and the reasons why it is not generally adopted are that it would necessitate extensive operation on the tongue in every case, however small and limited the cancer, and that the large wound in the neck would almost invariably become septic owing to its communication with the mouth. In spite of these disadvantages, which mean a larger mortality due to the operation and much greater permanent impairment of the mobility of the tongue, a decided leaning towards this method on the part of some of the surgeons who were at the Congress of the International Society of Surgeons at Brussels in 1908 was observed. Sir Henry Butlin was very much opposed to the practice, and would only employ it in those cases in which the primary disease passes deeply down into the floor of the mouth and involves the bone, the salivary gland, and other structures. The operation in separate parts is at present justified by the results and by the infrequency with which cancer is found in the lymphatic vessels of the intervening tissues.

CHAPTER III

OPERATIONS UPON THE TONSIL

By George E. Waugh, F.R.C.S.

That the general consensus of opinion at the present time is that the complete removal of the tonsil is the end to be attained whenever operative measures are necessary, is testified to by the large number of new tonsil-holding forceps, new blunt dissecting instruments, and ' new ' operations of tonsillectomy that have been described in print during the last five years. References in the literature previous to this date are confined almost exclusively to descriptions of modifications of the guillotine for the purpose of tonsillotomy, to the value of the snare and the galvano-cautery, with here and there an allusion to the operation of tonsillectomy as a major and sanguinary procedure to be undertaken as a last resource. This complete revolution of opinion is probably due to two reasons. The recognition of the extreme gravity and the far-reaching consequences of oral sepsis, of which tonsillitis is merely a variety, is one. The other is that complete removal of the tonsil can now be effected as a simple surgical procedure which is neither bloody nor difficult.

The operation of tonsillectomy by dissection is a simple and rapid procedure, but demands for its success a rigid attention to detail. The preparation of the patient is important. A preliminary visit to the dentist is essential for the stopping or extraction of carious teeth, and no operation upon the tonsils should be undertaken until the mouth is quite healthy in this respect. Starvation immediately before the operation must be avoided. Its influence upon the occurrence of post-operative acetonæmia has already been determined, and that influence is immeasurably greater in operative procedures which are likely to be followed by a forced abstention from food for about 48 hours. Before an operation to be performed at 9 a. m. the writer is accustomed to give his patients a small cup of tea and a piece of dry toast at 7.30 a. m., and at 8 a. m. three lumps of loaf sugar or a tablespoonful of glucose. Purgatives and enemata are strictly forbidden, whilst a hypodermic injection of a small dose of morphine and atropin is given one hour before operation. Chloroform anæsthesia must be used to ensure an immobile field of operation.

oughing reflexes by engorging the
morrhage from the tonsillar bed
ie operator but may prove a source
ist therefore abolish these reflexes
pplied over a large series of cases
ly absent whilst the conjunctival
e is not evidence of a dangerous

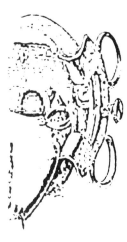

A small embedded tonsil is here seen
al ring forceps.

of the pulse and respirations are
tement.

the recumbent position a small
oulders, so that the head slopes
)od shed to trickle into the naso-
oid congestion by gravity of the
ied O'Dwyer's gag is inserted bend the tongue is held and drawn
thread passed through the tip. In
tened against the gag on the cheek,
ers of the same hand hold up the
clipping the silk thread between
other hand is free to continue the
)ugh a Junker's apparatus, which

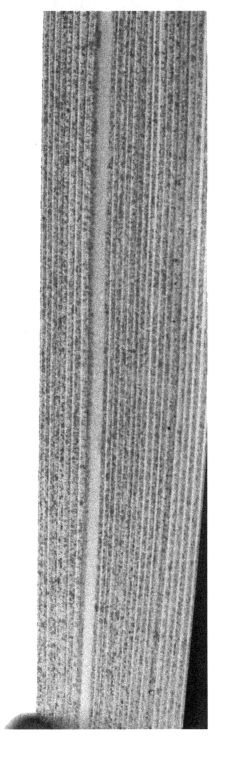

is fitted with a flexible lead tube to hang unaided from the corner of the mouth. The tonsil is then seized in a special pair of ring forceps and drawn inwards towards the middle line so that it bulges beneath the glosso-palatine fold, which is thereby made tense. A closed pair of long-handled finely-toothed forceps is then driven through the glosso-palatine fold as close to its free edge as possible, and by a rapid movement from the uvula to the base of the tongue a small strip of the fold is removed, thus revealing the capsule of the tonsil to the same extent. The

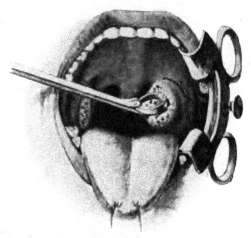

Fig. 247. Tonsillectomy by Dissection. The tonsil has been pulled towards the middle line of the pharynx so that the size of the embedded portion is now seen bulging beneath the glosso-palatine fold. The dotted line indicates the incision made by the closed finely-toothed forceps, and corresponds to the free edge of the glosso-palatine fold, which becomes temporarily obliterated when the tonsil is drawn inwards.

tonsil is then steadied by the toothed forceps whilst a firmer grasp is obtained of it by the ring forceps. The fold is now pulled outwards and the tonsil inwards at the same time so that the whole of the anterior surface of its capsule is exposed. The capsule properly seen is a clear bluish membrane and the blunt dissection should not be proceeded with until this appearance is evident (see Fig. 248). If the tonsil is dissected out with a yellowish layer containing fat overlying the capsule sharp hæmorrhage will be the consequence, as this is not the proper stratum in which the dissection should be conducted. The separation from the pharyngo-palatine fold is effected by blunt dissection with the closed

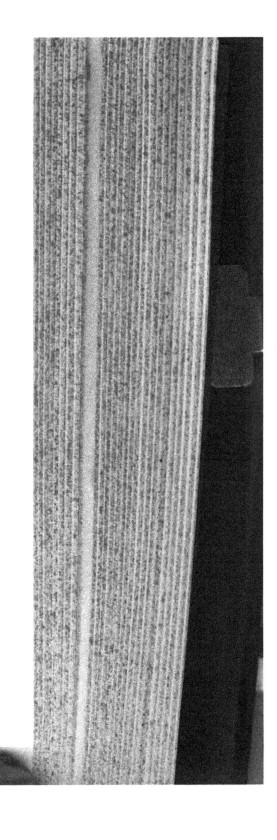

495

ɪg them down between the
d the fold itself. The dis-
e tongue and if necessary
sil is removed in one piece.
the muscular wall of the
t it is no unusual event to
ar bed in the course of an

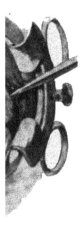

The capsular surface of the
the glosso-palatine fold out-
s the tonsil is drawn inwards

ɪ tonsillectomy is due to a
tails of procedure already
is not properly identified
h an imperfect anæsthesia
ements of the patient pour
ɪous plexus. This in turn
ɪereby further augmenting
cases no primary hæmor-
t, whilst secondary hæmor-
ɪlts or those with thickened
eps the main artery of the

tonsil before severing it. This enters the convex surface of the tonsil at the level of the junction of the upper and middle thirds. On drawing the tonsil inwards and the glosso-palatine fold outwards after the first incision, the site of the artery is easily identified by looking for the tortuous veins by which it is constantly accompanied (see Fig. 249). The total duration of time necessary to remove both tonsils in uncompli-

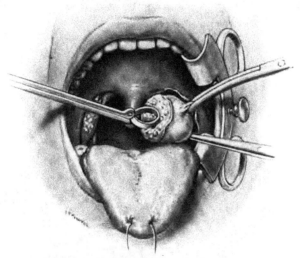

FIG. 249. TONSILLECTOMY BY DISSECTION. The tonsil is here seen with its capsular surface exposed after blunt dissection by the closed finely-toothed forceps. The main artery is indicated at the junction of the upper and middle thirds of the convex surface, secured in the grasp of specially curved artery forceps.

cated cases is 90 seconds. To state the average duration as 5 minutes is probably slightly to over-estimate it. Slight difficulty will be encountered in the removal of tonsils with dense fibrous adhesions around them as the result of previous operations with the guillotine or galvano-cautery, or of frequent attacks of suppuration. But even the densest adhesions are not a source of real difficulty. Between the posterior surface of the capsule and the pharyngo-palatine fold an isolated dense band of fibrous tissue will often be encountered as the result of previous abscess formation when the pus from the tonsil has made its way through the fold. This band can be cut safely by scissors if necessary. Direct traction upon the pharyngo-palatine fold should be avoided as much as possible, since reflex spasm of the glottis is often started in that way. This may be relieved almost instantaneously by relaxing the gag.

Patients should be kept in bed for the next few days after the operation. The mouth should be washed out frequently with a weak antiseptic mouth wash, and a mixture containing chlorate of potash and salicylate of soda may be given every four hours after the first day. By these means the temperature seldom reaches 100° F. even when pus has been present in a tonsil. An additional small dose of morphine should be given hypodermically at the end of the operation while the patient is still on the operating table under the influence of the anæsthetic, to a child ⅟₆₀ gr. and to an adult ⅛ gr. This is far more effective in relieving the after-pain than is the administration of a much larger dose after the patient has regained consciousness.

Ballenger, of Chicago, has consistently advocated the complete removal of the tonsil in its capsule for several years as the only procedure of value. His own method entails the use of a sharp scalpel or hooked knife for the purpose of dissection. He records six cases of ' moderately severe hæmorrhage ' in 3,000 operations. Another slight disadvantage is the use of an écraseur or snare to remove the base of the tonsil. Pynchon removes it by cautery dissection—a method with little to recommend it.

To Sluder belongs the credit for pointing out that with a modified Mackenzie guillotine the tonsil can be removed entire in its capsule in a certain number of cases. Ballenger states that this method is applicable to only 75 per cent. of all cases and that it is accompanied by considerable hæmorrhage. Pybus and Willis have extended the scope and improved the details of Sluder's method, so that in their own words, ' By a special method of using the guillotine we are able in nearly 50 per cent. of all cases to enucleate the tonsil complete in its capsule in one piece. In other cases it is possible to remove the tonsil in two or more pieces. In some few cases removal has been incomplete.' They estimate their total number of failures to effect complete removal at 3 per cent. For these cases and for adults they advocate the dissection method as described by the writer.

In post-operative hæmorrhage Ballenger advocates the local application of styptics, of a special pressure clamp, or, if necessary, ligature of the external carotid artery. In no instance in the writer's experience have any of these measures been necessary. One case of post-operative hæmorrhage in which the tonsils had been inadvertently removed from a hæmophiliac by another operator came under his notice. The child was admitted to hospital some six hours after the operation, having bled steadily all the time. An anæsthetic was immediately administered so as to abolish the pharyngeal reflexes and to enable the site of the operation to be carefully reviewed. It was then quite easy to see that a steady oozing was occurring from both tonsillar beds over their entire surface, and that the hæmorrhage was not due to the spouting from a solitary vessel. The folds of the fauces were transfixed by mattress sutures of stout catgut and then firmly approximated by tightening the stitches. The bleeding stopped immediately and the patient made a rapid recovery. To attempt to control hæmorrhage after operations upon the tonsils under a local anæsthetic or under a light general anæsthetic is a waste of time and a grave danger to the patient, likely to lead to disaster.

CHAPTER IV

OPERATIONS FOR PHARYNGEAL ABSCESS

By George E. Waugh, M.D., F.R.C.S.

A CAREFUL recognition of the type of pharyngeal abscess present is an essential preliminary to its treatment by surgical measures. These abscesses may arise as the sequel of disease of the vertebral column or independently. Their clinical characteristics are quite distinct, so that it is not a matter of difficulty to assign any abscess to its proper group. The importance of a correct classification is emphasized by the need of the different types of abscesses for diametrically opposed surgical procedures.

OPERATIONS FOR PHARYNGEAL ABSCESSES ARISING FROM DISEASE OF THE VERTEBRAL COLUMN

These are the only abscesses of the pharynx which occupy a truly median position upon the posterior wall, with a free edge on either side, equidistant from the lateral walls of the pharynx. Nearly all abscesses of spinal origin are of a tuberculous nature. The successful surgical treatment of a tuberculous abscess, apart from the natural resistance of the patient to the spread of the disease, depends upon the complete removal of the lining of the abscess cavity, together with its liquid contents, and upon the avoidance during the process of the introduction of other pathogenic organisms. To comply with this last condition, all operations upon these abscesses must be performed through the tissues of the neck with scrupulous attention to the details of surgical cleanliness.

An incision is made along the anterior border of the sterno-mastoid muscle through the deep cervical fascia until the carotid sheath with its contents has been exposed above the level of the omo-hyoid muscle. The sheath is pulled aside, either outwards or inwards, so that the transverse processes of the cervical vertebræ are exposed with the rectus capitis anterior arising from them. The lateral wall of the pharynx is then evident, and a pair of sinus forceps thrust into the interval between it and this muscle will readily enter the abscess cavity. The opening must be enlarged and the cavity scraped out gently with a Barker's flushing gouge, taking care not to perforate the pharyngeal wall. Sometimes a sequestrum can be removed in this way from one of the bodies of the vertebræ. The cavity may be filled with a sterilized emulsion of iodoform or with Beck's bismuth paste, and the wound in the neck must be closed without drainage. This procedure must be repeated whenever the abscess re-forms, and provided that sinus formation is avoided, a cure is likely to result. If the abscess has been allowed to reach such a size that it is pointing in the neck, either in the anterior or posterior triangle, the surface incision must be modified to suit the necessities of the case. Otherwise the method of treatment is the same.

OPERATIONS FOR ACUTE RETRO-PHARYNGEAL ABSCESS

Acute retro-pharyngeal abscess is the name applied by tradition to those abscesses of the pharynx which do not arise from the vertebral column. These abscesses must further be subdivided into those of intra-pharyngeal origin and those of extra-pharyngeal origin, a distinction of importance in determining the type of operation to be undertaken. The former are the result of the spread of infective material from a tonsil through the pharyngo-palatine arch into the lateral wall of the pharynx. Quite rarely they arise high up on the lateral wall of the pharynx as the result of inflammatory changes occurring in relation with a mass of adenoids. The extra-pharyngeal abscesses are the result of inflammatory changes occurring in the deep cervical glands leading to abscess formation in the deepest gland of the set lying against the pharyngeal wall. As a consequence the lateral pharyngeal wall is pushed inwards by a fluctuating swelling, which bulges into the cavity of the pharynx on one side. Intra-pharyngeal abscesses must therefore be treated by incision through the mucous lining of the pharynx, and extra-pharyngeal abscesses by external operation through the tissues of the neck. At the earliest sign of the appearance of fluctuation an operation must be performed. Under a light general anæsthesia, an incision is made into the abscess by means of a guarded scalpel. The patient is placed in the recumbent position with a sand-bag under the shoulders, allowing the head to rest slightly backwards upon the operating table. A gag is inserted behind or between the last molar teeth and the tongue is held out by means of a silk thread passed through the tip. With the index finger of the left hand as a guide, an incision into the abscess is made from below upwards, so as to open its cavity over the whole length of its vertical axis. It is important that the incision should be made of this length, otherwise a ' watch-pocket ' is formed by the lower part of the unopened abscess cavity, which subsequently is drained imperfectly, and by permitting suppuration to continue, may lead to the spread of the inflammation down the wall of the pharynx, with the possibility of infection of the mediastinum as a remote complication. If the abscess is very large, a small incision into its wall should be made first of all to allow the pus to escape, and it may be necessary to hang the head and neck of the patient over the edge of the table to prevent flooding by the amount of septic fluid liberated. When this has all been carefully mopped away, the incision must be extended to the proper length by introducing the blunt ends of a pair of curved scissors through the opening in the wall of the abscess, and then cutting upwards and downwards to the extreme limits of the abscess cavity. Subsequently, the throat should be syringed out two or three times daily with warm boric lotion, and the patients may be given any food which they feel inclined to swallow. At the end of about a fortnight the tonsils should be dissected out and the adenoids removed to prevent any repetition of a similar trouble.

It is quite obvious that the method of operating described above is unsuitable to abscesses of extra-pharyngeal origin, when their mode of formation is considered. In these cases, the enlarged glands in the neck must be removed by dissection until the abscess cavity in the deepest gland is reached. This may sometimes be removed entire without bursting; but as a rule it is so adherent to the constrictor muscles of the pharynx as to render that impossible. The lining cavity should therefore be removed systematically with a sharp spoon or with a pair of Lane's biting forceps, and the wound in the neck then closed with a small drainage tube inserted down to the site of the abscess. As a rule this can be removed at the end of forty-eight hours, resulting in the healing of the wound by first intention.

In a large number of cases under the care of the writer, between seventy and eighty altogether, no complications have ever followed the adoption of these procedures for the operative treatment of pharyngeal abscesses. The old controversy as to whether such an abscess should be opened through the mouth or through the neck clearly arose from an imperfect classification of the types of pharyngeal abscesses to be dealt with. With a proper classification the method is obvious.

CHAPTER V

OPERATIONS FOR MALIGNANT DISEASE OF THE ORAL AND LARYNGEAL PARTS OF THE PHARYNX

By Wilfred Trotter, M.S. (Lond.), F.R.C.S. (Eng.)
Captain R.A.M.C.(T.)

The oral and laryngeal parts of the pharynx present such resemblances as to the treatment of the diseases to which they are subject that they are conveniently treated together. The term pharynx as used in this article will refer to these two parts only unless otherwise specified. The surgery of malignant disease of the pharynx presents many special difficulties which may be classified under the headings of (1) the eradication of the disease; (2) the danger of the operation; and (3) the mutilation and disability due to the operation.

As to the *eradication of the disease*, it may be stated that as regards the epitheliomata—by far the most frequent form of disease—the ordinary methods of surgery are as adequate here as elsewhere. That is to say, the removal of early or only moderately advanced tumours with a margin of ½ to ¾ in. of healthy surrounding tissue will, in the great majority of cases, secure freedom from local recurrence. Advanced tumours do not follow this rule and always demand special treatment, if they are to be attacked at all. A systematic gland operation should be done in every case. It is sometimes found that a unilateral gland dissection proves to be adequate; extended experience, however, indicates that a bilateral dissection must be looked upon as the normal procedure.

There are two causes of failure in eradicating the primary disease which are special to the pharynx, viz. *recurrence by implantation* and *retro-pharyngeal lymphatic recurrences.*

Implantation recurrences are not very uncommonly seen in cases of carcinoma of the epiglottis when a growth appears on the posterior wall of the pharynx exactly opposite the primary one. Another manifestation of what appears to be a somewhat similar process is the appearance of one or more growths scattered along the pharynx or œsophagus below the primary one. It is difficult to be sure that such growths have not been due to spread in the lymph vessels, but many have an appearance suggestive of implantation and resembling the similar well-known occurrence of multiple growths in the colon secondary to ileocæcal tumours.

Lymphatic recurrence behind the pharynx is rather prone to occur.

It may be a good deal higher up than the primary growth, and in such a situation as to suggest that there have been infected lymph glands which could scarcely have been reached by the most radical gland dissection.

The *dangers of the operation* are almost entirely those of infection. Pneumonia is, of course, invariably and solely due to aspiration of infective material into the lungs. The only precaution against it which has any value is the performance of laryngotomy or tracheotomy at the earliest possible moment of the operation and the plugging of the windpipe above. Direct infection of the wound is undoubtedly the most serious danger. Essentially it is dependent on the normal presence of virulent organisms in the mouth, for wounds of the naso-pharynx are very little liable to serious infections, whereas wounds of the mouth, the oral and laryngeal parts of the pharynx, and the œsophagus are all liable to such. The anatomical features of the pharynx make infections in these regions much more serious than similar infection in the mouth.

The primary source of infection is the mouth, but secondarily the ulcerated surface of the growth becomes a further source. Consequently the degrees of sepsis in the mouth and the extent and foulness of the ulceration are important factors in determining the dangers of a given operation. A clean edentulous condition of the mouth undoubtedly influences the prospect of success more favourably than any other feature of the case, and conversely the presence of teeth, even if apparently quite healthy, is a decidedly unfavourable influence. It is doubtful whether an operation should be undertaken, at any rate in an elderly person, without a preliminary clearance of the mouth.

A wound exposed to contact with oral mucus always becomes infected, and the infection runs a fairly well defined course. It causes sloughing of the raw surface and a good deal of inflammatory reaction in the surrounding tissue. If the surface is quite open there is little tendency to spreading of the inflammation. For the first three or four days there is sloughing and serous discharge; in about a week suppuration is well established and by the tenth day the sloughs have usually separated, leaving a clean granulating wound which seems quite immune from reinfection.

The dangers occurring in the process of healing are as follows:

1. **Acute septicæmia.** This is not very uncommon, and is especially likely to occur when a very large wound is left exposed to infective material and when the mouth and tumour are highly septic. It seems especially common after operations during which, on account of imperfect access or want of care, the wound is grossly befouled during the actual operation. It is a wholly irremediable complication and is often fatal in forty-eight hours.

2. **Secondary hæmorrhage.** This is fairly common unless special precautions are taken. It occurs almost invariably between the eighth and tenth days, while the sloughs are separating and everything seems to be progressing well. It is a very fatal complication—usually through flooding of the air-passages with blood.

3. **Spreading cellulitis.** This is the most serious danger of operations on the laryngeal part of the pharynx. Any pocketing or imperfect drainage of the wound is likely to cause it. A diffuse sloughing cellulitis spreads along the areolar planes about the œsophagus and readily reaches the mediastinum. It is a very fatal complication, but occasionally can be checked by energetic treatment. As a rule it causes death in from ten days to a fortnight.

The question of mutilation and disability resulting from the operation can be dealt with only in relation to the different operative procedures.

PRINCIPLES GUIDING THE DESIGNING OF OPERATIONS

There are certain general requirements which are so important that they should receive individual consideration in dealing with each case. They need be stated here only in summary form.

(*a*) **Preliminary disinfection.** Cleansing of the mouth is the most important measure. By far the most efficient method is the removal of all the teeth, and whenever practicable this should certainly be done. To get the full advantage of it the tooth sockets should be allowed to heal before the main operation is undertaken, and during the extraction of teeth every precaution should be taken to inflict a minimum of injury. During the operation as soon as the growth is fully exposed its surface should be seared with the actual cautery. It is not usual for thorough disinfection to be possible by this means, but a good deal can often be done.

The wound throughout the operation must be as fully protected as possible from contact with mucus from the pharynx.

(*b*) **Freedom of access to the tumour.** A distinct step of the operation should be free exposure of the growth before any attempt to remove it is begun. This principle is absolutely cardinal in the provision of the best chance of eradicating the disease, preventing serious infection, and limiting mutilation. Nothing encourages failure more certainly than the confusion of the procedure of access with the procedure of removal.

(*c*) **Local removal of the tumour** in accordance with the pathological necessities of the case rather than in accordance with the supposed anatomical necessities of the part. An operation should never be undertaken with the design of removing a given organ, but always with that of eradicating a given tumour.

(d) **Closure of the wound or wounds in the pharynx.** This is by far the most efficient means of preventing serious infections. Sometimes it can be done by direct suturing, in other cases the loss of substance in the pharynx must be made good by a skin flap. In both cases the main object is the protection of the tissues from contact with pharyngeal mucus. Valuable as is wound closure as a method of limiting or preventing infection, it must be used carefully and with a knowledge of the necessary conditions, otherwise, by causing pocketing and imperfect drainage, it may actually increase the danger of serious infection.

The invariable effect of contact of pharyngeal mucus with any raw surface is to cause sloughing. Hence, if in closing the pharynx or stitching a flap of skin into it the ordinary edge-to-edge method of stitching is used, as in closing a skin wound, it will be found that a slough forms along each margin of the line of suture. To avoid this disappointing and sometimes very dangerous complication, wide surfaces must be brought together by mattress sutures, skin and mucous membrane, for example, being united very much in the same way as segments of bowel are brought together, end-to-end, the raw surface in the first case corresponding with the peritoneal in the second.

VARIETIES OF PHARYNGEAL TUMOURS

For the purposes of the operating surgeon the great majority of cases of malignant disease of the oral and laryngeal parts of the pharynx can be classified in four groups, according to the anatomical site of the tumour and the operation needed for the removal of it. Four principal standard operations are therefore to be described, and it will be found that practically every case of pharyngeal tumour that is met with can be satisfactorily attacked by one or another of them. A thorough grasp of these clinical types is extremely important, as a failure to recognize the true nature of a tumour and its actual place of origin may lead to the adoption of an unsuitable method which will prove a serious handicap to the surgeon and lead to unnecessary mutilation, or even failure to complete the operation.

The grouping of tumours which I have found of most practical value is the following :—

1. **Tumours of the oropharyngeal group.** This group includes endothelioma, lymphosarcoma, and epithelioma of the tonsil itself, and certain epitheliomata starting in the immediately adjacent parts, such as the glosso-palatine arch and the tongue at the attachment of the glosso-palatine arch.

The well-marked group of epithelioma of the base of the tongue falls anatomically into this group. It is not, however, dealt with in this article. (See Operations on the Tongue.)

2. **Tumours of the epilaryngeal group.** Experience shows that there is a fairly distinct class of tumours which start upon the epiglottis or arytæno-epiglottic fold. They are all epitheliomata, and, having no special tendency to invade the larynx, can in their earlier stages be dealt with by a local operation without laryngectomy.

3. **Tumours of the recessus piriformis.** These are among the most serious of all pharyngeal tumours because they are apt to escape diagnosis until a late stage. They are epitheliomata and, although primarily pharyngeal, always involve the skeleton and soft parts of the larynx very early.

4. **Tumours of the hypopharyngeal group.** This group is defined as including all tumours of the laryngeal part of the pharynx which do not in their early stages involve the larynx. They may begin on the posterior or lateral wall as high as the epiglottis or on the anterior wall behind the cricoid. Many of these tumours come within the group of so-called 'post-cricoid carcinoma.' This is not a good name, because operative experience shows that an exactly post-cricoid localization is not particularly common. In my own experience the lateral wall is as common a starting-place as any. All tumours of this group are epitheliomata. In their later stages they tend to involve the larynx, the whole circumference of the pharynx, and to extend along the œsophagus. The last mode of extension is very common, and soon puts the case beyond the reach of operation.

OPERATIONS FOR THE REMOVAL OF TUMOURS OF THE OROPHARYNGEAL GROUP [1]

Endotheliomata and lymphosarcomata of the tonsil are extremely difficult to cure by operation, unless they are dealt with at a stage when diagnosis is scarcely possible. Both tend to involve lymph glands at an early stage, and, once this has occurred, it is doubtful if cure is ever possible. In this respect these tumours contrast remarkably with epitheliomata, which quite frequently remain curable by operation long after lymphatic invasion has occurred. One feature which adds greatly to the difficulties of early diagnosis and successful treatment of the endotheliomata is their liability to inflammation and suppuration. It is per-

[1] The descriptions of operations in this and the subsequent sections refer only to procedures of which the author has personal experience. The scheme of operations presented has been found to contain methods suitable for attacking all forms of epithelioma of the pharynx which have been met with in the author's practice. In the interests of simplicity it has been thought undesirable to give alternative methods of dealing with tumours of the same group.

haps this which favours the early and extensive gland involvement which is so common.

Epithelioma is undoubtedly the commonest tumour, and the treatment differs according to the stage of the disease.

1. If the disease is strictly limited to the tonsil itself an intra-buccal operation should be done, followed, of course, by the bilateral gland operation. The choice of this method of treatment should not be made unless the limitation of the disease can be certainly established.

2. The operation usually necessary, and the one that should be chosen in all cases where it is doubtful if the disease is limited to the tonsil, is a much more serious one. Free longitudinal access is needed, and can only be obtained after the mandible has been divided just in front of the masseter. In many cases the cervical lymph glands will already be seriously involved.

INTRA-BUCCAL EXCISION OF TONSILLAR TUMOURS

Preliminary laryngotomy should always be done. The pharynx is then plugged and the cheek split backwards from the angle of the mouth parallel with the base of the jaw to the anterior edge of the masseter on the same side as the tumour. The latter can now be fully inspected and its extent made out. The tonsil should never be enucleated, but should be cut out with a margin of healthy surrounding tissues of $\frac{1}{4}$ to $\frac{1}{2}$ inch. Great care should be taken to get the full margin below. It is not necessary to remove much of the soft palate, and care should be taken to avoid inadvertently cutting at all widely into this, as a permanent modification of the voice may be thereby and unnecessarily produced.

The wound in the pharynx left by such an operation can always be completely stitched up. The stitches should be of catgut and should pick up the base of the wound so that broad surfaces are brought together and no cavity is left behind.

The cut surfaces of the cheek should have been protected during the operation by having gauze stitched over them or by the temporary suturing of skin and mucous membrane. The final stitching up of the cheek needs care if rapid union is to be obtained and scarring minimized. For the latter purpose it is essential that no cavity be left between the skin and mucous membrane; hence two or three mattress sutures are necessary on both the skin and the mucous aspects. By these stitches the surfaces of contact of the wound are made very broad and the subsequent cicatrization cannot produce a depressed scar. The laryngotomy tube is removed at the end of the operation. No dressing is applied to the cheek, but the wound is left to dry. Healing is usually very rapid, and the gland operation can be done in a week.

TRANSMANDIBULAR EXCISION OF TONSILLAR TUMOURS

In cases where this is necessary the question of whether the primary growth or the glands should be attacked first always arises.

The patients are usually elderly men subjects of arterial and renal disease and frequently of the effects of chronic alcoholism; the growth is the seat of a deep and extremely foul ulcer, which, owing to the tendency to downward extension, is probably very close to the upper opening of the larynx. The consequence is that a prolonged gland operation before the primary growth has been removed is extremely likely to be followed by pneumonia, which is practically always fatal. In my experience an extensive preliminary gland dissection is much more likely to be the cause of pneumonia than is the removal of the primary growth. The gland operation can scarcely ever be carried out without considerable and persistent impairment of the airway during the procedure. Restriction of the airway of course greatly increases the force of aspiration at the upper opening of the larynx, and this leads to the inhalation of septic matter from the ulcer, and consequent pneumonia. Nevertheless, it is necessary that the glands should be done first, because the division of the jaw and the almost necessary infection of some part of the wound left by removal of the primary growth usually delay healing for several weeks, during which, of course, the glands cannot be touched. Again, the scarring following such a wound interferes with the clean dissection which is so desirable in the gland operation.

There are two practical solutions of the problem either of which may be chosen: (*a*) a partial gland operation and removal of the primary growth as a first stage; (*b*) the gland operation as a first stage *in combination with a preliminary laryngotomy* as a precaution against pneumonia. The laryngotomy need only be used during the operation.

When a very large mass of glands is present in the neck and the case is still judged to be suitable for operation, the gland mass will certainly have to be removed first. In such a case the bilateral gland operation will almost certainly not be possible. This involves either dispensing with the dissection on the sound side or carrying out a third operation.

The *operation on the primary growth*, whether done first or second, should always begin with a laryngotomy and the plugging of the pharynx.

Exposure of the jaw by reflection of a flap gives the best access and the least conspicuous scarring. The incision begins in the median line of the lower lip and is carried down vertically over the chin to a point ½ inch below the jaw; it then turns backwards horizontally to the edge of the sterno-mastoid; at this point it will be 1 to 1½ inches below the angle of the jaw. The flap is reflected backwards till well beyond the anterior edge of the masseter and the facial vessels are divided. If the glands have not already been removed and a partial dissection is to be done, the contents of the submaxillary triangle and the tissues over the carotid sheath are now isolated and left attached above. The jaw is cleared immediately in front of the masseter, drilled in two places near the lower border, and divided; the saw-cut should be directed downwards and slightly forwards to prevent upward displacement of the posterior fragment later on.

From the moment the jaw is divided great care should be taken to protect its cut surfaces from contact with infective material. The floor of the mouth is now incised from a point near the section of the jaw backwards and inwards to the lingual attachment of the glosso-palatine arch. The jaw can now be widely separated and the growth examined. The deep, crater-like ulcer usually present in the growth should be plugged, as it cannot be cauterized adequately; the pharynx plug should be renewed and the whole region mopped over with an antiseptic.

The actual removal of the tumour is now undertaken, and the object of the surgeon should be to get a margin of healthy tissues of ¾ inch beyond the palpable induration. The growth has a special tendency to spread downwards into the recussus piriformis, alongside the upper opening of the larynx, and very careful attention should therefore be given to this part of the excision. When the tumour is large it is often necessary to remove the great cornu of the hyoid bone. Bleeding is never serious, and I have never had to divide either the internal carotid or jugular in dealing with an operable tumour.

Closure of the wound is often difficult and tedious, but if it is thoroughly done will repay the time spent on it. The gap to be closed is usually very extensive. As a rule a considerable part of the soft palate and the lateral, and even some of the posterior wall of the pharynx in the tonsillar region, have been removed, as well as a considerable part of the tongue and the pharyngeal wall down to the thyreoid cartilage. The wound usually stitches up in a triradiate form, consisting of (1) an upper vertical part in the region of the tonsil and palate; this usually comes together well enough and is the least important; (2) a lower vertical part in the lateral wall of the pharynx below the level of the tonsil; this is most important, but closes easily; two rows of stitches at least are necessary and must bring broad surfaces together; (3) a horizontal part between the other two; this is closed by bringing the tongue to the internal pterygoid muscle and to the inner side of the cheek; in order to effect this latter the alveolar border of the jaw may be cut away, and thus a thick covering of soft parts can be brought over the line of division of the bone.

The bone is firmly fixed by a wire during the suture of the soft parts. The skin wound is closed except for a large drainage opening in the submaxillary region. The laryngotomy tube should generally be left in for twenty-four or forty-eight hours.

The greater part of the pharynx wound usually heals by direct union. Rarely primary union throughout is obtained. Commonly there is some slight leakage from the pharynx after a day or two, at the point where the three limbs of the triradiate line of suture meet.

The chief technical defect of the operation is the liability to infection of the suture line of the jaw. Even in the exceptional cases where primary union occurs, the wire has practically always sooner or later to be removed. Usually union is considerably delayed by the presence of the wire and often by some superficial necrosis as well. In spite of this disadvantage I believe the operation to give by far the best means of dealing with all cases of malignant disease of the tonsil except the very early ones.

Results. Malignant disease of the tonsil is not quite so formidable a condition as is often supposed. Of eleven cases I have operated on myself, only one of which was in an early stage, three were free from any return of the disease more than three years after the operation. Epithelioma is more amenable to treatment than endothelioma and lymphosarcoma, for it can be cured even when fairly advanced.

The mortality of the operation, considering the nature of the procedures and the condition of the patients, is not very great. Of my own eleven cases two died from the operation. Of these deaths one was due to a complicating condition unconnected with the operation, and the other to shock following difficulty in breathing consequent upon the laryngotomy tube having been left out too soon.

OPERATIONS FOR TUMOURS OF THE EPILARYNGEAL GROUP

It has been generally assumed that malignant disease of the upper opening of the larynx cannot be dealt with without laryngectomy. There is a certain amount of evidence against this view, and consequently such cases should be approached by the surgeon with the intention of removing the tumour by a local operation rather than a formal laryngectomy.

Definite enlargement of glands is usually present at the time of the operation, at least on one side of the neck. As the approach to the primary tumour is to be a lateral one, and as in these cases there is usually already difficulty in breathing, the best course is to combine the unilateral gland operation with the removal of the primary tumour. This makes the operation very long, but if a satisfactory tracheotomy is done early very little shock is to be expected. The operation by which the upper opening of the larynx can be most conveniently exposed I have called lateral transthyreoid pharyngotomy. It is carried out as follows :—

Lateral transthyreoid pharyngotomy for a tumour of the epilaryngeal group. A tracheotomy is done as soon as possible, and the tumour examined carefully with the finger, so that its exact extent and distribution can be made out. The incisions are now made as for a unilateral gland operation, that is, along the anterior border of the sterno-mastoid and at right angles to this. As soon as the skin is reflected the deep fascia is incised about an inch in front of the sterno-mastoid and turned back as a separate layer. The gland operation is now done in the usual way, with removal of fat and glands from beneath the sterno-mastoid as far as its posterior border and from the anterior triangle up to the base of the parotid. In order the more securely to shut off from infection the large posterior part of the wound, which contains the carotid vessels fully exposed, the flap of deep fascia above described is turned forward and stitched to the prevertebral muscles behind the pharynx. In this way primary union of the gland wound can be ensured. A separate drainage tube should be put into it through a puncture behind the sterno-mastoid.

The exposure of the primary growth is now proceeded with. The infra-hyoid muscles are turned back from off the larynx and hyoid bone, the superior pedicle of the thyreoid gland is divided and, if necessary, part of the lateral lobe is removed. The great cornu of the hyoid bone and the ala of the thyreoid cartilage are now freed from the structures deep to them. This can be done very easily without wounding the mucous membrane of the pharynx. The posterior two-thirds of the ala are now removed, and the great cornu disarticulated from the body of the hyoid. The wall of the pharynx at the level of the upper opening of the larynx is now fully exposed and the tumour can be palpated through it. The wound is packed round with gauze, leaving the pharyngeal wall uncovered. The latter is incised longitudinally and held aside with threads so as still further to protect the wound from pharyngeal mucus. The upper opening of the larynx and the growth are now laid bare. The larynx is then securely plugged.

The removal of the tumour is now undertaken. Generally its primary seat is the epiglottis, but occasionally it is the arytæno-epiglottic

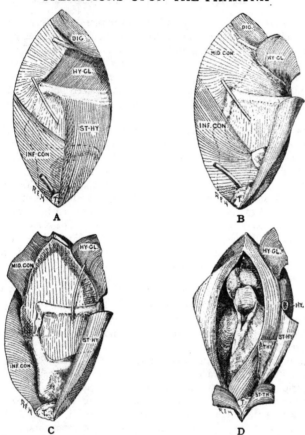

FIG. 250. THE OPERATION OF LATERAL TRANSTHYREOID PHARYNGOTOMY.
Diagrams of four stages in the exposure of the upper opening of the larynx. In
A the preliminary gland dissection has been done; in B the infra-hyoid muscles
have been reflected; in C the skeleton of the larynx has been laid bare. The ex-
posed parts of the hyoid bone and thyreoid cartilage are now to be removed. In
D the pharynx has been opened and the upper opening of the larynx is exposed.

fold. In either case, unless the disease is far advanced, an adequate
margin of healthy tissue can be obtained without difficulty. If the
tumour is epiglottic and of any size, the transverse incision isolating it
below should be only just above the vocal folds. Extension forwards
into the tongue is common and should be looked for. It is unusual for

the growth to be anywhere near the hyoid bone or thyreoid cartilage. Bleeding is never troublesome.

The large gap left between the tongue and larynx must now be closed by strong and deep mattress sutures of catgut. The mobility of the tongue allows this to be effected without serious difficulty. A large number of stitches should be used and care be taken to leave no cavity. Accurate suturing of the mucous membrane is of little importance compared with the bringing together of broad surfaces. The lateral wall of the pharynx must now be closed with at least two rows of suture. The skin wound can be closed except for an opening for a plug going down to the pharyngeal wall.

After-treatment. The drainage tube behind the sterno-mastoid is removed after twenty-four hours. The plug going down to the wall of the pharynx is changed daily. Usually its neighbourhood shows evidence of some infection at the time of the operation, but in the majority of cases there is no leakage at all from the pharynx and the wound may be practically healed in two or three weeks. The patient is fed through a soft rubber catheter of moderate size passed into the upper part of the œsophagus. The tracheotomy tube is necessary for a week or ten days, as there is usually a good deal of swelling about the glottis.

It is as well not to allow the patient to attempt to swallow for at least a week, but it is desirable to let him begin before the tracheotomy tube is left out, in case there should be uncomfortable spasm.

The mouth should be cleansed very frequently as long as swallowing is not allowed.

The re-establishment of normal deglutition usually takes two or three weeks, during which time the patient is very apt to become depressed and discouraged unless the surgeon is particularly careful to reassure him. The difficulty is often in getting the act to assume its normal automatic character again, and patients often find for a time that they can swallow quite well in solitude but are apt to choke in company.

A common difficulty during convalescence is coughing. The altered relations of the upper laryngeal opening and the irritative effect of the wound involving it lead to a greatly increased sensitiveness to stimulation. Consequently paroxysmal coughing is very apt to occur and disturb the patient a great deal. This tendency always passes off sooner or later, usually within about four weeks. It can be controlled, if much disturbance is being caused, by occasional small doses of morphine.

Results. Epilaryngeal growths have proved in my experience the least discouraging of all pharyngeal tumours. Out of ten cases, four were cured, one by laryngectomy and three by local excision without laryngectomy. These three latter were all serious cases on account of the size of the growth and extensive gland involvement. They recovered a practically normal voice and perfectly normal deglutition.

Of the ten cases, two died from the operation. This would represent a considerable death-rate per cent., but it may be remarked that it is only half the rate per cent. of cures.

OPERATIONS FOR TUMOURS OF THE RECESSUS PIRIFORMIS. LARYNGO-PHARYNGECTOMY

The peculiar clinical course of these tumours leads, as I have shown elsewhere,[1] to the diagnosis being made only at a late stage, when the lateral wall and skeleton of the larynx are already extensively involved. Such cases, therefore, stand alone amongst all the tumours of the pharynx in invariably necessitating a total laryngectomy. Doubtless many other pharyngeal tumours as met with in practice can be dealt with only by an operation which includes laryngectomy; nevertheless, such cases are always late ones, and have passed through a stage in which diagnosis was not difficult and would have saved the patient from the mutilating operation. I have never seen a case of tumour of the recessus piriformis in which there was the least possibility of treatment without laryngectomy.

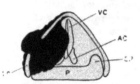

FIG. 251. DIAGRAM OF MODE OF SPREAD OF AN EPITHELIOMA OF RECESSUS PIRIFORMIS. The features to be noticed are early involvement of the thyroid cartilage, absence of projection into lumen of pharynx, and the presence of a bulging inwards of the lateral wall of the larynx without any ulceration there. At this stage the diagnosis can usually be made by external palpation of the larynx.

By the time the case comes to operation it will usually be found that the growth has extended beyond the actual recess and involved at least the lateral wall of the pharynx. Sometimes it will have encircled the pharynx completely. A mode of extension not uncommon is downwards to the œsophagus. When this has occurred, a satisfactory operation is impossible. The invasion of the pharynx renders the operation a much more serious matter than a simple laryngectomy, because a gap is left in the pharynx which cannot be closed. This adds so greatly to the seriousness of the operation that it would save confusion if the latter were always referred to as laryngo-pharyngectomy, in order to mark the distinction from laryngectomy in which, since none of the lateral pharyngeal wall is removed, the operation

[1] Hunterian Lectures, 1913, *Lancet*, April 19, 1913.

in the pharynx can be completely closed and primary union of the whole wound usually obtained.

The removal of any considerable amount of the wall of the pharynx renders necessary a type of operation differing essentially from those already described. Away from the neighbourhood of the tongue, simple suture does not suffice to close gaps in the pharyngeal wall that involve any considerable amount of the circumference. It is therefore necessary to provide something to take the place of the part which has been re-

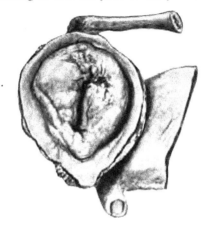

Fig. 252. Epithelioma of Lateral Wall of Pharynx removed by Lateral Transthyreoid Pharyngotomy. The tumour was adherent to the thyreoid ala and was removed with it. The gap in the pharynx was closed by simple suture, and there was no leakage from it. The figure is intended to show the maximum amount which can be removed from this part of the pharynx without the provision of a skin flap being necessary to close the resulting gap.

moved. Such a substitute is to be found in a flap of skin. The skin is completely tolerant of the pharyngeal contents and readily heals into the pharynx if it is turned in in the form of a flap.

The operation should begin with the exposure of the upper end of the trachea, transverse division of it below the cricoid and the suture of the lower end of the skin. Since an essential part of the operation is the cutting of an oblong flap from the front of the neck, the vertical tracheotomy incision should not go higher than the cricoid. If more room is wanted, a transverse cut may be made at this level, and will later form part of the flap incision. As soon as the trachea has been divided, its upper end should be securely plugged. The anaesthetic now being

given by the open end of the ţr
tumour is made through the m

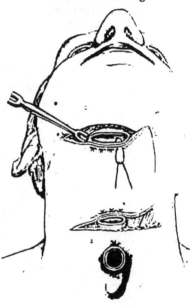

A

FIG. 253. LARYNGO-PHARYNGE
shows the reconstruction of the pha
larynx and the whole circumference
skin flap has been laid in position ar
pharynx above and to the œsophagus
are used is shown. The trachea has
the skin at an early stage of the opera
In ᴅ the skin flap has been folded
the pharynx. The flap thus forms p
the base of the flap an opening into t
in the figure to have been reduced
anterior edges of the flap for about ar
of the flap may be covered in by slidi
lateral aspect of the neck.

of the flap should be. If the los
the pharynx is to be extensive, t

teriorly. If the whole circumference of the pharynx must be removed the flap must obviously have length enough to form, when bent on itself, anterior and posterior walls. It is obvious that no detailed description can be given of the various modifications in the arrangement of the flap which may be necessary. The one general rule of essential importance is that the flap must be of ample size to fill the gap without the least tension. As soon as the flap has been reflected the muscles are turned off the larynx, and the pharynx is isolated as much as necessary before being opened. In clearing the larynx it must be remembered that the growth has almost certainly penetrated the ala of the thyreoid; on this side, therefore, the infra-hyoid muscles cannot be reflected off the larynx, but must be sacrificed with the tumour. When the time comes when opening the pharynx cannot be postponed, every precaution is taken to prevent escape of mucus into the wound. Substitution of pharyngeal wall by skin of course renders necessary the leaving of a temporary fistula at the pedicle of the flap. This is useful for feeding purposes at first, and will usually be found later not to interfere with normal swallowing. No attempt should be made to close it until the wound is thoroughly sound and the raw surface whence the flap was taken has healed. The stitching of skin to pharynx, as already said, should be surface to surface by mattress sutures and never edge to edge.

Results. The results of operations for tumours of the recessus piriformis are extremely bad. I have never seen a case cured by operation, and the operative mortality is still very high. Nevertheless, when the disease, as it might very well be, is recognized in its early stages I have no doubt that the operation of laryngectomy with reconstitution of the pharynx by skin will give at least moderately good results. The disease is not inherently incurable, and a patient and enterprising study of local pathological conditions and technique will, I am sure, sooner or later yield results as encouraging as those of operations for tumour of the oral and upper laryngeal parts of the pharynx.

OPERATIONS FOR TUMOURS OF THE HYPO-PHARYNGEAL GROUP

Tumours of this group are usually removable in their early stages without laryngectomy. Late cases become inoperable from diffuse extension to the œsophagus or through the pharynx to the structures of the neck.

The gap left by the excision can never be closed by simple suture, so that a flap must be provided for reconstituting the pharynx. The closure of the defect in the pharynx is especially necessary in this region for limiting sepsis and preventing stricture.

The operation should be begun with tracheotomy, and then the growth is explored through the mouth with the finger, so that the extent and situation of it can be made out and the nature of the flap decided upon.

After reflection of the flap, access to the pharynx is obtained by removal of the ala of the thyreoid cartilage and of the lateral lobe of

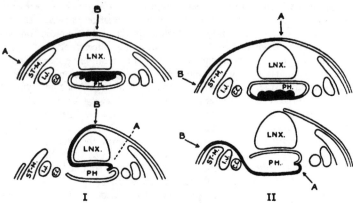

FIG. 254. DIAGRAMS TO SHOW THE ARRANGEMENT OF THE SKIN FLAPS USED IN RECONSTITUTING THE PHARYNX AFTER REMOVAL OF A TUMOUR OF THE HYPO-PHARYNGEAL GROUP. I. The tumour is on the anterior pharyngeal wall—so-called ' post-cricoid carcinoma '—and the skin flap must therefore have its attachment anteriorly. The upper diagram shows the skin flap marked but not reflected; the lower diagram shows the state of affairs after removal of the growth and suture of the flap in position. The skin flap and the growth are shown in solid black.

II shows the arrangement of the skin flap used in reconstituting the pharynx after removal of a tumour of the posterior wall. The flap in this case is attached posteriorly. In each diagram B points to the base of the flap, and A to its free edge. LNX, larynx; PH, pharynx; STM, sterno-mastoid; IJ, jugular vein; CC, common carotid.

the thyreoid gland or part of it. The growth can be felt through the pharynx wall, and the freeing of it from surrounding parts is carried as far as possible before the mucous membrane is opened. When this is done the larynx is at once plugged. The escape of mucus is prevented as much as possible by plugging until the flap has been stitched in place.

Feeding is best done through the fistula at the pedicle of the flap by means of a soft rubber catheter. After about the first week, the patient may begin to swallow through the mouth. As a rule, very little food escapes at the fistula. The latter need not be closed for several weeks.

Results. I am not able to record a case of permanent cure of a growth of this group. Experience, however, of the technique sketched above shows that the great obstacles to successful treatment, viz. infection of the wound and subsequent stricture, can be surmounted. It would seem, therefore, that the submission of the cases to earlier operation would yield a satisfactory number of cures. It is not sufficiently realized that epithelioma of this type is characteristically a disease of adult and even young women, and hence the number of cases which come to operation in a stage too late for successful treatment is deplorably large. Of all forms of epithelioma this is the one which is most frequent in relatively young people, and our efforts to deal with it should therefore be especially strenuous and persevering.

SECTION V

PART II

OPERATIONS UPON THE ŒSOPHAGUS

BY

C. H. FAGGE, M.S.(Lond.), F.R.C.S. (Eng.), Major R.A.M.C.(T.)
Assistant Surgeon to Guy's Hospital

CHAPTER VI

OPERATIONS UPON THE ŒSOPHAGUS

EXCISION OF ŒSOPHAGEAL DIVERTICULA

ŒSOPHAGEAL diverticula most commonly occur immediately below the level of the cricoid, at the junction of the pharynx with the œsophagus. They project from the posterior aspect of the œsophageal tube on the left side, and vary in length from a mere depression to a definite narrow-necked pouch several inches long. The lumen of the œsophagus is usually unaltered at the level of the pouch, though a definite constriction may be met with immediately below its orifice: a good example of this is reported and depicted by Richardson (*Ann. of Surg.,* May, 1900, p. 529). Halstead (*Ann. of Surg.,* 1904, vol. i, p. 192) has recorded a case in which the lower border of the neck of the diverticulum formed a valve-like projection into the lumen of the œsophagus, demonstrating one method by which obstruction to the natural passage is produced.

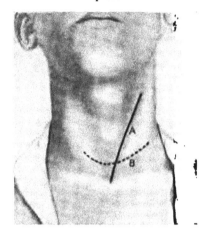

FIG. 255. INCISIONS FOR OPERATIONS UPON THE ŒSOPHAGUS IN THE NECK. A, Guattani's; B, Kocher's.

Examination with the X-rays is sometimes a useful preliminary to operation, as in a case of Landauer's (*Centralb. f. Inn. Med.,* April, 1899), where a photograph taken with leaden sounds passed into the pouch accurately indicated its situation. Or it may be possible after one or more doses of bismuth oxycarbonate to distend the pouch so that an X-ray photograph may be obtained.

Many cases have now been recorded of successful operations for this condition. Richardson (*loc. supra cit.,* p. 525) collected 56 cases, of which 18 had been dealt with by operation, viz. 16 by excision and 2 by Girard's method. Butlin (*Brit. Med. Journ.*, 1903, vol. ii, p. 65) published a second series of 8 cases, making 12 in all, of which he had operated on 8, and it is to the latter, who was the first surgeon in

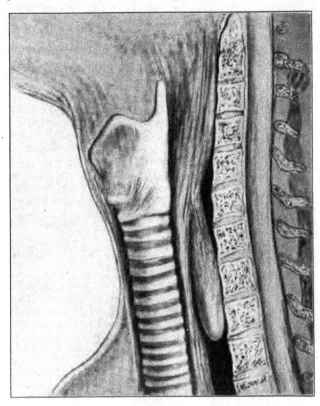

Fig. 256. An Œsophageal Diverticulum. This and the four following figures are from Richardson's paper in the *Annals of Surgery*.

England to undertake operation for this condition, that we are indebted for much of our knowledge relating to the symptomatology and to the indications for operation.

Operation. The patient is placed under the influence of a general anæsthetic, chloroform preceded by a hypodermic injection of morphine being the most suitable for such cases. A preliminary gastrostomy may then be carried out as recommended by Goldmann. An oblique incision is made along the anterior border of the left sternomastoid from the upper border of the thyreoid cartilage to the suprasternal notch (see Fig. 255, A). The deep cervical fascia is divided and the anterior jugular vein secured between ligatures, when the depressors of the hyoid bone are exposed. Of these the omo-hyoid is divided, while the sterno-hyoid

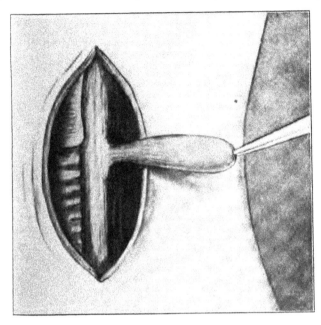

FIG. 257. EXCISION OF AN ŒSOPHAGEAL DIVERTICULUM.
(Richardson, *Annals of Surgery.*)

and sterno-thyreoid are retracted, or, if necessary, cut through as recommended by von Bergmann (*Arch. f. Klin. Chir.*, 1892, vol. xliii, p. 1). At the upper end of the wound the branches of the superior thyreoid artery are ligatured, and the dissection is carried deeply on the outer side of the thyreoid gland, which with the larynx is both drawn inwards and rotated on its long axis to the right: the carotid vessels are carefully defined and drawn outwards with a large blunt retractor. At this stage of the operation help in the definition of the diverticulum will be

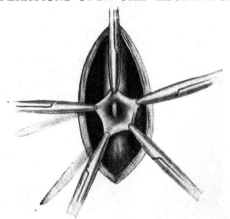

FIG. 258. REMOVAL OF THE DIVERTICULUM. The bougie is seen in the lumen of the œsophagus.

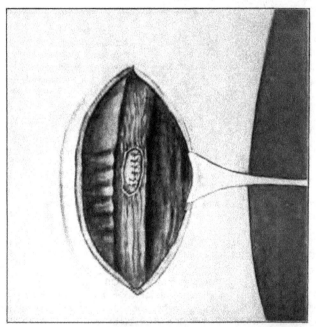

FIG. 259. SUTURE OF THE ŒSOPHAGUS AFTER EXCISION OF THE DIVERTICULUM. (Richardson, *Annals of Surgery*.)

obtained, as suggested by Butlin, by the passage of a curved pliable bougie into the diverticulum; also the œsophagus is defined, so as to avoid opening it inadvertently, by the passage of a long bougie from the mouth into the stomach.[1] Careful dissection should now expose the wall of the pouch lying to the left of the œsophageal tube, and traction upon it with forceps as it is separated from the other

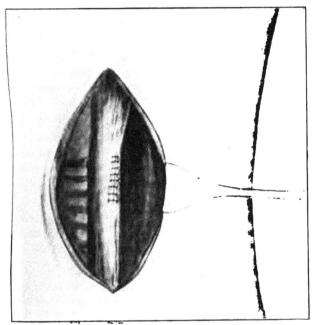

FIG. 260. EXCISION OF AN ŒSOPHAGEAL DIVERTICULUM. The operation completed. (Richardson, *Annals of Surgery*.)

tissues will enable the fundus to be drawn out of the wound, leaving the pouch connected with the œsophagus only by its neck. Butlin recommends that the pouch be now cut away at its neck from above downwards, and, as this is being done, the margins of the wound in the œsophagus be brought together by interrupted sutures. If these are inserted in a vertical row, so as to draw the lateral edges of the neck

---

[1] This may not be possible until the pouch has been freed and withdrawn from the wound, as the œsophagus is often pushed aside by a large distended diverticulum (Butlin).

of the pouch together, slight stenosis of the œsophagus at this level may result, so that when practicable it is better to cut gradually through the neck of the diverticulum transversely, and suture the upper to the lower margins of the incision, so as to form a transverse line of sutures upon the œsophageal wall.

In order to avoid opening the œsophagus and to eliminate the consequent risk of infecting the wound or of producing an œsophageal fistula, Girard of Berne twice invaginated the pouch into the œsophagus, and sutured the external aspect of its neck by three layers of sutures. This procedure was probably followed by atrophy of the pouch, as no obstruction resulted after these operations. Halstead (*loc. supra cit.*) treated a case by a somewhat similar method. The sac was isolated, and a purse-string suture of catgut was inserted around its neck. The sac was then invaginated into the œsophagus and the purse-string suture tightened. Over this three layers of sutures were inserted, the first two drawing together the longitudinal muscular layer of the œsophagus transversely, while the third layer, by which the lower fibres of the inferior constrictor were brought down so as to cover the œsophageal wound, was introduced at right angles to the first two layers of sutures. Halstead points out that this method is only adapted to diverticula of small size and to cases where the lumen of the œsophagus is not constricted at the level of the diverticulum. In cases where a constriction of the œsophagus is present immediately below the orifice of the diverticulum a more elaborate plastic operation may be necessary in order to overcome it. Richardson (*loc. supra cit.*) met with a case of this kind, and as he overcame the œsophageal stenosis by an ingenious plastic operation, a brief account in his own words may be here inserted :—

' The index-finger was passed carefully through the neck of the pouch into the œsophagus, and met with a constriction surrounded by friable mucous membrane. As this was done a longitudinal tear of this constricted portion resulted, and it was seen that the œsophagus below the opening had only the diameter of a lead pencil. The tear in the œsophagus was converted into a longitudinal slit by extending the incision downwards in the posterior wall through the lower border of the neck of the sac and through the constriction. The pouch was then cut off, leaving a considerable crescentic margin of its wall above the opening. The lower margins of this flap were then brought downwards and sutured together in the gap made by the divided posterior wall of the œsophagus. by which method the lumen of the œsophagus was slightly increased transversely. The subsequent effect of this plastic operation demonstrated its advantages, for afterwards the probang could be passed into the stomach without the least obstruction.'

Whatever method is adopted for suture of the œsophageal wall, there is great risk of leakage and infection of the cellular tissues of the neck, so that drainage should be provided in every case by the insertion either of a drainage tube or of gauze, packed right down to the external aspect of the œsophageal wound. The upper half of the wound in the neck may be closed with interrupted sutures, but the remainder of the wound must be left open for the purposes of drainage.[1] Butlin (*loc. supra cit.*), in dealing with this question, recommends that drainage with a soft tube should always be employed. He draws attention to the importance of opening up the cellular tissue of the neck as little as possible in the course of such an operation, owing to the risk of septic infection travelling downwards into the posterior mediastinum.

After-treatment. With regard to after-treatment, Butlin recommends that an œsophageal tube should be passed from the mouth into the stomach and retained for feeding purposes until the œsophageal wound is firmly closed. As a less desirable alternative a tube may be introduced into the stomach through the cervical wound, and retained until the wound is healing by granulation. Though in many of the recorded operations, as in Richardson's case quoted above, a temporary œsophageal fistula resulted, this eventually healed by granulation, and the patients are reported to have regained the power of normal deglutition without any evidences of constriction of the œsophagus at the site of the diverticulum.

CERVICAL ŒSOPHAGOTOMY

Indications. (i) For the removal of foreign bodies, usually large and irregular, such as tooth-plates, which have passed easily through the pharynx only to become impacted at or within a short distance of the upper end of the œsophagus. Killian (*Zeitschrift für Ohrenheilk.*, 1908, vol. l, p. 120) states that in his experience it is at this level that foreign bodies are usually retained, unless they are soft and smooth and glide easily. Should a foreign body pass the upper orifice of the œsophagus, it will probably readily traverse the mediastinal portion of the tube, which is easily dilatable, yet may become fixed within 2 inches of the cardiac orifice.

(ii) For the excision of benign œsophageal growths, *e.g.* polypi, when removal by the snare, aided by œsophagoscopy, is impossible.

---

[1] Cellulitis is less probable than after operation for foreign body when it is due to already existing infection (Richardson).

(iii) For the division of deeply situated fibrous structures of the œsophagus, which Gussenbauer has undertaken by this method.

(iv) For the suture and drainage of external wounds, stabs, and bullet wounds.

Œsophagoscopy, as introduced by Mikulicz, under cocaine in adults or a general anæsthetic in children, will enable a surmise as to the localization of an impacted foreign body founded on the symptoms and the position of pain to be confirmed, and through Killian's tube the large majority of smooth regular foreign bodies, e.g. coins, may be removed by long suitably curved forceps. This method of examination is, however, contra-indicated when severe pain in the neck, rise of temperature, and subcutaneous emphysema are present, suggesting that the foreign body has perforated the œsophageal wall; it is also inadvisable and may be impossible when secondary inflammation, possibly increased by ineffectual attempts at removal of the foreign body with a probang or coin-catcher, has extended to the larynx, causing dyspnœa which may urgently call for œsophagotomy.

Coins, tooth-plates, or any body partially composed of material opaque to X-rays may be localized in the œsophagus by radiography, and comparison of plates exposed at intervals of twenty-four hours will yield valuable evidence that the foreign body has either become impacted or is being steadily carried on towards the stomach. Gentle passage of a bougie will, when the aids to diagnosis mentioned above are not available, indicate at what level the foreign body is lodged, though on meeting with any obstruction the bougie must be at once withdrawn, as the use of force may cause a rigid sharp foreign body to penetrate the œsophageal wall.

Œsophagotomy is indicated for the removal of a foreign body which is seen by radiography or through Killian's tube to be large and irregular, as removal with forceps is likely to lacerate the œsophagus, when there will be great risk of cellulitis of the neck.

Œsophagotomy is imperative when symptoms of perforation of the œsophagus are present, e.g. intense pain at the seat of perforation, rise of temperature, and subcutaneous cervical emphysema; here, as pointed out above, the passage of Killian's tubes or forceps either for purposes of diagnosis or treatment is likely to make matters worse. Operation must be quickly undertaken, and the infected cellular tissues of the neck must be freely opened up, and if possible the point of perforation must be discovered. With this object in view it is best to leave the foreign body in situ, and to cut down upon it by an incision either on the right or left side as may seem most convenient after consideration of an X-ray photograph; in such cases suture of the œsophageal wall is inadvisable, and the superficial wound must be packed with gauze and drained. The prognosis under such conditions is more favourable when the perforation is situated high up in the cervical part than when it is in the mediastinal portion.

Before operating it is well to make certain by a second X-ray examination that the foreign body is impacted, as it is remarkable that many irregular foreign bodies, such as tooth-plates, with sharp projections upon them, may pass through the entire alimentary canal without danger to the patient. Lediard (*Clin. Soc. Trans.*, vol. xviii, p. 297) conscientiously records a case in which œsophagotomy was performed for a tooth-plate thought to be impacted below the thyreoid cartilage. An œsophageal tube was passed into the stomach, which was thought to impinge upon the plate as it was withdrawn. As the patient was still unable to swallow water, cervical œsophagotomy was performed, and a bougie was passed from the wound into the stomach. When this was done the operator ' believed that the plate was felt near the cardiac orifice of the stomach, but without giving the impression that the plate had been pushed into the stomach.' The plate appeared at the anus nineteen days from the date of impaction.

Similarly in the writer's practice examination of a five months' old baby detected a safety-pin brooch just below the level of the cricoid. Extraction with forceps was impossible, but a later examination with the X-rays showed that the brooch had passed into the stomach, and a week later the brooch, widely open, was passed without injury to the child.

At the same time all writers upon this subject have insisted that œsophagotomy, to give good results, must be promptly undertaken when other means of extraction have failed. The conclusion arrived at by Dr. Church (*St. Bartholomew's Hospital Reports*, vol. xix, p. 67), ' that there is very little risk in the operation itself, and that a good result may be fairly expected if the operation is done shortly after the foreign body becomes impacted,' still accurately defines the position.

Hæmorrhage, ulceration, and suppuration extending under the cervical fascia into the posterior mediastinum are likely to be early complications of impaction of a foreign body, and when septic infection of the tissues around the œsophagus has ensued, operation becomes a much graver matter.

Jacobson (*Operations of Surgery*, vol. i, p. 724), in discussing the question as to how low down in the œsophagus a foreign body can be extracted by cervical œsophagotomy, points out that the most accessible part is at its junction with the pharynx, opposite the cricoid cartilage, and for the first two inches below this point. In his knowledge the lowest point from which a foreign body has been removed by cervical œsophagotomy occurred in the practice of Mr. Bennet May. Here a halfpenny, which had ulcerated through the œsophagus and opened the right bronchus, was removed successfully by œsophagotomy.

Fullerton (*Brit. Med. Journ.*, 1904) extracted by cervical œsophagotomy a halfpenny which was shown by the Röntgen rays to lie opposite the third and fourth thoracic vertebræ. At the operation it lay 4½ inches below the opening in the œsophagus, to which it was drawn up by a bent probe.

Richardson (*Lancet*, 1887, vol. ii, p. 707) contends that all portions of the œsophagus are in the cadaver accessible either from above or below, for he states that if the left fore and middle fingers are introduced through the cardia by means of a gastrotomy, and passed upwards into the œsophagus, they can be touched by the right forefinger introduced from above by a cervical œsophagotomy. Richardson points out that the lowest three inches of the œsophagus are just within the range of gastrotomy. He says that the right forefinger, introduced through the cervical wound, cannot reach quite so far on account of the sternum and clavicle. He therefore argues that, if the obstruction be less than 6 inches from the cricoid, an attempt may be made to remove it from above, but if the distance is more than this gastrotomy should be performed.

The writer's experiments on the cadaver do not at all coincide with Professor Richardson's conclusions, as in his experience at least two, and usually three, inches of the mid-thoracic portion of the œsophagus cannot be explored by the methods detailed above. And further, it is well to realize, as Richardson himself points out, that deductions drawn from the cadaver by no means hold good in dealing with the living subject.

Operation. The head is extended over a sand-bag placed under the lower cervical vertebræ, the face turned to the right, and an incision is made over the lowest part of the left anterior triangle. This may be either an oblique incision along the anterior border of the left sterno-mastoid, 4 inches long, terminating below at the upper border of the sternum (Guattani's incision) (see Fig. 261, A) ; or, as recommended by Kocher, a rather longer curved incision, convex downwards, so placed in the line of cleavage of the skin of the neck that it crosses the mid-line an inch above the sternum (see Fig. 261, B). The superficial fascia, platysma, and deep fascia are divided in the line of the skin incision, when the anterior jugular vein is divided between two catgut ligatures if necessary. The sterno-mastoid is drawn outwards, and the omo-hyoid being divided, the sterno-hyoid and sterno-thyreoid muscles are retracted inwards. The pretracheal layer of deep cervical fascia, from which the capsule of the thyreoid gland is derived, must now be freely opened, the gland itself being drawn inwards, and the structures within the carotid sheath held as far outwards as possible by the same retractor that controls the sterno-mastoid. The lateral surface of the trachea is now defined, when the anterior surface of the œsophagus will be seen lying behind it, and projecting rather more to the left.

Difficulty in identifying the œsophagus may be overcome by the recognition of its red muscular wall or by distending it with a bougie introduced from the mouth. At this stage of the operation careful dissection with a Durham's elevator is necessary to isolate and avoid the recurrent laryngeal nerve and the inferior thyreoid artery, which pass upwards across the œsophagus from without inwards to lie in the groove between this structure and the trachea. These, after identification, may be drawn downwards and inwards, or if unavoidable the artery may be divided between ligatures.[1] Should the foreign body be impacted at this level, it can now be felt lying behind the cricoid or the upper rings of the trachea, and its location will determine the level of the incision to be made for its extraction: this

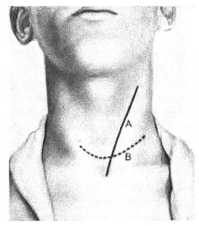

Fig. 261. Incisions for Operations upon Œsophagus in the Neck. A, Guattani's; B, Kocher's.

must be vertical, and, if the foreign body be within the field of operation, should be rather placed above than immediately over the foreign body. When the latter cannot be felt, a longitudinal incision 2 inches long, placed as far back as possible upon the œsophageal wall, so as to avoid the recurrent laryngeal nerve, is made upon the end of the bougie which has been withdrawn, and so manipulated as to distend the œsophagus at this point.

Bleeding from the muscular tissue of the œsophagus, which is at

[1] It may be easier to dislodge the recurrent laryngeal nerve outwards, as in Mr. Lawson's case quoted below.

first free, is controlled by Spencer Wells's forceps, which serve as retractors to keep open the incision in its wall.

It will now usually be possible to remove the foreign body with long curved forceps if within three or four inches of the opening. But it is well to bear in mind that the very foreign bodies which defeat attempts at their removal through the mouth are, owing to their irregularities, often firmly impacted in the walls of the tube. The greatest care must be exercised in avoiding injury to the œsophageal wall, and when the foreign body is embedded at both ends in the mucosa it may require division with cutting forceps before it can be dislodged.

Mr. George Lawson (*Clin. Soc. Trans.*, vol. xviii, p. 292) records an instructive case of removal of a tooth-plate impacted in the œsophagus. Œsophagotomy was performed, but the plate was so firmly fixed into the wall of the œsophagus by the sharp clips which had retained it in the mouth that it required division with bone-forceps before its removal was possible.

When a clean incision has been made in the œsophagus, and there is no reason to suppose that its walls have been damaged by the foreign body or during its extraction, the margins of the wound should be brought together with interrupted catgut sutures, so passed as not to include its mucous lining. The deeper parts of the wound must now be carefully dried, and the cut surfaces of the omo-hyoid brought together. Sutures should also be inserted so as to bring together the fascial layers of the upper two thirds of the wound, the lower third being left open for a drainage tube passed right down to the surface of the œsophagus. This will occupy the lower angle of the skin incision, which otherwise should be brought together with sutures.

Difficulties. The chief of these are: a short neck in a fat subject; an enlarged thyreoid gland; cellulitis or suppuration already present. Firm impaction of the foreign body may increase the danger of laceration or perforation of the œsophagus, or the foreign body may be beyond the reach of the longest available forceps.

After-treatment. Rectal feeding is to be carried out for the first forty-eight hours, though sufficient water to ally thirst may be given by the mouth from the first. Should there be no tendency for fluids taken by the mouth to escape through the wound, enemata may be replaced by milk, meat juice, and other fluids given by the mouth, and at the end of the first week the patient may be allowed to take semi-solids. Kocher recommends that the patient be fed through a soft œsophageal tube passed from the wound and retained in position, and Lawson, quoted above, left his wound completely unsutured, and fed the patient for three weeks through an œsophageal tube. In discussing the desirability of suturing the œsophagus he draws attention to the irritation of the wound which results from the constant flow of saliva over it, and which may, as in his case, produce some local cellulitis.

Dangers. The chief immediate danger is septic infection of the tissues of the neck owing to leakage from the œsophagus, sometimes resulting in mediastinitis or septicæmia. This may be best avoided by the establishment of drainage in all doubtful cases.

CERVICAL ŒSOPHAGOSTOMY

Indications. The establishment of a permanent opening into the œsophagus may be undertaken as a palliative operation for the relief of dysphagia due to obstruction from—

(i) An epitheliomatous growth at the junction of the œsophagus with the pharynx; or

(ii) Cicatricial stenosis, the result of syphilitic or traumatic ulceration at the same level.

At the present time this operation has fallen into disuse and has been replaced by gastrostomy, owing (1) to the greater difficulty of cervical œsophagostomy and the danger of injury to important structures, such as the recurrent laryngeal nerve; (2) the difficulty of making the artificial orifice so far below the growth that it may not become involved at a later date; (3) the constant discomfort to the patient from saliva flowing over the wound, and the risk of local infection of the cellular tissue from this source.

Operation. This is carried out exactly as has been detailed above in the performance of cervical œsophagotomy, but after the œsophagus has been opened its margins are secured to the edges of the skin wound with numerous interrupted sutures, or a rubber tube is inserted and the wound packed with gauze.

After-treatment. The after-treatment is similar, except that on the cessation of rectal alimentation fluids are passed into the stomach through a long œsophageal tube passed downwards from the wound.

CERVICAL ŒSOPHAGECTOMY

Indications. (i) This operation may be called for for the removal of a localized growth in the cervical portion of the œsophagus.

(ii) It may have to be undertaken as part of the operation of laryngectomy when a malignant growth primarily affecting the larynx has involved the œsophagus.

(iii) It has also been carried out when the œsophagus has been found involved in malignant tumours of the thyreoid gland.

In this article operation for cases of primary epithelioma of the œsophagus alone will be considered, and when the comparatively large number of conditions requiring partial œsophagectomy as part of a larger operation are excluded, it will be found to have a very narrow application. For clinically it is true that by the time that the cardinal symptom of œsophageal malignant disease, dysphagia, is so marked as to cause the patient to come for treatment the growth is so extensive that the whole lumen of the tube is usually involved for so considerable a distance that its radical removal is impossible.

Acting upon experiments made by Billroth on dogs, Kapper made two unsuccessful attempts to carry out the operation in 1875-6, but it was not until 1887 that the operation was successfully performed, when Czerny removed 6 centimetres of the whole circumference of the œsophagus for carcinoma.

Operation. A gastrostomy should be done as a preliminary to resection of the œsophagus, so that the patient may be built up, and also to prevent wound soiling about resected area. The cervical portion of the œsophagus is exposed by the same method as has been detailed for œsophagotomy (see Fig. 261), but it will often be necessary to divide the left sterno-hyoid and sterno-thyreoid muscles, as well as the omo-hyoid. When the œsophagus is reached, its posterior aspect is freely detached from the prevertebral structures with a blunt dissector, after which it will usually be possible to locate the growth and to define its limits: if, however, this cannot be done, it may be necessary to open the œsophagus for this purpose. Careful dissection is necessary to separate the trachea from the anterior œsophageal wall, and in doing this great caution must be exercised, so as to avoid injury to the recurrent laryngeal nerves on both sides. When the whole circumference of the œsophagus has been isolated, it is cut through at least half an inch below the growth, and when there is any doubt as to the exact level to which it is involved it will be wise to sacrifice additional tissue in order to render recurrence less probable, even though by doing so greater difficulty will be experienced in carrying out the later stages of the operation. The whole circumference of the œsophagus is now isolated and the ring-like portion occupied by the growth removed by dividing the œsophagus well above and below the growth.

If the œsophagus has, as is always desirable, been divided so wide of the growth that recurrence is unlikely, it is almost always impossible to restore the œsophageal channel, and therefore it is often necessary to bring the cut ends to the surface. Great difficulty may be experienced in suturing the lower end to the skin, both on account of its shortness and of the fact that the sutures are not well held by the œsophageal wall.

Butlin (*Operative Surgery of Malignant Disease*, p. 223) points out that even when this can be done stenosis of the œsophageal fistulous opening is extremely likely; whereas when the œsophagus cannot be drawn to the level of the skin stenosis is inevitable. Kocher suggests the employment of a rubber tube, retained in position during the cicatrization of the wound, but even this is unlikely to prevent stenosis.

Results. De Quervain, in 1899, collected fourteen cases in which portions of the œsophagus had been removed, and though several of these were complicated by implication of adjacent important structures, such as the pharynx, larynx, thyreoid gland, &c., the immediate mortality from hæmorrhage, shock, posterior mediastinitis, and septic pneumonia in five cases shows that the immediate risks are excessively grave. In addition to this, recurrence rapidly followed in six of the other cases, and none of these survived the operation more than thirteen months. Further, it must be remembered that the patient's life, even if prolonged for a few months by such an operation, is one of considerable discomfort, owing to the extreme probability of stenosis of the œsophageal opening in the neck, which must render the life of the patient one of great misery. Difficulty may also arise in connexion with the upper end of the œsophagus, where a salivary fistula is likely to form, which, as in a case reported by de Quervain, tends to close and to cause infection of the cellular tissues, so that repeated dilatation with bougies may be necessary for this also.

OPERATIONS UPON THORACIC ŒSOPHAGUS

At the outset a number of problems confront the surgeon in resection of the thoracic œsophagus for carcinoma. The fact that after fifteen years of work by such men as Sauerbruch, Mikulicz, Rehn, Torek, Willy Meyer, and others, but one successful resection has been reported is sufficient evidence of the operative difficulties that present themselves.

The diffidence which surgeons feel in attacking a carcinoma of the thoracic œsophagus has been due to the unsatisfactory solution of these problems. Exploration of the pleural sac has only within very recent years been frequently attempted. Operative shock has been extremely high. Until the advent of intra-tracheal insufflation in 1909 there was no satisfactory method of maintaining differential pressure save by the cumbersome chamber of Sauerbruch. No really satisfactory method of uniting the proximal stump with the stomach has been devised. Lastly, carcinoma is the usual indication for the operation, and most cases coming to the surgeon are so far advanced as to be beyond the stage of positive cure.

There are two methods of approach to the thoracic œsophagus: the trans-mediastinal route and the trans-pleural route. The trans-mediastinal route as suggested by Ach and Rehn, while not much used at present, still has its adherents. The chief object of this route has been the avoidance of the pleural sac. Nevertheless accidental opening of the pleura has been the catastrophe most feared in this operation, and has been the commonest cause of death, either through pulmonary collapse or suppurative pleuritis.

The second and usual method of approach is the trans-pleural route. This method has been made possible by the use of intra-tracheal insufflation first suggested by Meltzer and Auer. Since it is now possible for every clinic to possess a relatively simple apparatus for maintaining positive intra-pulmonary pressure in the open chest, the trans-pleural route is by far the better of the two. First, it offers by far the best means of exposure of the entire thoracic cavity; second, it is a most ideal means of respiratory control.

TRANS-MEDIASTINAL OPERATIONS UPON THE ŒSOPHAGUS

ŒSOPHAGOTOMY

Indications. The indications for œsophagotomy are:—

(i) The presence of a foreign body so fixed within the thoracic portion of the œsophagus that it cannot be removed through Killian's tube, and at such a level that it cannot be reached either from above by cervical œsophagotomy or from below by gastrotomy.

The exact localization of an impacted foreign body or of a malignant stricture within this tube is now more definite, owing to the increasing use of Killian's method of œsophagoscopy, and in many cases of foreign bodies help may be obtained by means of an X-ray photograph.

If Richardson's deductions (see p. 532) from his experiments on the cadaver are correct, it is clear that mediastinal œsophagotomy for the removal of foreign bodies has very little place in surgery, as the dangers and difficulties of this operation far outweigh those of cervical œsophagotomy or of gastrotomy. But it seems probable that mediastinal œsophagotomy would be necessary for the removal of a foreign body impacted between a point 4 inches below the cricoid and a point 2½ inches above the cardiac orifice, that is, more than 10 and less than 12½ inches from the teeth. It is fortunate that this, the least accessible portion of the œsophagus, corresponding to the bodies of the fourth, fifth, and sixth dorsal vertebræ, is very rarely indeed the site of impaction of a foreign body, for, as pointed out above, if it passes the narrow portion of the tube opposite the cricoid it will usually pass freely down to the level of the diaphragm.

(ii) The removal of a benign œsophageal growth, *e.g.* polypus.

The steps of the operation are those of the first stages of œsophagectomy (*vide infra*).

ŒSOPHAGECTOMY

Indications. This operation may rarely be required for the removal of œsophageal epithelioma, and has been carried out by this route by Rehn and others: hitherto no successful case has been recorded, but it is well to reserve judgment on the value of these procedures, as the surgery of the mediastina is still in its infancy.

The technique of these operations was first described by Nasiloff in 1880, and his method was adopted by Quénu and Hartmann in 1891. Nasiloff suggests that the upper part of the œsophagus is more easily reached on the left side, but on the right in the lower part of its course; while Potarca, after carefully studying the technique, advocated operation upon the right side only because of the danger and difficulty of dealing with the aorta on the left, though the way in which the right pleura naturally dips behind the œsophagus makes damage of this structure more likely when an operation is carried out on the right side. Rehn, in performing this operation on the living subject, followed Potarca's route through the right thoracic wall. Bryant (*Trans. of Amer. Surg. Assoc.*, 1895) states that the œsophagus should only be attacked on the left side above the aortic arch; below this point he exposes it on the right, and considers that below the ninth dorsal vertebra it is not accessible to surgical interference.

Clinical experience has shown that cases of œsophageal malignant growth which can be dealt with radically by excision of the growth very rarely occur. Sauerbruch (*Verhandl. d. Deutsch. Ges. f. Chir.*, 1905, vol. xxxiv, p. 140), after experimental operations upon dogs, is of opinion that the anatomical conditions in man are more favourable than in these animals. The results of operation would also be influenced by the nature of the obstruction, especially if it were carcinomatous. Statistics usually divide œsophageal carcinoma into that of the upper, median, and lower third of the œsophagus. From an investigation of 17,000 post-mortem inspections at Breslau, he found that during twenty-two years 204 were carcinoma of the œsophagus, 26 being in the cervical portion, and 163 in the thoracic portion, exclusive of the cardia. Of the latter, 117 were between the hilus of the lung and the cardia, 3 involved the entire œsophagus, and in 12 the site was not stated. Thus, out of 192 cases of carcinoma, 117, that is to say 60%, were favourable for operation, at least so far as position was concerned, and 70, that is 36%, were absolutely favourable, as Sauerbruch's invagination operation was possible. The results are naturally influenced by the general condition of the patient, and above all by the presence of adhesions or metastases. He points out, however, that pathological anatomy and statistics indicate that metastases occur comparatively late in œsophageal carcinoma, but when they do occur are very numerous and affect the posterior mediastinal glands, so that operative interference is of very little use.

Operation. The patient is anæsthetized, and placed in the semi-prone position on the left side. A longitudinal incision 8 inches long is made midway between the spines of the vertebræ and the inner border of the right scapula (see Fig. 262). This is carried down to the ribs, and a rectangular flap, fashioned by carrying horizontal incisions from the two ends of the vertical incision inwards to the mid-line, is reflected inwards. The exposed ribs are resected subperiosteally within the limits of the wound, 2 to 3 inches being removed from each. Heidenhain points out that easier access to the posterior mediastinum may be obtained by resecting the transverse processes of the corresponding vertebræ, and completely removing the posterior portion of the ribs from the heads outwards. Kocher considers that it is usually necessary to resect more than four ribs, the second to the seventh or the fourth to the ninth according to the situation of the disease, and advises that 4 inches of these ribs be resected subperiosteally.

Sauerbruch ('Die Chirurgie des Brustteils der Speiseröhre,' *Beiträge zur klinischen Chirurgie,* 1905, vol. xlvi, p. 405) recommends as an alternative a long intercostal incision, as giving adequate room and avoiding severe hæmorrhage and damage to nerves and muscles: its chief disadvantage would appear to be that it entails manipulation of the deeply seated œsophagus through a narrow wound; this may be partly avoided by the use of Mikulicz's rib-retractor.

After dividing the intercostal muscles the intercostal vessels and nerves must be defined, and the former divided between ligatures. The parietal pleura should now be freely exposed, and its attachments over the heads of the ribs and upon the lateral surfaces of the vertebræ carefully separated outwards with the finger or with a blunt instrument. In doing this it must be remembered that the sympathetic chain passes down over the heads of the ribs, and great care must be taken to avoid this structure.

As the posterior surface of the œsophagus is exposed, the vena azygos major, with the right vagus, comes into view, and the latter must be pulled aside and the vein ligatured. The œsophagus, unless adherent to surrounding structures, can now by further careful dissection be drawn into the wound, and if the operation has been undertaken for the removal of a foreign body it should now be possible to locate it. For the purpose of its removal the œsophageal wall is incised, and the foreign body removed; in doing this branches of the vagi must be carefully avoided. If it be necessary to excise a portion of the œsophageal wall for

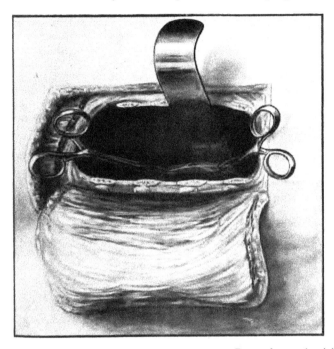

FIG. 262. TRANS-MEDIASTINAL ŒSOPHAGECTOMY. Parts of seventh, eighth, ninth, and tenth right ribs resected; œsophagus pulled up with Spencer Wells's forceps.

the removal of a malignant tumour, this may now be done, when both ends of the œsophagus must be drawn into the wound, and drained by means of rubber tubes carefully sutured in position. The lower end of the œsophagus may be used for feeding purposes, and for this a long œsophageal tube should be passed through it down into the stomach. Or if, owing to its depth from the surface of the thoracic wall, this be considered impracticable, gastrostomy should be undertaken.

Mikulicz (*Deutsch. Med. Wochenschrift*, April 14, 1904) drew atten-

tion to the difficulty of reuniting the two ends after resection in the following words: ' The straight muscular tube which we call the œsophagus
is but little stretchable; hence, even simple division and reuniting of the
cut ends is not easily accomplished, as the œsophagus is slightly shortened thereby, and the consequent tension is apt to cause the divided ends
to retract. In resections, of course, this difficulty is far greater.'

He pointed out that resection of the lower portion is far easier than
resection of the upper portion of the œsophagus, for the reason that in
the former the cardiac portion, as well as the fundus of the stomach, can
be drawn up through the enlarged orifice in the diaphragm sufficiently
to allow it to be sutured to the upper part of the tube so as to make
up for the defect caused by the resection. Again, different operations
are required in his opinion for resections in these positions, for in resection of the upper thoracic portion of the œsophagus he recommends posterior thoracotomy in the third to the fifth intercostal spaces. Here
the tube is exposed behind the hilum of the lung, and the vena azygos
major, which crosses the œsophagus at this level, must be pushed aside
or may require to be doubly ligatured after division.

Although it is feasible to stretch the two ends of the resected œsophagus so as to perform an anastomosis, it was, in his opinion, doubtful
whether the sutures would hold on account of tension. Mikulicz, therefore, no longer attempted to reunite the œsophagus after high resections,
but closed the gastric end and dropped it back into the wound, and the
patient was fed by means of a gastrostomy previously carried out. The
pharyngeal end of the œsophagus was pulled out through an incision
made along the anterior border of the left sterno-mastoid, which, as he
stated, is easily done because it is only loosely held by connective tissue
at this level; the wounds in the thorax and neck were now closed, and
the upper end of the œsophagus was drawn downwards under a bridge
of skin and fixed to a new incision over the second intercostal space after
the manner of a Frank's gastrostomy: von Mikulicz intended to unite
this latter to the stomach so that mouth-feeding might be again possible.
For resection of a growth in the lower end of the œsophagus anterior
intercostal thoracotomy in the fifth or sixth space was recommended.

Up to 1905 three resections carried out in Sauerbruch's chamber at
the Breslau Clinic had ended fatally, and this writer (*Journal of Amer.
Med. Assoc.*, Sept., 1908) says that he has employed this method in nine
fatal cases.

Sauerbruch (*München. Med. Wochenschr.*, 1906, vol. liii, p. 1) has
further elaborated the methods of operation by experiments on dogs.
These experiments and five operations performed on the human being for
the resection of œsophageal carcinomata were all carried out under

negative thoracic pressure within his pneumatic chamber (see Fig. 263). The incision was placed over the fifth or seventh intercostal space, and was followed by removal of the adjacent ribs or their temporary resection. The pleura was widely opened and the growth exposed after the vagi had been carefully isolated.

Experimentally Sauerbruch has devised two operations, which will be indicated under different conditions. In the first an œsophagogastrostomy with a Murphy's button is performed, after which the

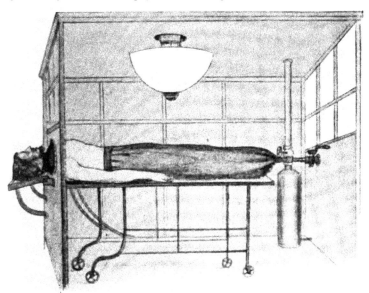

FIG. 263. SAUERBRUCH'S CHAMBER. By permission of Dr. Sauerbruch.

required portion of the œsophagus is resected. In the second operation, especially suitable for growths near the cardiac end of the œsophagus, the affected portion of this tube is invaginated into the stomach, and secured in this position by sutures connecting the circumference of the œsophagus above the growth to the stomach-wall. At a second operation gastrostomy is performed, and the invaginated portion of the œsophagus bearing the malignant tumour is excised.

Of the first five operations performed by Sauerbruch, all of which ended fatally, two cases, in which inoperable carcinoma was present, were complicated by perforation of the malignant growth, owing to which an empyema resulted, with death in fourteen days; in a third case the cause of death was undiscovered. A fourth operation consisted in resection of the lower portion of the œsophagus for carcinoma of the cardia. In a fifth case, in which there was a large tumour of the cardia, resection was abandoned owing to the general condition of the patient, and anastomosis performed, the patient dying twenty-four hours after the operation. Sauerbruch states that during the entire intrapleural operation the pulse and respiration remained normal.

Dangers and difficulties. *Hæmorrhage.* During the resection of the thoracic wall this will be severe, and must be dealt with by promptly seizing all bleeding points with Spencer Wells's forceps; the intercostal arteries must be taken up and ligatured before they are divided. Bleeding from one of the venæ azygoi or from a tributary may be troublesome on account of the depth of the wound, and in securing these with forceps care must be exercised that only the bleeding vessel is taken up; otherwise damage to important structures, such as the thoracic duct or the vagi, may result.

Injury to the Pleura. This is by far the most important danger of these trans-mediastinal operations, and the risks of injury to the right pleura will be appreciated when it is borne in mind that it is necessary for the patient to lie in the semi-prone position on the left side, so that while movements of the left lung are impaired entry of air into the right pleura may be followed by an immediately fatal issue. For this reason von Mikulicz made use of Sauerbruch's negative air-pressure chamber, and his example has been followed by the general use of a similar apparatus in the performance of such operations.

This chamber (see Fig. 263) is large enough to receive five persons if required, and in it the operator works at a negative air-pressure of 3 to 5 millimetres of mercury, which is increased to 7 or 8 mm. towards the close of the operation. According to Sauerbruch, opinion is now in favour of decreasing the thoracic pressure, the bronchial pressure remaining normal, as opposed to the alternative of increasing the pressure within the lungs while the thoracic cavity is exposed to normal atmospheric pressure as is done in most physiological experiments. (For further interesting details see Sauerbruch, ' Zur Pathologie des offenen Pneumothorax und die Grundlage meines Verfahrens zu seiner Ausschaltung.' *Mitteilungen aus den Grenzgebieten der Medizin und Chirurgie*, 1904, vol. xiii, p. 461.)

Empyema and infection of the mediastinal cellular tissues. Avoidance of injury to the pleura and drainage in all cases are the best means of avoiding the above, but it must be borne in mind in estimating the risks of these operations that the pleura has little of the tendency so favourably exercised by the peritoneum of limiting infection by the rapid formation of adhesions, so that even when drainage is employed infection may be carried in from without and an empyema may result.

Modifications. Several ingenious plastic operations have been devised in order to obviate the discomfort of a permanent gastric fistula after resection of the œsophagus, and of these the following are the most suggestive.

Roux (*Sem. Méd.*, January 23, 1907) operated upon a child suffering from simple stenosis of the œsophagus which had resisted all attempts at mechanical dilatation. He freed a sufficiently long portion of the jejunum, and ligatured four to five arteries leading to it at suitable distances from the intestine. Owing to the conditions of vascular supply in the jejunum the blood was not cut off from it, but was received from the vasa recta. The portion of intestine was sufficiently long to be brought to the abdominal wound. The anal end of the portion of jejunum was inserted into the wall of the stomach, the upper end being drawn out of the abdominal wound. The skin of the thorax was then undermined from a longitudinal incision over the upper end of the sternum, and the portion of jejunum drawn through the cutaneous bridge from the abdominal wound to the wound above. The twisted end of the jejunum was sutured to the skin in the thoracic wound, and nourishment given through an œsophageal tube. There was always good pulsation in the arteries supplying the jejunum. The abdominal fascia and rectus abdominis were slightly cut so as to allow plenty of room for the passage of the intestine, and the skin wound was closed. The result was favourable, the portion of intestine being seen to contract under the skin, and there was no difficulty in suturing the œsophagus to the upper end of the portion of jejunum at a later operation.

In carcinoma of the œsophagus Bircher (*Centralb. f. Chir.*, 1907, vol. xxxiv, p. 1479) devised another procedure, in order to restore the defect in the alimentary canal by forming an artificial œsophagus. He performed the operation in a very emaciated woman with stenosis of the œsophagus 31 centimetres below the teeth : the patient's history pointed to the presence of carcinoma. Two parallel skin incisions were made, from the submaxillary region to the costal margin, that on the left being somewhat outside the median line, while the right one lay just inside the nipple line. The margins of this median strip of skin were turned over and united by interrupted sutures, forming a tube covered internally by epidermis. The skin on each side of the turned-over portion was undermined and the edges approximated and sutured over this tube, so that it was covered completely by skin, and had an opening only above and below.

Three days later the patency of the tube was tested, and it was found to allow of the passage of a very large stream of water. Some suppuration occurred, and a sinus formed over the clavicle, leading into the newly formed œsophagus, and six weeks later there was a gastric fistula, the margins of which were adherent to the lower opening of the skin tube. Secondary sutures were therefore placed in the newly formed tube near the clavicle, and the skin over the fistula sutured. The stricture in the œsophageal tube was impermeable. A week later thin fluid nourishment was introduced into the artificial œsophagus from above, and entered the stomach without difficulty. The external skin sutures over the tube had to be removed owing to tension, the sutures around the fistula between the stomach and artificial œsophagus being well retained. Three days later pulmonary embolism occurred, terminating fatally. *Post-mortem examination* showed that the sutures were not retained at some points in the artificial œsophagus, and that there were small openings through which water flowed. Death was due to carcinoma of the œsophagus, mesentery, and uterus, embolism of the right pulmonary artery, œdema of the lung, and degeneration of the heart. In another case in which the procedure was employed the patient also succumbed to intercurrent complications. Failing this, definite closure of the wound might have been obtained by secondary operation and union have been established with the œsophagus, so that an artificial œsophagus would have been formed from skin. Bircher thinks that though peristalsis could not be obtained in the artificial tube, fluids would easily pass through it, and he believes that eventually it might be possible to form an artificial œsophagus in this way, especially if strict asepsis were maintained.

ŒSOPHAGO-PLICATION

Reisinger (*Verhandl. d. Deutsch. Ges. f. Chir.,* 1907, vol. xxxvi, p. 86) performed the following operation on a patient in whom dilatation of the œsophagus was diagnosed :—

The X-rays showed that almost the entire thoracic portion of the œsophagus was enormously dilated. The posterior mediastinum was opened from the right side, according to the method of Rehn, Nasiloff, and Bryant. A flap of skin and muscle was formed, with its base upon the spinous processes of the third to the eighth thoracic vertebræ, and its apex extending to the median border of the scapula. Portions of the fourth to the seventh ribs, 6 to 7 centimetres in length, were resected, the intercostal musculature removed, and the pleura loosened from the vertebral column. Practically the entire thoracic portion of the œsophagus was laid bare, carefully avoiding injury to the neighbouring structures, especially the pleura, and the œsophagus was seen as an enormously dilated thick-walled tube. An attempt was made to carry out œsophago-plication by folding the tube longitudinally so as to reduce its calibre, but the collapsed condition of the patient rendered it necessary to interrupt the operation. A few weeks later the œsophagus was freed from its adhesions, and narrowed by cutting away a longitudinal strip of its wall, and subsequently suturing the aperture in the tube by two rows of sutures. The strip removed was 15 centimetres in length, and varied in width from 2 to 3 centimetres. Considerable improvement in the condition of the patient resulted from the operation, and he was able to take solid and fluid nourishment without pain or any feeling of oppression.

TRANS-PLEURAL OPERATIONS UPON THE ŒSOPHAGUS

The only successful case of resection of the œsophagus has been reported by Torek. He succeeded in resecting a carcinoma by a trans-pleural œsophagectomy. The operation was done under intra-tracheal insufflation.

Intra-tracheal insufflation consists in introducing ether vapour under a tension of 20 to 30 mm. into the main bronchus by means of a tracheal catheter inserted down to the bifurcation. The apparatus consists essentially of an air pump, an apparatus for vapourizing ether, and a tracheal catheter connected to the latter by means of a rubber tubing. The entire apparatus is very simple. After the patient has been anæsthetized in the usual manner, the catheter is introduced by means of a Jackson laryngoscope.

The patient is now put in position for the operation. Both Richter and Torek emphasize the importance of approach from the right side where the lesion is in the upper portion of the œsophagus. Torek points out the fact that the œsophagus stands out more prominently on the right than on the left, because the right pleura partly covers it and the aorta is not in the way. But Torek also draws attention to the fact that approach to the lower third of the œsophagus from the right side is unfeasible because of the liver. When in doubt as to the exact location of the lesion he makes a left-sided incision.

The operation is done in two stages. First, either a Witzel or a Kader gastrostomy is done; and second, the resection is performed. A preliminary abdominal exploration for metastases precedes the gastrostomy. The patient is now placed upon his side; if it be on the right, the left arm is held upward and forward to pull the scapula out of the line of incision. The patient is held in this position by the use of sandbags.

Torek makes the following incision, which he feels is the one always to be used in exploration of the thorax. It is made in the seventh intercostal space and is carried over the entire length of the space. At its posterior end it is carried vertically upward to the third interspace (see Fig. 264). The skin flap is turned backward and protected carefully by towels pinned to the wound edges. Great care must be used

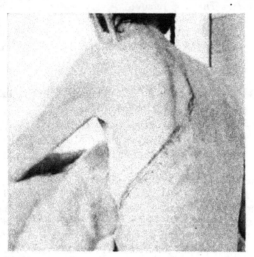

Fig. 264. Skin Incision. The dark line is a nitrate of silver mark made the day before operation. (*Torek.*)

to avoid soiling so large a wound surface. The fourth, fifth, sixth, and seventh ribs are resected, the pleura opened and the wound margins retracted by means of a rib spreader. By means of upward traction on the ribs and gauze pressure, Richter performs this stage of the operation without the use of a single clamp and with no bleeding. When the resection is completed, the bleeding intercostals are clamped and ligated. This saves time.

The thorax is now exposed. Quoting Richter: ' The structures in the field of operation are readily defined. The gullet stands out prominently; the pneumogastric nerve is plainly visible. It comes down from above in a single trunk and lies behind the azygos vein just as the latter turns in to meet the vena cava. Just below the azygos anterior it divides into numerous branches much after the manner of the pes anserina of the facial nerve. Viewing the parts as seen during the operation, with the lung retracted, the plexus so formed lies to the right, the ascending part of the azygos to the left and the transverse part of the azygos above the field of operation. From the pneumogastric plexus, and made up of it in part, the main trunk of the pneumogastric dips down to the side of the gullet ' (see Fig. 265).

The lung is now freed from adhesions, and laid over toward the front part of the mediastinum. Then, qutoing Torek, ' the œsophagus is

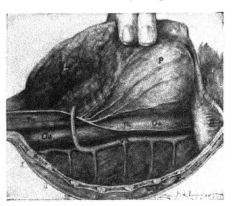

FIG. 265. NORMAL STRUCTURES AS SEEN WITH LUNG DRAWN FORWARD AND MEDIANWARD. L, lung; P, pericardium; Tr, trachea; Oe, œsophagus; Pn, pneumogastric nerve; VA, vena azygos; I, II, III, etc., ribs. (*Richter.*)

seen only as a slight bulging of the parietal pleura to the side of the aorta. The pleura and connective tissue covering the œsophagus are now divided at some portion where it is not involved, and the œsophagus is lifted out of its bed. A tape or strip of gauze is drawn through underneath it. This serves as a handle to draw the œsophagus forward or to the side, while the dissection proceeds (see Fig. 266).

' The œsophagus is liberated from the surrounding structures all the way up to the upper thoracic aperture and all the way down to the diaphragm, except in cases where the tumour is situated rather high up, when the diaphragmatic end need not be liberated. To determine the extent of the dissection of the diaphragmatic end, we decide at what place below the tumour the œsophagus is to be divided and allow about 3 cm. more for the invagination of the stump. The dissection is best done with the aid of a blunt instrument like Kocher's goitre sound, or a long Mayo dissecting scissors, which is inserted between the œsophagus and the tissues lying over it. The fact that some vagus branches crossing the œsophagus must be divided in the course of this procedure need not deter the surgeon.'

At this point it becomes necessary to digress for a moment to

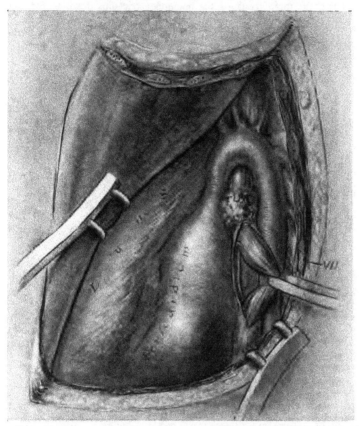

FIG. 266. BEGINNING OF DISSECTION OF THE ŒSOPHAGUS. After incision of the pleura covering it the œsophagus is lifted out of its bed and held by a tape passed underneath it. The two vagi have been detached. The tumour is seen below the arch of the aorta. The lung is fairly well collapsed. (*Torek.*)

emphasize the difference between the œsophagus and the intestine. The latter being covered by a serous coat, a plastic exudate immediately follows division and end-to-end union and prevents leakage.

Not so with the œsophagus; even though the resected ends can readily be brought together, end-to-end union must be attained by accurate apposition of the cut mucosa and muscularis, a very difficult thing to do. A suppurative pleuritis or mediastinitis has been the usual result of this procedure.

The dissection of that part of the œsophagus lying beneath the aortic arch is the most difficult. The œsophagus crosses the left bronchus at this point and it must be freed from both by blunt dissection. Great care must be used not to kink the aortic arch because of the danger of a

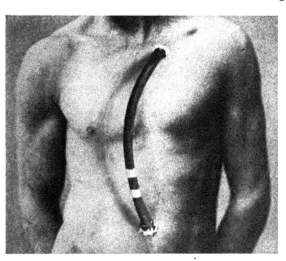

FIG. 267. TUBE CONNECTING LOWER END OF ŒSOPHAGUS WITH GASTROSTOMY OPENING. The two light stripes on the rubber tube are remnants of adhesive plaster which were removed before taking the picture. (*Torek*.)

sudden cardiac collapse. At the level of the upper thoracic aperture the finger or dissecting instrument is pushed by blunt dissection until the anterior border of the sterno-mastoid muscle is reached. At this point an incision is made through which the œsophagus is afterward to be pulled.

After a double ligation has been done, the œsophagus is divided and the end of the lower stump invaginated in the usual manner. When the tumour is close to the diaphragm the cardiac end of the stomach may have to be used to cover in the stump should the latter not be long enough.

The distal end, the mucous edge having first been cauterized, is drawn up and out through the neck wound. This is readily done because the œsophagus is only supported by loose connective tissue in its pharyngeal end. The œsophagus is brought up by means of tape passed down through the skin wound and tied at its end.

The chest is now closed by bringing the ribs together by means of Sauerbruch's pericostal sutures, the sutures either going around the ribs or through them. Intra-pulmonary pressure should be sufficiently increased during the last stages of the closure to keep the lung in contact with the chest wall. A slight pneumothorax will do no harm. After the free end of the œsophagus has thoroughly healed to the skin, the upper end of a gastrostomy tube is inserted into it when the patient wishes to take nourishment (see Fig. 267). During the act of swallowing a little pressure is brought to bear on the skin at one side of the tube to prevent leakage. The swallowed food passes from the œsophagus into the rubber tube and thus into the stomach.

Torek closes the pleura without drainage. At this point he differs with Willy Meyer, who feels that the pleura should always be drained. Meyer attributes the death of his seventh case directly to lack of drainage. Sauerbruch, who describes and has done the same operation, closes the pleura without drainage.

A plastic procedure worthy of mention for repair of defects of the lower end of the œsophagus is the Beck-Jianu operation. This consists in constructing a tube from the greater curvature of the stomach, drawing it through an opening in the diaphragm, and uniting it to the proximal portion of the œsophagus. No living case following this procedure has as yet been reported.

SECTION VI

OPERATIONS UPON THE STOMACH AND INTESTINES

PART I

OPERATIONS UPON THE STOMACH

BY

B. G. A. MOYNIHAN, M.S. (Lond.), F.R.C.S. (Eng.)
Lieutenant-Colonel R.A.M.C.(T.)
Surgeon to the Leeds General Infirmary

CHAPTER I

PREPARATION AND AFTER-TREATMENT OF PATIENTS OPERATED UPON FOR DISEASES OF THE STOMACH

No insignificant part of the successful treatment of patients operated upon for diseases of the stomach depends upon the care exercised in the preparation and in the conduct of the case subsequent to operation.

PREPARATION OF THE PATIENT

The usual precautions necessary to secure asepsis are more than ever necessary here. It is not seldom that one hears the remark that the 'margin for error' is greater in abdominal surgery than it is in the surgery of other parts. And it is quite true that the peritoneum has a great capacity for dealing with any infection introduced into it. But there can be no question that the more sedulously the details of an aseptic operation are observed, the speedier is the recovery of the patient. Many of the troublesome after-effects of an abdominal operation—pain, flatulence, hiccough, vomiting—are due to infection. They are evidence of a slight peritoneal response to an infection. The patient upon whom such an operation as gastro-enterostomy has been performed should suffer almost no discomfort after he has recovered from the anæsthetic. There should be no pain except a 'catch' in the wound on coughing or sneezing.

The chief infection in an operation comes from the patient's skin. If this be carefully prepared it may be rendered sterile, so that a little piece of the skin snipped away at the beginning of the operation, and dropped into a culture-medium, displays no evidence of infection. But an examination of the skin, similarly conducted, at the middle or end of the operation will show that infection is present. The surface of the skin is infected from the depths. It is my practice therefore always to cover the skin by fixing up to the edges of the wound with a special forceps the 'tetra' material, which consists of many layers of compressed gauze. When the stomach or omentum is taken from the abdomen there is no chance of any infection occurring from contact with the skin.

It is of great importance to secure before operation the cleanliness of the stomach and the jejunum. Some of the cases submitted to gastrectomy or gastro-enterostomy have enormously enlarged stomachs in which food lies stagnant. The discharge from an ulcer or a growth makes such retained material foul and intensely infectious. In these cases, indeed in all cases, every endeavour should be made to get the stomach thoroughly clean before the abdomen is opened. Lavage secures this end more certainly than anything else. The stomach, if stasis be present, is washed out twice a day for several days, and time and pains are spent on each occasion. It may be necessary to use many gallons of fluid—sterilized saline solution is the best—before the water returns clear. If there be no evidence of stasis the stomach need not be washed more than twice, once twenty-four hours before the operation, and the second time an hour before. The opportunity should be taken to give test-meals, when the stomach is washed, for purposes of investigation. Some of the patients who have suffered long from vomiting are very thin, emaciated, parched for lack of water. In them the continuous administration of saline solution by the rectum, or hypodermically, may prove very beneficial. It is most important also to attend to the condition of the patient's mouth. In almost all cases of stomach diseases the mouth is in an unsatisfactory condition; indeed oral sepsis not improbably plays a part in the causation of many organic diseases of the stomach or intestine. The teeth should be thoroughly cleaned several times daily, and a fragrant mouth-wash used at frequent intervals.

SUTURE OF THE ABDOMINAL WOUND

A few transverse scratches are made with a fine needle in the skin at right angles to the line of the intended incision. The abdominal incision is carried through the right rectus muscle in gastro-enterostomy, in the middle line usually for gastrectomy. The fibres of the rectus are split, the nerves being preserved, if possible, or the whole belly of the muscle is displaced outwards. As soon as the peritoneum is reached, and before it is opened, ' tetra ' cloths are fixed over the edges of the wound, and fixed at each side and at each end by the special forceps made for me by Down Bros. The wound is sutured in several layers. A continuous catgut stitch is taken from one end of the wound to the other, picking up the posterior sheath of the rectus and the peritoneum together. The needle is then laid aside. Then with a long straight needle interrupted sutures of silkworm-gut are passed through skin and rectus muscle on each side. The needle is introduced on one side and brought out on the other through one of the faint scratches made in the skin before the incision was started. About six or eight of these sutures are passed, and the ends of all are then seized by a clip on each side.

The needle carrying the catgut suture, which has just been laid aside, is again taken up, and is made to return along the incision; it now picks up the anterior sheath of the rectus on each side. On the left side it is introduced about ½ inch from the cut edge of the sheath, and is brought out just clear of the cut margin; it therefore picks up a transverse piece of the anterior sheath. On the right side the needle passes from the deep to the superficial aspect of the sheath. On pulling the suture tight it will be found that the right edge of the fascia overlaps the left edge. The fascia is approximated therefore by flat surfaces, and not by edges only, and this makes for sounder healing. When the end of the wound is reached, the catgut is tied to the original end of the suture which had been left long. Then at each end of the skin incision a small volsella is placed, and one or two along the wound, bringing the scratches accurately together. A row of Michel's clips are then put in and the skin edges thus accurately brought into contact. The silkworm-gut sutures are now tied rather loosely, and cut short. The dressing I use consists of four layers of gauze laid along the wound (the skin being previously washed over with spirit). Over this a large square of gauze is placed; a piece of stout gauze bandage is the best. This bandage is then fixed to the skin by a solution of formalin and gelatine applied hot. In a test tube an ounce of gelatine (20% in water) has been previously sterilized on three successive days by heating to 100° C. Just before use the test tube is put to stand in very hot water until the gelatine is liquefied. To it then are added ♏ 20 of a 4% solution of formalin. The solution is then rapidly applied to the gauze bandage, which it attaches firmly to the skin. The dressing dries in about one minute; over it a thin layer of wool is applied to prevent the blankets or the clothes from sticking to it. No bandages are used. I never use any abdominal bandage now unless a drainage tube is left in the wound. The dressing I have described is very comfortable; it covers only the wound, and leaves the rest of the abdomen open to inspection or palpation.

The Michel's clips are removed in forty-eight hours. The deep stitches remain ten days or longer according to the case. In malignant cases I often allow them to remain for three weeks.

AFTER-TREATMENT

As soon as the operation has been completed the patient is placed in a warm bed, lying on the back with one pillow. After an hour or two, as soon that is as the effect of the anæsthetic is passing off, the patient is propped up in bed with a bed-rest or five or six pillows. This position is one of great comfort to the patient, but it is difficult to maintain. There is a very marked tendency, for a heavy man particularly, to slide down in the bed. A most useful device for keeping the patient in the sitting position is that suggested by Dr. Cairns Forsyth. A hard round pillow covered with mackintosh and a pillow-slip is placed beneath the patient's thighs, immediately below the buttocks. To each end of this pillow a stout strap is attached, terminating in a

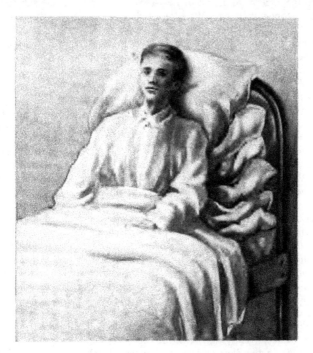

FIG. 268. POSITION OF THE PATIENT AFTER OPERATIONS UPON THE STOMACH.

buckle. A second strap is fixed to the upright end of the bed, and its lower end engages with the buckle attached to the pillow; by pulling this strap tight and fixing it, the position of the pillow is made secure. The patient is supported by this pillow quite comfortably, and is prevented from slipping down in the bed. About five or six hours after the operation the feeling of nausea caused by the ether will have passed off, and the patient begins to ask for fluid. At once water is given, an ounce or more at a time to begin with, and in two or three hours a cup of tea. Most patients like tea better than any other drink; during the first twenty-four hours three or four cups, made to the patient's liking, may be given. I do not restrict the quantity of water allowed to patients. They rarely drink more than 20 or 30 ounces in the first twenty-four hours, but it is their own desire which regulates the quantity given, not any order of mine. There is no harm done by giving fluids freely. If a patient can vomit without injury to the suture line, it is quite certain that the passage of fluids through the anastomotic opening will do no hurt. For the last three or four years I have put no restraint upon patients in this matter even from the first. Thirst is the most intolerable of all sufferings after abdominal section, and there is no justification for allowing a patient to suffer from it. Fluid taken by the mouth has to pass to the large intestine to be absorbed. The intestines are kept active, therefore, and this is entirely an advantage. I do not order solid food until a patient himself asks for it. In the early days milk, soups, tea and cocoa are given freely, but solid food is not desired by a patient until eight or ten days have passed. As soon as the request is made I grant it, ordering sweetbread, fish, bread and butter, mince, and so on, and the quantities taken are not restricted. In eighteen or twenty days ordinary food can be taken and enjoyed. I discourage pastry, fresh fruits, and green vegetables in all cases for some time, for these things are without value as foods.

On the night of the operation the patient may be allowed ⅙ gr. of morphine hypodermically. There is usually not much pain after the operation involving the stomach, but if the patient complains of pain I do not hesitate to give one hypodermic injection of morphine. It is extremely rare for a second dose to be asked for or to be given. In all cases a simple enema, with or without turpentine, is given twenty-four hours after the operation. Flatus is brought away, and the patient is more comfortable. An aperient, castor oil or calomel, is given about the first day. The patient is allowed up sometimes during the second week, usually on the ninth or tenth day. In malignant cases I get the patients out of bed earlier than this, often on the day after operation.

CHAPTER II

GASTROTOMY: GASTROSTOMY: PARTIAL GASTRECTOMY

GASTROTOMY

Indications. In the operation of gastrotomy the stomach is opened for the purpose of exploring its interior, for the removal of a foreign body, or for obtaining access to the cardiac orifice when retrograde dilatation of an œsophageal stricture is to be attempted. When the purpose of the operation has been fulfilled the opening in the stomach is closed, and the viscus is returned within the abdomen.

Operation. The abdomen is opened in or near the middle line, according as access to the cardiac or the pyloric extremities of the stomach is to be obtained. The rectus muscle, when a lateral incision is used, is split or displaced in the usual manner. When the stomach is exposed, it is drawn well into the ample wound. The peritoneal cavity is then protected by two layers of gauze swabs introduced into it. Those swabs first packed away are of large size, and remain unmoved throughout the operation; a more superficial layer consists of smaller swabs which are changed when necessary. The edges of the abdominal incision are also well protected by gauze packing or by 'tetra' cloths. In addition to the stomach the transverse colon should be drawn well into the wound, for it may be necessary to tear through the gastro-colic omentum in order to reach the posterior surface of the viscus. The stomach is then opened either by a vertical or by a transverse incision. The latter is to be preferred as it gives a better exposure of the stomach, though, since more vessels are necessarily divided, the hæmorrhage is more severe. As the vessels are divided they are seized and ligatured at once with fine catgut. A fine volsella then seizes each edge of the wound and the stomach cavity is open to inspection. A good deal of frothy viscid mucus may be found in the interior; it is to be mopped away with gauze. The foreign body (a dental plate, or a hair ball or other intruder) is to be removed, or the intended procedure carried out, and the wound in the anterior wall closed. If a close inspection of the stomach be necessary, one or two fingers are passed through a rent in the gastrocolic omentum immediately below the stomach, a bloodless spot being chosen, and the posterior wall protruded through the anterior opening.

One portion after another of the stomach-walls may thus be passed in review, and may be dealt with as is necessary.

The opening in the stomach is closed by two layers, an inner suture of catgut introduced by the 'loop on the mucosa stitch,' and an outer sero-muscular suture of Pagenstecher's thread. The stomach is then cleansed by wiping with moist sterile swabs, the gauze packing and the protecting swabs are removed and the abdomen closed.

GASTROSTOMY

Indications. The operation of gastrostomy is performed in those cases where there is stenosis of the œsophagus, or at the cardiac orifice of the stomach, to a degree which renders the passage of nourishment so difficult that life cannot long be maintained.

Operation. A great variety of procedures have been adopted in the search for a perfect method. There is at present a choice of several operations which fulfil well the necessary conditions. These are that the operation should be simple and speedy, for the vitality of patients needing the operation is small; that it should give adequate access to the stom-

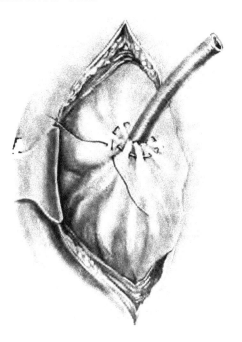

FIG. 269. GASTROSTOMY BY SENN'S METHOD.
The suture placed.

ach; that it should not permit the regurgitation of fluids or of gastric juice; and that the external opening should show no great tendency to spontaneous closure.

Senn's method. In my judgment this is the most satisfactory of all methods, for it best fulfils the necessary conditions which have been already enumerated. It consists in the infolding of a cone of the anterior wall by a series of purse-string sutures around a central tube which passes into the cavity of the stomach. The abdomen is opened by a vertical incision 2 to 3 inches in length through the outer part of the left rectus immediately below the costal margin. The muscle fibres are split, care being taken not to fray them, and the peritoneum incised.

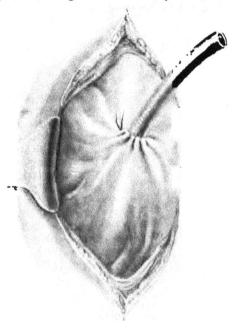

FIG. 270. GASTROSTOMY BY SENN'S METHOD.
The suture tied.

The stomach is then exposed; it is often, indeed usually, found small and shrunken, and hidden beneath the hollow of the ribs under the shelter of the left lobe of the liver. It is pulled well up into the wound, and a point upon it selected for the introduction of the tube. This point should be as far away from the pylorus as is convenient, and it should be approximately midway between the curvatures. The stomach is now surrounded with small gauze packs, to prevent soiling of the wound. At the point chosen a small incision is made into the anterior wall of the stomach, through all the coats. Through this opening a rubber catheter (Jaques's No. 12) or a piece of small drainage tube is passed towards the pylorus for a distance of 2 or 3 inches. The edge of the incision and the tube are now both caught up in a needle which carries a catgut thread; the stitch when tightened fixes the tube to the opening in the stomach. A series of purse-string sutures of fine Pagenstecher's thread are now passed in circles around the tube where it enters the stomach. The first of these is about ½ inch from the tube; as it is tightened an assistant pushes the tube inwards to the stomach so that the stitch comes to lie close against the tube. A second stitch about ¼ inch from the tube is then passed and tied in the same manner; then a third, and if need be, a fourth; each suture is tightened snugly round the tube and is then cut short. Finally, the stomach is secured to the anterior abdominal wall by a suture above and below the tube. The parietal wound is closed in layers and the operation is complete. A meal of peptonized milk may be given at once. As a rule the stomach is so small that it cannot comfortably hold more than 6 or 7 ounces, but

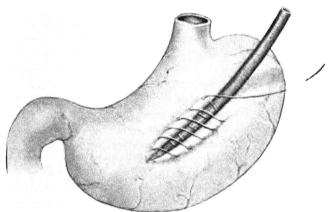

FIG. 271. GASTROSTOMY BY WITZEL'S METHOD.

in a few days its capacity increases. I prefer to give a meal every four hours, and between each meal to pour a few ounces of water into the stomach, for it is fluid that these patients mainly want.

Kader's method. The principle of this is similar to that just described. A tube is introduced into the stomach at the same point as in Senn's operation. Then transverse sutures are passed which raise up vertical folds on each side of the tube. By means of the stitches, which pick up only the sero-muscular coats, two longitudinal ridges are brought together, and at the mid-point of the ridge the tube passes vertically into the stomach. As the sutures are tightened they are cut short. There are usually two above the tube and two below. A second layer of stitches, and then a third, are passed in a similar manner; and finally the stomach is fixed to the anterior abdominal wall as before.

Witzel's method. This ingenious method is useful not only in the stomach, but also in the jejunum, and its analogue is used in other regions of the body. The method consists in introducing a tube into

the stomach and fixing it by a suture, as in the two methods already
described.   The tube is then laid flat upon the anterior wall of the
stomach and is buried in a groove or furrow there, by means of a
continuous suture which picks up the sero-muscular coats, as in a
Lembert's suture, first above and then below the tube.   As the stitch is
tightened a ridge is lifted up on each side of the tube which .is thus
entunnelled.   The suture begins a little distance beyond the point of entry
of the tube into the
stomach and con-
tinues for about 2½
inches to 3 inches.
Finally, the stomach
is fixed by a few
stitches to the ante-
rior abdominal wall.

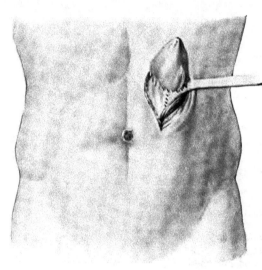

Frank's method.
(S b a n ajew-Frank-
Albert-Kocher me-
thod). This is prob-
ably t he   method
most employed at the
present time, and it
is   certainly   that
which has been sub-
jected to the greatest
variety of modifica-
tions,   by   Kocher,
H a r t m a n n, and
others.

FIG. 272. GASTROSTOMY BY FRANK'S METHOD.
The stomach sutured to the peritoneum.

The operation is
thus performed: A
vertical incision over the upper part of the left rectus muscle is made.
The rectus fibres are split, or the anterior sheath of the rectus muscle
dissected up to the middle line and the whole muscle displaced outwards
(Kocher). The peritoneum being opened, the stomach is sought, and a
cone-shaped piece of its anterior surface is brought well out of the
wound. The base of this cone is then fixed by a running suture to the
margins of the parietal peritoneum in the wound (see Fig. 272). A
second incision is now made parallel to the costal margin and 1 inch
beyond its free edge; that is to say, on the wall of the thorax. Between
the two incisions the subcutaneous tissue is then cut through by scissors,
in such manner as to raise up a bridge of skin, which, as it were, roofs

in a tunnel in the subcutaneous tissue. Through this tunnel and beneath this bridge of skin the cone-shaped piece of the stomach is passed until the apex of the cone pouts through the thoracic incision. It is there fixed by a hare-lip pin or a few sutures, and the original abdominal wound is then closed completely (see Fig. 273). This method is one which is in my opinion distinctly inferior to Senn's operation. For in all cases of œsophageal obstruction the stomach is small; it is accordingly by no means an easy matter to bring so much of it out of the abdomen as is necessary to make a good subcutaneous fold. Moreover, so much of the stomach as is employed in the operation is put out of use, as it were, so far as any digestive or other function is concerned; whereas in Senn's and Kader's operations the stomach-wall being infolded is not deprived thereby of its function. The efficacy of the 'valve action' is certainly not one whit better than in Senn's operation; indeed it is not, I think, quite so consistently secure. Finally, the time con-

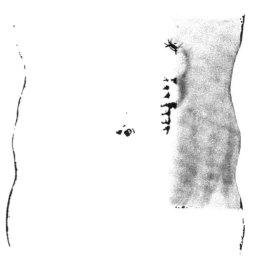

FIG. 273. GASTROSTOMY BY FRANK'S METHOD. The stomach sutured to the skin and the wound closed.

sumed in the operation is a little longer, and in patients who are seriously ill this is a factor not to be disregarded.

Tavel's method. This most ingenious method consists in fastening a tube—an œsophagus, so to speak—between the anterior abdominal wall and the stomach by utilizing a resected portion of the small intestine.

A free incision is made through the left rectus muscle, reaching to the umbilicus. The stomach is sought, and then the omentum is lifted up and the jejunum brought up into the wound for examination. A piece of it is then selected which is well supplied with blood (any chance piece will not do) and is then clamped by two pairs of clamps above and below. Between the clamps the bowel is cut, and the ends above and below the resected length are united by suture. The intestinal continuity is thus restored, and a piece of the jejunum some inches in length, still attached by its mesentery, which contains a free blood-supply, is available for the purposes of the new 'œsophagus.' This piece of the bowel is now united at one end to the stomach and at the other to the abdominal wall, and the parietal wound is closed around it. The description of this operation is enough to convince any surgeon that for most cases requiring gastrostomy it is quite inadmissible. It is too severe and too prolonged a measure for a weakly and wasted patient to bear. But for cases of simple œsophageal obstruction it may occasionally be useful. A very striking use of the method has been made by Roux of Lausanne, who, in the case of a boy aged about eight who had an impermeable stenosis of the œsophagus due to the swallowing of a caustic fluid, brought a long piece of the jejunum (attached at the lower end to the stomach) upwards beneath the skin of the abdomen and chest to a point a little below the manubrium sterni. The boy, whom I saw many months after the operation, was fat and well, and the new œsophagus acted perfectly.

After-treatment. After the operation of gastrostomy has been performed the patient should be fed at frequent intervals. At first about 5 ounces should be given every one and a half to two hours. Peptonized milk with a little brandy is given at first, and between the meals a little water is allowed to run into the stomach. It relieves the patient's thirst and prevents coagulated milk from blocking the tube. During the first few days no more than 6 or 8 ounces at one time can be received into the stomach with comfort; a quantity larger than this causes distress, and the fluid may regurgitate if the stomach be over-distended. After a few days the stomach may be washed out through the tube, and a dose of castor oil administered. Patients often express a desire to have something in their mouths, the flavour of which they can appreciate. I usually allow them to sip any favourite drink, for after gastrostomy has been performed the power to swallow is often much improved and a fair quantity of fluids can be given by the mouth. But I prefer to give all the necessary food by the tube, allowing by the mouth only those well-flavoured drinks for which the patient has a special liking. Some days later meat may be chewed and spat out into a funnel, and washed thence into the stomach. The tube can usually be removed at the end of eight or ten days; it is boiled and replaced, or a new one used. The patient should be instructed not to remove the tube except for cleansing purposes. The tube is brought through an opening in a pad affixed to a belt which encircles the abdomen; this is the most convenient method of fixing it. Patients should not be allowed to remain in bed for more than three to five days after this operation; as a rule the sooner they are up the better, and they should early receive instruction in the details of feeding, so that they may depend entirely upon themselves for this. The most distressing complication after this operation is hiccough. It occurs to a greater or less degree in about one-fourth of the cases; it is relieved by washing out the stomach, and by small doses of morphine or cocaine.

PARTIAL GASTRECTOMY

In planning an operation for the removal of a cancer beginning in or near the pylorus the lines which the procedure must follow are determined by a consideration of certain factors. These are—

1. The lymphatic system of the stomach.
2. The mode of spreading of the growth in the stomach.
3. The involvement of the duodenum.

1. *The lymphatic system of the stomach.* The lymph vascular supply of the stomach is free. For convenience of description certain territories are marked out upon the stomach, which may be looked upon as watersheds, each draining into a separate group of glands. Cunéo describes three such areas, which are marked out by drawing two lines upon the stomach. The first line extends from the apex of the fundus to the middle of the pylorus and passes across the stomach at the junction of its upper two-thirds with the lower third. The second line extends from the mid-point of the greater curvature vertically upwards to meet the first line. In this way three areas are marked out: from the upper all the lymph-vessels flow to the glands along the lesser curvature and to those around the cardiac orifice; from the left lower area the vessels pass to the spleen, and from the right lower area they run obliquely downwards to glands which lie along the greater curvature close to and beyond the pylorus. The glands into which these vessels run direct are called 'primary.' When a gland receives vessels which have already passed through other glands it is called 'secondary.' It is clear that if good is to be done by any surgical procedure involving the removal of a cancer, not only must the growth itself be taken away, but also all the lymphatic vessels which drain the region in which the growth lies and the primary glands which drain that area. The primary glands are—

(a) Those which lie along the coronary artery.

(b) A gland or glands lying above the pylorus, by the side of the pyloric artery, the 'suprapyloric' gland.

(c) Glands which lie along the upper border of the pancreas, to the right of the cœliac axis, the 'right suprapancreatic' glands.

(d) The glands which lie along the greater curvature in association with the right gastro-epiploic artery.

(e) Retropyloric glands.

All these glands must be removed therefore as well as the stomach.

2. *The local increase of the growth in the stomach.* The apparent size of a growth in the stomach is no guide to its actual size; for all around the palpable growth an extensive invasion of the submucosa has occurred. This invasion in cases of pyloric growth extends for at least an inch on the cardiac side. The growth, moreover, shows a striking tendency to invade the curvatures, especially the lesser curvature. It is not uncommon to find a solid cord of growth extending from a small pyloric growth quite up to the cardiac end of the stomach along the lesser curvature. It is therefore necessary in all cases of resection of the stomach to take away the whole length of the lesser curvature.

3. *The involvement of the duodenum.* As a general rule a pyloric cancer seems to stop abruptly at the duodenum, and comment has been made by a multitude of authors upon the integrity of the intestine in cases of gastric cancer. But as a result of the work of Cunéo and Borrmann we have been brought to realize that an invasion of the duodenum is by no means infrequent. Borrmann examined sixty-three specimens removed by operation and found that in no less than twenty was it evident that the cut surface of the duodenum was involved in the growth. At least one inch of the duodenum must accordingly be removed.

The lines therefore which a resection of the stomach should follow may be indicated. The whole growth with a wide margin should be taken away; all the lesser curvature and one-half of the greater curvature must be removed, and all the primary glands must be sacrificed.

Operation. The operation is carried out in the following manner: An ample incision is made in the middle line, reaching as a rule from the ensiform cartilage to the umbilicus. The central incision is more convenient than the lateral incision which is commonly employed for the operation of gastro-enterostomy; it gives easier and more immediate access to all parts of the operation area. An inspection of the extent of the cancerous invasion of the stomach itself, of its adhesion to the pancreas or abdominal wall or liver, of the number and position of any glandular enlargements, and finally of the liver, peritoneum, and parts immediately in the neighbourhood to discover if secondary growth be present, is made. Neither adhesions nor the involvement of lymphatic glands preclude removal of the stomach, though they may render the mechanical difficulties rather more serious. When a resection has been decided upon, flat gauze swabs, wrung out of hot saline solution, are packed round the stomach so as to afford a barrier between the field of work and the general peritoneal cavity. As a rule two layers of swabs are introduced, the first consisting of very large ones, which are unchanged throughout the operation, and the second of smaller ones, which when soiled are changed at once. No care is too punctilious so long as absolute security of the peritoneal cavity is ensured.

It is best to begin the operation by ligature of the principal arteries of supply so as to render the operation comparatively bloodless. I formerly began by ligature of the coronary artery, but now prefer to leave this vessel until a later stage of the operation for reasons presently to be mentioned. The gastro-hepatic omentum is first torn through, and if need be ligatured close to its attachment to the liver, beginning near the cardia, and the omentum stripped down to the stomach, and to the right until the pyloric and gastro-duodenal branches of the hepatic artery are exposed. These vessels may arise together or separately from the hepatic stem. They are best defined by stripping along the hepatic artery with gauze wrapped round the finger. Each vessel is surrounded by an aneurysm needle carrying a double thread; between the ligatures each artery is divided. The gastro-epiploica sinistra is now tied in a similar manner at the point on the greater curvature of the stomach at which its section is to be made. The index and middle finger of the left hand are now passed from above downwards through the opening made in the gastro-hepatic omentum, behind the pylorus, where they are made to project below the duodenum, through the great omentum. In this way any adhesion of the growth to the pancreas is felt. If such adhesion be firm, a thick fibrous mass welding the two together, it is better not to endeavour to separate the stomach, but to deal first with the duodenum. The finger which projects below the duodenum indicates the point at which a clamp is introduced at the place where the bowel is to be divided. As a rule two clamps are introduced, a rubber-covered distal one and a bare proximal one; between them the duodenum is divided, a full inch beyond the pylorus. The proximal cut end of the duodenum may show a tendency to slip away from the clamp; this is prevented by passing a couple of sutures through the stomach and tying them over the clamp. The distal end of the duodenum may be closed by one of several methods. I prefer a running suture of catgut taken from top to bottom and drawn tight; its two ends are tied together in such manner as to pucker up the suture line to a small knot. Outside this a continuous Pagenstecher's suture is passed until it is quite certain that a perfectly secure closure of the duodenum has been effected. I generally use a third layer of stitches, for the records of cases show that leakage from the duodenum is one of the common causes of disaster. I have never had any trouble from this source, but I perform this part of the operation with the most sedulous care. If need be, a part of the pancreas is stitched over the end of the duodenum to make assurance doubly sure.

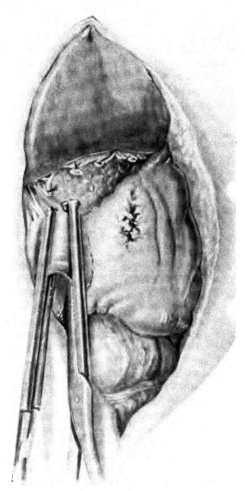

FIG. 274. PARTIAL GASTRECTOMY.
Gastro-hepatic omentum ligatured; division of duodenum.

The proximal cut end of the duodenum is now lifted up with the clamp, the whole being held in a large moist swab. If only slender adhesions to the pancreas be found they are torn through, but if the stomach seems rather to have grown into the gland it is better to slice away a thin layer from the surface. The pancreas may be safely cut

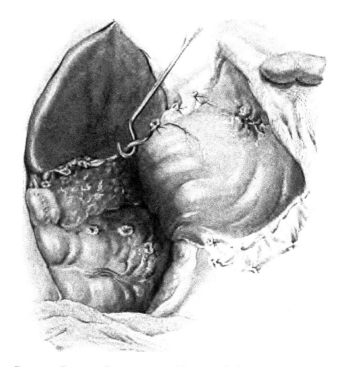

FIG. 275. PARTIAL GASTRECTOMY. Ligature of the coronary artery.

in this way, but the shaving must not be carried too deep lest the duct be opened. Bleeding is free at the first, but is readily checked by firm pressure, or by a few ligatures.

It is now the time to see that all the glands along the greater curvature of the stomach are removed. The subpyloric glands are often grossly enlarged, but not always so. It is important to see that all the fatty tissue which bears them, in the angle between the first and second parts of the duodenum, is taken away. On the greater curvature of the stomach the glands are also numerous in the pyloric half. They show a great tendency to drop down in the omentum; not seldom being found 1½ to 2 inches from the stomach. As these are removed it is necessary to see that no damage is done to the middle colic artery. To prevent this most serious mishap the transverse colon and omentum should be withdrawn from the abdomen and the under surface of the transverse

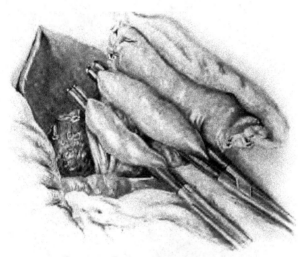

FIG. 276. PARTIAL GASTRECTOMY.
The clamps applied, preparatory to gastro-enterostomy.

mesocolon, whereon the arterial arch is easily to be seen, constantly examined. The great omentum well below the greater curvature of the stomach is then ligatured in bundles and divided. As each part of the omentum is displayed care must be taken to see that the ligature lies well below all glands to be removed. This process of tying the omentum in bundles is continued until a point an inch or more beyond the middle of the greater curvature, well beyond the left of the glandular chain, is reached. It is at this point that the left gastro-epiploic artery has already been tied.

The stomach is now free and mobile in its pyloric half—for the gastro-hepatic omentum has been divided, the duodenum severed, and the great omentum ligatured. This mass of the stomach held in a large hot swab is now turned well over to the left, so that its posterior surface is exposed. The time has come for ligature of the coronary artery. This is best done now by cleaning with a little gauze, which soon clearly displays the cœliac axis. The coronary artery is surrounded with an aneurysm needle close to its origin, tied and divided. The stomach is at once much looser, for its chief remaining anchor has been cut. The advantages of dividing the coronary at this stage are, that it is easier,

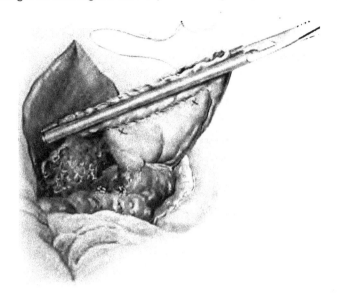

Fig. 277. Partial Gastrectomy.
Closure of the wound in the stomach. X X, the gastro-enterostomy suture.

being displayed in a few moments, and that it is divided at a higher point, so that the upper coronary group of glands can be removed completely. The artery being divided, the glands are stripped down with gauze until the œsophagus and the beginning of the lesser curvature are clear. The line of division of the stomach from the highest point of the lesser curvature to a point about the middle of the greater curvature is now determined, and a clamp may temporarily be laid along this line, and lightly clamped to indicate its direction. But before the stomach is divided along this line the anastomosis with the jejunum should be made. At this stage it is easily done, for the loosened part of the stomach gives one a handle with which to manipulate the remainder, the part, that is, which is to be engaged in the anastomosis. If the stomach be first divided, the part that remains is sometimes so small, and handled with such great difficulty, that the performance of the gastro-enterostomy becomes very difficult, and the anastomosis when completed looks anything but shapely. By performing the short circuiting operation now it is easier, speedier, and therefore safer. I prefer in performing this anastomosis to make the jejunum lie to the left, on Mayo's line, as this is undoubtedly an advantage in cases of partial gastrectomy.

Clamps are therefore now applied to the posterior surface of the stomach, and to the jejunum, close to the flexure, drawn up through a rent in the transverse mesocolon. The lines of suture and all the details of the operation are the same as those described on p. 604. When the gastro-enterostomy is completed, Kocher's long clamp is applied to the stomach along the line already indicated. A second clamp is applied distal to it, and between the two the stomach is divided. In doing so it is well to cut first through the serous and muscular coats back and front and to strip these back a little way before dividing the mucosa: so that when this is divided and sutured it can be well covered by the exuberant outer coats. After division of all the coats the mucosa is sutured with catgut and the serosa and muscularis with Pagenstecher's thread. The only points of difficulty are at the curvatures, and here especial care must be taken to see that the closure is secure. At the point of section of the lesser curvature the stomach may sometimes seem likely to slip away from the clamp; if so, it is sutured at once, and an extra Halsted's suture may be useful to hold it secure. The time has now arrived to clear away the only remaining primary glands, the right suprapancreatic, which lie along the hepatic artery above the pancreas. This is best done by careful dissection, and the constant stripping of the parts with gauze. It is best to begin at the cœliac axis and work to the right; the pancreas may possibly have to be sacrificed in some small degree, but this does not signify. What is important is the security of the hepatic artery, and this must throughout be jealously guarded. It now remains only to clean the operation area, arrest any chance leakage of blood, to remove the swabs, and to close the abdominal wound. Drainage is not as a rule necessary unless the pancreas has been exposed; it is then desirable.

PARTIAL GASTRECTOMY FOR SIMPLE ULCER OF THE STOMACH. RESECTION OF THE ULCER-BEARING AREA. RODMAN'S OPERATION

There are occasions upon which it may be necessary to perform a resection of the pyloric region of the stomach for simple disease. The indications for this operation are chiefly two: firstly, when there are multiple ulcers in the stomach; secondly, when the ulcer is so much indurated that an accurate discrimination between simple and early carcinomatous disease is very difficult, or even impossible. The advocacy of resection for such conditions began with Dr. W. L. Rodman of Philadelphia, and the name of this distinguished surgeon is now generally

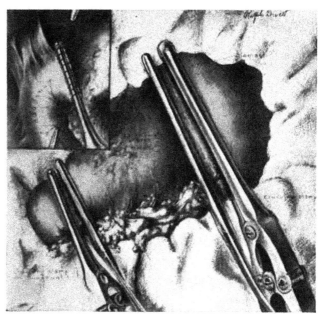

FIG. 278. BLOOD-VESSELS TIED, GLANDS SEPARATED, CRUSHING CLAMPS IN PLACE AND ALSO CLAMPS TO PREVENT LEAKAGE FROM PART TO BE REMOVED. Upper left drawing shows stump of duodenum in crushing clamp with suture placed for closing. (*Mayo.*)

given to the operation for removal of the ' ulcer-bearing area.' The procedure in such cases is very similar to that which has already been described in cases of carcinoma. The chief differences are—

(a) It is not necessary to remove the stomach very wide of the growth; an interval sufficient to allow of the easy application of the clamps is all that is needed.

(b) The removal of the whole of the lesser curvature is not necessary.

(c) The sacrifice of the glands is not necessary.

(d) The duodenum need not be removed unless ulcers are found there also.

(e) The performance of an end-to-end anastomosis or of Kocher's gastro-duodenostomy may be possible; Rodman himself prefers, I think rightly, to perform gastro-enterostomy.

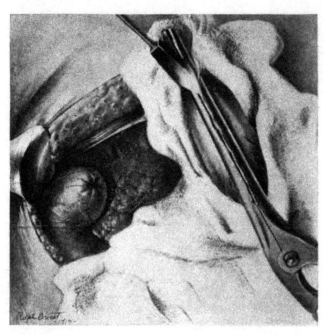

Fig. 279. Crushing Clamp on the Stomach. Cautery used to sterilize and prevent carcinomatous implantation. Stump of duodenum closed. Sutures placed to turn the duodenal stump into the denuded head of the pancreas. (*Mayo.*)

Pólya operation. The Pólya operation, as described by Mayo, is as follows:

The diseased portion of the stomach is removed in the usual way and the stump of the duodenum closed and buried (see Figs. 278 and 279). An opening is made in the avascular arcade of the transverse mesocolon and the jejunum pulled through until it can be easily brought into contact with the stomach, which is held in the crushing clamp of Payr, and united by suture to the loop of jejunum (see Fig. 280) quite as the ordinary gastro-enterostomy is made. If the diameter of the end of the stomach be very large, it can easily be diminished by placing the sutures in such manner as to take a proportionately greater bite in the stomach than in the intestine, thus reducing the lumen of the stom-

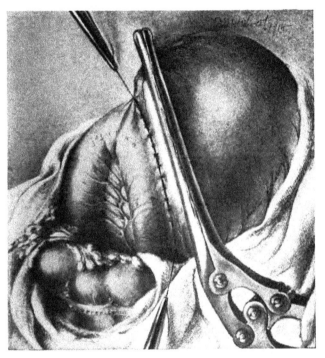

FIG. 280. UPPER JEJUNUM SIX TO TWELVE INCHES FROM ORIGIN BROUGHT THROUGH AN OPENING WHICH HAS BEEN MADE IN THE TRANSVERSE MESOCOLON AND UNITED BY OUTER ROW OF SEROMUSCULAR SILK SUTURES TO THE POSTERIOR WALL OF THE STOMACH. (*Mayo.*)

ach as the suturing progresses. The stomach is anastomosed to the jejunum at a point where the jejunal blood-supply is extraordinarily good, and the jejunum can be depended upon to do more than its share in the healing process. Before the inner through-and-through sutures are placed, the stomach and intestine are grasped with elastic holding clamps to prevent soiling; the inner row of sutures is then run entirely around and the outer row completed. The entire anastomosed end of

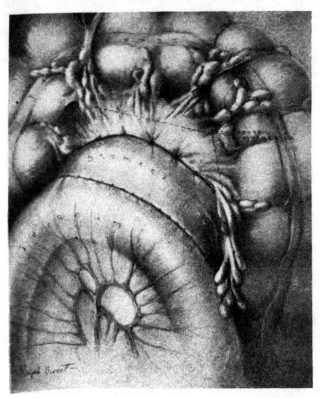

Fig. 281. Anastomosis completed by an Anterior Row of Seromuscular Sutures. Anastomosed end brought through the opening in the transverse mesocolon and margins of opening sutured to the stomach. (*Mayo.*)

...ch is then drawn down below the transverse mesocolon and ... of the opening in the transverse mesocolon carefully at-... number of sutures to the wall of the stomach (see Fig. 281). ... used for the peritoneomuscular sutures and chromic catgut ... through-and-through inner row.

Balfour operation.   Balfour, of the Mayo Clinic, has described a modification of the Pólya operation, the technique of which is as follows:

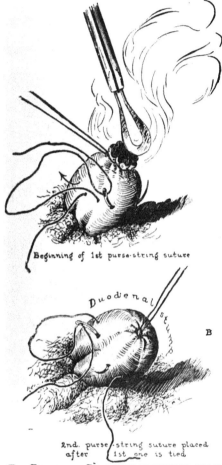

Beginning of 1st purse-string suture

Duodenal stump

B

2nd. purse-string suture placed after 1st one is tied

Fig. 282. A, The End of the Duodenum transfixed and tied with Catgut. The actual cautery used for sterilizing stump beyond ligature. The purse-string suture in place. B, The stump inverted and first catgut purse-string suture tied. Second catgut purse-string suture in place below the first. A few interrupted silk sutures may be placed to draw together the sheath of the pancreas and omenta in the vicinity, thereby burying the end of the duodenum. (*Balfour.*)

The resection is carried out in the ordinary way with especial attention to such important parts as the wide removal of gland-bearing tissue, the avoiding of injury to the middle colic blood-supply of the transverse colon, the resection made well beyond the cancer limits, the cauterization of all cut mucous surfaces to prevent cancer-cell transplantation,

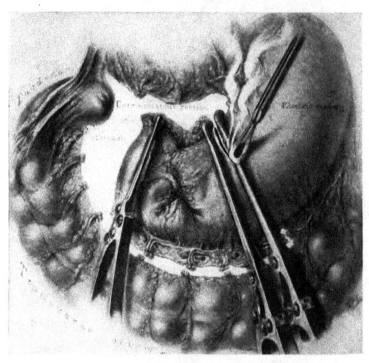

FIG. 283. END OF DUODENUM CLOSED, VESSELS LIGATED AND FAT AND GLANDS ISOLATED WITH THE CARCINOMATOUS PORTION OF THE STOMACH. Section being made with an electric cautery knife. (*Balfour.*)

and the secure inversion and burial of the duodenal stump. The operative field is inspected and carefully isolated by fresh packs and the second stage is carried out as follows (see Figs. 282 and 283):

The first loop of jejunum is procured and a point about 14 to 18 inches from the duodeno-jejunal angle is marked. The jejunum is then carried up in front of the transverse colon and omentum and a

segment of suitable size is chosen at the point already marked. This
section of jejunum is lightly grasped with rubber-covered forceps, and

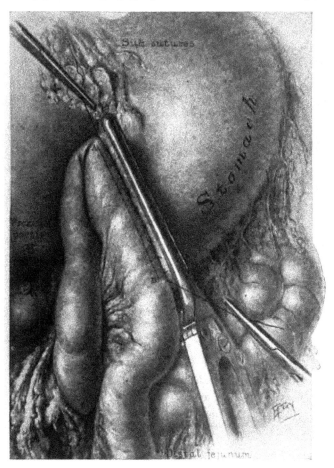

Fig. 284. First Row of Interrupted Silk Sutures uniting the Proximal
Portion of the Jejunum to the Posterior Wall of the Stomach. Anticolic.
(*Balfour.*)

directed so that the proximal end of the loop will be approximated to
the lesser curvature of the stomach. A series of interrupted silk sutures

in the serosa is used for the first line posteriorly, beginning at the greater curvature. All these sutures are placed before any are tied, and the ends of the top and bottom sutures may be conveniently left as guides. The first suture line is about ½ inch below the clamp on the cut-end of the stomach, and on the side of the jejunum about ¾ of an inch from the summit of the loop. In extensive resections it is extremely important to get the best possible exposure of the lesser curvature, for at this point it is occasionally difficult to make a secure anastomosis, and it is along the lesser curvature that inflammatory products frequently extend, rendering the gastric wall friable and a distinct source of danger. Any measure in such cases which will prevent retraction of the lesser curvature should be utilized. We still find the right-angled rubber-covered clamp of greatest service for this purpose. The jejunum is now incised on the line (see Fig. 284) and the crushing clamp removed from the stomach. (If it has been possible at any previous stage in the operation to place without difficulty a straight rubber-covered clamp at a higher level on the stomach, soiling by unevacuated gastric contents will be prevented.) Any actively bleeding vessels are ligated. The posterior row of the anastomosis uniting the posterior wall of the stomach to the inner cut-edge of the jejunum is of chromic catgut. The stitches on the gastric side should be taken after the edge which has been crushed by the clamp has been trimmed with the scissors. A second row of finer catgut may be used to advantage in the posterior line. The first chromic catgut suture is continued in front in the usual way to complete closure. An interrupted silk suture line similar to that used posteriorly is placed anteriorly, particular care being taken to reinforce the angle of anastomosis at the lesser curvature. A few interrupted silk sutures are placed where necessary further to protect the anterior suture line and the suture at the lesser curvature, the stump of gastrohepatic omentum which contains the ligated gastric artery being utilized as a support to the gastro-jejunal angle at this point.

CHAPTER III

OPERATIONS FOR GASTRIC ULCERS AND THEIR SEQUELÆ

EXCISION OF AN ULCER FROM THE LESSER CURVATURE

Indications. Experience has shown that when chronic ulcers are found upon the lesser curvature, in the cardiac half of the stomach, the relief from gastro-enterostomy is slight or transitory, and my practice has now been, for some time, to excise such ulcers. As a rule an ulcer so placed is solitary, and when it is removed the stomach performs its work as well as ever before, but there are cases, very exceptional I believe them to be, in which such an ulcer is found together with a chronic ulcer in the duodenum. In such circumstances the choice before the surgeon lies between the performance of gastro-enterostomy well on the cardiac side of the ulcer and the excision of the gastric ulcer followed by gastro-enterostomy. I have excised many of these saddle-shaped ulcers of the lesser curvature, but have never yet found it necessary to perform gastro-enterostomy also.

Operation. The operation may be extremely difficult, for the ulcer may be firmly adherent to the pancreas or to the liver, or it may lie so close to the cardiac orifice of the stomach that it is almost inaccessible. I have on one occasion found the operation quite as difficult as a complete gastrectomy: the case concerned a man who had been very stout, but was much wasted, and the ulcer was close to the cardia and very adherent. The ultimate result was, however, very good.

The abdomen is opened by an ample incision through the right rectus muscle and the stomach exposed. The ulcer is then investigated, and the extent and density of any adhesions carefully noted. The first step consists in the division of the gastro-hepatic omentum above the ulcer and the inclusion within the part to be removed of any glands (the 'sentinel gland' of Lund) that lie along the lesser curvature. The coronary artery on each side of the ulcer is then ligatured; this is best done by surrounding it by an aneurysm needle, which is threaded with stout catgut and withdrawn. When ligatured above and below the ulcer the artery and vein are divided. A finger is then passed behind the stomach into the lesser sac, and the part of the viscus which is involved

in the subsequent manipulations pulled upwards into the wound. A
secure packing of large swabs is then introduced. The area of the
stomach which has to be excised is then mapped out, and clamps are
applied above and below. As a rule a bayonet-shaped clamp will be found
very convenient to apply on the cardiac side; an ordinary straight

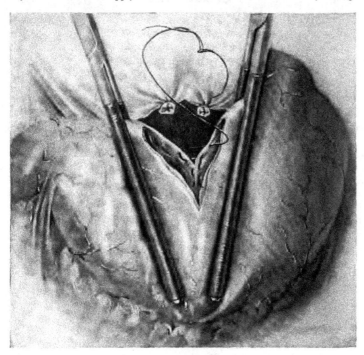

FIG. 285. EXCISION OF AN ULCER FROM THE LESSER CURVATURE.

clamp suffices for the pyloric side. Between these two clamps a triangular
area of the stomach, bearing the ulcer, is isolated. Care must be taken
to see that the tips of the clamp blades do not extend too far downwards
towards the greater curvature, for if too long a wedge is removed from
the stomach the puckering which results may be unsightly, and may
lead to stenosis. As much as possible of the healthy stomach-wall on
the side towards the greater curvature is therefore left.

When the clamps are secure, the ulcer, with the triangular portion
of the stomach which carries it, is excised, by snipping a little distance

from the clamp blades with large straight scissors. The clamps prevent any escape of blood or of stomach contents. The two clamps are now approximated and the suturing begins. A curved needle, which bears either chromic catgut or fine Pagenstecher's thread, is passed on the

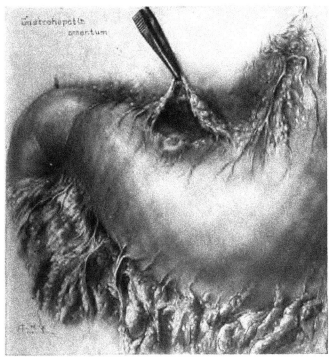

FIG. 286. ULCER ON ANTERIOR WALL WITH GASTROHEPATIC OMENTUM DIS-
SECTED FROM LESSER CURVATURE. (*Balfour.*)

posterior cut surfaces of the stomach at the part nearest the greater curvature from the mucous surface of the one side through all the coats to the mucosa of the opposite side, and then returns again through all the coats to the mucosa of the lower side, which is pierced about ⅛ inch from the original point of entry. The thread is now knotted, and a continuous suture begun. The needle passes as before from mucosa to serosa of the lower side through serosa to mucosa of the upper side, and then returns from mucosa, through the two apposing layers of serosa, to the mucosa of the lower side. A 'loop on the mucosa' (see p. 608) is thus left at each passage of the stitch. This stitch continues up towards the lesser curvature along the posterior margins of the incision, and then descends along the anterior surface of the stomach from the lesser curvature, to the end of the incision which lies nearest the greater curvature. As soon as this suture is completed it is seen that it has

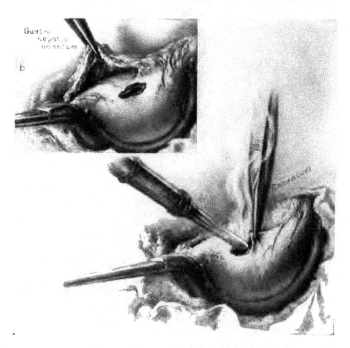

FIG. 287. a, BURNING OUT ULCER. b, ULCER COMPLETELY BURNED THROUGH.
(*Balfour.*)

infolded the mucosa, and has secured accurate serous apposition on both anterior and posterior aspects of the stomach. The clamps are then removed, and if any vessel bleeds it is secured by a ligature or by a separate stitch. The whole line of sutures is then reinforced by a continuous Pagenstecher's suture which begins on the posterior surface at the lower end, and continues along the whole line to the end of the suture line on the anterior surface.

The aperture in the gastro-hepatic omentum is then closed, the swabs removed, and the abdomen closed.

If excision of the ulcer in this way should seem impossible, or very difficult, the centre—the 'core,' so to speak—of the ulcer may be excised, and the aperture which remains closed by interrupted suture. In this

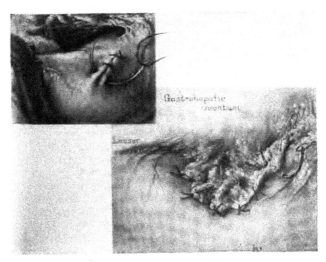

FIG. 288. a, FIRST ROW OF SUTURES CLOSING OPENING FROM WHICH ULCER HAS BEEN EXCISED. b, ULCER AREA COVERED BY GASTROHEPATIC OMENTUM. (*Balfour*.)

way an artificial perforation is produced and closed. When perforation of an ulcer in this situation occurs we know that its closure results in the permanent relief of the patient in almost every case.

Treatment of gastric ulcer by cautery (Balfour). The technique as described is as follows:

The portion of the gastrohepatic omentum in the region of the ulcer is carefully dissected free from the lesser curvature (see Fig. 286). The ulcer is carefully palpated and with a Pacquelin cautery maintained at a dull heat the point is slowly carried through the ulcer until an artificial perforation is produced. The moderate burning is continued until the actual area of the ulcer is entirely destroyed (see Fig. 287). Closure of the opening is then made by interrupted sutures of chromicized catgut reinforced by mattress sutures of silk. The reflected gastrohepatic omentum is then replaced over the site of the ulcer and fixed by superficial interrupted sutures of fine silk (see Fig. 288).

OPERATION FOR PERFORATING ULCER OF THE STOMACH OR DUODENUM

It is in cases of this class that the speed and dexterity which come to the surgeon as the fruit of long practice are of the greatest service. The operation should of course be thorough, and all its details must be observed with the most sedulous care; but the more speedily these things are done the greater is the chance of success. As a general rule the position of the ulcer can be localized to one or other side of the middle line before the operation is begun, and accordingly the incision should fall upon the abdomen to right or left of the middle line. If this be done there will be no need for any other incision than the vertical one; a transverse division of one or other rectus muscle is then unnecessary, and is at all times most undesirable.

Operation. The abdomen being opened, fluid will escape at once; if the fluid be bile-stained a perforation will probably be found in the duodenum, and it is there that a search should first be made. If the fluid be clear or turbid, containing the remnants of food recently taken, the perforation may be sought in the stomach. This fluid is usually sterile, and is inodorous. The ulcer may be difficult to discover. It may be covered over by adherent masses of thick lymph; to where these are abundant the search should be especially directed. At times the sizzling or the bubbling of gas may lead the surgeon to the point from which the leakage is occurring. The ulcer, as a rule, is found quite readily by searching along the lesser curvature, close to which it usually lies. As soon as it is found I think it best to secure its opening by a single catgut suture taken across it. By this means that constant leakage from the stomach, which is nearly always full, is prevented. My own practice then is to request the anæsthetist to pass the stomach tube, which is ready for use, in order to empty the stomach. This makes the subsequent suturing very much easier; and when the stitches are complete the stomach may be washed out with advantage. The single catgut suture, together with the ulcer, is now infolded by a double layer of stitches of thin Pagenstecher's thread, passed with a fine curved intestinal needle. This infolding and suture may be easy or may be extremely difficult. It is made difficult by the induration and stiffness which surround the ulcer. The hard œdematous margins of the ulcer do not hold the sutures easily. As soon as the stitch is passed it may cut through; or the attempt to bring the edges together may be rendered impossible by the inflexible nature of the stomach-wall at this part. If these difficulties be encountered they can only be overcome either by taking a much wider hold of the stomach, or by covering over the gap in the stomach by a layer of omentum. The former is to be preferred. The stiffness and brittleness, as a rule, do not extend over a large area, and sutures passed wide of this hold firmly enough. A double layer is used, and each layer extends well beyond the ulcer at each extremity. A flap of omentum may then be placed over the suture line and fixed there by one or two interrupted stitches.

The toilet of the peritoneum must now receive attention. The views of all surgeons as to how this may best be accomplished do not coincide, and my own practice has from time to time been modified as my experience increased, and as the time which had been allowed to lapse between perforation and operation by degrees became curtailed. In most cases a little local wiping is all that is necessary; a hot moist swab is used, and is gently patted on to the parts immediately in the neighbourhood. There should be no rubbing or ungentle handling. The abdomen is then closed without drainage. If there be more extensive soiling of the peritoneum, the process of cleansing must extend further. Hot swabs are passed to one or both kidney pouches, where fluid is prone to trickle and to lodge, or into the iliac fossa or into the pelvis. If there be a general infection of the peritoneum, the whole cavity being full of fluid, and the pelvis overflowing, then anything like a complete cleansing by mechanical means is impossible. I am then content to cleanse, as best I can, hurriedly, with swabs, which are packed away in the abdomen while the suturing of the ulcer is being done. When these are removed, a hand is passed down into the pelvis and a median incision immediately above the pubes is made, and a very large drainage tube is passed to the bottom of the pelvis. I do not practise, nor do I approve of, lavage. It probably does little to cleanse the cavity, and it is not seldom a cause rather than a preventative of shock. Drainage, though rarely necessary, when used should be ample. A split rubber tube in the suprapubic wound may be enough, but other openings may in very late cases be needed to drain the iliac fossæ or kidney pouches. A drain may also be left in the original wound. I find that I have drained only two cases in the last twelve upon which I have operated, and in these two only suprapubic drainage was necessary.

A further and perhaps the most important point is concerned with the necessity of performing gastro-enterostomy at once. When, for example, there has been a perforation of a duodenal ulcer, the infolding and suture will, of necessity, have caused some narrowing of the lumen of the gut. This lessening of the lumen is certain to become worse as

time passes and cicatricial contraction occurs in the area of the stomach
or duodenum involved in the operation. Again, not a few cases are
recorded in which two perforating ulcers have simultaneously, or almost
simultaneously, occurred; or in which, after the secure closure of one
ulcer, a second has perforated a week or more later, involving death or a
second operation. It is a consideration of cases such as these which has
drawn attention to the question of the advisability of gastro-enterostomy
as an addition to the closure of the rupture in the base of the ulcer. My
own practice is to perform gastro-enterostomy when stenosis has been
caused at or near the pylorus, or in the isthmus of an hour-glass stomach
by the closure of the ulcer; when stenosis is likely to result in the future
as a result of the healing of the parts engaged in the operation; or when
a second ulcer is present. The performance of gastro-enterostomy as
a routine procedure is certainly not necessary, and in some cases—as, for
example, when a solitary ulcer near the cardia on the lesser curvature
has ruptured—it is quite unnecessary. Inasmuch as it adds appreciably
to the length of an operation, every minute of which is of importance,
it is then positively dangerous.

After-treatment. The operation being completed, the patient is
propped up in bed, and continuous rectal infusion is given. This lessens
the thirst of the patient, and also the need for giving much fluid by the
mouth for the first thirty-six or forty-eight hours. I allow the patient
to drink as soon as the nausea due to the anæsthetic is over.

OPERATION FOR HOUR-GLASS STOMACH

In the condition known as hour-glass stomach there is a division of
the stomach into two cavities by a constriction which may be placed
at any point between the cardiac and pyloric orifices, but which lies
usually closer to the latter. This constriction is always acquired, and
is always pathological. It may be due to the cicatricial constriction of
a simple ulcer, to compression of the stomach by external adhesions
which probably have their origin in an ulcer, or to a new growth.

When the narrowing of the body of the stomach is due to a chronic
ulcer, there is not seldom evidence of the existence of a second ulcer
at or near the pylorus. This circumstance may add gravely to the
surgeon's task in devising an appropriate operation. For the pyloric
complement of such a stomach is often dilated, by reason of the obstruction at its outlet. If then gastro-enterostomy be performed between
the cardiac pouch and the small intestine, the pyloric pouch remains
undrained; if the distal pouch be engaged in the anastomosis, the cardiac
pouch is unaffected and the chief disability from which the patient

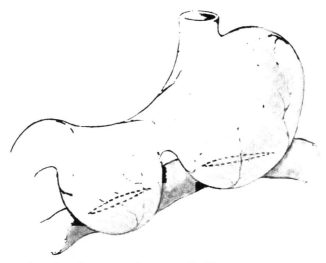

FIG. 289. HOUR-GLASS STOMACH. Double gastro-enterostomy.

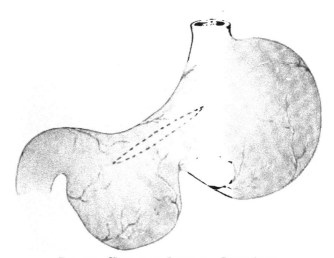

FIG. 290. HOUR-GLASS STOMACH. Gastroplasty.

suffered remains unrelieved. It is accordingly sometimes necessary to
perform a double operation.

The following operations may be needed :—

1. Gastro-enterostomy : anterior or posterior.

2. Double gastro-enterostomy, a junction of the intestine being made
with each sac : Weir and Foote's operation.

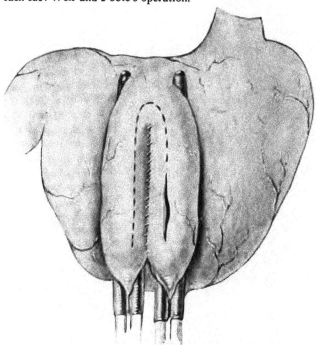

FIG. 291. HOUR-GLASS STOMACH. Kammerer's method of Gastroplasty.

3. Double gastro-enterostomy in **Y** : Monprofit's operation.

4. Gastroplasty.

5. Gastro-gastrostomy.

6. Partial gastrectomy.

7. Stretching of the constriction, as in Loreta's operation.

8. Duodenostomy or jejunostomy.

1. In the majority of cases *gastro-enterostomy between the cardiac
pouch and the jejunum* will be the operation of choice. When there

is only the single constriction present, the ulcer which has caused it lies as a rule in the prepyloric portion of the stomach.   The cardiac pouch is therefore very large—larger, indeed, than the whole stomach ordinarily is—whereas the pyloric pouch is not more than 2 or 3 inches in length, has undergone no dilatation, being unobstructed at its outlet, and is in no need of direct surgical treatment.   The problem then with

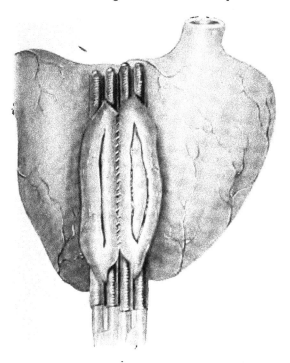

FIG. 292. HOUR-GLASS STOMACH.   Gastro-gastrostomy.
The clamps applied, one on each pouch.

which the surgeon has to deal is precisely that which confronts him in a case of simple pyloric stenosis, and gastro-enterostomy is the chosen procedure.   It is rare to find a difficulty in the performance of the posterior operation, but there may be an adhesion of the stenosing ulcer to the pancreas, with so many surrounding adhesions that the hinder surface of the stomach cannot easily be reached, and the anterior operation has to be performed.   These procedures are carried out in the manner described elsewhere.

2. *Double gastro-enterostomy.*   Weir and Foote in one case adopted this method.   Considering it desirable to ensure the emptying of both pouches, they attached the jejunum to each, the two openings in the bowel being near to one another.   I have never adopted this method. To perform it, it is necessary that both pouches should be large (they would otherwise not be in need of separate drainage); if they are large, then the operation of gastro-enterostomy would seem to be preferable.   There are no indications for this procedure which are not, as I think, better met by other operations.

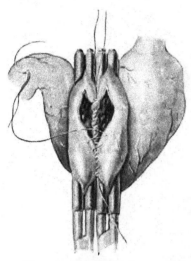

FIG. 293.   HOUR-GLASS STOMACH.
The inner suture.

3. *Monprofit's operation.* This is an application of Roux's method of gastro-enterostomy to hour-glass stomach.   The jejunum is divided at a point about 6 inches below the flexure; the distal cut end is attached to the cardiac pouch. and the proximal to the side of the distal about 3 inches below this point; so the cardiac pouch is drained.   A second division of the jejunum is made about 10 inches below the first division: the distal end here is attached to the pyloric pouch, and the proximal end again to the side of the distal: in this way the pyloric pouch is drained.   The objections to this operation are that it is necessarily tedious and prolonged, four separate anastomoses having to be made, and that the indications for its performance are more appropriately met by a different procedure.

4. *Gastroplasty.*   Gastroplasty is the application to the body of the stomach of a similar procedure to that which is followed in cases of pyloric stenosis in the operation of pyloroplasty.   And just as the latter operation, at first sight attractive, has proved in its results extremely unsatisfactory, so with gastroplasty has a secondary operation been too often necessary.   A modification of pyloroplasty introduced by Finney. and since known by this name, has given better results.   Kammerer has

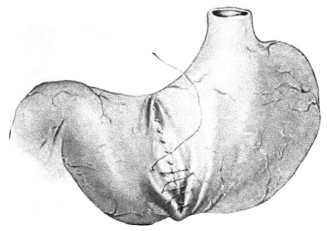

FIG. 294. HOUR-GLASS STOMACH. The outer suture nearly complete.

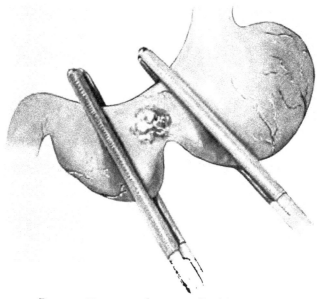

FIG. 295. HOUR-GLASS STOMACH. Partial gastrectomy.

adopted Finney's procedure in a modification of gastroplasty, which converts the operation almost into one of gastro-gastrostomy. The operation is carried out exactly as in Finney's method. Clamps are applied to the two compartments of the stomach close to the isthmus; a sero-muscular suture is applied from the isthmus to the greater curvature; an inverted U or V shaped incision is made in front of this, passing above through the isthmus and laterally down each complement of the stomach to the greater curvature. The inner through-and-through suture is then introduced, and finally the anterior sero-muscular suture is completed. (For details see Finney's operation, p. 623.)

5. *Gastro-gastrostomy or gastro-anastomosis,* first suggested by Wölfler, is indicated in those cases in which there is a tight stenosis in the centre of the stomach, with a surface of healthy stomach-wall on each side of it sufficient for a wide anastomosis. There must be no second narrowing in the pylorus or in the duodenum, so that when the obstruction in the body of the stomach has been relieved there is no further impediment to the onward passage of food. This operation in its general lines follows the method already described for gastro-enterostomy. The two pouches are drawn well up into the wound, isolated by large gauze swabs, and seized by a clamp which embraces the whole breadth of the stomach on each side of the constriction from the lesser curvature to the greater. The two clamps are then laid side by side, and every detail of the operation carried out as in gastro-enterostomy. When the clamps are removed a few additional stitches are needed to ensure that there shall be no tension on the suture lines.

6. *Partial gastrectomy* is not often necessary in the treatment of hour-glass stomach. The indications are chiefly two: first, in cases of carcinoma of the stomach, a central cylinder being removed and the stomach on each side being then united, or the stomach removed as in the ordinary operation of partial gastrectomy for carcinoma at or near the pylorus; and, secondly, in all those cases in which an indurated mass in the body of the stomach, though almost certainly a chronic ulcer, is yet possibly a malignant growth. The principle upon which to act here is that which Rodman has emphasized when urging his operation of excision of the ulcer-bearing area in multiple ulcers, or in ulcers suspected of malignancy. In a case upon which I recently operated I preferred to remove the greater part of the stomach in the manner described under the title Partial Gastrectomy (see p. 568).

7. *Digital divulsion* can only be very infrequently needed. In one case, however, it served me very well. The case was one of hour-glass stomach with a very large tumour at the isthmus. On opening the abdomen the mass was found to be adherent everywhere, to the abdomi-

nal wall in front, and the pancreas behind, so that access to the small cardiac pouch, sheltered under the costal margin, was impossible. Removal of the growth was equally out of the question. I therefore passed one, two, three, and finally four, fingers through the tight constriction from the distal to the cardiac pouch. The patient recovered, and now, several years later, is quite well. The tumour has entirely gone.

8. *Duodenostomy, or jejunostomy,* is only needed in cases of irremovable carcinoma when the cardiac pouch is too small or too inaccessible to permit of an anastomosis being attempted.

CHAPTER IV

GASTRO-ENTEROSTOMY

THE performance of gastro-enterostomy consists in the making of an anastomosis between the stomach and the small intestine. The jejunum is now always selected for attachment to the stomach, and the name 'gastro-jejunostomy' is therefore commonly used for this operation. Two methods of performing the operation are practised: in one the anterior surface of the stomach is engaged in the anastomosis, the operation being described as 'anterior gastro-enterostomy' or 'Wölfler's operation'; in the other the posterior surface is selected, the operation being known as 'posterior gastro-enterostomy' or 'Von Hacker's operation.'

Indications. The following are the indications for this procedure:

(i) *In certain cases of gastric or duodenal ulcer.*

(*a*) In cases of perforating ulcer of the pyloric portion of the stomach, or of the duodenum, when the closure of the perforation causes such narrowing of the outlet of the stomach that it would be difficult or impossible for food to pass.

(*b*) In cases of perforating ulcer of the stomach when other ulcers in or near the pyloric region are disclosed, ulcers which are causing, or are likely to cause as they heal, some hindrance to the free onward passage of food, or are themselves likely to perforate.

(*c*) When perforation has occurred at the isthmus of an hourglass stomach, and the closure of the perforation has narrowed the passage through the isthmus to a dangerous degree.

(*d*) In cases of hæmorrhage, recurrent and increasing, from either gastric or duodenal chronic ulcers.

(*e*) In all cases of chronic ulcer of the prepyloric or pyloric portions of the stomach or of the duodenum. If however, as is explained elsewhere, the ulcers are multiple, or are possibly becoming malignant, Rodman's operation of excision of the ulcer-bearing area may be preferable.

(*f*) In cases of fibrous stricture at or near the pylorus, due to a healed ulcer, the symptoms of whose activity have long been in abeyance. The condition in such cases is one of simple pyloric obstruction.

(*g*) In cases of perigastritis or periduodenitis in which the adhesions, due probably to ulcer in the first instance, but possibly to other causes, such as cholecystitis, are offering a mechanical impediment to the proper emptying of the stomach.

(*h*) In those rare cases of obstruction of the pylorus or duodenum due to biliary calculi which have ulcerated through from the gall-bladder (I have operated upon two such cases in which at the first glance the diagnosis of malignant disease seemed irresistible).

(*i*) In certain cases of hour-glass stomach, when the constriction is not far from the pylorus; or when gastroplasty has been performed. In the former the cardiac, in the latter the pyloric, complement is engaged in the anastomosis.

(ii) *In cases of carcinoma of the stomach,* or in the rare cases of cancer of the duodenum, in which the growth is already causing obstruction, or is likely soon to cause obstruction by its increase in size, provided always that the growth cannot safely be removed. The operation may also be performed as a preliminary to gastrectomy in cases where a cancerous growth is still limited to the stomach, but the patient is so wasted and ill that an immediate reaction has every prospect of being fatal. In such cases gastro-enterostomy permits a patient to take a great quantity of fluid nourishment, and very rapidly to gain strength for the more formidable operation which is performed two or three weeks later.

(iii) *In cases of congenital (infantile) hypertrophic stenosis of the pylorus.* In such cases, if any surgical treatment is necessary, and in my judgment it very rarely is so, gastro-enterostomy is to be preferred to all other operations. It is, however, only fair to add that pyloroplasty in the most capable hands of Mr. Clinton Dent has proved very successful.

(iv) *In cases of corrosion of the gastric mucosa* by caustic fluids, acids or alkalies, carbolic acid, nitric acid, soap-lye, or the like. If the pyloric part of the stomach only be affected gastro-enterostomy must be performed, and it may be advantageously combined with temporary gastrostomy.

(v) *In certain cases of acute dilatation of the stomach,* where there is obstruction at or near the pylorus or in the duodenum at the crossing of the superior mesenteric vessels.

Such are briefly the indications for gastro-enterostomy; but it is at least of equal importance to mention the conditions in which the operation must not be performed. In the first place, it cannot be too strongly asserted that this operation must not be done for the relief of symptoms unless there is a demonstrable organic cause for them in the stomach or duodenum. Symptomatic gastro-enterostomy, if one may use the expression, cannot be too strongly condemned. The surgeon will no doubt be asked at times to operate upon patients who suffer much from vomiting, for which an ulcer of the stomach is assumed to be responsible. Unless a definite organic cause can be discovered, a cause fully adequate to evoke the symptoms, this operation must not be practised. The surgeon, moreover, should not be satisfied with a few fine strands of adhesions or a doubtful thickening or roughening of the stomach-wall. If symptoms are caused by a chronic ulcer of the stomach its demonstration calls for no effort of imagination upon the part of the surgeon or the onlookers. The operation is valueless in cases of atonic dilatation of the stomach and in cases of gastroptosis, for both of which it has been warmly recommended, and not seldom performed. It is not in my opinion admissible in either condition. When an ulcer is found upon the lesser curvature near the cardiac end of the stomach excision of the ulcer is preferable to gastro-enterostomy. But excision is not always possible on account of adhesions to the liver or (chiefly) to the pancreas. In such circumstances gastro-enterostomy on the proximal side of the ulcer will be necessary.

POSTERIOR GASTRO-ENTEROSTOMY

The operation of posterior gastro-enterostomy is performed in the following manner :—

The abdomen is opened by a vertical incision 4 to 5 inches in length, about 1 inch to the right of the middle line between the ensiform cartilage and the umbilicus. The anterior sheath of the rectus is opened and the muscle fibres split, or the body of the muscle displaced outwards, and the posterior sheath and the peritoneum then incised together. The outer displacement of the muscle probably leaves a rather firmer abdominal wall when healing is complete, but I have only once seen any weakness of the scar after the separation of the rectus fibres, and that was in a case several years ago, in which Pagenstecher's thread was used to suture the various layers of the abdominal wound, and suppuration subsequently occurred.

The abdomen being opened, an inspection of the whole stomach and of the duodenum and gall-bladder is necessary. This examination must not be omitted, nor may it be only perfunctory. Unless it is carefully observed an hour-glass stomach may be overlooked, as in several recorded cases, or a duodenal ulcer, or old-standing gall-bladder changes due to calculi may escape recognition, and the patient's recovery be thereby seriously prejudiced. The few minutes expended in this investigation are well spent, for if the surgeon has begun the operation in the expectation of performing gastro-enterostomy he may find that other operations are necessary,—gastro-gastrostomy, gastroplasty, gastrectomy, or cholecystotomy alone or in addition to gastro-enterostomy. The stomach is

then withdrawn from the abdomen, together with the transverse colon
and the omentum, which are turned upwards so that the under surface
of the transverse mesocolon is exposed.   At the same time the duodeno-
jejunal flexure and the jejunum at its origin are recognized, and the
direction which the jejunum takes is noticed.   A thin peritoneal fold
usually attaches the first ½ inch of the jejunum to the under surface of

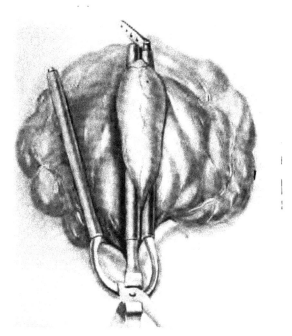

FIG. 296. POSTERIOR GASTRO-ENTEROSTOMY.
Application of the clamp to the stomach.

the mesocolon.   At the point where this leaves the mesocolon a pair of
forceps is applied and the mesocolon drawn well away, by means of them,
from the posterior surface of the stomach.   The mesocolon is then incised, or a snip made through it with the scissors, and the lesser sac thus
opened.   The rent in the mesocolon is then enlarged until it is 3 inches
in length.   The opening of the lesser sac is not always an easy matter, for
there may be adhesions of the upper surface of the mesocolon to the
posterior wall of the stomach, or a separation between the layers may be

made in the erroneous belief that the lesser sac has been opened. By
seizing the under layer with forceps in the way I have mentioned a clear
space is made upon which the incision may fall. Occasionally a vessel
may be wounded; if so, it is ligatured at once with very fine catgut. An
avascular area is of course chosen for the incision, and any vessel
wounded is therefore insignificant in size and quite unimportant.

The stomach is then inspected again from the front, and with the
left hand that exact portion of the viscus which it is desired to engage in
the anastomosis is pushed from above downwards through the opening
in the mesocolon in such manner that the posterior surface can be

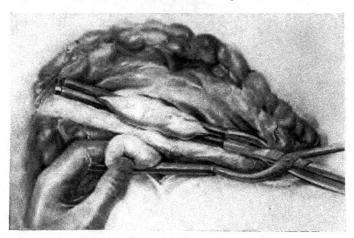

Fig. 297.   Posterior Gastro-enterostomy.
Application of the clamp to the jejunum.

grasped by the surgeon's right hand and pulled well through, in a bulk
sufficient to allow of the easy application of the clamp. A fold is then
made upon the stomach from the lesser curvature to the greater along
a vertical line. To do this the clamp is applied with the handle on the
surgeon's right side, and the tip of the blades pointing towards the
patient's head. With the three-bladed clamp, the two upper blades grip
the stomach (the uppermost blade bears the loose flange). The clamp
is now turned until it lies horizontal and transverse, the handle towards
the assistant, the tip of the blades towards the surgeon. The uppermost
part of the jejunum is now pulled taut from the duodeno-jejunal flexure
in readiness to be clamped by the two lower blades of the three-bladed
clamp; but before it is so seized two points must be observed.

The whole of the transverse colon, stomach, and omentum must be pushed backwards into the abdomen through that part of the incision which lies above the clamp; when this is done a large hot flat swab is placed over the wound, coming close up to the clamp, and at each end underlying it a little. Then between the stomach and the jejunal fold as it is pulled up to be grasped by the clamp a long thin strip of hot moist gauze is placed, to lie beneath the centre blade of the clamp so as to catch any possible discharge which may chance to trickle backwards. The jejunum is now clamped. In doing this the gut is pulled up very

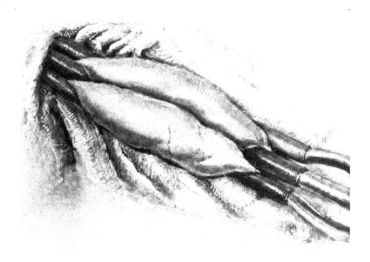

FIG. 298. POSTERIOR GASTRO-ENTEROSTOMY.
The viscera clamped and surrounded by gauze.

tightly from the flexure, and care is taken to see that its proximal end is not twisted or kinked. In a few cases the upper end of the jejunum is adherent to the under surface of the mesocolon, or more rarely to the posterior abdominal wall. It chances that I have noticed this condition of mesocolic adhesion more especially in cases of intractable duodenal ulcer. It is worth noting that the adhesion invariably in my experience fixes the jejunum to the right of the flexure. These adhesions must be freed completely up to the flexure before the gut is embraced by the clamp. When it is secured the flange on the top of the upper blade is closed over the middle and lower blades so as to pull the blade-tips well together. A second large moist swab is placed below the clamp, covering in the lower part of the wound.

All that is now seen outside the abdomen is the clamp, which carries the folds of the stomach and jejunum to be anastomosed, each about 3 to 4 inches in length, closely surrounded in all parts by the substantial gauze swabs. There is, of course, no 'exposure of viscera' throughout this operation, if these steps be properly observed; though it is no uncommon thing to hear this supposed detraction from the merits of the operation discussed. The union of the two viscera is now begun. Two sutures only are used, both continuous. The outer suture is sero-

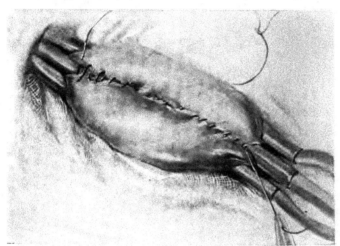

FIG. 299.   POSTERIOR GASTRO-ENTEROSTOMY.
The first line of suture; sero-muscular.

muscular; the inner includes all the coats. The needle I prefer is a curved needle of my own pattern; it is slender, five-eighths of a circle in its curve, has a slot eye, and is of such a diameter that it is the slightest degree thicker than the finest Pagenstecher's thread when doubled. These needles are made by Down Bros. This needle picks up almost automatically the exact amount of the viscera that is necessary, and because of the relationship between its thickness and that of the thread which it carries there is no 'pull' necessary when the thread is to be drawn through the puncture which the needle has already made.

The first suture introduced is a sero-muscular suture. It is begun at the left end of the viscera engaged in the clamp (that nearest the assist-

ant) and is brought directly along in a straight line until the tip of the
blade is reached.   It is here that the greater curvature lies, and care is
necessary to see that the lowest part of the curvature is engaged in the
suture.   The large vessels which at this point lie along the curvature
and send off their branches to the stomach may readily be avoided.   As
the suture is introduced it is pulled fairly tight so as to bring the apposing
surfaces snugly together.   The part of the thread between the last stitch
and the needle when drawn upon raises up a little hillock on each viscus,

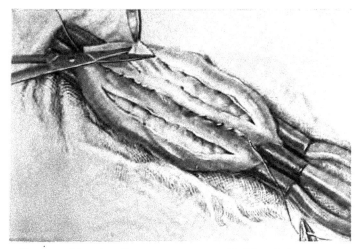

FIG. 300.   POSTERIOR GASTRO-ENTEROSTOMY.   Excision of the mucosa.

showing where the next insertion of the needle is to be made, and making
that insertion easier.   The number of introductions of the needle is
usually about eight to ten to the inch, and at least $2\frac{1}{2}$ inches should be
included in this suture.   When this first line is completed the needle is
laid aside for a time.

An incision is now made about $\frac{1}{4}$ inch in front of this suture into
both stomach and intestine.   The serous and muscular coats only are
incised, and the mucous coat then pouts into the wound.   An ellipse of
this mucosa is then excised from both the stomach and the jejunum;
from the stomach it is removed easily in one piece; from the jejunum it
is almost impossible to take all that is necessary away in one piece, for
after removing a large ellipse it is found that a small additional piece
at each end requires to be snipped away.   The inner suture is now introduced.   It embraces all the coats of both viscera, and is hæmostatic.   The

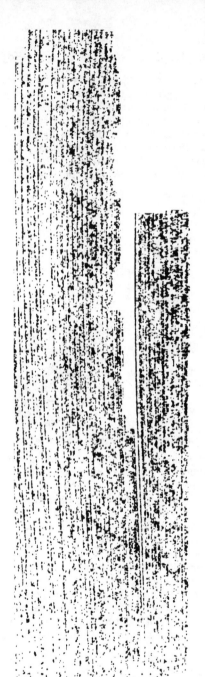

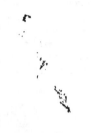

FIG. 301.
The inner su

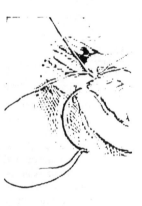

FIG. 302.
The inne

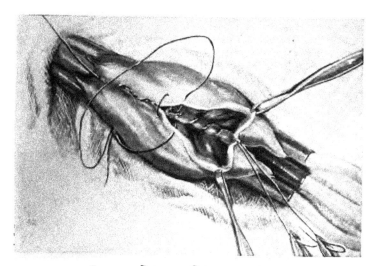

FIG. 303. POSTERIOR GASTRO-ENTEROSTOMY.
The inner suture, showing the loop on the mucosa.

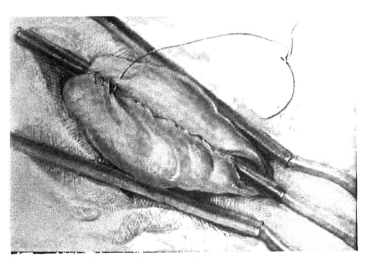

FIG. 304. POSTERIOR GASTRO-ENTEROSTOMY.
The inner suture complete; continuation of outer suture.

needle is first introduced through the extreme left end of the jejunum, passing from the mucous to the serous surface; then from the serous to the mucous surface at the extreme left end of the stomach; when the knot is tied it lies therefore upon the mucosa. The stitch is now carried along the posterior (in this position) margins of the opening, passing from mucosa to serosa on the jejunal side and from serosa to mucosa on the stomach side, continuously. It is drawn so tight that any vessel opened by the incision is secured, and the same gentle pull upon the

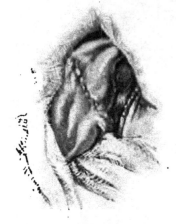

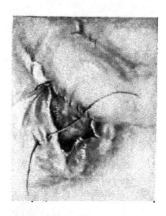

FIG. 305. POSTERIOR GASTRO-ENTEROSTOMY. Removal of gauze strip.

FIG. 306. POSTERIOR GASTRO-ENTEROSTOMY. Attachment of great omentum to suture line.

thread raising up a fold for the next introduction of the needle will be found of great service.

When the greater curvature of the stomach is reached the type of stitch may well be changed. I now frequently adopt for the return half of the suture line the stitch best described as the ' loop on the mucosa ' stitch. It is, I believe, identical with the old ' pillow-maker's stitch.' The change to this stitch is made when the extreme right end of the suture line is reached. The needle at its last passage has penetrated from the mucosa of the jejunum to the mucosa of the stomach, from which the thread now emerges. In the next passage the needle is made to traverse from the stomach mucosa to the serosa. It is now passed through the anterior margin of the jejunum twice, first from serosa to mucosa, then from mucosa to serosa, so that a ' loop on the mucosa '

is left.   Then the needle engages the stomach, passing from serous to
mucous and from mucous to serous coats at each separate passage of
the needle.   As the suture is drawn tight, the edges of the incision will
be seen to infold themselves so that the serous surfaces come accurately
into apposition.   This is the prettiest stitch in all surgery; to see the
inversion ·of the two edges occurring as each turn of the suture is
tightened is quite pleasing.   The suture is continued along the whole

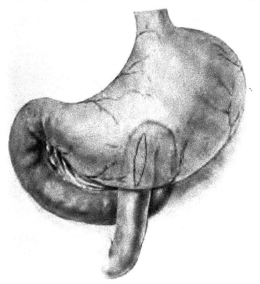

Fig. 307. Posterior Gastro-enterostomy.   Completion of the operation.

length of the anterior margins until the original starting-point is reached,
and here the needle is made to emerge at the last on the mucosa, and the
thread is tied to the end originally left long; the knot therefore lies on
the mucous surface.   This inner suture may be of thin chromic catgut,
or of Pagenstecher's thread; it is immaterial which is chosen.

The parts are now wiped over with a. moist swab, and the clamp
loosened, the terminal flange being first undone.   The clamp is, however,
left in position until the final suture is complete.   The hands of the
surgeon and assistant are thoroughly rinsed, as both have been in contact
probably with the mucosa, which, though generally sterile, may be infected.   All instruments which have been used up to this stage are discarded and a clean sterile towel is placed below the wound, upon which

the fresh instruments may lie. Before the final suture is introduced the
suture line is carefully inspected to see that there are no bleeding points.
The needle used for the first suture, temporarily laid aside, is now taken
up again, and the sero-muscular suture continued from the greater curvature, which it had just reached, back again, in front of the inner through-
and-through suture just completed, to the original starting-point at the
lesser curvature. The final turn of the needle at this point is introduced
after the original end of the suture, which was left long, has been drawn
up in the surgeon's left hand, so that the parts embraced by it are clearly

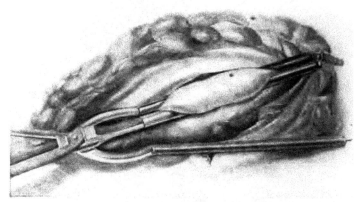

FIG. 308. POSTERIOR GASTRO-ENTEROSTOMY. Antiperistaltic anastomosis.
Application of clamp.

seen. The needle is then passed just beyond this first suture, to secure
accurate closure at this point, and the suture knotted and cut short.

The parts are again cleaned, the clamp removed, and the strip of
gauze which lay behind it pulled out towards the surgeon so that the first
line of sutures can be inspected. The next step is to secure the edges of
the opening in the mesocolon to the suture line. The transverse colon
and omentum are pulled out from the upper part of the wound, wherein
they have been lying, and with the surgeon's left hand the transverse
colon is lifted away from the abdominal wall until the mesocolon is made
taut. An edge of the mesocolon is then seized with a clip and a suture
introduced. The needle picks up the mesocolon at some distance from
the edge, and then passes through the stomach and jejunum at the line of
suture, or through the jejunum alone just as close as possible to the
suture line. When this stitch is tightened the roughened cut edge in

the mesocolon is rolled inwards to the lesser sac. Three or four more sutures of the same kind are introduced, all round the opening in the mesocolon, until this peritoneal layer fits closely round the line of anastomosis. The reasons for these sutures are chiefly two: they close the opening into the lesser sac, leaving no gap through which the gut may pass and be strangled, and they ensure a smooth peritoneal fold over all the lines of suture so that no rough edges or tags remain to which adhesions may form. The stomach, colon, omentum, and jejunum are now returned within the abdomen, care being taken to see that the first six or eight inches of the jejunum are directed aright in continuation of the line of anastomosis.

Mayo's modification of this method consists in making the attachment of the jejunum to the stomach along a line which is oblique from above downwards and to the left. Mayo supposed that this was the 'natural direction' of the jejunum; but I have elsewhere given rea-

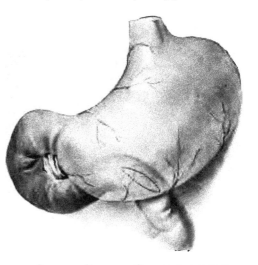

Fig. 309. Posterior Gastro-enterostomy.
Antiperistaltic anastomosis. Operation complete.

sons to show that there is no 'natural' direction of the jejunum at its origin, for it is there free to move to any position in accordance with the position of the body. The vertical position is consequently that most commonly occupied, and it is that which it is best to maintain in the operation of gastro-enterostomy.

The method of applying the clamp and the position of the operation in Mayo's modification are shown in the figures (see Figs. 308, 309) ; all the other details of the operation are the same as those already described.

Roux's operation. A most ingenious, and in certain cases a most satisfactory, method of performing gastro-enterostomy has been suggested by Professor Roux of Lausanne. It is described as the 'gastro-enterostomy in Y'. The intention of the operation is to reproduce artificially at the new anastomosis the conditions which exist at the pylorus. To give effect to this, the jejunum is divided at a spot about 10 or 12 inches below the duodeno-jejunal flexure; the distal end is implanted into the stomach (making a new pylorus), the proximal end is attached to the side of the distal 3 to 4 inches below the junction with the stomach (making a new diverticulum of Vater). The anastomosis with the stomach is made on the posterior surface close to the lowest point of the greater curvature. The following is the method of procedure: The posterior surface of the stomach is exposed and clamped as in the usual posterior operation. The jejunum is then brought up into the wound, and a point on it about 10 inches below the flexure is selected as the apex of a loop about 8 inches in length, the base of which is gripped with a clamp. This loop, being securely held, is now divided at about 2 inches below the upper clamped extremity. The division continues a little way into the mesentery so as to allow the distal limb to be drawn away from the proximal. The distal open-

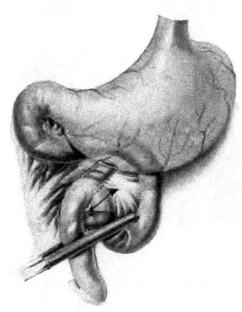

FIG. 310. POSTERIOR GASTRO-ENTEROSTOMY. Roux's operation. Application of clamp, division of gut.

ing is now united by suture to that portion of the stomach-wall which is gripped by the clamp. Two layers of suture only are necessary, and they are passed in exactly the same manner as in the procedure already described; Roux himself, however, uses three layers of stitches. This anastomosis being completed, the divided proximal end of the jejunum is now united to the side of the distal limb about 3 inches below the stomach. The opening in the transverse mesocolon is then closed by suture to the stomach around the anastomosis and the operation is complete.

ANTERIOR GASTRO-ENTEROSTOMY

The abdomen is opened by an incision through the right rectus muscle, as in the former method, and the stomach examined in all its parts. The decision to perform anterior gastro-enterostomy having been made, the transverse colon and the omentum are drawn out of the lower part of

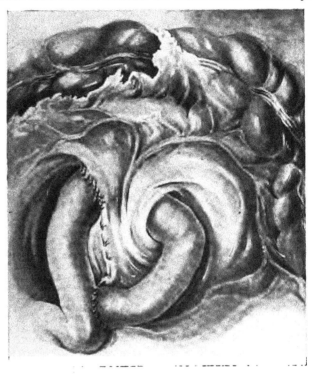

FIG. 311. POSTERIOR GASTRO-ENTEROSTOMY. Roux's operation completed.

the wound, and are displaced upwards sufficiently to allow the discovery of the uppermost part of the jejunum as it comes off from the duodeno-jejunal flexure. The jejunum is lifted into the wound, and passed through the fingers until a point on it about 16 to 18 inches from the flexure is reached. This is the part which is to be engaged in the anastomosis. A clamp is now applied, embracing about 3 to 4 inches of the gut at this part, the proximal end being to the left, the distal to the right, that is, towards the operator. A similar clamp is now applied to the stomach, in such a manner that the portion of the anterior wall of the viscus which is grasped lies obliquely from above downwards and to the right. The lowest part of the fold lying in the blades must be that point on the greater curvature of the stomach which lies vertically below the right margin of the œsophagus; it is the lowest point of the greater curvature. The two clamps being applied, all the viscera not grasped by them are returned within the abdomen. A long thick gauze strip is now laid between the clamps, which are brought together, and around

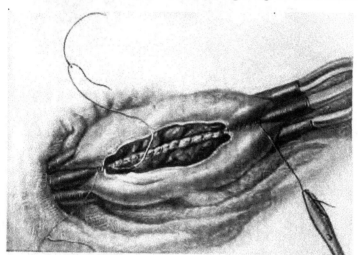

Fig. 312. Anterior Gastro-enterostomy. Clamp applied.

them are laid flat gauze swabs wrung out of hot saline solution. Nothing, therefore, can now be seen except the clamps, the parts of the viscera they hold, and the flat swabs which fit closely round them.

The union of the two viscera is now begun, and the exact details which are given in the description of the operation of posterior gastro-enterostomy are followed, with a slight exception. When the first line of sutures has been introduced, the incision in the stomach and the intestine is not made to the full extent of this, but lies along only the lower two-thirds of the line. The result is that when the suturing is complete the outer suture extends upwards along the stomach and jejunum for some distance beyond the opening which connects them. There is a suspension therefore of the jejunum above the anastomosis, the suspension being caused by the upper extremities of the outer line of suture. Another point worthy of attention is this: the opening in the jejunum should lie not at the part exactly opposite the line of mesenteric attachment, but rather on that side of the gut which lies nearest the stomach, in such manner as to secure that the lateral aspect of the bowel lies flat against the anterior surface of the stomach.

The suture being completed the clamps are withdrawn. One or more additional suspension sutures may be placed between the stomach and jejunum at the upper end, if thought desirable. When the viscera are replaced within the abdomen, care should be taken to see that the transverse colon and the omentum are well placed, and that the proximal limb of the jejunum does not seem to constrict the transverse colon.

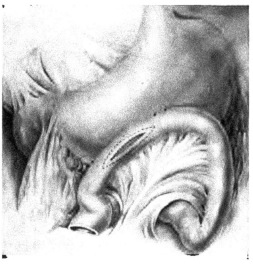

If it be thought desirable to perform an entero-anastomosis between the afferent and efferent limbs of the jejunum, this may readily be done about 3 inches below the stomach. The two jejunal lengths

FIG. 313. ANTERIOR GASTRO-ENTEROSTOMY. Complete.

to be united are embraced by clamps, isolated by gauze swabs, and united by suture in exactly the same manner as has been already observed in the making of the union between the stomach and the bowel.

COMPLICATIONS AND SEQUELÆ OF THE OPERATION

The experience of the last decade has shown that the operation of gastro-enterostomy, however brilliant its immediate results, is not free from certain risks, which, though perhaps tardy in appearance, are yet directly attributable to the operation. It is true that the majority of these complications are now abolished, or have had their frequency much lessened by recent improvements in technical details; but their consideration here is none the less incumbent upon me.

Hæmorrhage. The occurrence of bleeding after the operation of gastro-enterostomy may be of every grade of severity. If a patient vomits at all after this operation, a very unusual circumstance in my own experience, the ejected matter is almost always just tinged with altered blood. This blood has probably escaped into the stomach at the time the anastomosis was made, and in quantity it is not more than one or two teaspoonfuls. But there are cases in which the hæmorrhage may be considerable, and at least three cases have been reported in which it has proved fatal. The blood may come from two sources: from the ulcer or ulcers for which the operation has been performed, or from the incisions made into the stomach or jejunum at the line of anastomosis. It is only rarely that the ulcer is the source, but the fact that it some-times is so should compel the surgeon to exercise great gentleness in handling the ulcer itself, or the part of the stomach or duodenum in which it lies. Furthermore, the policy of infolding all ulcers of the duodenum or of the pyloric portion of the stomach, which I have so long advocated, should be adopted, for thereby the vessels going to the ulcer are carefully secured, and the risks both of perforation and of hæmorrhage are annulled. The hæmorrhage may occur also from the suture line, and it is probable that it does so in the majority of cases. I have had two cases in which fresh blood, to the quantity of about one pint, was vomited within twenty-four hours of the operation; in both the hæmorrhage came, no doubt, from the incision in the stomach, for in both the ulcers were small, and had never bled before. These two cases were in my early experience; since I learnt to suture better I have had no cases of hæmorrhage, for the securing of all vessels by a well-applied stitch will effectually prevent even the slightest risk of bleeding. This untoward complication may therefore be avoided by the handling of all parts during the operation with the most sedulous care, and by so applying the inner suture that all vessels are well secured.

When hæmorrhage occurs in any quantity it is desirable at once to cease giving fluids by the mouth, except perhaps adrenalin (30 minims of 1 in 1,000 solution in a dessert-spoonful of water every half-hour, or every hour, till six or eight doses have been taken); lavage of the stomach with water as hot as can be comfortably borne is sometimes useful.

Regurgitant vomiting. No small part of the literature dealing with operations upon the stomach is concerned with this question of regurgitant vomiting. The ' vicious circle ' has proved the most terrible and the most frequent of the serious complications of gastro-entero-stomy. I well remember that of the first thirteen cases of gastro-entero-stomy that I saw as a resident officer, no fewer than nine died as a result of regurgitant vomiting. Vomiting comes on as a rule within the first few hours or days of the operation. In quantity the ejected matters vary considerably, but in the severer cases two or three pints are vomited every twenty-four hours. The ejected matters are bile-stained; in some cases they consist of pure bile, in others the colour may be brownish and the odour offensive. As a rule, the act of vomiting is painless, a great gush of fluid pours from the mouth, with little or no straining on the part of the patient.

Regurgitant vomiting is due to high intestinal obstruction. The obstruction may be at the anastomosis, either afferent or efferent opening being implicated; or it may involve the jejunum a few inches below the anastomosis. As a rule, the obstruction is at the afferent opening, and is probably due to the fixation of a piece of intestine, weakened by the division of its circular muscular coat, in such conditions that a loop remains between the duodeno-jejunal flexure (a fixed point) and the anastomosis. As a result of a kink at the weakened spot the loop becomes ' waterlogged '; it is found greatly distended and overfull when the abdomen is opened. Relief is afforded by entero-anastomosis, by the union of the engorged loop to the empty and collapsed intestine distal to the obstruction. The efferent opening also may be obstructed by kinking, or the jejunum may be compressed by adhesions immediately beyond its attachment to the stomach. Regurgitant vomiting is avoided by adopting the posterior no-loop operation. Nevertheless, in some cases after this method has been practised there may be vomiting of bile, irregularly and painlessly. This condition may appear weeks or months after the operation; it is distressing and troublesome, but not a serious menace to health. It is almost certainly due to some slight obstruction at the duodeno-jejunal flexure or at the upper end of the anastomosis to the stomach, the result of an improper application of the intestine rotated around its axis; or to the selection of a piece of intestine an inch or more too low down on the jejunum, so that a very short loop is left which may kink either at the upper or at the lower end. When vomiting of this kind occurs, recourse should quickly be had to lavage of the stomach. It is remarkable how effectual this may be in lessening or even in entirely abolishing this most distressing symptom. If the stomach be emptied and washed out once or twice daily, the vomiting may disappear, never to return. If, however, in spite of lavage, regurgitation still continues, then the abdomen must be reopened and the mechanical defect, which is generally easily recognizable, repaired at once. Entero-anastomosis between the proximal and distal jejunal limbs, or the division of the afferent limb and the performance of Roux's gastro-enterostomy in Y at another part of the stomach, will usually be indicated.

Jejunal ulcer. The occurrence of this, perhaps the most serious, certainly the most interesting, complication of gastro-enterostomy was first observed by Braun, and recorded in 1889. Since then some forty cases have been related.

The ulcer is found in the jejunum bordering on, or within a short distance (usually within 1 inch) of the opening from, the stomach. As a rule, it is solitary, but two, three, or in one case four, ulcers have been found. The investigation of the recorded cases has shown me that four types of this disease may be recognized.

(a) The ulcer develops rapidly and perforates shortly after the operation. There are only three cases which can be included in this group. The circumstances in all are similar: gastro-enterostomy was performed for an ulcer at or beyond the pylorus, associated with hyperacidity, which in two cases was intense; the progress for the first few days was satisfactory, then suddenly there was an acute onset of pain followed by peritonitis and death. In all cases an ulcer just beyond the anastomosis was found, and perforation had occurred into the general peritoneal cavity.

(b) The ulcer develops within a few weeks or months of the operation, and the symptoms suggest a recurrence of the ulcer for which the operation was performed. The cases in this group are many. The symptoms are very similar to those which were caused by the original ulcer, in the stomach or in the duodenum, for which the gastro-enterostomy was performed. These complaints are attributed to a supposed 'recurrence' of the ulcer. Secondary operations were performed for disabling symptoms or for perforation and peritonitis. In these instances acute perforation had occurred in a chronic ulcer.

(c) The ulcer develops languidly, and insidiously undergoes a 'subacute' perforation, with the result that a tumour forms in, or abutting upon, the epigastrium. About two-fifths of all the recorded examples fall in this category. There are not usually any symptoms of which the patient takes serious notice. As a rule only some trivial discomfort after meals or indigestion is noticed; on examination of the patient a distinct tumour is felt. When the abdomen is opened the jejunum at or near the anastomosis is found adherent usually to the parietes. On separating the viscera a perforation into the intestine at the site of an ulcer a little below the anastomosis is discovered. The condition, it will be seen, is precisely analogous to that of 'subacute perforation' in the stomach (see *Annals of Surgery*, 1907, vol. xlv, p. 223).

(d) The ulcer perforates into a hollow viscus. The ulcer is of the chronic type, and perforation occurs after adhesion to a hollow viscus, either the stomach or the colon.

A careful examination of all recorded cases has shown that jejunal ulcer occurs only after operation for simple ulcer of the stomach or duodenum. I have found no instance in which the operation was performed for cancer. This absence of jejunal ulcer in malignant cases may be due to the short duration of life after operation—the patient has not time, as it were, to develop an ulcer; or it may be due to the absence in most cases of free HCl from the gastric juice. Peptic ulcer has occurred more often after the anterior operation than after the posterior, though probably the latter has been, and now certainly is, far more frequently performed for non-malignant conditions. All forms of gastro-enterostomy have, however, furnished examples; the anterior and the posterior with or without entero-anastomosis, Roux's operation and the no-loop method. More cases have occurred in men, and in most instances free HCl has been found in excess.

The fact that peptic jejunal ulcer may occur after gastro-enterostomy should urge the surgeon to see that the greatest care is exercised by the patient in the matter of diet for several months after operation. In a patient who for years has been unable or unwilling to take food, the swift return after operation to health and a good appetite which can without discomfort be appeased, leads not seldom to over-indulgence in both food and drink. It is probable that the same conditions are being repeated which were responsible for the development of the original ulcer in the stomach. It is most desirable that all patients who have been submitted to operation upon the stomach should report, or present themselves, to their medical men for some months after operation.

Intestinal obstruction. Several cases of intestinal obstruction following gastro-enterostomy are recorded. As I have mentioned, regurgitant vomiting is due to obstruction of the jejunum very high up, close to or at the anastomosis. Several other forms are described. I have myself lost a patient from an internal hernia, the small intestine having passed through the opening made in the transverse mesocolon into the lesser sac, and having become obstructed by the margins of this opening. This accident may be prevented by closure of the opening, its margins being sutured to the stomach, jejunum, or suture-line, after the anastomosis is complete. Other cases have shown obstruction of a length of gut which has passed through a loop left between the duodeno-jejunal flexure and the anastomosis. This loop, together with the meso-colon, forms a ring, and through this ring intestine has passed from right to left in some cases, from left to right in others, to become strangulated; in one case a volvulus of the bowel was also found (Barker). In anterior gastro-enterostomy the loop of jejunum, if pulled too tight (by selection for the anastomosis of a part too near the flexure), may constrict the colon. One case of obstruction due to the adhesion of a piece of small intestine to the abdominal incision is also recorded (Newbolt, *Lancet*, 1907, ii. 1461).

Diarrhœa. In some few cases diarrhœa after operation has been observed; as a rule it is transient and easily relieved; in some cases, however, it has been continuous and uncontrollable and has caused the patient's death. Kelling has described two forms. Firstly, that in which the diarrhœa is due to the escape into the intestine of acid contents which are not neutralized by the bile or pancreatic juice. Secondly, that in which it is due to ' fermentation '. The latter he considers is not serious, and is seen only in patients suffering from carcinoma, or in those cases where HCl is deficient or absent. There is no convincing evidence of the existence of the first form. Indeed, a survey of one's own experience and of the recorded evidence available has shown that it is almost exclusively in cases of carcinoma that diarrhœa occurs, and that it is only in them that it is at all serious. The motions are always offensive. Anschütz believes that the chief cause is the extreme exhaustion of the patient, by a long-standing disease, at the time the operation is performed; and he remarks that exactly the same type of intestinal uncontrol is found when there is carcinoma or advanced tuberculous disease in other parts than the intestine.

There is, however, no acceptable explanation which is applicable to all cases. So far as treatment is concerned we must attend to the diet, giving only sterile foods (not necessarily fluid) and administering antiseptics (isoform preferably), magnesia usta, and opium or other astringents in large doses.

THE RELATIVE MERITS OF ANTERIOR AND POSTERIOR GASTRO-ENTEROSTOMY

The gradual transference of the allegiance of the surgeons of largest experience from the anterior to the posterior operation is not due to mere caprice, but to a confident belief that the latter operation, both in its immediate and remote results, is the better procedure. The points which are to be discussed in this connexion are concerned with—

(*a*) Regurgitant vomiting.

(*b*) Peptic jejunal ulcer.

(*c*) Intestinal obstruction due to internal hernia.

Regurgitant vomiting. The causes of this most disastrous complication are elsewhere discussed. It is only necessary here to say that it is an evidence of intestinal obstruction occurring at or near the anastomosis. It occurs far more commonly after the anterior than after the posterior operation; indeed in many of the early cases of the former method it was the direct cause of death. It is now recognized that it is the existence of the ' loop ' which is responsible for the onset of this symptom. The jejunum, attached normally at the duodeno-jejunal flexure, and fixed by suture to the stomach at a point 15 or 18 inches lower down, forms a loop, which is apt to become ' waterlogged '. At the point where the anastomosis to the stomach occurs, not only is there an abnormal fixed point, but the gut at this part is weakened by the division of circular muscular fibres in its wall. That the obstruction occurs at the anastomosis (either afferent or efferent opening being blocked) is shown by the fact that relief from the vomiting is promptly ensured when the limbs of the bowel are united by the performance of entero-anastomosis. The ' loop ' is the responsible factor. If posterior gastro-enterostomy is performed with a loop, regurgitant vomiting is as likely to occur as after the anterior operation. It is in the abolition of the loop, by performing the anastomosis close to the flexure, that safety lies. The posterior operation, therefore, is better than the anterior, not merely because it is posterior, but because, being posterior, it allows the jejunum close to the flexure to be engaged in this anastomosis, and the loop, consequently, to be eliminated.

Peptic ulcer. This condition has only been found to occur after operations for non-malignant diseases; it has never followed upon gastro-enterostomy for carcinoma. The number of recorded cases shows that the ulcer is found more frequently after the anterior operation than after the posterior; perhaps because the lower opening into the bowel exposes a mucosa which is more sensitive to acid contact.

Internal hernia. Several forms of internal hernia are recorded. In the posterior operation it may be caused by the escape of the small intestine upwards into the lesser sac, through the opening into the transverse mesocolon. I have myself lost one case through this accident. The attachment of the mesocolon by a few stitches to the stomach, or to the stomach and jejunum along the line of suture, will, however, close the aperture into the lesser sac and prevent the occurrence of this form of hernia.

In the anterior operation two forms of obstruction have occurred. In one the loop of jejunum, being drawn up tightly from the flexure to the stomach, has constricted the transverse colon and occasioned an obstruction sufficiently severe to prove fatal. In the other loops of the small intestine have passed from right to left, or from left to right through the ring formed by the under surface of the transverse meso-

colon and the jejunal loop as it passes from the flexure to the anastomosis, and have become strangulated.   In both cases it is the loop of
jejunum which is the factor responsible.

Taking these points into consideration there can, I think, be no doubt
that the posterior no-loop operation is that which is, on all counts, the
most satisfactory.   It is sometimes argued that the posterior operation
is not so suitable in many cases as the anterior method, on account of
its difficulty and because of the necessary ' handling ' and ' exposure ' of
the viscera.   Those who argue thus have but little experience of the
posterior operation, or employ a technique which is not satisfactory.
The one operation is as easy as the other; there is very little handling
of the viscera in either case, and nothing more than a momentary and
quite harmless exposure.   I have a considerable experience of both
operations, having performed the posterior operation over five hundred
times and the anterior over seventy times.   The results in the immediate
after-history of the two operations differ sensibly.   After the posterior
operation the patient is at once quite well.   He has no sickness, no feeling
of nausea, is comfortable, and is soon eager for food.   After the anterior
operation there is sometimes a feeling of nausea, occasionally a little
vomiting, and appetite returns less rapidly.   We should, however, consider the results of the anterior method decidedly good (as indeed they
are) were it not that they suffer by comparison with those achieved by
the posterior operation.

GASTRO-DUODENOSTOMY (FINNEY'S OPERATION)

The operation of gastro-duodenostomy was introduced into surgery
by Jaboulay, who first performed it in 1894.   He made two incisions of
equal length, one in the stomach, the other in the duodenum, and united
these by suture, the pylorus being displaced backwards, as it were, to
allow of the approximation of the two openings in front of it.   Kümmell
adopted a different method; he divided the duodenum completely across
and implanted the distal end into the anterior wall of the stomach after
closure of the proximal end.   The operation of pyloroplasty suggested
by Heinecke and Mikulicz consisted in dividing the pylorus transversely.
in cases where an ulcer has caused cicatricial stenosis, the wound then
being sutured in a vertical direction.   The results of this operation at the
first were very remarkable, but the lapse of months or of years did not
bear out the early promise.   Patients who had for a time enjoyed perfect
health and normal appetites began to have a recurrence of their former
symptoms, and many of them submitted willingly enough to the operation of gastro-enterostomy in order to obtain relief from their renewed

sufferings. Pyloroplasty, indeed, fell very properly into disuse. Dr. J. M. T. Finney of Baltimore introduced what he termed a 'modified form of pyloroplasty,' to which the names of 'gastro-duodenostomy' and 'gastro-pyloro-duodenostomy' have been given. The simplest and most generally accepted title is 'Finney's operation,' which is thus performed :—

The abdomen is opened by an incision to the right of the middle line, as in gastro-enterostomy. The pyloric region of the stomach is exposed and examined. Ad-
hesions which at first sight would appear to negative any plastic procedure being performed will yield readily to careful and persistent stripping with gauze. The free division of all tethering adhesions is the first and perhaps the most important of all the steps in the operation. The second portion of the duodenum is well stripped upwards by incising, as Kocher directs, the peritoneum along the outer side of the gut, and working the fingers in towards the middle line on the inner side of the incision until the duodenum

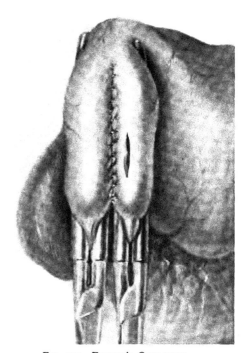

FIG. 314. FINNEY'S OPERATION.
The first suture; the stomach opened.

is rendered movable and can be lifted upwards and forwards into the abdominal wound. The pyloric part of the stomach, the pylorus and the first and second parts of the duodenum—the parts, in fact, which are to be engaged in the operation—being thus made free, are then carefully surrounded by hot moist swabs, which isolate them from the rest of the peritoneal cavity. The purpose of the operation is now to anastomose the stomach to the duodenum, and to this end clamps are applied to each, gripping those portions of the viscera in which the openings are to be made. The clamps are then laid side by side and surrounded with gauze. At the top of each there is a portion of the stomach and of the duodenum which is not embraced, as will be seen by reference to Fig. 314.

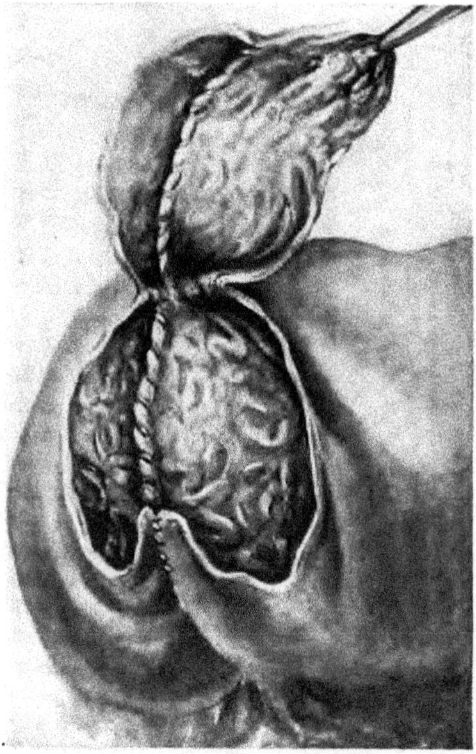

The sutures are now introduced. They are of the same material, and are similarly applied, as in the operation of gastro-enterostomy. A double layer is used, as in that case—an outer sero-muscular, and an inner which embraces all the coats. When the first sero-muscular suture has been introduced, the viscera are opened by two incisions, which are continued into one another at the upper extremity, so that a single inverted U-shaped incision is made, instead of two separate incisions, as in gastro-enterostomy. The details of the operation do not differ further from those already described in the chapter dealing with that operation.

FIG. 315. FINNEY'S OPERATION.
Showing new disposition of the parts.

I have rarely used Finney's operation, believing that the indications which are held to call for its performance are better met by the operation of gastro-enterostomy.

CONGENITAL PYLORIC STENOSIS

The pyloric-stenosis baby is one of the poorest of operative risks. Consequently it is of the greatest importance that a uniform technique in the handling of these cases be adopted. The high mortality of many excellent surgeons who have operated upon only a small series of cases bears out this point.

The following method of care in these cases is the one employed by H. M. Richter, whose series represents 25 gastro-enterostomies and 4 Rammstedt operations.

The extremities and body of the child with the exception of the abdomen are wrapped in cotton batting held on by bandages; the arms are bandaged to the sides; the legs are bandaged together. This conservation of body heat is of the utmost importance. In his entire series of cases Richter had one operative death, a fact due to two conditions: conservation of body heat and a highly developed gastro-intestinal technique. The anæsthesia is begun only when the skin is prepared and sterile linen is on. Ether is always the anæsthetic of choice. Preliminary catheterization of the stomach to relieve over-distension is usually necessary.

An incision 2 inches in length a little to the right of the midline gives the best exposure. The pyloric tumour, which is instantly recognizable, because of its size and firmness, is delivered through the incision by means of the thumb and index finger.

Of the various operative procedures resorted to only two have given sufficiently satisfactory results. One is the posterior no-loop gastro-jejunostomy, and the other the pylorotomy of Rammstedt, a modification of Weber's operation.

Gastro-enterostomy possesses the advantages of being an operation familiar to surgeons and offering a certain method of getting around the tumour. The operation is identical to that in the adult. The small size of the structures, however, makes it exceedingly more difficult. Richter uses the finest obtainable silk and a No. 10 cambric needle for every layer. He uses no clamps.

A smooth, clean, and rapid technique is nowhere more necessary.

Until the operation of Rammstedt was generally adopted some four years ago, gastro-enterostomy offered the only satisfactory surgical cure. The operation of Rammstedt, however, occupies about one-half of the time required for a gastro-enterostomy, involves less operative

U. S. Sup., Jan., 1920.

work, and has resulted in a much lower mortality rate. However, with the exception of Alfred Strauss's series the mortality average of the Rammstedt operation has been higher than Richter's mortality average in gastro-enterostomy, which was 3 deaths in 26 or 11%. Strauss reports 54 cases, with 3 deaths. Downes reports 35 cases, with 8 deaths.

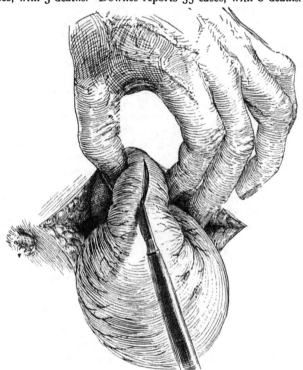

FIG. 316. SITE OF INCISION OVER HYPERTROPHIED MUSCLE.

Rammstedt's operation is based upon the fact that the hypertrophied circular muscle compresses and obliterates an otherwise normal mucosa and lumen. Therefore, a simple incision, cutting transversely the circular fibres and allowing sufficient separation of these fibres, would restore the normal lumen. The operation is as follows:

The tumour is delivered as described above. It is firmly grasped by the thumb and index finger; the stomach itself is not delivered, save for an inch or so of the pyloric end.

A longitudinal incision the full length of the tumour is now made (see Fig. 316). The latter is often of almost cartilaginous hardness. The incision is carried through the circular muscle down to the mucosa. As the tense fibres separate a plane of cleavage between muscle and mucosa may be seen.

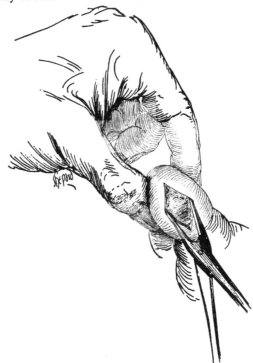

Fig. 317. Shows Method of separating Hypertrophied Muscle from Mucosa. Great care must be used at duodenal end since that is where rupture is likely to occur.

The incision is now spread by means of a pair of sharp-nosed hæmostats in order that the muscle be made to retract and to separate from the mucosa (see Fig. 317). As the edges of the muscle are stretched apart the mucosa herniates through as a redundant fold. Bleeding is slight, as the tumour is practically bloodless. The operation is now completed. The pylorus is now replaced into the abdomen and the latter closed.

In spreading the incision extreme care must be used to avoid tearing the mucosa. A large tear would necessitate a gastro-enterostomy. Otherwise nothing need be done to cover the mucosa, as there seems to be no danger of leakage. Moreover, the tumour is so rigid that it is impossible to suture it.

Downes, feeling that simple division of the hypertrophied circular muscle would not meet the indications in all cases, added a modification. Through a small incision in the anterior wall of the stomach he passed a sound (No. 20 French) and introduced the sound into the pylorus and beginning of the duodenum for the purpose of stretching any remaining constriction.

Another recent modification of the Rammstedt operation is the pyloroplasty of Alfred Strauss. After completely separating the mucosa from the muscularis, Strauss closes in the defect with a pedicle flap made from the cut circular muscle. Where there is insufficient muscle he uses a free transplant of rectus fascia and muscle. He restores the peritoneal defect by means of an omental transplant. Strauss has reported a large series with the lowest mortality to date.

The post-operative care of these babies is most important. They are usually in urgent need of fluids and feeding should begin in the first two or three hours after operation. Richter passes a catheter into the stomach immediately upon completion of the operation and puts in two ounces of water.

Complete recovery from anæsthesia usually occurs in from one to two hours, after which the child may be given a bottle or put to the breast. In all cases the post-operative care should be directed by a pediatrician.

Post-operative convalescence is rapid. Bowel movements become normal and weight rapidly increases. Post-operative vomiting is less frequent following the Rammstedt operation than after gastro-enterostomy.

The sutures are removed on the tenth day. Strips of adhesive are placed between every two or three sutures just previous to their removal to prevent any accidental separation of the skin wound.

CHAPTER V

GASTROPEXY

GASTROPEXY is the operation by which a stomach which is prolapsed, is brought up into its normal position and there fixed by sutures which engage either the stomach or its upper or lower omental attachments.

Indications. The value of the operation, or rather the need for its performance, is very differently estimated by various surgeons. There are some, Rovsing for example, who consider that the falling downward of the stomach is by no means an infrequent event, that the displacement is attended by symptoms of such severity or of such persistence that its repair by operation is not seldom necessary. There are other surgeons, of whom I count myself one, who do not attach much importance to this one deformity, but consider it rather as a part, and by no means always the most important part, of a more widespread disorder; they consider accordingly that operative treatment of the condition is rarely necessary.

Rovsing (*Trans. Int. Soc. de Chir.,* i. 338) recognizes two forms of gastroptosis. In the first and less common form, which he describes as 'virginal,' the descent occurs in young women who have not borne children, and in whom, therefore, the abdominal wall is firm and strong. The second form occurs in multiparous women with lax and perhaps pendulous abdominal walls; the prolapse of the stomach is associated with a general descent of all the viscera. In the former type operative treatment is indicated; there is no fault in the abdominal wall and the pressure of a belt does little or nothing to help the muscular support, which is neither weak nor insufficient. In the latter type a well-fitting belt, whose greatest pressure is below (this is effected by means of a triangular air-pad, the base being at the pubes and the apex above the umbilicus), will suffice to give that support to the stomach and to the other viscera, of which they have been deprived by the relaxation of the abdominal wall. Rovsing, in his last report, gave details of forty-nine cases upon which he had operated. Forty-four of these were of the virginal type, five of the multiparous. In six of the cases stasis of the stomach contents was noticed. The results of the operations were very satisfactory; there were no deaths; the only patient who was not relieved was one in whom, at a second operation, duodenal ulceration and adhesions, which had previously escaped notice, were discovered. In two cases displacement of the liver was also found.

Operation. The surgical treatment of gastroptosis was first advocated by Duret of Lille.

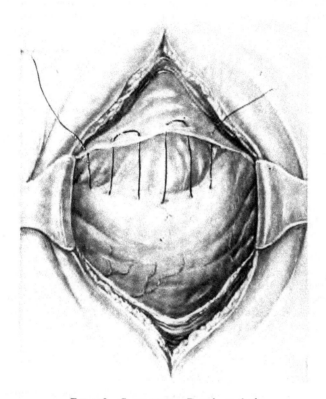

FIG. 318. GASTROPEXY. Duret's method.

Duret's operation. The abdominal wall is incised from the ensiform cartilage to the umbilicus until in the whole length of the wound the posterior sheath of the rectus and the peritoneum are exposed. These layers are incised only for a short distance at the lower end; the fingers introduced through this opening into the peritoneal cavity manipulate the stomach during the subsequent stages of the operation. The purpose of the steps which follow is to replace the stomach and to fix it by suture against the layer of undivided peritoneum in the upper part of the wound. A continuous suture of silk was used by Duret, but probably a strand of chromic catgut or of kangaroo-tendon would be preferable. The recti muscles are separated as widely as possible at the upper part of the incision. Through the edge of the left rectus muscle the needle passes from before backwards into the abdomen, where it is seized by the fingers of the left hand passed upwards through the lower part of the incision. The needle is then passed horizontally through the stomach-walls close to the lesser curvature, at its left extremity. The needle then returns from behind forward through the undivided peritoneum in the upper end of the abdominal wound, being brought out about three-quarters of an inch from the point of its original introduction. The stitch therefore forms up to this point a single mattress suture. The needle is now passed in a similar manner several times into the abdomen to engage the stomach, and out again through the peritoneum. The last stitch comes out through the edge of the right rectus muscle. When the whole length of the thread is tightened the lesser curvature of the stomach is drawn into intimate approximation with the anterior abdominal wall.

The first patient upon whom Duret operated was a married woman who had suffered acutely for three years. The result of the operation was perfectly satisfactory; the patient was completely relieved of all her symptoms and gained 25 lbs. in three years.

Beyea's operation. This is, in my opinion, the most satisfactory of all the methods; in six cases I have adopted it either alone, or, when organic disease of the stomach has been present, in addition to gastro-enterostomy, and I have been satisfied that the principles and the details of the operation are sound. I prefer to give Dr. Beyea's own description of the operation (*Phil. Med. Journ.*, 1903, i. 257) :—

' An incision about three inches in length was made through the linea alba, midway between the xiphoid cartilage and umbilicus. The tissues were separated in the usual manner, and the peritoneal cavity opened, exposing a small portion of the lesser curvature and cardiac end of the stomach, the gastro-hepatic ligament or omentum, gastro-phrenic ligament, and the lower portion of the left lobe of the liver. The table was then elevated to the Trendelenburg position, and the stomach displaced still further downward and out of the wound by means of gauze sponges. This procedure caused the gastro-hepatic and gastro-phrenic ligaments to be slightly stretched and separated from the underlying structures, which permitted an accurate determination of the length of these ligaments and very much facilitated operative manipulations. The gastro-phrenic ligament was seen well developed, and evidently formed a strong support to the cardiac end of the stomach. The adjoining portion of the gastro-hepatic ligament was composed of thin, delicate peritoneum, increasing in thickness and strength towards the right or pyloric end of the stomach. Retractors were introduced and the liver held aside by placing a gauze sponge beneath a retractor. Three rows of interrupted silk sutures were then introduced so as to plicate and thus

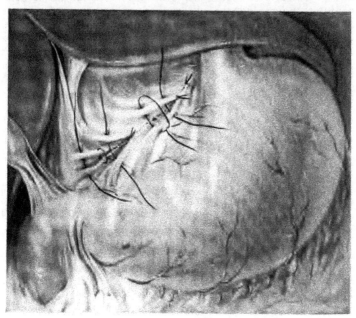

FIG. 319. GASTROPEXY. Beyea's method.

shorten the gastro-hepatic and gastro-phrenic ligaments in the following manner. The first row, beginning in the gastro-phrenic ligament, and extending across the gastro-hepatic ligament to almost opposite the pyloric orifice and hepatico-duodenal ligament, was introduced so as to form a plication in the centre of these ligaments, and included from above, downward or vertically, about 4 cm. of tissue (row No. 1). They were practically mattress sutures, including sufficient of the delicate tissue (1 cm.) to insure against their tearing out. Five sutures, about one inch apart, were introduced from right to left and caught in hæmostatic forceps. The next row (row No. 2) of sutures was introduced in the same manner, but 2.5 cm. above and below the first two. Then a third row (row No. 3) was introduced just above the gastric vessels and a short distance below the diaphragm and liver. The suturing was strictly confined to the normal ligamentary supports, and the distance between the rows from left to right was increased with the length of the ligaments, being greater towards the right. The gauze sponges were then removed, and the first, the second, and finally the third row of sutures were secured, the stomach, particularly the pyloric end, being elevated to a little above the normal position.'

In the cases in which I have operated I have usually included in the final row of ligatures a portion of the stomach close to the lesser curvature.

Coffey's operation. This also, in my judgment, is a sound surgical procedure, which I have once adopted. Dr. Coffey writes (*Phil. Med. Journ.*, 1902, x. 506) :—

'The stomach is suspended in a hammock made of the great omentum. When the abdomen is opened the stomach is freed from adhesions and pushed gently upward into its normal position. A series of chromicized catgut sutures are then passed transversely across the abdomen, picking up on the one side the great omentum one inch below the stomach, and on the other the anterior abdominal wall. As to the technic, I think this can well be varied to suit the case in hand. If only the stomach is displaced and not much dilated, it will probably be sufficient to put one row of sutures across, about an inch below the attachment of the stomach. If the abdomen is much relaxed and the colon shows a decided tendency toward the prolapse in splanchnoptosis, it will be probably well to put two rows of sutures across, penetrating the entire thickness of the omentum just below its attachment to the colon. In this way such a broad line of adhesion will be constructed that it will practically be impossible for the organs to become prolapsed.

'In my first case I placed three interrupted chromicized catgut sutures, covering a space of about 2 inches, near the centre of that portion of the omentum attached to the dilated portion of the stomach. In my second case I used eight chromicized catgut sutures, covering a space a little more than 6 inches. In a case of a very much dilated stomach I would suggest extending the suture still further, taking in 8 or 10 inches across the omentum. The stitches have been passed about 2½ inches above the umbilicus and have been passed from a large longitudinal incision.'

Rovsing's operation. By this method the stomach is supported by three or four sutures passed horizontally through its outer coats. These stitches at each end are passed through the abdominal wall, where they are tied over a glass rod. The sutures are of silk and are allowed to remain four weeks, by which time the stomach is 'united solidly' to the anterior abdominal wall.

CHAPTER VI

COMPLICATIONS OF OPERATIONS UPON THE STOMACH AND INTESTINES

WOUND INFECTION

THE steady decrease in percentage of wound infections among surgeons of wide experience is another example of the advances made possible by perfection of organization and close attention to details of technique. With numerous possible atria of infection,—the patient's skin, the hands of the surgeon or his assistants, the operating-room linen, basins, instruments, suture material, the germ-laden particles of moisture constantly present in the air,—nothing short of eternal vigilance will suffice to prevent infection of clean wounds.

Beckman (¹), in a review of 6,825 surgical cases at the Mayo Clinic in 1913, found postoperative wound infections in 117 cases, 1.7%. Of the total number of operations 1,494 were operations upon the stomach or intestines. Of these, 53, 3.6%, showed postoperative wound infection. (Every case in which there was an escape of fluid from the wound following operation was considered as possibly infected. In 35 of the 117 cases no growth developed upon culture of the discharge.) Since almost every organism identified in the bacteriological examination of the discharge from infected wounds was of the group commonly found in the body tissues, and of the type readily destroyed by ordinary methods of sterilization, he also concluded that the most important source of contamination was the patient's skin.

To obviate the possibility of the organisms which are constantly present in the superficial tissues from entering the wound it has already been suggested that the skin be covered to the edges of the wound with several layers of gauze held in place by forceps. Tuffier makes his initial incision before donning rubber gloves, lays aside the knife used for cutting through the superficial tissues, and then, after putting on his gloves, fixes gauze to the edges of the wound without permitting his fingers to touch the skin. In this way neither the surgeon's gloves nor his instruments have the opportunity of coming in contact with the skin. Cushing lays sterile gauze over the operative field and makes his initial incision through the gauze.

The incidence of wound infections has been noted by many observers to be greater during the winter months, due, it is inferred, to the greater prevalence at such times of infections of the upper respiratory passages. The rapidity and ease with which air-borne infections may be transmitted was impressed upon the medical profession with terrible force during the influenza epidemic of 1918. To safeguard the patient from infection from healthy individuals who may be harboring virulent organisms in the throat and nasal passages, especial care must be taken to cover the mouths and noses of the operating-room personnel with double layers of gauze, and to provide face masks for visitors and spectators.

The presence of fever over 99.6°, persisting for more than twenty-four hours in uncomplicated cases, suggests the possibility of wound infection. The treatment rarely offers difficulty. The early removal of one or more sutures may permit the escape of a localized collection of fluid, and prevent the spread of infection beneath the superficial layers of the abdominal wall. In the event of an infection, dichloramine—T in oil may be instilled with advantage into the infected wound. In cases with widely spreading infection the application of hot, moist dressings for forty-eight or seventy-two hours, followed by the use of Dakin's fluid, will hasten the process of recovery. The greatest possible care in the changing of dressings is necessary to prevent the addition of fresh infection from the patient's skin, or from outside sources, to that already present. A persistent wound discharge with a tendency toward sinus formation should suggest the possibility of foreign material, such as necrotic tissue or infected suture material, in the depth of the wound.

PERITONITIS

Peritonitis, if one of the least frequent of complications which may follow operations upon the gastro-intestinal tract, is by all odds the most serious. In addition to the potential sources of infection present in undertaking any surgical procedure there is the additional danger of introducing septic material from the stomach or intestines. This danger is especially acute in cases of prolonged stasis in the gastro-intestinal tract, such as occurs in the partial obstruction caused by carcinoma at the pylorus, or near the flexures of the large bowel, and in those cases in which because of their urgency adequate preoperative preparation is impossible.

Cushing, Gilbert and Domenici, Miller and others have shown that the presence of bacteria in the stomach and upper bowel depends upon the time of administration of food, its character, and upon the ability of the stomach to empty itself; that the organisms ingested with food steadily decrease in number with the process of digestion until, at its completion, the empty stomach and upper intestine are sterile. If emptying is prevented at the pylorus or in the intestines, the dammed-up intestinal contents contain organisms whose number and virulence are greatly increased. It is in these cases that careful gastric lavage before operation, repeated until the stomach is washed clean, is of especial importance in lessening the danger of peritoneal infection from the stomach or intestinal contents. Given an adequate and complete preparation before operation, the prevention of peritoneal infection becomes chiefly a question of surgical technique.

With pain persisting after operation, with increasing abdominal distention, and with a rising pulse rate, the presence of peritonitis is strongly suggested. The pain gradually becomes generalized, due to the pressure of the distended, paralyzed bowel. The pulse is the surest indication of the patient's condition. If it remains below 100 the condition is usually not serious; if it rises steadily and becomes progressively poorer in quality the outlook is grave. The temperature may be only slightly elevated, and give little indication as to the seriousness of the situation. The leukocyte count is usually high; a low leukocyte count is an ominous symptom. As the infection progresses the patient's expression becomes anxious and careworn. He lies with his hands above his head, and his knees drawn up to relax the tension upon the abdomen. Vomiting and hiccough may persist. The former is relieved temporarily by gastric lavage, but tends to return.

The treatment of diffuse peritoneal infection is taken up in detail in a later chapter. The essential features are absolute rest and warmth, maintenance of the body fluids by proctoclysis or hypodermoclysis, and elimination by gastric lavage, enemata, and by intramuscular injections of pituitrin in 10-15 minim doses.

The question of reopening the abdomen in cases of general peritonitis is one that will tax the most skilled surgical judgment. The futility of such a procedure in the majority of cases is self-evident from the picture presented at autopsy. In a very few cases where the source of infection may be traced with reasonable certainty to a definite source, such as leakage of the gastro-intestinal contents at the site of anastomosis, or soiling of the peritoneal cavity at the time of operation, it may be absolutely necessary to reopen the abdomen and repair the damage, cleanse the soiled parts, and establish drainage.

POSTOPERATIVE PULMONARY COMPLICATIONS

Pneumonia has been called ' the friend of the aged ' by Sir William Osler. To the surgeon it is a danger the possibility of which must be weighed in every case before operation, and the likelihood of whose occurrence increases with the patient's advancing years. With bronchitis, pleurisy, empyema, lung abscess and pulmonary embolism, it forms a group of pathological conditions which results in a mortality of approximately 1% of all cases undergoing major surgical operations (Cutler and Morton, [2]). In a series of 3,490 cases, operated upon at the Massachusetts General Hospital and reported by the authors mentioned, 65, or 1.8%, developed definite postoperative pulmonary complications, and of these 33, or 50.7%, were fatal. Of 65 cases, 40 were classified as pneumonia, divided about equally between lobar and diffuse types. Of a total of 52,581 cases, gathered by them from the statistics of various clinics, 1,043, or 1.9%, developed postoperative pulmonary complications. Of a total of 37,989 cases 386, or 1.01%, developed pneumonia. Of 344 of these in which the final outcome was recorded, 182, or 52.9%, were fatal. Following 17,219 operations upon *the abdomen alone* 742, or 4.7%, developed pneumonia. Following operations upon *the upper abdomen* the percentage of postoperative pulmonary complications in Cutler and Morton's series was 7.7%, and as high as 8.1% in the statistics of one clinic.

Various causes have been suggested as responsible for this morbidity: pre-existing lung pathology; the administration of the anæsthetic; its irritating effect upon the bronchial mucous membrane; the inhalation of septic material during anæsthesia; chilling of the patient during and after operation; stagnation of bronchial secretion in the dependent portion of the lungs, because of diminished respiratory excursion following operation; septic emboli; and extension of infection through the diaphragm.

It seems reasonable to believe that any of these causes may be the chief factor responsible in any given case. The danger of giving an anæsthetic in the presence of a pre-existing bronchitis, of bronchiectasis, or of incipient pulmonary tuberculosis has been repeatedly shown by disastrous experience. In Cutler and Morton's series, 20 of 65 cases showed some definite lung pathology at the time of operation. A careful examination of the lungs before operation, checked by a fluoroscopic examination if necessary, should be a routine procedure in every case.

The administration of the anæsthetic itself was for many years held responsible as the chief factor until it was found that postoperative pneumonia occurred not infrequently following operations under local anæsthesia. In spite of this fact, its importance should not be minimized. The careful administration of the anæsthetic, given without haste, without struggling and cyanosis on the part of the patient, and in such a quantity that the patient is beginning to awake at the close of the operation, is an extremely important factor in assuring a normal postoperative course.

The inhalation of septic material from the mouth during anæsthesia is emphasized by many writers, especially by Otte ([3]) and Pfannenstiel ([4]). Their advice as to thorough cleansing of the mouth before operation, with removal of all carious teeth and infected roots, is of particular importance, since they report an entire absence of postoperative pulmonary complications in their clinics. Various observers (Poppert,[5] Hoelscher,[6] and Gatch[7]) have shown the danger of aspirating mucus during anæsthesia and the greater likelihood of so doing with the administration of a concentrated vapor by the closed method. Kelly ([8]) has stated that there is constant aspiration of mucus during anæsthesia. If the aspirated mucus is constantly contaminated by the addition of septic material from infected teeth the danger of oral sepsis for patients about to undergo operation is self-evident. That septic material may be inhaled from an infected anæsthetizing apparatus should not be forgotten.

Chilling of the patient by bringing him to the operating room with a minimum of clothing, covering him with a thin sheet while administering the anæsthetic, perhaps drenching him with cleansing solutions, and finally, after he has been perspiring profusely in the operating room, permitting him to return through draughty corridors to a distant part of the hospital, surely conduces to a lowered resistance and the development of pneumonia. The incidence of this complication was almost abolished in the clinic of the Peter Bent Brigham Hospital ([9]) by providing warm recovery rooms adjacent to the operating rooms, where the patients might recover from the effects of the anæsthetic under the constant supervision of competent nurses.

Prolonged operation, chilling and trauma of the diaphragm, injury of the vagus and sympathetic nerves, and infection of the field of operation are factors which come directly within the province of the operator, and which are of particular importance in operations upon the upper abdomen. Kelling ([10]) has laid especial stress on chilling of the diaphragm, and advocates careful walling off of the subdiaphragmatic space with hot packs during epigastric operations. Armstrong ([11]) has emphasized the ease with which infection may extend from the upper abdomen to the pleural cavity and lungs through the diaphragm   The dislocation of septic emboli from the site of operation is an accident whose likelihood must surely be lessened by careful hæmostasis and gentle handling of the tissues at the time of operation.

Following operation every effort should be made to induce deep breathing in order to get rid of the excess of absorbed anæsthetic, and to prevent the stagnation of accumulated bronchial secretions. To this end alternate friction of the chest and extremities with ice-cold cloths, followed immediately by the application of warm clothing and blankets, will prove of great value. Mikulicz pointed out the value of forced deep breathing for a few minutes three or four times daily, more especially following operations upon the upper abdomen where there is every tendency for the patient to 'splint the wound' and prevent full expansion of the lungs by holding the abdomen rigid.

The rather indiscriminate use of intravenous salt solution after operation has been followed in some cases by acute œdema of the lungs. The strain on an already enfeebled heart, caused by the rapid addition of a considerable quantity of fluid to the circulation, should not be too lightly estimated, especially in view of the rather transient value of physiological salt solution when given intravenously. Where indicated it should be given slowly, and preferably in a quantity not exceeding 750 c.cm. at one time.

The treatment of postoperative pulmonary complications does not differ from that of similar conditions under ordinary circumstances. Support of the heart and free elimination are the essential factors. The use of the steam inhaler may afford the patient great relief, especially when the sputum is particularly tenacious and expectoration difficult.

ACUTE DILATATION OF THE STOMACH

Acute dilatation of the stomach is a comparatively rare complication of operations upon the stomach and intestines, but an extremely grave one. It occurs also, though less commonly, following operations upon other parts of the body, during the course of an acute illness, such as pneumonia or typhoid, or during the course of a chronic illness such as tuberculosis. It has been known to develop following the ingestion of an excessive amount of food or fluid.

The symptoms develop rather insidiously, most frequently throughout the first forty-eight or seventy-two hours after operation. Increasing pain due to abdominal distention, intolerable thirst, and repeated vomiting, which may at first be mistaken for the vomiting which commonly follows the administration of an anæsthetic, are the first symptoms to draw attention to the patient's condition. On removing the dressings the epigastrium will be found to be distended and tympanitic, the outline of the dilated stomach may even be distinguished through the muscles of the abdominal wall. Passage of the stomach tube results in the evacuation of a considerable amount of gas and fluid with temporary relief, but the condition tends to recur rapidly, and within an hour the vomiting and distention may be as marked as before. Vomiting is often effortless. The vomitus may be brought up 'in great gulps without straining.' At first it is watery and bile-tinged. Later it becomes dark red or brown from the admixture of blood, and of an unpleasant fetid odor. In spite of continued vomiting passage of the stomach tube will always result in the evacuation of additional, sometimes surprisingly large, amounts of fluid. As the gastric dilatation becomes extreme the abdominal distention may be more marked on the left side and in the lower half of the abdomen. In other cases the entire abdomen is affected. Percussion over the distended area yields a tympanitic note. Very often a succession splash may be obtained.

The patient's general condition is recognized as serious from the first, and unless relieved develops rapidly into one of collapse. The pulse becomes fast and thready, the respiration rapid and shallow. The patient looks desperately ill, his expression is anxious, his features pinched and drawn, due to the excessive dehydration. The skin is cold and covered with perspiration. Thirst is intolerable, and unrelieved by large amounts of water. There may be obstipation or diarrhœa. The urine is scanty or suppressed. If the stomach is emptied regularly and frequently the general condition may appear less serious, but fatal collapse may develop in a few hours.

On opening the peritoneal cavity the tremendously dilated stomach is found to occupy the great portion of the abdomen, compressing and shutting off from view the small and large intestine. Its walls are tremendously thinned, in some places appearing like tissue paper. Frequently there are hæmorrhagic erosions of the mucous membrane. The duodenum is often dilated as well. (That this is not constantly observed is due, in the opinion of some investigators, to the fact that the involvement of the duodenum is not considered, and therefore its condition is overlooked.)

The etiology of acute dilatation of the stomach has been the subject of considerable controversy, and a brief résumé of the opinion of different observers will be of interest because of its bearing on the treatment. Various causes have been suggested: paralysis of the gastric musculature (Brunton, Braun and Seidel [12]); constriction of the duodenum by the superior mesenteric vessels (Rokitansky, Kundrat, P. Müller [13]); primary paralysis of the stomach, followed by pressure upon the third portion of the duodenum by the distended stomach (Box and Wallace [14]) ; gastric hypersecretion (Fagge, Morris [15]) ; as well as other causes.

Borchgrevink ([16]) was able to collect 29 cases, including one of his own, in which an occlusion at the duodeno-jejunal junction was shown at autopsy or operation. He suggested that the primary paralysis and distention of the stomach forced the small intestine before it into the pelvis, and this in turn, by traction on the mesentery and superior mesenteric vessels, caused an occlusion of the duodenum. It seems probable that the condition is brought about by a combination of factors, in which a temporary paralysis following manipulation, or acute overdistention from food, fluid, possibly even from swallowing of air, permits the enlarged stomach both to force the intestines downward, and thus change the mesentery into a constricting band, and to produce in some cases as well direct mechanical pressure upon the duodenum just over and to the left of the lumbar spine. As the stomach enlarges it pushes its way downward, chiefly on the left side of the abdomen, in the position that has come from radiographic examination to be recognized as normal for a somewhat enlarged, ptotic stomach. There it forms a U-shaped tube, with the left or cardiac limb somewhat larger than the pyloric limb. With the cardiac and pyloric ends remaining fixed, increasing distention causes a sharp angulation at the bend of the ' U ' on the lesser curvature, and at the pylorus. The marked constriction thus produced may well be an important factor in preventing recovery once the condition is established. Simultaneously with the increase in size there is an increase in secretion of the gastric and duodenal mucosa. Vomiting of tremendous amounts of fluid—a half bucketful in Borchardt's case—has been reported.

With reference to the rapid collapse, the results of experimental work on dogs, carried out by Whipple, Stone, and Bernheim ([17]), are of especial interest. They found that in cases of high intestinal obstruction, the normal secretion of the duodenum is altered by reason of changes which take place in the mucosa, so that it becomes intensely toxic; and that if a small amount of the duodenal content from dogs with obstruction is injected into normal dogs rapid collapse and death follow.

Treatment. Early recognition of the condition is the most important factor. Gastric lavage, continued until the stomach is washed clean, should be followed by placing the patient in the prone position, with the hips elevated by placing a pillow or sandbags underneath. Occasionally a more extreme elevation of the pelvis, such as the knee-chest position, is of benefit, but it is usually not necessary. The relief afforded by this simple measure is immediate and striking. In one of

Borchgrevink's cases the picture changed in a few moments from that of impending death to one of comparative comfort. At the same time tap water by rectum or salt solution subcutaneously is essential to restore the body fluids. In few conditions is there such rapid and extreme dehydration of the tissues as in acute gastric dilatation. Further gastric lavage is usually unnecessary. Once the obstruction is relieved the fluid does not tend to reaccumulate. Operative procedures such as gastro-enterostomy, gastrostomy, etc., have been suggested, and carried out in a number of instances. They usually result fatally because of the patient's condition, and because they fail to afford prompt and permanent relief of the pathological condition.

BIBLIOGRAPHY

1. Beckman, E. H. Complications following surgical operations. Surg., Gynec. & Obst., 1914, xviii, 551-555.
2. Cutler, E. C., and Morton, J. J. Postoperative pulmonary complications. Surg., Gynec. & Obst., 1917, xxv, 621-649.
3. Otte, A. Ueber die postoperativen Lungenkomplikationen und Thrombosen nach Aethernarkosen. Münch. med. Wchnschr., 1907, liv, 2473-2476.
4. Pfannenstiel, J. Ueber die Vorzüge der Aethernarkose. Zentralbl. f. Gynäk., 1903, xxvii, 8-15.
5. Poppert. Experimentelle und klinische Beiträge zur Aethernarkose und zur Aether-Chloroform Mischnarkose. Deutsche Ztschr. f. Chir., 1902, lxvii, 505-523.
6. Hoelscher, R. Experimentelle Untersuchungen über die Entstehung der Erkrankungen der Luftwege nach Aethernarkose. Arch. f. klin. Chir., 1898, lvii, 175-232.
7. Gatch, W. D. The use of rebreathing in the administration of anæsthetics. Tr. Am. Surg. Ass., 1911, xxix, 196-216.
8. Kelly, R. E. Intratracheal insufflation of ether. Brit. M. J., ii. 617-618.
9. Boothby, W. M. J. Am. M. Ass., 1916, lxvii, 539.
10. Kelling, G. Ueber Pneumonien nach Laparotomien. Verhandl. d. deutsch. Gesellsch. f. Chir., 1905, xxxiv, 136-160.
11. Armstrong, G. E. Lung complications after operations with anæsthesia. Brit. M. J., 1908, i, 1141-1142.
12. Braun, W., and Seidel, H. Klinisch-experimentelle Untersuchungen zur Frage der akuten Magenerweiterung. Mitt. a. d. Grenzgeb. d. Med. u. Chir., 1907, xvii, 533-578.
13. Müller, P. Ueber postoperative Magendilatation hervorgerufen durch Arterio-mesenteriale Duodenalkompression. Deutsche Ztschr. f. Chir., 1900, lvi, 481-511.
14. Box, C. R., and Wallace, C. S. A further contribution on acute dilatation of the stomach. Lancet, Lond., 1901, ii, 1259-1260.
15. Morris, H., cited by Thompson, Campbell. Acute Dilatation of the Stomach. London, 1902.
16. Borchgrevink, O. J. Acute dilatation of the stomach and its treatment. Surg., Gynec. & Obst., 1913, xvi, 662-693.
17. Whipple, G. H., Stone, H. B., and Bernheim, B. M. Intestinal obstruction. J. Exper. M., 1913, xvii, 286-323.

CHAPTER VII

COMPLICATIONS OF OPERATIONS UPON THE STOMACH AND INTESTINES—*CONT'D.*

SHOCK

Postoperative shock is especially likely to develop in those cases which, because of their urgency, do not permit of adequate preparation before operation, or which, because of their difficulty, involve a prolonged anæsthetic and extensive manipulation of the bowel. It is an ever threatening danger in patients, who, after a prolonged illness, with all their forces of resistance at a low ebb, come to the surgeon as a last resort. It is essentially a progressive failure of the circulation, manifested especially by a pulse which becomes progressively weaker and more rapid, and by a constantly falling blood pressure. With circulatory failure the respiration also becomes more rapid and shallow, and the temperature frequently falls below normal. As death approaches the skin becomes cold and covered with perspiration. The mental condition varies : some patients may be very restless, so that morphine is apparently without effect, and the mentality may remain unclouded, even hyperacute; others are deathly quiet, and imperceptibly lapse into a fatal coma.

The symptoms usually supervene rapidly after an operation. In severe cases they develop as the effect of the anæsthetic disappears. The treatment is essentially prophylactic, and is directed toward preventing its occurrence, rather than combating it after it appears.

The etiology of shock has been the subject of much investigative work during recent years, especially throughout the war, by reason of the high percentage of its incidence among the wounded at the front. That the causes of shock are of pre-eminent interest to the surgeon because of their bearing upon the treatment is self-evident. A number of *predisposing* factors have been shown to be of especial importance : prolonged exposure to cold and dampness; fatigue; pain; loss of body fluids; prolonged anæsthesia with ether or chloroform; trauma and exposure of the peritoneum and bowel; infection.

The most important of these in the opinion of all observers is the occurrence of hæmorrhage. Indeed, among the wounded the occurrence of shock unaccompanied by hæmorrhage was questioned by some observers, notably of the French medical services. The rare appearance of shock in the trenches and advanced dressing stations except in 'severe surgical cases,' or in cases in which severe hæmorrhage was self-evident was pointed out by Cowell ([1]), Vincent ([2]), Roux-Berger ([3]), Santy ([4]), and others. It is interesting to note also that in a series of notable experiments carried out by the Medical Research Committee ([5]) on the experimental production of acidosis and its relation to shock, the explanation of several apparently contradictory experiments in which the blood pressure of decerebrated animals continued to fall after the infusion of a relatively small amount of acid was that 'more hæmorrhage had occurred in the process of decerebration than was realized at the time.'

Robertson and Bock ([6]), in an investigation of blood volume after hæmorrhage, showed that the amount of blood lost by wounded patients was surprisingly large; that cases with a history of bleeding tended to show a loss of 40% or more of the total blood volume, and that cases with no positive history of severe bleeding often showed a diminution of blood volume of 20% to 30%. Bazett ([7]) estimated the loss of blood during operation in ten cases and concluded that in none was it less than 7% of the total blood volume, while in one case it was 27.5%. He concluded that the loss of blood, even in comparatively bloodless operations, was always considerably more than was realized. This conclusion doubtless holds in civil practice as well, especially so in prolonged and difficult operations.

The importance of cold and exposure in the production of shock has been frequently emphasized. The depressant effect of chilling upon the circulatory system is one of the most commonly observed of physiological phenomena. One of the simplest means of producing experimental shock is by opening the peritoneal cavity and exposing the bowel. The gradual appearance of shock in slightly wounded patients following exposure and delay in getting to the rear, and their prompt recovery upon the application of warmth, has been frequently commented upon. The development of shock accompanied by acidosis upon immersing rabbits in an ice-cold bath was shown experimentally by Wright and his colleagues ([8]).

The relation of anæsthesia to shock has long been recognized as of importance. The danger of subjecting patients with a low blood pressure to an anæsthetic was especially emphasized by workers interested in the problem of shock throughout the war. Fraser and Cowell ([9]), Cannon ([10]), and others showed that with the blood pressure at the critical stage, viz. 80 to 90 mm. of mercury, administration of ether or chloroform was frequently accompanied by a further rapid fall of pressure and a fatal outcome. The fatal effects of even small doses of ether or chloroform, with the blood pressure near the critical stage, has been repeatedly shown by laboratory experiments. The relatively slight depressant effect of nitrous oxide and oxygen, as compared with ether and chloroform anæsthesia, on the circulatory mechanism has been pointed out by many observers.

Finally, the importance of infection as a predisposing factor has been frequently emphasized, especially with reference to anaerobic infections, by Wright and his colleagues ([11]). Doubtless in cases of prolonged sepsis the gradual destruction of blood, with a corresponding decrease in blood volume, is quite as important a factor as the direct toxic effect of the absorbed poisons upon the circulatory mechanism.

With any or all of these factors present the question of the mechanism of the development of shock assumes especial interest. Experimentally, shock has been produced by exposure and trauma of the peritoneum and bowel; by pain, for example by exposing large nerve trunks and subjecting them to the tetanizing effects of an electric current; by the injection of foreign substances, such as peptone, oils, histamine, etc.; and in numerous other ways.

The presence of fat emboli in the lungs and other viscera of patients dying with all the symptoms of acute surgical shock has been reported by Bissell ([12]), who also remarked upon the large amount of fat in the venous blood of such patients, as well as in the blood of patients with broken bones. The frequency of shock in the wounded among patients with broken bones, or with multiple wounds of the soft parts, was also pointed out by Porter ([13]) as evidence of the part played by fat embolism in the production of shock.

A number of theories have been suggested as to the starting point in the breaking down of the circulatory mechanism. Henderson ([14]) suggested that the decrease in the carbon dioxide content of the blood following the hyperpnœa induced by pain caused a fatal apnœa; or failure of the heart through cardiac tetanus. Other observers ([15]), in attempting to confirm his findings, stated that only by such extreme hyperpnœa as to cause a venous obstruction in the lungs were they able to reproduce a condition of shock. Adrenal exhaustion ([16]) with consequent hypotension, impairment of the vasomotor mechanism ([17]), paralysis of the cardio-inhibitory centre, lowering of the alkali reserve (acidosis) ([18]), have all been shown to be of secondary importance, and the result rather than the cause of the failing circulation. Recent investigative work ([19, 20]) has tended to confirm the earlier suggestions of Delbet and Quénu that the primary fall of blood pressure is due to the absorption into the blood stream of the toxic products formed at the site of tissue injury. Cannon ([20]) suggests that 'traumatic toxemia' may be closely allied to peptone shock in which there is an increased permeability of the capillary walls and a marked escape of plasma from the blood vessels into the tissues.

We must admit that the question as to what initiates the circulatory failure is still unsettled; but nevertheless we may not lose sight of certain well-demonstrated facts:

1. Hæmorrhage, with consequent diminution of blood volume, is a factor constantly to be reckoned with. The blood volume is further decreased by the decreased intake of fluids which so frequently precedes emergency operative procedures, and by the profuse perspiration which follows injuries, and which is invariably present during prolonged operations. As a result of the decreased blood volume the blood pressure tends to fall, due to the diminished volume of blood delivered to the heart.

2. With increased concentration of the blood there is present an increased viscosity, in other words, an increased peripheral resistance for the heart to overcome. The effect of cold upon the peripheral circulation, whether from exposure or from the loss of heat associated with profuse perspiration, still further intensifies this peripheral resistance, causing an increase in internal friction and stagnation of blood within the capillaries. That the presence of fat in the blood stream greatly increased its viscosity was demonstrated by Gauss ([21]).

3. The stagnation of blood in the capillaries, and in the splanchnic veins under certain conditions, has been shown by various observers. Dale and Richards ([22]) pointed out that in histamine shock more than 50% of the blood plasma passed into the tissues. Henderson showed that the increasing acidity of the blood resulted in increased osmosis into the tissues, and, therefore, in a higher concentration of the blood.

Here then are a number of factors that help to make up a vicious cycle: diminished blood volume; falling blood pressure; increased viscosity, throwing additional work upon the heart; stagnation of blood in the capillaries; exudation of plasma into the tissues. These various factors intensify one another, and are themselves intensified by the various predisposing factors mentioned above. The 'critical stage,' a systolic pressure of 80-90 mm., probably represents the lowest level to which the blood pressure may fall and still insure an adequate blood supply to the vasomotor centre. Having once dropped beyond that point a further decline is rapid and inevitable.

Treatment. Before attempting operation upon cases not demanding immediate interference, the patient's nutrition should be carefully investigated, and if necessary, high caloric feeding maintained for an appropriate interval. The body fluids should be restored to a normal level by increased fluid intake, by proctoclysis with a solution containing 5% glucose and 3% sodium bicarbonate, by hypodermoclysis if necessary, or by intravenous injection of a 6% solution of gum acacia.[1] With subcutaneous or intravenous injections care must be taken not to overload the heart by too rapid administration. If the patient has lost a large amount of blood, as for example in cases of chronic gastric ulcer with repeated small hæmorrhages, blood transfusion from an appropriate donor is indicated.

During and after operation the body warmth must be maintained by artificial means. Anæsthesia with nitrous oxide and oxygen in the hands of an expert is much to be preferred to ether or chloroform. Crile has found that the blocking of afferent impulses by local anæsthesia is an important factor in preventing shock.

The administration of tap water or glucose solution by rectum, or of physiological salt solution subcutaneously, will maintain the fluid content during the first twenty-four or forty-eight hours, more particularly during the period of postoperative nausea. Morphine given hypodermically during the first twenty-four or forty-eight hours will help greatly to bring the rest and freedom from pain which is absolutely essential. The use of caffeine, camphorated oil, or strychnine is rarely indicated. The heart should not be whipped up, but rather supported by reducing its work to a minimum.

If the patient enters the hospital in shock, such as, for example, follows a severe contusion of the abdomen with injury to a viscus, treatment of shock must be coincident with preparation for operation. The application of external heat, the use of morphine, the subcutaneous or intravenous administration of fluid in a suitable form will help to restore the blood pressure to a level of safety. If intra-abdominal hæmorrhage is in progress it must be stopped as quickly as possible. The determination of this fact may be very difficult. The concentration of blood cells in the capillaries may give a misleading picture when

---

[1] Bayliss' ([23]) solution is made up as follows: The requisite quantity of "turkey elect" gum acacia for a 6% solution is dissolved in tap water on a water bath. After cooling, 2% sodium bicarbonate in powder form is added. The solution is allowed to stand for twenty-four hours, then filtered through Chardin paper or centrifuged to remove the precipitate of calcium carbonate. The solution, after being sterilized in sealed bottles to prevent the escape of carbon dioxide, is ready for use.

Another solution ([24]) widely used in France, without the addition of sodium bicarbonate, is made up as follows: sodium chloride, 2 gms.; potassium chloride, 0.05 gms.; calcium chloride, 0.05 gms.; powdered gum acacia, 5 gms.; distilled water, 100 c.cm.

The solution is filtered through paper pulp under pressure, and then autoclaved. It may be made up in five times the strength desired and diluted with sterile water when ready for use.

estimating the number of red cells and the hæmoglobin. In case of doubt, blood transfusion or intravenous injection of gum acacia solution carried on simultaneously with operation may help to tide the patient over the critical period.

BIBLIOGRAPHY

1. COWELL, E. M. The initiation of wound shock. J. Am. M. Ass., 1918, lxx, 607-610.
2. VINCENT, C. Shock. Arch. d. mal. du cœur, 1918, xi, 394.
3. ROUX-BERGER, J. L. Shock in the wounded. Progrès méd., 1918, xxxiii, 49.
4. SANTY, P. Le traitement à l'avant du choc chez les grands blessés. Lyon chir., 1917, xiv, 54-62.
5. Acidosis and shock. Reports of the Special Investigation Committee on Surgical Shock and Allied Conditions. No. 7. Medical Research Committee, London, 1918
6. ROBERTSON, O. H., and BOCK, A. V. Blood volume in wounded soldiers. J Exper. M , 1919, xxix, 139-172
7. BAZETT, M. C. The value of hæmoglobin and blood pressure observations in surgical cases Reports of the Special Investigation Committee on Surgical Shock and Allied Conditions. No. 5. Medical Research Committee, London, 1918.
8. WRIGHT, Sir A. E, and COLEBROOK, L. On the acidosis of shock and suspended circulation Lancet, Lond., 1918, i, 763-765.
9. FRASER, J., and COWELL, E. M. A clinical study of the blood pressure in wound conditions. J. Am. M. Ass , 1918. lxx, 520-526.
10. CANNON, W. B. Acidosis in cases of shock, hæmorrhage, and gas infection J Am. M. Ass., 1918, lxx, 531-535.
11. WRIGHT, Sir A. E, and FLEMING, A. Acidæmia in gas gangrene. Lancet, Lond., 1918, i, 205-210
12. BISSELL, W. W. Pulmonary fat embolism,—a frequent cause of postoperative surgical shock. Surg., Gynec. & Obst., 1917, xxv, 8-22.
13. PORTER, W. T. Shock at the front. Boston M. & S. J., 1916, clxxv, 854-858.
    Idem: Further observations on shock. Boston M. & S. J., 1917, clxxvii, 326-328
14. HENDERSON, Y. Acapnia and shock. Am. J. Physiol., 1908, 1909, 1910.
15. JANEWAY, H. H., and EWING, E. M. The nature of shock. Ann. Surg., 1914 lix, 158-175.
16. CORBETT, J. F. The suprarenal gland in shock. J. Am. M. Ass., 1915, lxv, 380-383
17. CRILE, G. W. An Experimental Research into Surgical Shock. Philadelphia, 1899
    Idem: Blood Pressure in Surgery. Philadelphia, 1903.
18. CANNON, W. B. A consideration of the nature of wound shock. J. Am. M. Ass., 1918, lxx, 611-617.
19. TURCK, F. B. The primary cause of shock. Med Rec., 1918, xciii, 927.
20. CANNON, W. B. The course of events in secondary wound shock. J. Am. M. Ass., 1919, lxxiii, 174-181.
21. GAUSS, quoted by BISSELL.
22. DALE. H. H., and RICHARDS, A. N. The vaso-dilator action of histamine. J. Physiol., 1918, lii, 110.
23. BAYLISS, W. M Proc. Roy. Soc., Lond., 1918, 89B, 381.
    Idem: Intravenous injection in wound shock. Brit. M. J., 1908, i, 553-556.
24. DRUMMOND, H., and TAYLOR, E. S. The use of intravenous injections of gum acacia in surgical shock. Reports of the Special Investigation Committee on Surgical Shock and Allied Conditions. No. 3. Medical Research Committee London, 1918.

SECTION VI

OPERATIONS UPON THE STOMACH AND INTESTINES

PART II

OPERATIONS UPON THE INTESTINES

BY

SIR G. H. MAKINS, K.C.G.M., C.B., F.R.C.S. (Eng.)

Surgeon to St. Thomas's Hospital and President of the Board of Examiners for the Naval Medical Service

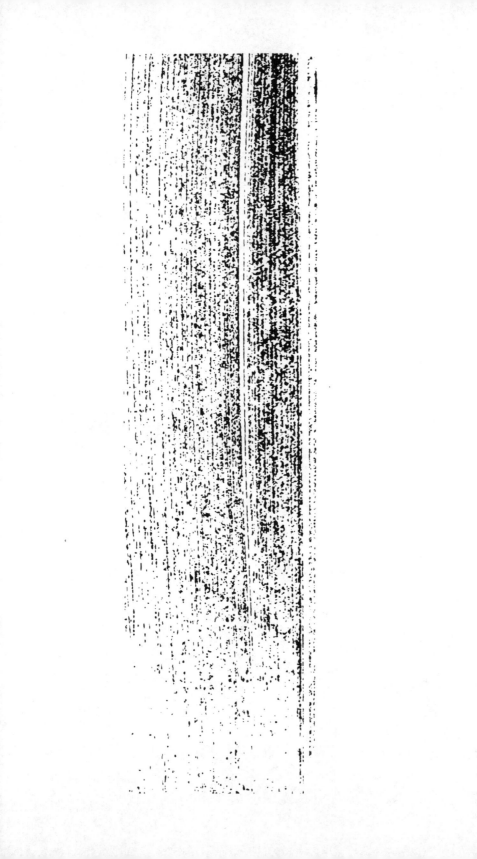

CHAPTER VIII

GENERAL REMARKS ON THE TECHNIQUE OF OPERA-
TIONS UPON THE INTESTINES

THE continuous widening of the field of intestinal surgery that has taken place during the last twenty years has been accompanied by a steady tendency to simplification in the methods employed. Experience has shown the technical success of any particular procedure to depend primarily on the sufficiency of the suture employed, and the sufficiency of the latter to be in direct ratio to its simplicity. The first great advance from the through and through stitches employed by Astley Cooper was made in the introduction of the principle of plane apposition of peritoneal surfaces by Lembert, and the further adaptation of the same principle to the continuous stitch by Dupuytren; thus the technique of the French School may be said to have dominated all subsequent developments.

Methods of suture. The chief requirements for a successful method of suture may be summed up under the following headings:—

1. Security.
2. Even coaptation of a sufficient peritoneal surface.
3. Adaptability to rapid insertion.
4. The avoidance of the production of obstruction in the lumen of the bowel by too free inversion of its wall.

The first question arising out of these requirements is the comparative advantage of a continuous or interrupted stitch. The advantages offered by the former method are so manifest that it has to-day been adopted by the great majority of surgeons. It is the more rapid, secures the more even coaptation of the surfaces, provides for reliable hæmostasis without necessity for the ligature of individual vessels, forms a circular line of support to the suture itself, should the bowel subsequently become distended (Jacobson), and allows of the use of as few knots as possible, thus eliminating the most dangerous element in a line of suture as far as infection by imbibition is concerned.

The alleged disadvantages may be briefly dealt with: the old established notion (founded on the behaviour of suppurating wounds of greater magnitude), that the giving of the suture at one point results in a loss of sufficiency of the whole line, has been definitely exploded by practical experience; also the assertion that a continuous line injuriously affects the nutrition of the tissues included. The latter danger is readily avoided by not drawing the thread too tightly, while the same precaution suffices to ensure that the line of suture is not a source of greater narrowing at the point of union than is inseparable from the inclusion of the amount of bowel-wall necessary for purposes of coaptation.

Allowing these advantages of the continuous stitch, occasions arise on which an interrupted suture is advisable or even necessary, and its employment either in the simple or the mattress form is attended by excellent results. For general application, however, the following objections may be urged against the interrupted stitch. It takes more time to introduce, coaptation is not so exact, hæmostasis may not be ensured without the individual ligature of vessels, and, lastly, the number of knots necessary is an obvious disadvantage, since it has been definitely shown by Chlumsky that the direction of the flow in the thread by imbibition, and consequently the line of extension of infection, is towards the knot. The last objection may be eliminated by the use of one of the ingenious methods devised by Maunsell, Connell, Bishop, Wiggin, and others, in which the suture is so introduced that all the knots are tied within the lumen of the bowel; but none of these methods have up till now obtained any very general favour.

The general question of how great a thickness of the intestinal wall should be included in the suture may be said to be fairly definitely agreed upon. When two tiers of suture are employed the inner is very generally passed through the entire thickness of the intestinal wall, with a view to increase in the strength of union and the ensurance of reliable hæmostasis. It has, moreover, been shown by the successful employment of the methods of Connell and others that a single tier of stitches may be safely passed in this manner. When healthy intestine has to be dealt with, however, sufficient strength of union may be looked for from the outer tier of sutures, and, if the surgeon prefers, the inner tier may be made to include the mucous membrane only. The writer has for many years employed this method without cause to regret it, especially in lateral anastomoses. When combined with excision of superabundant mucous membrane, it has the advantage of producing less projection inwards of the line of union towards the lumen of the bowel than is the case when the whole thickness of the wall is included in the stitch.

The outer tier should dip deeply into the submucous layer, as so strongly enforced by Halstead and Gross.

Of the numerous methods of suture in use, the following may be mentioned as the most generally useful, and as comprising all that are necessary for successful intestinal union.

Lembert's suture. Originally devised as an interrupted stitch extending through the peritoneal coat only, this stitch has undergone various modifications, as in the substitution of continuous introduction, the inclusion of the muscular coat, and later, of the submucous coat also (see Fig. 320).

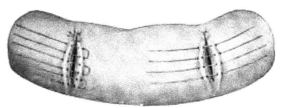

Fig. 320. INTERRUPTED LEMBERT'S SUTURE. Right hand, six Lembert's stitches, two tied. Left hand, four mattress stitches, one tied.

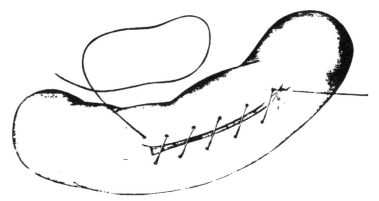

Fig. 321. CONTINUOUS LEMBERT'S SUTURE. Thread not drawn tight to show the course of the stitches and the folds raised by them.

As employed at the present day, the needle is introduced about a quarter of an inch from the margin of the wound to be closed, made to penetrate to the greater part of the depth of the submucous layer, and is then brought out about a tenth of an inch from the opening in the bowel and made to emerge on the free surface, having penetrated a similar depth and distance of the bowel-wall as on the first side; succeeding stitches are passed at intervals of three-sixteenths of an inch until the required length of suture has been attained.

When this suture is employed as a running stitch, it is a modification of Dupuytren's (see Fig. 321).

The method of introduction has been modified by Cushing by the passage of the needle parallel to the line of the wound instead of transversely to it.

In order to prevent a too great approximation of the two ends of the line of union, the blanket stitch or the tying of a knot in the line of suture at one or two places is sometimes employed, but neither of these methods is usually necessary.

Mattress suture. In this method (see Fig. 320) each suture encloses

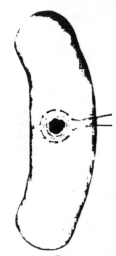

a small square of tissue. The most important result of its adoption and advocacy by Halstead has been a thorough appreciation of the advantage of penetrating to the submucous coat, but the method itself has the disadvantage of procuring a somewhat less even adaptation, since a series of short puckers is unavoidable. It is, moreover, an interrupted stitch. The advantage of the mattress suture is, however, sometimes great, as by its use a very firm hold is obtained, and this is especially the case when gut thickened by inflammatory infiltration has to be dealt with.

Purse-string suture. This method is of frequent utility in closing perforations of the intestinal wall, sinking the stump of the appendix, or closing the cut ends of the bowel when lateral union is made after an enterectomy. It can be applied with great rapidity, and is readily strengthened when necessary by the introduction of a more superficial line of Lembert's stitch. As in the case of Lembert's

FIG. 322. PURSE-STRING SUTURE OF THE LEMBERT TYPE.

stitch, the needle and thread should be made to pass deeply into the submucous coat, or under certain conditions, it may be passed through the whole thickness of the bowel.

A description of Connell's suture will be found on p. 726.

Sewing materials. For general employment no material is more useful and satisfactory than *silk*. Either Chinese or Japanese twist is usually chosen; the latter has the advantage of being the more tightly woven, hence it is finer and a given calibre possesses greater strength and less absorbent power than the corresponding size of Chinese twist. Equal tensile strength is possessed by Japanese twist two sizes smaller than that of Chinese twist.

Celluloid thread, in the form known as Pagenstecher's thread, is strong, smooth, and less absorbent than silk; its use is strongly recommended by Moynihan and others.

Catgut is also employed by some surgeons, especially for the inner lines of suture. It has the disadvantages of needing to be somewhat thicker than is necessary with silk or linen thread, its surface is less smooth, and it is more difficult to sterilize in emergencies. Its chief virtue, ready absorbability, can scarcely be said to be necessary, since the use of silk or linen thread seldom carries any troublesome complication with it from want of this property.

Needles for intestinal suture should be round bodied. The needle with a cutting edge not only makes a larger wound than is necessary, but also prepares the way for further cutting by the thread when the latter is tightened.

For the passage of Lembert's stitches a straight needle is the most convenient, as it most readily pierces the base of the small fold raised by the tightening of the last passed element of the stitch. When sutures need to be so introduced as to enter by the inner aspect of the bowel, or at a depth from the surface, a curved or semicircular needle is necessary.

Needles of the split-eyed variety are convenient; the only disadvantage is the occasional accident of slipping of the thread from a calyx eye when the tissue is hard or resistant, or when the double thread is considerably larger in calibre than the needle carrying it. In such circumstances an ordinary eye may be preferable, or the needle designed by Paterson may be used. The latter has the eye somewhat widened at the distal part, while the proximal end is so narrowed as to allow the thread to hitch firmly in this part. The hole made by the needle is slightly increased in size, but not more so than is necessary for the easy passage of the double thickness of thread at the needle's eye.

Clamps. For purposes of coprostasis some form of clamp is to be regarded as a necessity. A very slight degree of pressure suffices to entirely control the escape of fæcal contents from the bowel; hence the principle of elastic compression by the metal of the instrument itself embodied in the clamps of Doyen renders the use of any form of rubber sheathing unnecessary. The rubber sheathing increases the bulk of the blades, and interferes with the accuracy with which the necessary compression is applied.

No clamps are more generally useful than those introduced by Doyen. They possess the advantage of exerting an equable and sufficiently light elastic compression, while the length of the handle and blades serves the useful purpose when laid across the abdominal wound of retaining the bowel readily in the required position, and preventing its retraction into the abdominal cavity. These clamps may be obtained of varying size and weight, and fulfil all ordinary requirements (see Fig. 323).

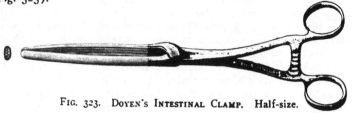

FIG. 323. DOYEN'S INTESTINAL CLAMP. Half-size.

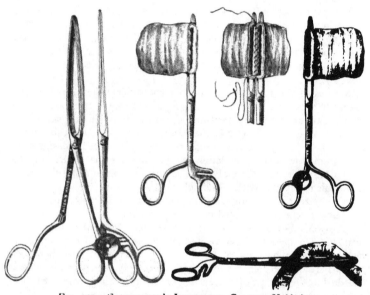

FIG. 324. CARWARDINE'S INTESTINAL CLAMP. Half-size.

Various modifications have been introduced, such as the fenestration of the blades, to allow the introduction of sutures before the removal of the clamp, and, perhaps the most useful, that of Carwardine, which allows for the accurate fixation in proper relative position of the two portions of intestine to be united (see Fig. 324).

In Carwardine's clamp, by a simple arrangement, the handles are capable of fixation by a screw, so as to allow of exact parallelism of the pairs of blades; further, the blades themselves are light and elastic, and exert an equable compression on the whole width of the included gut.

The gastro-enterostomy clamp of Roosevelt is useful in lateral anastomoses, especially when the large intestine is included. The broad metal

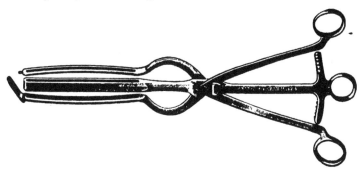

FIG. 325. ROOSEVELT'S CLAMP, AS MODIFIED BY MOYNIHAN. One-third size.

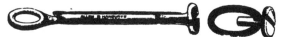

FIG. 326. LANE'S CLAMP. Two-thirds size.

FIG. 327. MAKINS'S CLAMP. Two-thirds size.

central fixed blade serves the purpose of the gauze plug ordinarily placed on the deep aspect of the anastomosis before commencing the suture. This clamp may also be used for axial enterectomies, if the surgeon be content to leave the closure of the mesenteric gap to be the last step in the operation (see Fig. 325).

When smaller clamps are for any reason desirable, as when several pairs are necessary, Lane's clamp or the modified Dieffenbach's forceps devised by the writer may be employed. Either form has the advantage of occupying little space in the field of operation, or in the bag of the surgeon (see Figs. 326, 327).

GENERAL ANATOMICAL CONSIDERATIONS

The small intestine affords the most favourable conditions of the alimentary tract as far as the manipulations of the surgeon are concerned. Smooth and regular as to its serous surface, more or less cylindrical in outline, varying but slightly in calibre, and furnished with an abundant blood-supply, every essential for the successful union of wounds is presented.

Although for the most part clad with peritoneum so intimately connécted as to allow the direction of the longitudinal muscle fibres to shine through the serous and tenuous subserous layer, yet at the attached margin where the true mesenteric layers allow the passage of the vessels and nerves to and from the structures of the bowel-wall a small interval exists, which in the early days of intestinal surgery proved the source of more disasters than any other single element in the field of operation. Again, in spite of the free blood-supply, the small intestine is singularly susceptible to gangrene if the mesenteric margin and arterial arcades be unduly interfered with.

The whole *length* of the tube is approximately 21 feet, but considerable variations occur (even 14 feet, Monks) : such variations may be of moment when long portions of intestine need to be resected.

The small bowel occupies roughly the central parts of the abdominal and pelvic cavities, covered for the most part by the great omentum, and surrounded by the colon. Only two fixed and certainly determinable points exist: the junction of the duodenum and jejunum at the side of the second lumbar vertebra, and the termination of the ileum in the right iliac fossa. Between these points the bowel is attached by a mesentery of somewhat variable length, and the position of any one coil differs in individual subjects, and even in the same subject under varying conditions, such as posture, the degree of distension of successive parts of the bowel, or the presence of ascites or tumours encroaching on the peritoneal cavity. Some broad lines may, however, be laid down as to the location of the different parts in normal bellies, the position of the various coils being dependent, as has been shown by Mall, on the length and direction of the mesentery. Mall's (*Bull. Johns Hopkins Hospital*, 1898, vol. ix. p. 197) investigations suggest that in a considerable number of cases the coils are arranged in four successive groups from above downwards, and assume regular positions: (1) Coils passing to the left, occupying a space partly covered by the transverse colon, and reaching to the splenic flexure; (2) Coils passing to the right, crossing the umbilical region to the hepatic flexure; (3) Coils passing to the left loin and iliac region; (4) Dependent coils dipping into the pelvis.

These general indications are supported by the investigations of Monks, who divides the abdomen into three zones limited by oblique lines, the centre of which is determined by the two points of fixation of the mesentery (see Fig. 328).

Monks has further drawn attention to the fact that the upper end of any individual coil may be determined by drawing it out, passing the hand beneath the mesentery to the spine to ensure the absence of any twist, and then placing it transversely on the abdominal wall. With the gut so placed, the end to the patient's right will be the lower. Beyond these broad lines we can only trust for localization to such points as the comparative thickness, calibre, tint, the apparent direction of the mesenteric pull, and perhaps the arrangement of the blood-supply. With regard to the latter, Monks has pointed out that in the mesentery attaching the upper four feet of the small intestine, the vasa intestina tenuis form simple arcades, while the vasa recta are comparatively long (3 to 5 centimetres); in the middle portion of the gut the arcades may be two or even three deep, while in the lower third a more and more irregularly arranged network takes the place of the symmetrical arcades, and the vasa recta are short, not exceeding 1 centimetre. It must, however, be allowed that in the change from the thick, wide, red upper jejunum, with its frequently

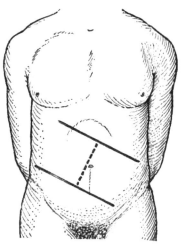

FIG. 328. ABDOMINAL ZONES. Three zones, containing in most instances the upper middle and lower thirds of the small intestine respectively. The dotted line indicates the root of the mesentery; the dark oblique lines cross the two extremities of this at right angles. (Monks, *Ann. of Surgery,* 1903, vol. xxxviii, p. 574.)

obviously distended lacteals, to the narrow, pale, thin lower part of the ileum, the alterations are so gradual that the formation of a certain opinion under the disadvantageous conditions often present from pathological causes is practically impossible.

The large intestine in anatomical arrangement, structure, and function differs widely from the small, each anatomical segment possessing special characters of its own which influence surgical procedures to so great an extent that they are most conveniently considered together with the special operations which may require to be performed upon them. Certain general characteristics only will therefore be mentioned here.

The average normal *length* in males has been computed at 4 feet 8 inches, in females at 4 feet 6 inches, with extremes of 6 feet 6 inches and 3 feet 3 inches (Treves). Pathologically, the length may be greatly increased when chronic distension has existed, such increase in length affecting particularly the more mobile portions, *e.g.* the transverse colon and the sigmoid flexure.

The general position of the large intestine in the abdominal cavity is marginal around the mass of the small intestine; this position, with the exception of the splenic flexure, facilitates access to the bowel, while taken together with the comparative fixity of the large intestine, it diminishes the danger of diffusion of infection from colic lesions to the general peritoneal cavity.

The different segments of the colon are fairly constant in position, the main element in their fixation being the peritoneal investment. As the most common arrangement, the ascending and descending colons are not only devoid of a mesentery, but the posterior surfaces have an area of some width in contact with the posterior abdominal wall, the extent of which varies with the amount of the distension of the bowel. The degree of fixation increases the difficulty of successfully uniting the bowel in enterectomy, or fixing it to the surface for the purpose of performing a colostomy, while the deficiency in the peritoneal investment affects the probability of effecting axial union safely, beyond affording the additional risk due to opening up the cellular tissue of the retro-peritoneal space. Again, the uncovered area opens up the possibility of wound or rupture of the bowel without the confines of the peritoneal cavity. On the other hand, the mobile portions of the colon are exposed to dangers of their own; thus, kinking at the junction of the transverse colon with the hepatic or splenic flexures, or volvulus of the sigmoid.

The special arrangement of the muscular coat affects surgical measures. Thus, the tenia are useful in providing a firm grip for sutures, and the even surface afforded by them is that best fitted for approximation when a lateral anastomosis is made, while the inequalities dependent on the presence of the haustra are inconvenient in making lateral unions.

The vessels of the large intestine for the most part form but one simple arcade, except those for the flexures and the pelvic colon.

Common morbid conditions of the bowel. In connexion with these general anatomical points it must be borne in mind that, while in cases of injury or strictly local disease the surgeon may have comparatively normal tissues and anatomical arrangements to deal with, yet in disease these conditions may be enormously disturbed.

The position of mobile portions of the bowel may be altered either as the result of simple distension, the weight of growth, habitual location in a false position, as in the sac of a hernia, or as a result of the pull of adhesions. On the other hand, the mobility of any portion may be decreased as a consequence of infiltration, either inflammatory or specific, of its mesenteric attachment (mesenteritis), by the spread of bowel growths to the surrounding parts, or by the presence of adhesions.

The condition of the bowel-wall itself may be such as to cause embarrassment. Simple distension may result in extreme tenuity and lowered vitality, increasing the difficulties of manipulation, and decreasing the chances of obtaining a successful union.

Compensatory hypertrophy in the presence of some source of obstruction may give rise to an opposite condition, the wall of the proximal portion of intestine being enormously thickened by tissue through which sutures readily cut, and of which the vitality is low; to which troubles incongruence in size of two segments to be joined may be added. Where a portion of intestine has been for a time unused the condition of atrophy and contraction may equally be a source of embarrassment, and the question of mere incongruence in size is here often much complicated by the presence of large masses of fat in the appendices epiploicæ and the mesentery, which commonly develop especially in connexion with portions of the large intestine which have been for any time cut off from performing their normal function.

In the neighbourhood of gangrenous gut a spreading cellulitis may extend over long lengths of the bowel, necessitating the removal of even some feet in order that a part capable of safe union may be obtained. Chronic œdema, or stiffening from chronic inflammatory infiltration, may give rise to much trouble in the closure of perforating ulcers, or in the performance of enterectomy in the neighbourhood of inflammatory tumours of the bowel; and, lastly, operations may have to be performed in the presence of specific disease, such as tubercle, widely disseminated in the peritoneum or bowel.

CHAPTER IX

THE REPAIR OF INJURIES, AND PERFORATIONS
OF THE BOWEL

DEFECTS in the continuity of the wall of the intestine demanding surgical repair may be the result of either injury or disease. The multiplicity of causes which may lead to such defects necessitates numerous variations in detail, and even in general principles in their operative treatment.

Traumatic defects may be the result of wounds by sharp instruments accompanied by no serious destruction or loss of tissue, or by gunshot injury in which the same characters are more or less maintained; or they may be lacerations such as those produced by a fragment of a fractured rib or portion of the pelvis. Again, they may be inflicted by the surgeon in the process of separating adhesions, and then often, in bowel in conditions of varying degrees of inflammation.

Injuries differing little in general characters may result from the infliction of blunt force. Thus, the bowel may be perforated or divided by compression between a strictly localized force, such as that applied by the point of a horseshoe or carriage pole, and the bony wall of the abdominal or pelvic cavity; or it may give way more or less completely at the point of junction of a fixed and movable portion as the result of being stretched beyond its potential elasticity. These accidents form a very considerable proportion of those liable to occur in the abdomen. A consideration of 8,153 injuries of all classes admitted into St. Thomas's Hospital showed that 292, or 3.59%, were located in the abdomen, and of the latter number 22, or 23.59%, were injuries to the intestine.

Pathological perforations may result from such varying causes as chronic ulcer of the duodenum, peptic ulceration of the jejunum, typhoid or tuberculous ulceration of the lower ileum, cæcum, or colon, acute or chronic intestinal distension, acute septic infection and gangrene of the bowel, ulceration in diverticula, either congenital or acquired, or the extension or degeneration of malignant growths.

Although the immediate and ultimate result of accidents of either class are similar, yet two important distinctions must be drawn as affecting the treatment of the traumatic and pathological varieties. First, in mechanical injuries the tissues bounding the defect in the intestinal

662

wall are more or less normal in character, while in pathological perforations the bowel-wall is the seat of varying degrees of inflammatory
change. Secondly, the escape of intestinal contents, either gaseous, fluid,
or solid, is much more free and widely diffused in the pathological perforations. These points affect the site of the abdominal incision, the
technicalities of suture, and the mode of dealing with the abdominal
cavity. Hence each condition needs special consideration.

THE REPAIR OF INTESTINAL INJURIES

Indications for exploration. No individual symptom or even
complex of symptoms can be regarded as certain evidence of a perforating injury to the intestine, but the following points may be set down
as those to be specially considered in cases of suspected abdominal
wounds or contusions.

1. *The process of exclusion of injury to other viscera.* Although a
combination of injury to the intestine is obviously a possibility, yet this
step is the most useful preliminary procedure in all cases of doubt.

2. *Consideration of the site of the injury, and of its nature.* In
many instances the violence may have been exerted in an area where an
injury of any other viscus than the intestine is unlikely, while ruptures
of the intestine due to strictly localized force are in the great majority of
instances to be found in the lower half of the abdominal cavity, where
the possibility of crushing of the intestine between the applied force
and the bony wall of the abdomen or pelvis is possible. A very large
proportion of the localized ruptures are caused by such forms of violence
as the kick of a horse or the impact of a carriage pole, while lacerations
in which the bowel is torn apart in its continuity follow such accidents as
the passage of a wheel over the abdomen or a crush between railway
buffers.

3. *The amount of shock.* This point is only of importance when
taken in connexion with other signs, since here, as in all serious abdominal injuries, the degree of shock is variable to a degree.

4. *A steadily rising pulse.* Although this sign in itself is really
only one accompanying the development of infection, it is to be regarded
as the most generally useful indication for exploration of the entire
complex. The same remark in a lesser degree applies to a marked
acceleration of the rate of respiration; but this sign as a later one is far
less useful.

5. *A rise in temperature.* In the earlier stages the temperature may
be depressed by existing shock, but occasionally an early rise may be
of use. As a rule a serious rise of temperature only occurs when septic

absorption has reached a degree calculated to render the chances of an exploration small; hence this sign is of little practical use.

6. A rupture is occasionally followed by *a sudden action of the bowels,* and, if the injury be in the lower segment of the canal, blood may be passed. These signs, though useful, if present, are so occasional as to rarely afford material aid.

7. *Extreme localized tenderness,* with corresponding rigidity and possible immobility of the abdominal wall, are very important indications; in fact, no less so than the same signs in the presence of a pathological intestinal perforation.

8. In the early stages *fluid in the flanks* may indicate the presence of blood, but this is comparatively rare in the absence of injury to the mesentery or omentum, and its presence should excite suspicion of one or other of these injuries, or of damage to one of the solid viscera.

9. Injuries to the duodenum or colon may lead to the development of *cellular emphysema,* but usually only at a comparatively late date.

10. A wound of the bowel may occasionally be *obvious* on examination should an extensive opening exist in the abdominal wall; and, rarely, gas or fæces may escape from an opening of lesser size.

11. *Blood* is occasionally vomited.

12. Later indications, of less value as being merely signs of severe infection rendering any chances of successful treatment slight, are the symptoms and signs of progressing peritoneal infection.

Method of operation. *Site of incision.* In cases of wound of the intestine the site of the incision in the abdominal wall will generally be determined by the position of the original injury, except in wounds due to gunshots, when a consideration of the course of the entire track may be necessary.

In cases of subcutaneous rupture, external evidence of the point of impact of the occasioning violence may lead to the same course being taken; or in some rare instances, when the patient is seen early, extreme sharply localized tenderness may serve the same purpose as a bruise or graze in indicating the most suitable site for the exploratory incision. Usually, however, such evidence is not forthcoming at the date at which the operation has to be undertaken, and in the absence of any guiding signs a paramedian subumbilical incision is the most generally useful. bearing in mind the fact that such injuries are more commonly situated in the lower than the upper half of the abdomen.

The main exception to this rule is met with in lacerations of the jejunum at the duodeno-jejunal junction, but this injury rarely occurs except where signs of injury to the upper abdomen, or a history of a fall on to the feet, exist.

During a period of eighteen years, 34 cases of rupture of the intestine were admitted into St. Thomas's Hospital; of these ruptures 26 were situated in the small intestine, 9 in the large; in one case both small and large intestine were implicated (duodenum and transverse colon). The injuries to the small intestine were distributed as follows: Duodenum, 5 (third part 4, first part 1); jejunum, 10; ileum, 8; small intestine, part not stated, 3. Of the injuries to the colon, we find cæcum, 1; ascending colon, 2; hepatic flexure, 2; transverse colon, 2; descending colon, 1; sigmoid flexure, 1.

The incision, wherever made, should be of sufficient length, or if made small at first for the purpose of preliminary exploration, should be lengthened if a wide area has to be overlooked, since the probabilities of diffusing infective matter are largely increased if the necessary manipulations for the search are made through a small opening.

When the abdomen has been opened, certain indications may at once give aid. Such are the escape of free gas, if the rupture be extensive; the presence of blood, or blood-clot; the local collection of fluid, due to reaction to infection by the peritoneum, and the development of plastic lymph; and lastly, the presence of intestinal contents. The amount of extravasation of intestinal contents is small, except in extensive lacerations; hence the detection of such matter usually at once leads to that of the opening by which it has escaped.

The search for the wounded spot will in the first instance be guided by any localizing evidence obtained from the history; failing this, or should the evidence prove elusive, the small intestine is best searched from below upwards, and the large from the cæcum downwards. When secondary reactionary peritoneal effusion has had time to take place, the fluid should be carefully mopped out as the search is proceeded with, since it is important not to effect its further diffusion during the considerable displacement of the bowels which may be necessary.

When the abdomen has been opened shortly after the infliction of an injury, the bowel in some cases of abdominal contusion may be in a state of spastic contraction in the area affected by the violence. This condition is not, however, of very great localizing importance, since in some individuals the intestine rapidly assumes this state when the abdomen has been opened and the bowel touched.

The local injury having been discovered, means should be taken, either by wrapping the affected coil in gauze and putting it into the hands of an assistant, or by the application of clamps, to prevent further extravasation of intestinal contents, and then the surrounding area should be as thoroughly as possible cleansed by dry mopping. The latter effected, the injured coil should be well drawn forward, the general peritoneal cavity protected from further contamination by the introduction of gauze plugs, and the process of suture proceeded with. In dealing with punctured wounds the fact that the bowel lesions may be multiple must never be lost sight of.

An incised wound needs only the most simple treatment. A double line of suture should be introduced, the inner including the mucous membrane only, or, if preferred, the whole thickness of the bowel; the outer layer being a continuous Lembert's stitch, including the serous and muscular coats and dipping well into the submucosa.

Should the wound be of the nature of a puncture, it may be closed by a purse-string suture, to which a line of Lembert's stitch should be superadded, preferably introduced in a direction transverse to the long axis of the bowel.

If the lesions assume the character of lacerations the margins may be unfit for immediate approximation. This point must be carefully investigated, and if it is decided that tissue must be removed, the procedure will vary with the amount of destruction present. In some cases it will be necessary merely to freshen the margins to a requisite degree, and then to approximate them in a direction more or less corresponding to the transverse axis of the bowel, in order to avoid narrowing of the lumen as far as possible. In others, where the surrounding contusion is more extensive, a portion of the whole circumference must be removed, and a typical enterectomy performed. In regard to the latter procedure, it is as well to emphasize the fact that a circular enterectomy is not to be undertaken as a mere alternative. Experimental study, and experience of the results following the performance of enterectomy in cases of gangrenous herniæ, &c., appear to show that the proximal portion of the intestine for long distances remains afterwards in a thinned and more or less dilated condition. This matter will be more fully discussed later, but it suffices here to lay weight on the fact that avoidance of a complete solution of continuity of the nervous plexuses is always to be aimed at, even if the more perfect cosmetic result is not obtained.

Repair of ruptures of the small intestine. The damaged portion of the bowel having been localized, three main types of injury may require to be dealt with.

1. *The laceration may not have extended to the lumen of the intestine.* Such injuries are usually the result of combined pressure and tearing. An illustration of them is given in Fig. 329. Here the serous and muscular coats have been ruptured and widely separated from the

mucosa and submucosa, the lesion being accompanied by a tear in the mesentery which led to the death of the patient from internal hæmorrhage. It is well to bear in mind that the latter combination is not infrequent, since injuries of this type usually result from the application of diffused violence such as the passage of a cart-wheel over the abdomen.

In dealing with extensive incomplete ruptures, special care must be devoted to the examination of the state of the mesentery, since, putting aside the danger of further hæmorrhage from the wound, the vitality of the portion of intestine involved may be hopelessly compromised by interference with its blood-supply.

Small serous or sero-muscular rents are treated by a single series of deep Lembert's stitches. Even when very small, if ununited, they afford the probability of the future development of undesirable adhesions. Extensive lesions demand the excision of the implicated length of bowel. The enterectomy, in the case of the small intestine, will be of the axial type. If the mesentery be not seriously damaged, it may be separated from the bowel and plicated, care being taken to so suture the freed margin as to close any opening likely to serve as a possible gap through which the intestine might travel later and become strangulated. The projecting fold should be sutured to the surface of the mesentery (see Fig. 330).

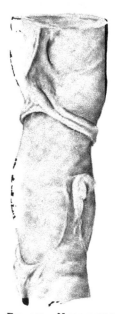

FIG. 329. NON-PERFORATING INJURY TO THE SMALL INTESTINE. The peritoneal and muscular coats are separated from the mucosa, in which no solution of continuity has occurred. (*St. Thomas's Hospital Museum*, No. 1001.)

2. *The lesion may consist of a limited perforation* more or less closed by eversion of the mucous membrane; a large example of this is illustrated in Fig. 331. In ruptures caused by strictly localized violence, as applied by the point of the shoe of a horse, the opening may be very small. This is the most satisfactory for the work of the surgeon; the local damage is limited, the lesions are usually single, and a simple suture meets every requirement. The margins seldom need any refreshment, and the openings may be closed by an inner layer of through and through sutures, either passed as a purse-string, in the case of small wounds, or as a continuous line, this layer being buried by a second line of deep Lembert's stitches. If

the opening is of material size, whether transverse or longitudinal in direction, it should be sutured in the transverse axis of the bowel.

3. *The lesion may implicate the whole circumference of the bowel.* In Fig. 332 an instance is illustrated in which three-quarters of the circumference was torn. In such injuries an axial enterectomy and reunion is indicated.

The cleansing of the peritoneal cavity is completed after the suture of the wound or rupture. The exposed coil may be washed with saline solution, and the immediate neighbourhood wiped with a moist sponge, care being taken to remove any blood-clot which may have escaped the preliminary sponging in the surrounding area.

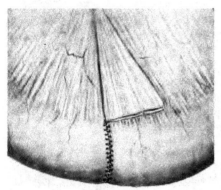

FIG. 330. PLICATED MESENTERY. Edge not sewn, and flap of mesentery loose.

The wound in the abdominal wall is then closed by suture in layers. The provision of drainage is to be avoided if possible, and is unlikely to be necessary in cases dealt with during the first twenty-four hours after the occurrence of the accident. If severe inflammation be met with, drainage must be provided for by the insertion of a tube and one or more gauze plugs, and the external wound should be left sufficiently open to give a free vent.

Repair of wounds or ruptures of the large intestine. Small wounds of the large bowel on the peritoneal aspect possess some special characteristics due to the small disposition of the more solid fæcal contents to escape. In many cases of small wounds this tendency is so marked that the amount of escape gives rise to little more than a mere local infection, which may be followed by the formation of protecting adhesions and the development of an abscess.

In this segment of the intestine another condition, shared by the second and third portions of the duodenum, has to be considered. In either situation a portion of bowel unprovided with a serous covering may be implicated. Some of the more important consequences of this circumstance should be mentioned. Thus, the great advantage of the rapidly agglutinating serous surface is lost, the wounds are often in very inaccessible situations, the openings are comparatively fixed and less liable to be closed by intestinal contraction, while, lastly, intestinal contents are extravasated into and infect loose cellular tissue far less easily cleansed than the smooth even surface offered by the peritoneum.

Extra-peritoneal wounds and ruptures then demand special treatment. Theoretically, suture of the wound is the proper course to follow; practically, it can rarely be effectively performed. In the first place, diagnosis is often made proportionately late, when serious infection of the tissue

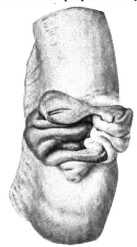

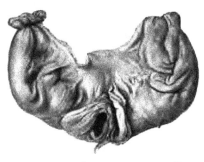

FIG. 331. RUPTURE OF THE SMALL INTESTINE, INVOLVING NEARLY HALF THE CIRCUMFERENCE OF THE BOWEL. Marked eversion of the mucous membrane. (*St. Thomas's Hospital Museum*, No. 1006.)

FIG. 332. A RUPTURE INVOLVING THREE-FOURTHS OF THE CIRCUMFERENCE OF THE INTESTINE. Moderate eversion of the mucous membrane. Inflammatory lymph on the neighbouring surface. (*St. Thomas's Hospital Museum*, No. 1007.)

has already developed; secondly, the results of direct suture have been far from satisfactory. Two alternatives exist: (1) The enlargement of the wound and its practical conversion into a temporary artificial anus, the bowel being brought to the surface and either sutured there or fixed by the insertion of a Paul's tube, efficient drainage of the surrounding wound being established; (2) the fæces may be temporarily diverted by the establishment of an artificial anus in a convenient proximal portion of the bowel, and the wound itself be drained.

Prognosis and results. The prognosis in cases of rupture of the intestine should not necessarily be bad when the lesions are unaccompanied by coexistent injury to other parts. The indifferent results obtained up to the present time are in great measure attributable to difficulties in diagnosis, from the fact that the initial symptoms are often quite incommensurate with the gravity of the lesion, and in consequence many operations are undertaken at a time too remote from the reception of the injury to afford reasonable chances of successful treatment. To ensure a reasonable chance, the operation must be performed during the first twenty-four hours.

Of 34 cases treated by operation in St. Thomas's Hospital, 9 recovered (mortality 73.5%), the first successful instance being the classical case of Croft. 24 of the cases implicated the small intestine; of these 5 recovered (mortality 79%); and 10 implicated the large intestine; of these 4 recovered (mortality 60%). Of the last 22 cases occurring between 1893 and 1907, 8 recovered (mortality 63.6%).

Berry and Guiseppi (*Proc. Roy. Soc. of Med.*, 1908, vol. ii, p. 1, Surg. Sect.) have analysed the results obtained in ten London hospitals during the last fifteen years, and find the mortality to have amounted to 87.2%.

So little weight can be placed on the results obtainable by collation of successful published cases that none are included.

Speaking generally, it is clear that wounds or ruptures of the small intestine, however caused, are more formidable injuries than those affecting the large bowel; but some exceptions must be made to this statement. Thus, certain segments of the large bowel, as the transverse colon and the sigmoid flexure, share with the small intestine the disadvantage of occupying an area in which intestinal movement is free and the conditions for the rapid spread of infection are favourable. Again, extra-peritoneal ruptures of the colon or duodenum lead to the occurrence of infection of the retroperitoneal tissue, a situation in which infection can be less successfully dealt with at the time of operation, and in which it is difficult to arrest the process by incision and evacuation.

OPERATIONS FOR GUNSHOT INJURIES TO THE INTESTINE

Although in their results these accidents differ little, if at all, from the corresponding injuries of civil practice, yet, both in regard to difficulty of diagnosis and to the question of treatment, they present features of their own which render a special consideration of them convenient.

Indications. The indications already set forth on p. 663 relating to the injuries of civil practice are of the same import in dealing with gunshot wounds, but certain special points need elaboration.

(i) *With regard to the site of the injury.* The military surgeon may be in the same position as the civil practitioner when no aperture of exit is present, but in a large proportion of cases a completed track through the body exists, and the advantage of the information as to the part of the abdominal cavity traversed may be considerable. Certain tracks have been observed to be especially unfavourable; thus wounds passing from flank to flank, the track of which crosses fixed portions of the colon and complicated coils of the small intestine. These wounds are particularly dangerous when situated between the eighth rib in the mid-axillary line and the crest of the ilium. Above this level, the liver or liver and stomach are often alone implicated, while wounds crossing the false pelvis have been observed to traverse the area occupied by the intestine without inflicting injury somewhat frequently. Antero-posterior tracks directly crossing the area occupied by the small intestine are especially dangerous; in such the bowel rarely escapes injury.

Wounds passing obliquely from the front of the abdomen to the loin, although dangerous to the colon, often miss the small intestine, and vertical tracks, either descending from the thorax and terminating high in the anterior abdominal wall, or ascending from the pelvis and opening in the subumbilical area, are comparatively favourable to the escape of the intestine.

(ii) *Nature of the violence.* Injuries caused by portions of large projectiles, as shells, do not differ from serious lacerated wounds in civil practice. In the case of bullet wounds the size of the projectile and the velocity it may possess at the time of impact with the body are of considerable importance. Bullets of the larger sporting variety of the Martini-Henry class (calibre 0.45 inch) may be regarded as never likely to enter or traverse the abdominal cavity without occasioning serious injury, and wounds of any part of the intestine caused by them can never be expected to heal spontaneously. The same remark applies in lesser degree to bullets of smaller calibre which have ' set up ' before or after impact with the body. Thus, a large irregular wound, or the fact that the bullet has pierced or comminuted bone prior to traversing the area occupied by the intestine, may be an important element in deciding on an exploration. High velocity at the time of impact, in my experience, is on the whole a favourable moment as far as abdominal injuries are concerned, provided that the soft parts only are struck. Bullets travelling with a low velocity are more liable to be retained; they may possibly turn over during their course across the abdomen, and the displacement of the bowel due to laterally distributed force is less likely to occur. Gas or fæces may occasionally be noticed to escape from the wound in gunshot injuries.

In speaking of the special indications for exploration in cases of gunshot wounds of the abdomen, certain *sources of fallacy* to which these injuries are liable must be mentioned. First of all, the intestine may actually escape in spite of the fact that the apertures of entry and exit indicate a track in the course of which injury to the bowel might be deemed inevitable. Many factors may contribute to this result. The apertures of entry and exit by no means always accurately indicate the actual course of the track. Thus, Cheatle has shown experimentally that the level of a certain portion of the skin may vary immensely in different attitudes of the body; thus, a point in the mid-axillary line may ascend not less than 5 inches when the arm is raised above the head. Lesser degrees of displaceability were noted in other parts of the body, as over the iliac crests and groins in varying relative positions of the trunk and lower extremities. Further, as Cheatle illustrates by reference to the surgical use of the Trendelenburg position, the portion of the bowel occupying any given area within the abdomen may be widely altered by changes in the position of the trunk. Again, the skin at the aperture of entry, and, to a lesser degree, at the aperture of exit, may be displaced by the bullet itself, when the latter strikes tangentially (G. L. Cheatle. *Journ. Roy. Army Med. Corps,* 1906, vol. vii, No. 1, p. 31).

The bullet in its course, although striking the intestine, may only cause contusion or a non-perforating abrasion. This form of escape is furthered by the general tendency of the travelling bullet to effect lateral displacement of the structures of the body without serious destruction of tissue, so well illustrated by the perforation of the peripheral nerves. A general consensus of opinion favours the assumption that when the bowel contains little beyond gas, it is more likely to escape perforating injury.

The injury or escape of any portion of the bowel is definitely influenced by the degree of mobility of the portion of intestine concerned. Thus, injuries crossing the fixed portion of the colon are usually perforating, and the same may be assumed for the more fixed segments of the small bowel, such as the duodenum and the upper end of the jejunum and lower end of the ileum respectively. The location of a wound in a fixed or mobile portion of the intestine is also of the first importance with regard to rapidity of spread and extent of the resulting infection.

Lastly, many surgeons are of opinion that perforations, when small. may be closed temporarily by the eversion of the mucous membrane. become rapidly sealed by lymph, and heal spontaneously. The writer has little belief in this assumption as far as the small intestine is concerned.

Mention should be made of the fact that the small intestine may be ruptured by a blow from a spent bullet, or at any rate a bullet which does not penetrate either the skin or the abdominal cavity. Watson Cheyne recorded such an instance during the South African War, in which the small intestine was found ruptured in two places.

This subject is dealt with more fully in Volume V.

THE REPAIR OF INJURIES TO THE MESENTERY

Wounds of the mesentery are usually limited in extent, and comparatively easy of treatment. Ruptures, on the other hand, are not rarely very extensive. Ruptures or lacerations are caused by injuries affecting the middle and upper parts of the abdomen; very often the patient has been run over. The mesentery is then crushed against the prominence of the spine, or the mesentery is torn, as a result of dragging from the violent displacement of the intestines. The cardinal indication for operation in these injuries is internal hæmorrhage.

Operation. A paramedian incision, the centre of which lies well above the umbilicus, is most convenient, and when the rupture is an extensive one the wound will probably need considerable enlargement. The bleeding vessels must be secured by forceps and tied, and the rent in the mesentery itself closed by suture. The method of closing the rent in the mesentery after enterectomy advocated by Moynihan, *i.e.* of approximating the edges by tying vessels on the opposite sides of the rent with the same ligature, is particularly appropriate here, since it is of the utmost importance that the stitches should not perforate uninjured vessels and still further prejudice the vitality of the bowel. In estimating the seriousness of any given vascular injury, it is obvious that the obliteration of even several of the trunk vasa intestina tenuis is of less importance than a comparatively limited injury completely severing the continuity of the vascular anastomotic arcades.

If the rent be extensive very free displacement of the bowel is necessary to thoroughly expose the field of operation, hence the abdominal wound must be large, and a considerable degree of evisceration may be unavoidable. Precautions must therefore be taken to protect the exposed bowel with warm towels. Suture is the proper method in either small or very large rents. When the rent is of moderate degree, but of such a nature as to entirely cut off some three or more inches of bowel from its direct blood-supply, it is safer to resect the affected portion of bowel as well as close the defect in the mesentery.

In connexion with this subject it may be pointed out that the prevailing belief as to the danger to the vitality of the bowel in mesenteric injuries is probably somewhat exaggerated. Evidence certainly exists to show that very extensive injuries may be recovered from. Thus the writer has seen a case in which, as the result of the handle of a wheel-

barrow being driven against the abdomen by a passing motor-car, almost the whole length of the base of the mesentery was torn across.
The rent was repaired by A. Y. Pringle and the patient made a good
recovery, some three months later being well, except for occasional attacks of diarrhœa.   Mayo Robson has recorded a case of successful
ligature of the superior mesenteric vein (*Brit. Med. Journ.*, 1897, vol. ii,
p. 77).   Again, the observation of Haberer (*Brit. Med. Journ.*, 1906,
vol. i, p. 882) that the obliteration of the inferior mesenteric vein by
thrombosis in the neck of a duodeno-jejunal hernia had not caused gangrene, bears upon this point.

Wounds or laceration of the great omentum are sutured in a similar
manner.   When the rent in the omentum is transverse in direction, it
is advisable to remove the distal portion and suture the margins of the
gap.   In wounds of either mesentery or omentum, the importance of not
leaving a hole through which intestine can pass and become strangulated is obvious, and in cases of injury to the omentum care should be
taken to avoid leaving raw stumps liable to form adventitious adhesions
with their attendant dangers.

OPERATIONS FOR PATHOLOGICAL PERFORATION OF THE INTESTINE

Perforations of this character may occur in patients with long-
standing symptoms of the disease which gives rise to them, or their
advent may be sudden, forming, to the patient at least, the first indication of anything seriously amiss.

Whatever the cause of the perforation, the subsequent course of
events is usually towards a fatal issue in the absence of operative treatment, except in the comparatively uncommon cases in which the process
of perforation is subacute and the diffusion of infection is limited by
protecting adhesions developing around the opening.

The site of the incision, made for the purpose of dealing with pathological perforations, is often determined by the conclusion arrived at as
to the primary nature of the disease, and on opening the abdomen
immediate confirmatory or other evidence may be furnished as to the
nature and locality of the lesion.   Free gas may at once be liberated
from the peritoneal cavity, pointing to the probability of the existence
of a perforated viscus, or the characters of the fluid effusion found may
afford useful aid.   Thus, if gruel-like fluid, odourless and accompanied
by the free deposition of lymph, be disclosed, we suspect the stomach;
if the matter be deeply bile-stained, the duodenum or upper jejunum;
if stinking, the vermiform appendix or a portion of the lower bowel;
or if sanguineous, malignant disease.

PERFORATIONS OF THE DUODENUM

Perforations of the duodenum may supervene on ulceration of an acute or chronic character, but the great majority are of the latter variety, although the ulcer may have been latent as far as symptoms are concerned. The disease is far more common in men than in women, some 70% of recorded cases occurring in the male sex. It is also more frequent in middle life or later, although cases have been met with in patients as young as ten years, and in one recorded case in an infant of ten weeks (Cecil E. Finney, *Proc. Roy. Soc. of Med.*, 1908, vol. ii, Sec. for study of Dis. in Child., p. 67).

Indications. Actual perforation is indicated by a sudden attack of severe pain, usually in the upper abdomen, accompanied by acute local tenderness above and to the right of the umbilicus; the patient may vomit, occasionally the vomit contains blood. The right rectus muscle becomes rigid, and the general respiratory movements decreased, sometimes markedly restricted in the upper segments of the abdomen. The liver dullness may become rapidly obliterated.

With time the area of physical signs widens, although it remains for long limited to the right half of the abdomen. Dullness in the right loin may develop, while extension of the area of pain and tenderness in the direction of the right iliac fossa has given rise, in a large number of instances, to confusion with a perforation of the appendix. In fifty-one cases of operation collected by Moynihan, a primary incision, intended to deal with the appendix, was made in no less than nineteen instances.

The occurrence of perforation is attended by signs of collapse, followed by a great increase in the pulse rate and elevation of the temperature; if the condition be not promptly attended to, signs of general peritoneal infection rapidly develop.

Operation. The operation is best commenced with the patient in the supine position. An incision is made over the right rectus muscle 1 inch to the right of the median line. The sheath is incised, and the anterior connexions having been carefully separated from its deep aspect, the muscle itself is displaced to the right. The freeing of the intersections is accompanied by some hæmorrhage from small vessels which needs to be controlled, or it may otherwise continue during the further part of the operation. The length of the incision should not be less than 5 inches, since not only has the perforation to be dealt with, but also a considerable area of the abdominal cavity to be cleansed.

The posterior layer of the sheath of the rectus is divided, and the peritoneum opened. The escape of gas and a variable amount of fluid often follow this step; the latter must be at once mopped up.

It is convenient for the further stages of the operation, either now to raise the shoulders of the patient by elevation of the upper half of the table, or to distend an air-cushion, previously arranged in a collapsed condition beneath the lower ribs. This procedure facilitates the retention of the lower abdominal contents, enlarges the field of exposure, and allows the duodenum to be more readily brought up to the surface.

The search for the perforation is now proceeded with; in early cases, when no previous peritoneal changes have occurred, this is usually readily found; if any difficulty arises, it is best met by tracing the duodenum from the pylorus downwards. When old peritoneal changes have occurred, or when operation has been deferred beyond twenty-four hours, adhesions may render the search much more difficult. The same method of exposure is, however, to be adopted; thus the liver is drawn upwards, the transverse colon downwards, and the stomach to the left.

The perforation is most commonly on the anterior aspect within 3 inches of the pylorus, the most manageable portion of the gut. Of thirty-two cases subjected to operation at St. Thomas's Hospital, the opening was found in the first part in twenty-eight, in the second part in three, and at the junction of the first and second parts in one. Of 131 cases collected by Collin, 119 perforations were in the first part, eight in the second part, and four in the third part.

The opening is commonly a small punched-out orifice with thin margins, forming the centre of an indurated area corresponding with the ulcer within the bowel. From it, gas and bile-stained contents escape freely on manipulation. In rare instances the opening may be large, and the escape of duodenal contents has then been abundant. It must also be borne in mind that occasionally more than one perforation is present. The perforation having been located, the further escape of contents is controlled by pressure with a plug, the immediately surrounding area is rapidly cleansed, and the surrounding viscera protected by the introduction of strips of gauze.

It is rare that excision of the ulcer should be taken into consideration, since experience has shown it to be unnecessary, and the removal of tissue necessitates eventual narrowing of the lumen, but, if thought advisable, the margins of the perforation may be refreshed. Usually the opening is closed by inversion, which may be effected by one of two methods. If the opening be small and the surrounding infiltration of the bowel-wall moderate in degree, an ordinary purse-string suture will suffice; if the bowel-wall be stiff and too brittle to give secure hold to the purse-string stitch, a single mattress suture, passed in a direction transverse to the long axis of the gut, gives a safer hold and inverts the perforation effectually. The closed opening is then further sunk by the introduction of a second line of continuous Lembert's sutures, also passed in a direction transverse to the long axis of the bowel. Should doubt still exist as to the efficiency of the closure, this is a position where the application of an omental graft is easy and open to no serious objection.

The opening closed, attention is turned to the permanent cleansing of the peritoneal cavity. When effusion has been moderate in amount, and is limited to the right half of the abdomen, the whole procedure may be effected from the existing wound, and, bearing in mind the common course taken by these effusions, especial care is extended to the hepato-renal pouch, the two margins of the ascending colon, the right loin, and to make sure that the sac of the lesser omentum is free. When the effusion has extended into the pelvis, or to the general peritoneal cavity, a second paramedian subumbilical incision, with displacement of the rectus muscle outwards, is needed to allow of these parts being reached.

The process of cleansing should be carried out by the careful intro-duction of long, soft, dry, sterile gauze plugs; the only part in which washing can come into consideration is the area immediately surround-ing the perforation itself, elsewhere it is unnecessary and harmful.

When the general state of the patient is such as to warrant the in-creased expenditure of time involved, and the local condition of the area of peritoneum in the immediate vicinity of the perforation is not such as to render the risk of diffusing infection too great, recent experience is strongly in favour of the immediate establishment of a gastro-enteros-tomy. This step is calculated to give relief to the sutured spot, and also to favour the ultimate cicatrization of ulceration present.

Lastly, the question of drainage has to be decided upon. In this relation it must be borne in mind that the duodenal contents may be sterile, or, at any rate, not highly septic, and if effusion has been only local and existent for less than twenty-four hours, no drainage is neces-sary. Even when the effusion is abundant, it is in the main a fluid the result of peritoneal reaction, and in favourable cases all drainage may be dispensed with. The insertion of a pelvic drain is, however, very gen-erally recommended, to be retained for the first twenty-four to thirty-six hours.

Local drainage is to be avoided, if possible, as unfavourable to the best chances for the intestinal suture, and is to be employed only in the presence of bad local conditions.

The abdominal wound is closed by suture of the posterior layer of the rectus sheath together with the peritoneum, replacement of the rectus muscle, suture of the anterior layer of the sheath, and, lastly, suture of the skin. If forceps have been left on the small vessels of the subcutaneous layer of fat, the latter may be approximated by using the same ligature to obliterate the opposite ends.

Operations for subacute perforations, and perforations of the posterior wall of the duodenum. When the process of perforation has been gradual and an abscess localized by firm adhesions has formed, primary interference with the opening into the gut is dangerous and not permissible. When the lesion is situated in a peritoneal clad portion of the bowel, the abscess will occupy some part of the area which accommodates the effusion in acute perforation; thus it may point below the costal margin, near the umbilicus, in the right iliac region, or it may even descend into the pelvis.

Should it be desired to expose the posterior non-peritoneal clad aspect of the duodenum in cases of injury or perforation, this portion of the bowel may be approached from the right loin, by an incision similar to that employed for exposure of the kidney, the lower pole of which latter organ forms a rallying point for the localization of the duodenum.

Such an incision is superior to that devised by Braune, since it affords more space for manipulation and allows the peritoneum to be more readily displaced. The method of mobilization of Kocher shows that the duodenum and pancreas are readily lifted for purposes of exploration. In this operation the position of the right colic artery and the relation of the vessels and ducts to the duodenum and head of the pancreas need to be borne in mind.

Prognosis and results. The results of these operations have undergone a steady improvement corresponding with the comparatively greater frequency with which they are performed. Experience has definitely shown that nothing short of an effectual closure of the perforation is of avail, since all recorded cases in which simple drainage has been resorted to have terminated fatally.

In a collation of fifty-one cases by Moynihan, published in 1901 (*Lancet*, vol. ii, p. 1685), seven recoveries only occurred, a death-rate of 86.27%. In a collation of 155 cases by Mayo Robson, published in 1906 (*Brit. Med. Journ.*, vol. i, p. 248), fifty-two recoveries are recorded. the mortality being reduced to 66%.

During the years 1890-1907 inclusive, twenty-three operations for perforated duodenal ulcer were performed at St. Thomas's Hospital. with eight recoveries, a result corresponding to Mayo Robson's table (65.2%). In five of the earlier operations the perforation was not closed. and if these cases be subtracted we have eighteen sutured perforations with eight recoveries, a reduction of the mortality to 55.5%.

The interval between the occurrence of perforation and the operation for its closure is of the same importance as in the case of gastric perforations. Weir, in commenting upon twenty-five operations, states that in thirteen in which an interval exceeding thirty hours elapsed before operation, all died; while of twelve in which the operation was undertaken after less than thirty hours, four died, a mortality of 33.3%. The same point is illustrated in Mayo Robson's collation. Thus, in sixty-one cases in which the operation was undertaken before twenty-four hours, the mortality was 37.7%, while in sixty-three in which more than twenty-four hours had elapsed, the mortality reached 82.5%.

Death most frequently results from peritoneal infection, and this has often commenced prior to the operation. Other causes of death are lung complications, which will no doubt be rarer with the general adoption of the ' almost sitting ' position after operation; the presence of a co-existent second perforation of the duodenum itself, or of the stomach; local abscesses, or abscesses in the subdiaphragmatic or perisplenic area.

PERFORATION IN ENTERIC FEVER

This accident accounts for a very large proportion of the mortality from enteric fever. In a series of 2,533 cases of enteric fever collated by Hector Mackenzie from the reports from four London General Hospitals (St. Bartholomew's, St. Thomas's, Middlesex, and Charing Cross), 346, or 13.4%, died. Perforation had occurred in no less than 117 of the fatal cases; thus, in a proportion of nearly one to three (*Lancet*, 1903, vol. ii, p. 863). A similar proportion was observed in 1,948 cases reported by J. Alison Scott from the Pennsylvania Hospital; thus, 153 deaths in which were 48 perforations (*Univ. of Penn. Med. Bull.*, 1905-6, vol. xviii, p. 81); and by Goodall in the Eastern Fever Hospital (*Lancet*, 1904, vol. ii, p. 9); thus, 1,921 cases, with 304 deaths, in 96 of which were perforations, all the patients dying but two.

Indications. These are of the same nature as in other pathological perforations, but they differ somewhat in their relative importance, and tend to be obscured by the coexistence of the severe symptoms of the primary disease.

Operation. The patient is placed in the supine position, and a subumbilical incision 4 inches in length is made through the right rectus sheath, exactly in the same manner as for dealing with an appendix in which pelvic suppuration is suspected. This incision has the great advantage of allowing subsequent drainage for a time, without the ulterior development of a ventral hernia.

The abdomen open, an immediate escape of sero-fibrinous exudation or possibly free gas may occur. If this be not the case, search for the perforation is commenced by finding the ileo-cæcal junction, and carefully following the gut in an upward direction. This part of the search should be made with circumspection, as the position of escape of gas or fluid is a valuable localizing indication of the site of perforation. In some 90% of all cases the latter will be found in the ileum within 2 feet

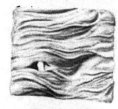

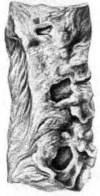

FIG. 333. TWO PIECES OF ILEUM FROM A CASE OF ENTERIC FEVER. In the upper is seen a perforation shelving from within; in the lower a large slough is seen in the process of detachment, and several depressions from which sloughs of varying depths have separated. (*St. Thomas's Hospital Museum,* No. 1044.)

of the ileo-colic valve, and in nearly four-fifths of the ileal cases within the first foot. In 264 cases collected by Hector Mackenzie (*loc. cit.,* p. 864) 2 perforations were seated in the jejunum, 232 in the ileum, 22 in the large gut, and 9 in the vermiform appendix. Fluid and escaped intestinal contents are mopped up with gauze sponges as the search proceeds, the possible situation of the perforation in the cæcum or the vermiform appendix being excluded or verified, as the case may be, at the commencement of the exploration. Adhesions rarely give rise to any trouble, as the operations are often performed at an early stage; and even when the perforation has existed longer, the deposition of plastic matter capable of localizing diffusion, as in appendix perforations, is rare, probably from the bad condition of the patient and consequent want of proper reaction on the part of the peritoneum.

The perforation may be one of two varieties; either a small opening at the free margin of the bowel, from about the size of a pin's head to 1/4 of an inch in diameter, forming the deepest part of the base of an ulcer, or an area sometimes involving the whole circumference of the bowel, may be the seat of a gangrenous cellulitis, one or more openings existing within the necrotic area (see Fig. 333). When the openings are of the small variety they are usually single, but it is not uncommon to discover one or more incipient perforations, the site of which is indicated by the presence of a small yellow area in the near neighbourhood of the complete one.

Should the search in the lower ileum prove fruitless it must be borne in mind that perforation may exist in the ascending, transverse, or even descending colon: also that in colic perforations there is more tendency to the formation of multiple openings.

When the perforation has been found, there is often room to apply clamps on either side of it, in order to prevent further escape of contents during the process of suture. This procedure is often unnecessary, as escape is not free and the opening small. The surrounding area is mopped as dry as possible, and it may be a convenience at this stage of the operation to raise the foot of the table to facilitate the packing away and retention of the intestines during the process of suture.

Small perforations may be closed by the introduction of a single mattress stitch, the closed spot being further sunk by a few Lembert's sutures passed in the transverse axis of the bowel. The same procedure must be adopted should incipient perforations be noted in the neighbourhood of the complete one. In larger perforations a through and through suture should be used, but again the mattress form of suture affords the firmest hold. In the rarer cases in which a large necrotic area is found, it may be necessary to perform an enterectomy, care being taken that the portions of bowel to be united are free from ulceration.

Perforations of the vermiform appendix are treated by removal of the same in the type manner, and the same course should be taken in the rare cases in which the perforation is situated in a Meckel's diverticulum. It should be borne in mind that suppurating mesenteric glands are occasionally met with in patients the subjects of perforation.

Should doubt exist as to the efficiency of the suture the perforation is usually so situated as to readily allow the application of an omental graft. In the right iliac fossa it is also possible to suture the omental apron in such a fashion as to shut off the greater part of the upper abdomen and even the pelvis, in order to minimize the dangers of possible ulterior leakage.

Lastly, should the bowel-wall be in such condition as to make the introduction of sutures futile, the last resources of establishing an enterostomy may be adopted, although with small hope of ultimate success.

The process of suture completed, attention is turned to the final cleansing of the peritoneal cavity. The sutured bowel itself, and the immediate neighbourhood, may be washed with normal saline solution; wider spread peritoneal exudation is better absorbed by dry gauze strips carefully introduced in all directions where its presence is suspected. The area of peritoneum most severely inflamed will be situated in the pelvis, and here intestinal contents will be most likely to have gravitated. A drain must always be introduced, since there is no chance that either the escaping intestinal contents or the consequent reactionary peritoneal exudation will be sterile, as in the case of a duodenal perforation. The bacillus coli-communis is usually present, and sometimes pyogenic cocci. A large india-rubber tube passing to the bottom of Douglas's pouch, supplemented by a gauze drain in one strip, so introduced as to be most ample in the right iliac fossa as deep as the pelvic brim, and emerging by the abdominal wound, is the most satisfactory form of arrangement. By this means both the capillary action of a gauze drain and the advantage of the more permanent channel afforded by a tube are obtained.

The wound is closed, leaving sufficient space for the withdrawal of the gauze drain, which latter process should be commenced on the second day, and be completed on the third or fourth.

Prognosis and results. When the general condition of the patients on whom this operation has to be performed is borne in mind, the recorded results are surprisingly good, and support the view originally advanced by von Mikulicz, that patients in whom a perforation is suspected should undergo an exploratory operation. Experience, however, has shown this course to be open to considerable danger. Harte and Ashurst (*Ann. of Surg.*, 1904, vol. xxxix, p. 39) give details of 26 cases in which the abdomen was opened and no perforation discovered, of which number 10 subsequently died. This mortality cannot be entirely attributed to the operation, since the latter has often to be undertaken in desperate cases of a disease which itself possesses a general mortality of 13–14%, but it suffices to give a useful caution against too free resort to exploration.

Recovery is usually slow, and the occurrence of both general and local complications is common; thus, exhaustion from the fever itself, pneumonia, secondary abscesses, iliac thrombosis, &c. The existence of coexisting intestinal hæmorrhage is a very bad prognostic element. The prognosis is naturally best in operations undertaken during the first twenty-four hours, and also in patients between ten and twenty years of age. Elsberg (*Ann. of Surg.*, 1903, vol. xxxviii, p. 71) has published 25 cases of perforation in children with 9 deaths, a mortality of only 36%. Sydney R. Scott records 9 cases operated upon at St. Bartholomew's Hospital (*St. Barts. Hosp. Rep.*, 1903, vol. xxxix, p. 131), including the first successful suture performed in London by Bowlby, with 5 deaths, mortality 66.6%. J. Alison Scott (*loc. cit.*, p. 86) records 39 operations performed at the Pennsylvania Hospital with 27 deaths, mortality 69.2%. Harte and Ashurst (*Ann. of Surg.*, 1904, vol. xxxix, p. 8) report 362 collected cases with 268 deaths, mortality 74%. Zesas (*Wiener Klinik*, 1904, vol. xxx, p. 317) records 255 operations with a mortality of 66%.

Zesas's statistics include 142 cases of simple suture with 89 deaths, mortality 62.6%; also 20 enterectomies with 12 deaths, mortality 60%. This would appear to show a margin in favour of the more radical method of enterectomy, but it must be remembered that the patients in whom it would be considered safe to undertake an enterectomy, are those whose general condition is the more promising at the time of the operation. Murphy reports 5 consecutive operations and recoveries (*Surg. Gyn. and Obst.,* June, 1908, p. 565).

The general results have therefore improved since the publication of Keen's list of 83 cases with 67 deaths, mortality 80.7% (*Surg. Compl. and Seq. of Typhoid Fev.,* 1898). Collected results gleaned from various sources are, however, open to the usual defect of statistics thus obtained, of not including the large number of unsuccessful cases remaining unrecorded, and against the numbers given above may be quoted those of Goodall (*Lancet,* 1904, vol. ii, p. 14), who reports four recoveries only in 49 operations performed at the Metropolitan Fever Hospital, mortality 91.8%.

PERFORATIONS OF AN INFECTIVE AND INFLAMMATORY NATURE

Such perforations are met with in their simplest form in the case of loops of bowel implicated in internal or external herniæ, then usually on the free convex margin of the bowel. They require to be sutured with some care, since the surrounding area is not so much the seat of inflammatory induration, as of defective vitality due to infection and distension of the intestinal wall dependent on interference with the blood-supply. Such sutured spots may remain weak and form the site of recurrent perforations; thus, an old woman, in whom a perforation was closed during the performance of an operation for strangulated femoral hernia, came again under treatment six months later for general peritonitis due to recurrence of ulceration at the sutured spot, the silk stitches of the former operation being found still in position on one margin of the opening.

PERFORATION OF STERCORAL ULCERS AND IN DIVERTICULAR DISEASE

Acute perforations of either nature are generally only diagnosed during an exploratory operation; they occur usually in subjects of chronic constipation, who are suddenly seized with symptoms of acute peritoneal infection closely simulating those of acute obstruction. The ulcers are situated in some portion of the colon, the diverticula, especially in the sigmoid flexure. Perforation of a diverticulum frequently results from the presence of a stercolith. If practicable, the opening should be closed by suture, and the peritoneal cavity closed and drained. In diverticular disease, when distal obstruction exists it is advisable to make a proximal colostomy in addition. The ultimate prognosis in these cases is bad.

When the process of perforation is subacute or chronic, localized suppuration results; here incision and drainage form the immediate treatment, to be possibly followed in diverticular disease by colectomy (see pp. 716–42).

PERFORATION IN MALIGNANT DISEASE

This condition offers little scope for credit to the operating surgeon. When the perforation is acute the majority of the patients die from acute peritoneal infection, whether operated upon or not. None the less, when brought into the presence of one of these cases the position of the surgeon is one of some perplexity. Laparotomy offers slight chance of recovery, and if no operation is decided upon the patient must be kept under opiates to relieve the misery which continues until death. If laparotomy be decided upon, closure of the opening should be accompanied by the performance of a proximal colostomy or unilateral exclusion, to divert the course of the fæces. Under these circumstances, if the patient be in good condition, and is dealt with within a few hours of the occurrence of the accident, a recovery may occasionally be obtained, and in any case the sufferings of the patient may be very materially relieved.

CHAPTER X

ENTEROTOMY AND ENTEROSTOMY

THE terms enterotomy and enterostomy naturally include operations on any part of the whole length of the intestinal canal. It has, however, long been customary to designate openings into the colon under the terms colotomy and colostomy, while later the convenient custom of specially designating any enterostomy by a name corresponding to the part of the tube opened has become general.

Indications. These operations have a somewhat wide application, either as temporary or permanent measures, and may be indicated under very varying circumstances.

(i) Enterotomy is employed as a convenience during the performance of operations where intestinal distension interferes with the necessary manipulations. When the bowel is in good condition, and readily contracts after the evacuation of its contents, the opening may be at once closed.

(ii) In other instances, when intestinal fermentation has reached an advanced stage, and either the muscular contractility of the bowel has suffered severely from the action of the toxins on the nervous plexuses (Barker), or from continued distension when in a septic condition, an enterostomy for a short period is often advantageous. Under these circumstances an enterostomy not only relieves the bowel-wall, but also allows nutriment to be introduced into the distal segment of the bowel.

(iii) In a similar manner a jejunostomy may be established to nourish the patient, and relieve the general condition, antecedently to the performance of a gastro-enterostomy.

(iv) In the large intestine an enterostomy may be used as a temporary measure prior to the removal of growths of the bowel, for purposes of lavage in morbid conditions of the colon, or as a safety-valve to prevent the collection of gas and fæcal matter in the case of short circuiting.

(v) Lastly, in one or other of the forms of colostomy, the issue of the fæces may be permanently diverted to a new aperture.

685

ENTEROTOMY

Operation. When enterotomy is used as a purely temporary measure its performance is one of great simplicity. A coil of bowel is drawn as far as practicable out of the wound, thoroughly surrounded by gauze plugs to protect the abdominal cavity, and then punctured.

In some cases where a single coil, as the sigmoid flexure, is locally distended, it may suffice to first introduce a purse-string suture, and in the centre of the included area to enter a large trochar and canula to evacuate the contents, which are often in a large measure gaseous.

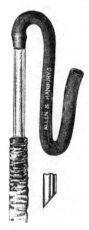

A rubber tube may be fitted to the canula to allow of the contents being collected in a vessel well away from the field of operation. When the coil is emptied the suture is tightened up as the canula is withdrawn, and the tied purse-string suture is sunk by the introduction of a short transverse line of Lembert's stitches.

When distension is more general, and a longer stretch of intestine needs to be emptied, it is preferable to make an incision with the knife, and several of these may be needed. In order to avoid multiple incisions, Moynihan employs a piece of glass tubing some 6 or 8 inches long, to which is applied a piece of india-rubber tubing to carry the intestinal contents well away from the area of the wound (see Fig. 334). When the contents in the immediate neighbourhood of the opening have escaped, the glass tube is introduced in nearly its whole length, a piece of gauze is wrapped around the point from which the tube emerges to prevent escape by the side, and it is entrusted to the hands of an assistant. The surgeon now slowly, and with care, draws on to the tube the intestine beyond; in this way as much as 8 or 10 feet may be brought into the field of operation and thoroughly emptied.

FIG. 334. MOYNI-HAN'S INTESTINAL DRAINAGE TUBE.

Moynihan further makes use of this tube either for washing out the intestine with saline solution, introduced by a hollow needle provided with a funnel and rubber tube, entered at the highest point to which the tube has penetrated, or, in certain cases, for the introduction of solution of sulphate of magnesia.

When the enterotomy opening has served its purpose, an inner line of suture, including the whole thickness of the bowel, is introduced, and this is sunk by the addition of a transverse line of Lembert's stitches, involving the serous and muscular coats.

The exposed loop is now thoroughly cleansed by washing with warm normal saline solution and returned.

ENTEROSTOMY

Operation. In cases where the wall of the bowel has suffered so much as to lose its tone and contractility, the incision in the bowel may be employed for the purposes of a temporary enterostomy. For this object it suffices to tie in a Paul's tube, and fasten the bowel in a lower angle of the wound with a few stitches; two, one at either end of the loop of bowel, will usually suffice. In using the Paul's tube for this purpose it is important to pass the retaining purse-string suture close to the margin of the wound in the bowel, including as little of the bowel-wall as can be safely employed, in order that the resulting loss of substance shall be as small as possible.

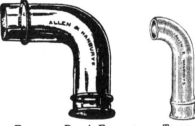

Fig. 335. PAUL'S ENTEROSTOMY TUBES.

If this precaution be taken, a lateral enterostomy opening only results, which, if it does not close spontaneously, may be occluded with ease by suture later. (See Closure of fæcal fistulæ, p. 773.) A temporary enterostomy of this nature, made in cases where the distension has been above a mechanical obstruction, and where the bowel below is in good condition, may be of considerable use later as a means of introducing nourishment in the early stages of the further treatment of the case.

In certain positions, *i.e.* the upper end of the small intestine, a permanent enterostomy for purposes of nourishing the patient is occasionally employed. In these operations, which are founded upon an exactly opposite principle to the so-called artificial anus, the object to be striven for is the prevention of the escape of intestinal contents, and, as might have been expected, the technical experience attained in perfecting the corresponding operation of gastrostomy has been freely drawn upon.

DUODENOSTOMY

Bearing in mind the object of these operations, it is natural that the duodenum should have been chosen as the most fitting site for the fistula, since the nourishment can be here introduced above the point of entrance of the biliary and pancreatic secretions, and some addition at least of the gastric secretion may be looked for; hence the conditions approach the normal as far as possible.   Experience has, however, shown that although the anatomical conditions allow the approximation and fixation of the duodenum to the abdominal wall without great trouble, yet the resulting fistula is exceedingly difficult to manage, escape of the secretions frequently occurring.   Hence this operation, although theoretically advantageous, has found little favour, and, in spite of the able advocacy of Hartmann, is seldom performed. Moreover, the technique of the operation of jejunostomy has been so much improved, that the latter may be said to offer practical advantages little inferior, even in theory, to those claimed for duodenostomy.

JEJUNOSTOMY

This operation was first performed by Surmay of Ham in 1878, as a means of dealing with a case of inoperable gastric carcinoma; that is, at a period prior to the introduction of gastro-intestinal anastomosis, an operative procedure which has rapidly restricted the employment of jejunal fistulæ as a route by which nourishment can be afforded to subjects of pyloric obstruction.   Conditions are met with, however, in which the procedure is still applicable, although the success attained by it has not brought many enthusiastic supporters to the method.

Indications.   Jejunostomy may be resorted to under the following conditions:—

(i) It may be employed in cases in which the coats of the stomach have received serious damage from the ingestion of caustic fluids, to ensure rest during the process of healing.

(ii) In certain cases of gastric or œsophageal carcinoma, where the stomach is so contracted as to render gastrostomy impracticable.   With regard to this indication it may be pointed out that since gastrostomy has been resorted to at an earlier date, such contractions of the stomach are far from common.

(iii) In cases of pyloric carcinoma, where the extent of the growth makes an anastomosis an impossibility.

(iv) Its employment has also been advocated as a means of securing physiological rest for the stomach in some cases of gastric hæmorrhage (von Mikulicz), or even in functional disorders (von Eiselsberg).

Operations. A paramedian incision, with displacement of the rectus outwards, is made, and the great omentum drawn up and pushed to the right. (Near the median line the above plan is preferable. A separation of the fibres of the right rectus for the permanent opening may be made when the muscle returns into position if desired.) The index-finger of the left hand is next passed along the under surface of the transverse mesocolon to the spine, and the finger hugging the left side of the second lumbar vertebra hooks up the commencement of the jejunum, which is brought into the abdominal wound. The bowel is then tested to make sure that one extremity of the loop is fixed, and the

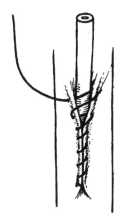 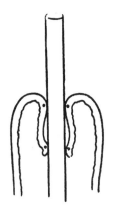

Fig. 336. JEJUNOSTOMY. Tube inserted by Witzel's method.   Fig. 337. JEJUNOSTOMY. Kader's method.

subsequent steps of the operation are proceeded with according to which method of arrangement and fixation is determined upon.

The simplest method is that of *von Eiselsberg*, who in 1895 modified the plan introduced by Witzel for gastrostomy. Two folds are raised on the wall of the intestine by the introduction of a Lembert's suture, including the serosa and muscularis, which marginate a groove in which a No. 10 rubber catheter can lie (see Fig. 336). At the distal end of this groove an opening is made and the tube pushed deeply into the lumen of the intestine. The Lembert's suture is now tightened, reinforced by the introduction of a few stitches beyond the point of perforation, and the intestine sutured to the parietal peritoneum in such a way as to lie transversely to the long axis of the abdominal wound. The external opening should be about on a level with the umbilicus.

Another simple method, *Kader's,* is founded on the gastrostomy of Fontan and Senn. An opening is made in the centre of an area surrounded by a purse-string suture, and the tube is secured in the opening made into the bowel by tightening and tying the suture. A second area is now enclosed by a further purse-string suture, the catheter pressed in to invert the bowel-wall between the two sutures, and the second string tied (see Fig. 337). The shoulder projecting around the tube is sutured to the parietal peritoneum and fascia transversalis at the lower angle of the abdominal wound, and the latter closed.

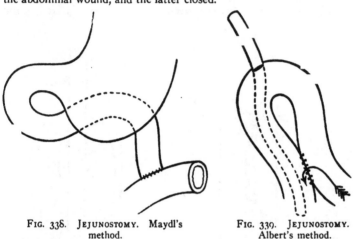

FIG. 338. JEJUNOSTOMY. Maydl's method.   FIG. 339. JEJUNOSTOMY. Albert's method.

Two other methods in which the aid of an anastomosis is invoked should be mentioned.

In *Maydl's method* the loop is well drawn out, and after the application of clamps, the intestine is completely divided, the incision passing from 4 to 5 inches into the mesentery.

The lower portion is now sufficiently drawn out of the abdomen to allow of the application of a third clamp some 6 inches down at its convex margin. Above this clamp an incision 1¼ inches in extent is made at the free margin of the bowel, and into the opening thus made the lower end of the proximal portion of the bowel is implanted (see Fig. 338).

The free open end of the distal portion of the jejunum is now drawn into the wound and so fixed as to allow the projection of some ¾ inch beyond the skin. This portion of the bowel, which is to serve as the permanent fistula, may be drawn obliquely through an opening in the right rectus obtained by separation of the muscle fibres.

Maydl's method is well devised for the prevention of the escape of the biliary and pancreatic secretions, while these fluids are also added to the nutriment given subsequently to its introduction, and thus the natural conditions pertaining to a duodenostomy are reproduced. The objection to the method is that its performance necessitates considerable expenditure of time, while the patients on whom the operation has to be performed are often in the last degree of exhaustion.

In *Albert's method* a loop of jejunum is well drawn out, and a lateral anastomosis is established at its base (see Fig. 339). After the loop has been drawn through the fibres of the rectus, and its base attached to the parietal peritoneum, an opening is made at its apex and a tube tied in. The tube in this case may well be fixed in by the double purse-string or 'inkpot' method.

The operation of jejunostomy has not been very warmly taken up in this country, and it does not appear likely, in spite of the commendation it has received from Maydl, von Eiselsberg, and others, that it will gain much ground. A consideration of the indications set forth shows that only in the rare cases of entire abolition of the cavity of the stomach can it be looked upon as the sole resource, while further experience is necessary before it can be recommended as a means of giving rest to the stomach. It has been claimed that the operation is slight, may be performed with local anæsthesia, that it can be employed in cases of carcinoma of the stomach in which the condition of the patient renders the risk of an anastomosis unjustifiable, and that it affords absolute rest to the stomach, which is not the case after an anastomosis. Further, that a jejunal fistula, by resting the pylorus, reduces the spasm of that sphincter and allows an increase of the amount of food which can pass by the normal route, hence it is employed as an antecedent to anastomosis by some surgeons. In a series of twenty-five cases reported from Garre's clinic by Loyel, the average duration of life after the operation amounted to eighty-seven days.

Of the four methods it is clear that physiologically Maydl's is the most perfect, but when the condition of the patients in whom this operation is indicated is taken into consideration, one of the simpler will usually be selected. Moynihan has devised and recommends an operation similar to von Eiselsberg's, while Mayo Robson recommends one on the principle of Albert's.

APPENDICOSTOMY

There are several conditions under which this operation is applicable.

Indications. (i) The canal of the vermiform appendix may be employed for the provision of a safety vent in cæcal distension, or to serve as a route for lavage, or for the introduction of medicaments into the large intestine, as proposed by Weir. The operation has found very considerable favour, no doubt in great measure on account of the ease with which it may be performed, and the neatness of the procedure.

Where a safety vent alone is required it has proved a satisfactory measure, since the fistula is easily maintained, easily closed, and, as a result of the facts that the normal direction of the peristalsis is towards the interior of the bowel, and of the valvular nature of the opening, it gives rise to no inconvenience by allowing the escape of the cæcal contents. Moreover, it has been shown that when the fistula requires to be used for lavage, the patient can be entrusted with the performance of the same.

(ii) As to the employment of the operation in cases of colitis, the measure of success to be expected must differ with the character of the disease. In simple mucous or membranous colitis it is an operation of minor severity, and appears to possess the great advantage over a lateral colostomy in the ascending colon of not closing spontaneously. In severe ulcerative colitis, where the benefit to be derived from the colostomy depends not upon the possibility of lavage, but on the complete diversion of the flow of fæces, no advantage can be gained by its employment.

(iii) The application of the operation has been greatly widened since its first introduction; thus, to the treatment of amœbic dysentery, and even of enteric fever, as a means of evacuating stagnating intestinal contents from the proximal side of the ileo-cæcal valve (Ewart).

(iv) Keetley (*Proc. Roy. Soc. of Med.,* vol. ii, Sec. of Surg., p. 67) has employed the appendical canal as an actual artificial anus in a case of malignant disease of the colon successfully, and he claims that the capacity of the appendix for dilatation warrants its use for this purpose.

(v) The operation has also been performed to allow of lavage in cases of chronic constipation of intractable nature. The good effect is often temporary.

(vi) Lastly, an appendicostomy opening has been employed for the introduction of fluids and nutriment into the cæcum and lower end of the ileum.

Operation. The operation is best performed by following the early stages of the procedure described for the removal of the appendix by McBurney's method (see p. 784). The appendix having been freed, it is brought either directly through the centre of the wound, or a small special opening may be made for its passage between the fibres of the internal oblique and transversalis muscles, at the lower end of the opening in the external oblique aponeurosis.

The appendix may be secured at its base by a few sutures; or it has been fixed, as has been done in the cases of some enterostomies in other portions of the bowel, by the passage of a couple of safety-pins. In anchoring the appendix, care should be taken that neither the tube nor its mesentery be damaged or unduly pressed upon, as in some instances undesirable sloughing has resulted from one or other of these causes. The tip of the appendix, or a convenient portion, is removed in the course of two or three days.

COLOTOMY AND COLOSTOMY

The operation of simply incising the colon is rarely undertaken except for the temporary reduction of distension during the performance of an operation. That of colostomy, on the other hand, is performed with great frequency in spite of the limitation of its field of application which has attended the improvement in methods of intestinal anastomosis.

Two factors in particular have served to increase both the popularity and success of the operation: firstly, the practical abandonment of the lumbar route, adopted in preaseptic days as a means of avoiding the risk of opening the peritoneal cavity; secondly, the introduction by Paul of the tube which bears his name, which has rendered it possible to open the bowel with ease and safety at the same time that it is exposed.

Opinions still differ as to the degree of comfort enjoyed by the patient after the performance of colostomy, and it must be allowed that the procedure is perhaps held in more favour by the operating surgeon than by the general practitioner, whose duty requires him to guard his patient to the end. With regard to this unpopularity, however, the forms of disease for which the operation is most commonly undertaken must undoubtedly take the chief blame, for in those cases in which colostomy is performed for conditions other than malignant disease the patient may live many years in comfort, and suffer little inconvenience from the artificial anus. A colic anus ensures the proper evacuation of the segment of the bowel lying above an obstruction, with consequent relief from the dangers of auto-intoxication, and those attendant on ulceration either of the distended bowel above the growth, or of the growth itself.

The patient is relieved from much pain, but in this particular it is necessary to discriminate as to the cause of the symptom; one of the most distressing forms, that due to flatulence, may be certainly relieved, also pain due to the passage of fæces over an ulcerated surface; but when pain of the neuralgic character, which indicates the implication of neighbouring bones or nerves, is present, the surgeon must be wary as to how far he promises relief to the patient.

Again, with regard to the diminution of discharge; an efficiently performed colostomy, which thoroughly eliminates undue retention of intestinal contents, at the same time tends to cure the catarrhal colitis, which is the main source of the offensive mucus, which forms a large proportion of the frequent stools; but where the source of the discharge is rapid degeneration and disintegration of a malignant growth, little is to be looked for in this particular from a colostomy, and the same remarks are pertintent in the case of hæmorrhage.

The colon may be opened in any part of its course, but since the left lumbar operation has fallen into disfavour, occasions on which the descending colon are opened, except at its lowest part, or junction with the sigmoid flexure, are rare, since the depth at which this portion of the bowel lies from the surface, and the practical absence of any mesentery, render it unsuitable for the formation of a satisfactory anus. The same difficulties, in a lesser degree, attend the formation of a colostomy opening in the cæcum and ascending colon, and here it may be impossible to perform other than what is known as lateral colostomy, *i.e.* an opening in the wall of the colon without the formation of an efficient spur. These openings are unsatisfactory for two reasons: firstly, they allow the passage of fæcal contents into the distal segment of the bowel, and secondly, they have a strong tendency to contract and close spontaneously. Where the opening is intended to be of a temporary nature this is of little importance, and indeed may sometimes be an advantage, but when a permanent complete diversion of the fæces is needed, such operations rapidly prove themselves unsatisfactory or useless.

Indications. (i) To afford a permanent artificial anus in cases of malignant growth of the rectum or pelvic colon, either alone or in combination with removal of the growth itself.

(ii) As a temporary expedient to relieve the obstruction due to the presence of a malignant or other stricture of the bowel, prior to radical treatment of the obstruction itself by colectomy.

With regard to these indications, some remarks will be found elsewhere as to the performance of colostomy in carcinoma and other conditions of the rectum (see p. 685); it suffices simply to point out here that colostomy is suited for some cases and not for all, and that the indiscriminate application of the operation in such diseases has been the most potent factor in such discredit as pertains to the operation.

(iii) As a temporary measure in cases in which obstruction is acute and accompanied by much distension, and due not to growth or stricture, but to the kinking of the bowel either by the tension of a normal band (*e.g.* costo-colic ligament at the splenic flexure) or by an abnormal adhesion.

(iv) A temporary colostomy may be rarely needed in cases of volvulus accompanied by great distension above the affected loop or loops.

(v) As a temporary measure in the treatment of some forms of colitis, or ulceration of the colon or rectum (*c.g.* tubercle and dysentery), for the diversion of the fæces and the lavage and application of medicaments to the bowel.

The treatment of ulcerative colitis by colostomy has become a somewhat frequent measure, and in considering this disease as an indication it is necessary to use some precision as to what is aimed at. Is the primary requirement that of an opening to allow of lavage and local applications to the bowel? or is the diversion of the fæces the primary object? There seems little doubt that here, as in many other instances, writers on this subject have somewhat obscured the question by dealing with cases of a very different nature under the same general heading. In cases in which the prominent symptoms are diarrhœa, the passage of mucus and blood in large quantities, fever, and rapid emaciation, there can be no doubt that diversion of the fæces is the first object to be aimed at, and that unless this be complete no advantage will accrue from the operation. Again, that in some cases in which pain, amounting to such a degree as to cause actual attacks of collapse, is the main feature, diversion of the fæces affords the only likelihood of relief.

In obstinate cases of mucous colitis, the complete diversion of the fæces is not so much the primary object, as the possibility of the direct treatment of the interior of the bowel by lavage and the application of various medicaments. Here, therefore, a lateral fistula into the colon, which is easy of closure, or an appendicostomy, meets the requirements. The same remarks apply to the treatment of amœbic dysentery, in which satisfactory results by these measures have been obtained in severe cases.

In true ulcerative colitis a complete colostomy is required, although performed in the anticipation of ultimate closure. This latter question of closure is fraught with grave difficulties, partly as to the suitable moment at which it should be undertaken, and partly from the danger to life with which the procedure is attended.

In some cases the beneficial effect of diversion of the fæces is prompt; the hæmorrhage and auto-intoxication from the ulcerated bowel are completely checked, and in the course of from three to six months the question of closure of the artificial anus may be safely considered. Many such cases have now been recorded, but in the experience of the individual surgeon they are none too common. A considerable improvement persists so long as the artificial vent is maintained, but the attempted closure of this is often followed by either the recurrence of symptoms or the death of the patient.

Further experience and improved methods of treatment, local and general, may render it practicable to lay down definite rules as to the period after which it is safe to attempt to close an artificial anus in this disease. A glance at Fig. 340 shows the condition which may exist in cases of any standing prior to the performance of the colostomy. When general and local symptoms have subsided, a preliminary examination with the sigmoidoscope, both from the natural and the artificial anus, may afford help as to the condition of the interior of the bowel, and this examination should be supplemented by the introduction of a Mitchell

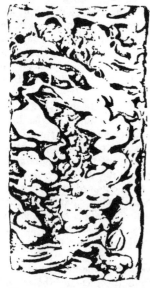

FIG. 340. ULCERATIVE COLITIS. Irregular ulceration exposing the muscular coat. The remaining mucous membrane forms under-mined and tumid islands. (*St. Thomas's Hospital Museum*, No. 1077.)

Banks's tube to observe the result of diversion of the fæces into the portion of the normal channel which has been excluded. If these tests afford satisfactory results, the closure of the anus may be attempted.

It must be borne in mind that the portion of bowel excluded after a time undergoes a process of cicatrization as well as contraction, which may render it quite unfit for purposes of anastomosis as a preliminary to closure of the artificial anus. When the bowel has been excluded for six months or more it may contract to such an extent as to resemble a tape, its wall assumes a singularly pale bloodless aspect, while the appendices epiploicæ gain a very large size, resembling considerable fatty tumours. Beyond this the tissue is brittle and friable and quite unsuitable for the safe introduction of sutures. In these particulars the contracted bowel is very different from that met with when the excluded portion of the colon is itself healthy, and should they be revealed by an abdominal exploration, the case is probably not only unsuited for the establishment of an anastomosis, but also for closure of the artificial anus.

(vi) The existence of a fistulous communication between the bladder and the rectum.

(vii) Obstruction due to pressure on the bowel from without, most frequently by pelvic tumours. Most commonly the source of obstruction is in connexion with disease of the female generative organs; less frequently, a tumour, springing from the pelvic wall, may be the source of pressure.

(viii) Certain congenital malformations of the lower end of the alimentary and genito-urinary tracts.

(ix) Occasionally spontaneous perforations of the colon from malignant or other disease, or injury to the bowel, especially on its extra-peritoneal aspect.

LUMBAR COLOSTOMY

The important part played by lumbar colostomy in the development of modern methods of enterostomy and the treatment of intestinal obstruction renders it almost impossible to exclude all mention of the method in a textbook of operative surgery. Many reasons, however, have led to the almost complete fall into desuetude of the operation; indeed it is difficult to lay down definite indications for its choice, a right lumbar colostomy as a substitute for a cæcostomy being almost the only situation in which the alternative measure can receive serious consideration. The practical disadvantages of the method are sufficiently obvious; the loin may be deep, or the space between the last rib and the iliac crest narrow, the gut itself when contracted may not be easily detected, the presence of a mesocolon may increase the difficulty of performing an extra-peritoneal operation, or as a result of congenital peculiarity the colon may not occupy its normal position. The presence of ascites may cause the peritoneum to bulge and obscure the colon, or an enlarged or abnormally-placed kidney may interfere both with the exposure of the bowel and its fixation to the surface. Again, the wound gives little scope for exploration, and affords no elasticity for further procedures if any of the enumerated difficulties be met with, or, if it should be found that growth actually occupies the situation destined to be the site of the artificial anus, the resort to a second incision in the right lumbar region could hardly be faced with equanimity at the present day merely for the advantage of an extra-peritoneal operation, so greatly valued by surgeons in bygone times. Lastly, the lumbar artificial anus is so situated as to be in a less convenient position than one in the iliac region.

CÆCOSTOMY, TYPHLOSTOMY, ASCENDING COLOSTOMY

The cæcum and commencement of the ascending colon are more frequently utilized as the seats of temporary than permanent colostomies. Thus this portion of the colon is sometimes opened in cases of obstruction due to stricture or growth of the ascending or transverse colon, where great distension exists, as a preliminary measure to further treatment when the distension shall have subsided. Again, the intestine is often opened in this position in case of ulcerative colitis.

The operation has always been unpopular for obvious reasons, the most important of which is the tendency of the resulting intestinal discharge to cause irritation of the surrounding skin; this trouble, although more marked in some cases than others, may be looked upon as a constant one. With regard to the consistence of the matter discharged from a cæcal anus, however, it may be pointed out that it by no means necessarily retains its primary fluid character. With time the fæcal matter tends to acquire more consistence and becomes less irritating; thus the condition in some degree conforms with what is seen in iliac colostomies, where the patients with time acquire very considerable regularity in the occurrence of actions of the bowels. A second objection, the loss of nutrition due to the early escape of the intestinal contents, is also a real one, but not of so marked a nature. It has been shown that patients with a cæcal anus may live for a considerable time, gaining flesh, and not unbearably uncomfortable. Thus two cases are recorded by Messrs. Goodsall and Miles, in one of which the patient had lived nine years, putting on 25 lbs. in weight, and another six years, during which the weight increased 10 lbs.

It cannot, however, be too strongly laid down, that the disadvantages resulting from an artificial anus in this situation steadily and rapidly decrease with every inch that the opening can be advanced towards the anus. It is well known that the tendency is for a certain stagnation of the intestinal flow to take place when the cæcum is reached, and that the fluid constituent is freely absorbed, and this fact has an important bearing on the consistence of the matter discharged. Moreover, with an ascending colostomy the direct transverse flow of small intestinal contents from the ileo-colic valve to the artificial anus is avoided. In cases of colostomy for ulcerative colitis in which it may be necessary to maintain the artificial anus for very considerable periods, these points are of special importance, and the anus should not be established below the level of the ascending colon.

Operation. The lines of operation are the same whether the cæcum or the ascending colon is to be the site of the colostomy.

If the conditions allow the ascending colon to be employed, an incision similar to that for appendicectomy by McBurney's method may be used. The question then arises whether the muscular fasciculi should be separated or divided across their course, and in this relation it should be remembered that a lateral colostomy is often either all that is, or can be, aimed at. Hence, considering the known tendency of such openings to contract and close spontaneously, it is better to divide the muscles to an extent of at least 2 inches. If this course be taken, in spite of the disposition to contract possessed by the opening of the bowel, considerable prolapse of the mucous membrane often occurs with the lapse of time, and the patency and efficiency of action of the artificial anus increases.

After the incision of the peritoneum, no difficulty usually presents itself in at once dealing with the colon which lies directly beneath the wound. The parietal peritoneum, together with the fascia transversalis, should be carefully sutured to the surface of the cæcum or colon, a proceeding which may necessitate some enlargement in the wound in the abdominal wall, and the external wound having been suitably reduced in size by the introduction of sutures, the bowel may be left to be opened two or three days later. When it is imperative to relieve the distension at once, the bowel must be drawn as prominently as possible into the wound, the central area is surrounded by a purse-string suture, within the limits of which an incision is made, and a Paul's tube is inserted.

In cases of obstruction the cæcum may be enormously distended, and the removal of the support previously afforded by the intact abdominal wall may be followed by the occurrence of distension rents of the peritoneal covering of the bowel. Under these circumstances great gentleness is required in the manipulation of the intestine, lest a rupture and escape of fæces should occur. The same condition may make the introduction of sutures, without perforation of the bowel-wall, very difficult, but every effort must be made to avoid this complication.

When the ascending colon is selected, the conditions may permit the bowel to be sufficiently mobilized for the introduction of a glass rod across the mesenteric aspect, if a complete colostomy be preferred. For this purpose it may suffice to divide one or more of the folds which frequently pass from the outer aspect of the colon to the abdominal parietes, or if these are not present a small vertical incision may be made through the parietal peritoneum just beyond its reflection from the bowel to the abdominal wall. In either case care must be taken not to compromise the integrity of the colic vessels.

TRANSVERSE COLOSTOMY

This operation offers some technical advantages over that upon the ascending colon, in that the length of the transverse mesocolon makes the performance of a complete colostomy an easy matter. The operation may often be utilized as a temporary measure in dealing with acute obstruction in the bowel beyond, and the transverse colon may sometimes be made use of in inguinal colotomy where the shortness of the mesosigmoid prevents the satisfactory extrusion of the sigmoid flexure (see p. 707). Unfortunately, transverse colostomy is seldom applicable to cases of ulcerative colitis, since the operation fails to fulfil the important indication of relieving as far as possible the whole colon from the duty of conducting the fæces.

Of late years there has been a tendency to extend the employment of this method, and the following advantages have been claimed for it: A complete colostomy is always possible; the position of the anus allows it to be readily employed by the patient by simply leaning forward over a suitable receptacle; the situation of the opening allows the separated fibres of the rectus abdominalis being utilized to form a sort of sphincter, such as is sought for in some of the operations of gastrostomy or jejunostomy. The resistance afforded by the costal arch and the portion of the rectus strengthened by the lineæ transversæ offers a better support for the retentive apparatus; gravity is not an important element in the occurrence of prolapse; there is no prominent anterior superior spine to make the application of retentive apparatus difficult; the fæces, although sufficiently consistent, are not so offensive as at the sigmoid flexure, and the opening, if established for temporary purposes, is more easy to close (McGavin, *Clin. Soc. Trans.*, 1906, vol. xxxix, p. 69).

The above merits of the transverse operation are fairly stated, except as to the implied suggestion that it is a preferable operation to inguinal colostomy for general use. Against this view it must be urged that, although it affects the nutrition of the body to a very small extent, yet the exclusion of a greater length of the intestinal canal than is actually necessary is inadvisable. It is also obvious that the anatomical arrangement of the mesocolon, especially beyond the mid-line, are such as to allow of prolapse more readily than in any other segment of the large intestine, and in fact this accident is more frequent and pronounced than in properly performed iliac colostomies.

Operation. The incision should be vertical, its centre above the level of the umbilicus, and carried through the separated fibres of the rectus muscle.

The further details of the operation do not differ from those described in the case of iliac colostomy, except in so far as it may be necessary to free the attachment of the great omentum, both as a matter of convenience in fixing the bowel, and to minimize the size of the opening in the abdominal wall.

ILIAC COLOSTOMY

An oblique incision 4 inches long is made, the centre of which impinges at right angles on the junction of the middle and outer thirds of a line carried from the umbilicus to the anterior superior iliac spine.

The skin and the subcutaneous tissue are divided, and the vessels
secured.   The aponeurosis of the external oblique is incised in the
direction of its fibres, and the fibres of the internal oblique and transversalis muscles are separated with a retractor and blunt dissector.   The
gap in the muscles thus obtained is stretched with a pair of retractors to
the desired size, and the peritoneum is opened.

When distended, the sigmoid colon often bulges into the wound; if
this be not the case and any difficulty arises, the small intestine must be

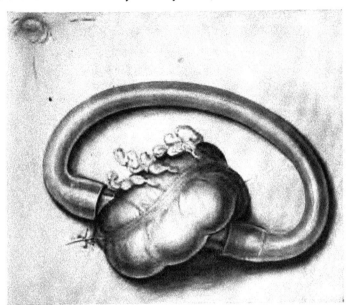

Fig. 341.   The Sigmoid Flexure supported on a Glass Rod.   A loop
of rubber tubing is applied to hold the rod securely in position.

displaced inwards with plugs, and the colon sought for in the iliac fossa.
The flexure is never absent except in the case of transposition of the
viscera, but shortness of the mesentery may make it difficult to get the
bowel into the wound.

When secured, the loop is followed upwards until its most fixed point,
the junction with the descending colon, is reached.   This portion is
employed for the purposes of the anus, the precaution being designed to
guard against the subsequent occurrence of prolapse, which is more likely
to occur if a part with a long mesentery be employed (Cripps).

The loop is drawn forward, and with a blunt instrument a gap is made in the mesentery between the vessels, through which a glass rod (see Fig. 341) is introduced to lie on the abdominal wall transversely to the long axis of the wound. A single stitch should be passed at either end of the loop, including the margins of the skin wound and the anterior longitudinal muscular band of the bowel. These stitches serve to support the loop, if necessary, when the glass rod has been removed.

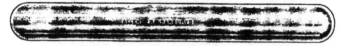

FIG. 342. GLASS ROD FOR COLOSTOMY. Full size.

Other methods of fixation may be employed in place of the rod, such as Burghard's pins (see Fig. 343), or a folded plug of gauze may be passed through the opening in the mesentery. If it be preferred, the use of any such appliances may be replaced by the passage of a single mat-

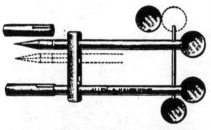

tress stitch across the centre of the wound, including the two skin margins and the intervening mesentery, so as to establish a cutaneous bridge in the concavity of the exposed loop of bowel (Ward).

The appendices epiploicæ may be ligatured at their base and removed. If the colon requires to be opened

FIG. 343. BURGHARD'S COLOSTOMY PINS. Half-size.

at once, the angles of the abdominal wound are sutured, and a gauze plug is carefully wound around the base of the projecting loop. A purse-string suture is made to surround a sufficiently extensive area, and in the centre of this the bowel is incised, an assistant seizing either edge of the opening as it is made. A Paul's tube is then rapidly inserted into the opening and the purse-string suture drawn up and tied. A second thick ligature of silk should then be tied around the portion of bowel surrounding the tube to reinforce the weaker purse-string thread. The Paul's tube is provided with a soft-rubber tube to convey the contents of the bowel into a suitable receptacle. The tube separates spontaneously on the third or fourth day. The support to the loop of bowel is better left until the fifth or sixth day, when it may be removed.

When immediate relief is not required, the exposed loop of bowel is left for three days, and then opened. The safest method of procedure is to remove as large an oval portion of the wall as possible. This method is preferable to complete division of the bowel on the rod. No anæsthetic is necessary, and bleeding is readily controlled.

The future control of the anus is effected by means of some sort of pad. The most generally useful apparatus consists in a cup with a pneumatic rim, which is fitted over the opening, and retained by a belt. The older fashioned plug is unsatisfactory, and indeed, when the artificial anus is of old standing, a simple pad of lint is comfortable and efficient. When the colotomy is upon the right side and the fæces fluid, a receptacle should be added to the cup. In the case of a left inguinal colostomy, if care be taken with the diet, it is usually possible to get the bowels to act at fairly regular intervals; thus on rising in the morning, again after breakfast, and later not more than once during the day. Too much care cannot be taken in the fitting and adjustment of the colostomy pad, since on its efficient action the comfort of the patient and the reputation of the operation will depend. In the after-treatment washing out of the distal portion of the bowel should be done at regular intervals, especially if an ulcerating growth is present. This is best done from above downwards. The advantages

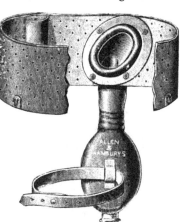

Fig. 344. Colostomy Cup and Belt with Receptacle attached.

gained by the possibility of this procedure are sufficiently great to render undesirable the method in which the colon is completely divided, and the lower end of the bowel sutured and allowed to drop back into the abdomen.

COLOSTOMY

To make an artificial anus over which the patient has absolute control Marro devised a method which consisted in causing the proximal end of the severed colon to cross a subcutaneous tunnel, so that a belt might be worn to constrict it.

Through a medial suprapubic laparotomy incision the sigmoid is brought up and clamped at the selected point. This first clamp passes from right to left (*e.g.* handle to the right). Likewise a second clamp is applied at a short distance, after emptying the intervening colonic segment by pressure. Marro then opened into the colon between these clamps with a cautery, cauterized the entire mucosa of the segment, and then cut the colon close to the proximal clamp. Next a 2-inch incision is made at the border of the left rectus with its upper extremity at the intercristal line, extending into the peritoneum. Through this a

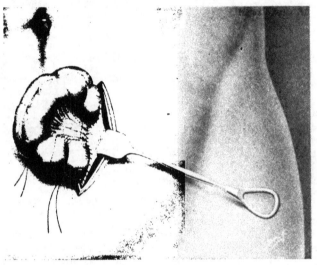

Fig. 345. The Dotted Line shows Line of Section. The blunt retractor holds outer third of rectus muscle together with skin and aponeurosis. (*Lilienthal.*)

clamp, passing of necessity from left to right, is applied behind the first forceps and mobilizes the proximal end, which is then drawn out of the abdomen. A third incision passing only through the skin is made in the upper half of the abdomen at the left rectus border. A forceps is thrust into this incision, spread, and made to emerge from the lower left rectus incision and creates a subcutaneous tunnel. This last forceps now grasps the end of the colon and aided by the forceps attached thereon draws the mobilized segment through this tunnel.

The distal segment of bowel may be invaginated and dropped back into the abdomen and the first laparotomy incision closed in layers.

The colon edges in contact with the lower left rectus incision are sutured to the peritoneum here and the skin closed over it. An excess of about 2 inches of colon has been drawn through the upper incision. To this a rubber tube may be temporarily attached to furnish continuous drainage until convalescence is established, when the excess length may be removed.

A modification of this operation consists in making the tunnel hori-

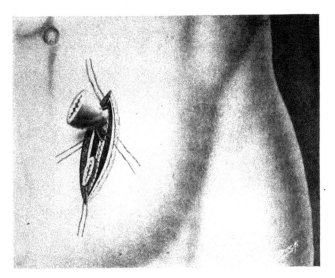

FIG. 346. TWIST COMPLETE AND MAINTAINED IN POSITION BY ANCHOR SUTURES HOLDING SIGMOID TO APONEUROSIS. (*Lilienthal.*)

zontal with its exit over the iliac crest, so as to make constriction by bands around the pelvis easier and more certain.

Lilienthal brings a loop of sigmoid through an incision in the outer one-third of the left rectus. The upper limb of the sigmoid loop is sutured to the peritoneum at the upper angle of the incision and the lower limb is likewise sutured at the lower angle. This is done with a continuous silk or linen suture, locking every third stitch. This completed, the intervening peritoneal gap is closed by a continuous stitch through and through the mesosigmoid (see Fig. 345). The lower limb is ligated and cut short. The upper limb is then freed from the mesosigmoid and should be about 3 inches long. Clamps are applied to its free edges and torsion of the stump is made so as to just occlude the lumen. The force used in this manœuvre is gauged by a finger in the bowel. This torsion is maintained by sutures in the fascia (see Fig. 346). A colon tube is inserted, anchored by sutures, and left in place about one week. At this time the redundant sigmoid may be removed by the cautery without anæsthetic.

The desirability of providing a substitute for the normal anal sphincters has led to numerous attempts to provide some muscular control of the artificial anus. When the fact is considered that no substitute for the tonic contraction of the internal sphincter can be found, it is evident that no more can be hoped for than is gained by the separation

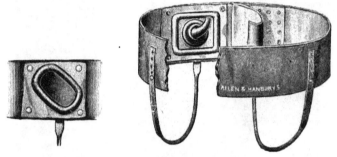

FIG. 347. COLOSTOMY CUP AND BELT.

of the muscular fibres of the abdominal wall, rather than incising them across their course.

Difficulties. In spite of the general ease with which iliac colostomy can be performed, yet certain difficulties and complications arise with sufficient frequency to need notice.

The most common technical difficulty experienced is dependent on the nature and condition of the mesosigmoid. The length of this fold may be deficient, as a result simply of individual conformation; more often the shortening is due to morbid conditions. Thus mesenteritis may have been the result of simple inflammatory change, or some form of specific infiltration, especially when ulceration has been in progress; or the shortening and rigidity of the mesentery may be due to the implication of the lymphatic vessels and glands, especially in cases of malignant disease. Again, adhesions may have formed, fixing the colon to other portions of the gut; thus the writer has had to deal with adhesions between the sigmoid colon and the stomach by removing a part of the stomach-wall. If there be adhesions between a growth of the pelvic colon and coils of the small intestine, the complication is liable to render the performance of a colostomy of very transient benefit, as secondary obstruction may soon develop. Great distension or great contraction of the bowel may also give rise to considerable technical difficulty.

Shortness of the mesentery has to be met in a variety of manners; thus the parietal peritoneum may be incised at its junction with the mesentery and the latter stretched. If this course be taken, care must be exercised to avoid too great tension on the vessels, and consequent interference with the vitality of the extruded loop. In some cases the difficulty may be got over by separation of the growth itself when the latter is in the immediate neighbourhood of the wound. The growth is then drawn outside the abdomen, the bowel fixed, a Paul's tube inserted well on the proximal side, and the growth is removed a day or two later. When dealt with in this manner the growth necroses unless soon taken away.

When operating for urgent obstruction, the colon may be sutured to the parietal peritoneum, and opened in the depth of the wound. Although this is sometimes expedient, it is a most unsatisfactory procedure, the artificial anus under such conditions seldom continuing to function more than a week or two, after which time the performance of a second operation has to be undertaken.

The proper procedure under the circumstances is to secure the transverse colon in place of the sigmoid. It is frequently possible to draw the transverse colon into the iliac colostomy wound, since the previous distension has often resulted in increase in its length, and correspondingly low position in the abdomen. If this be not possible, a second incision should be made in the abdominal wall, and a proper complete transverse colostomy performed.

Complications. *Peritoneal infection* may be said to be a rare event, even when the colon is at once opened. This happy circumstance is in some degree due to the fact that the subjects of the operation have been suffering from a varying degree of auto-intoxication for a long period before the operation, and thus have acquired a certain immunity and protection. In this particular, the advisability of exercising especial care when ascitic fluid is present should receive mention. Such fluid is difficult to retain if present in material quantity, and its leakage not only favours infection, but also interferes with the proper healing of the wound. It is best, therefore, to remove as much fluid as possible at the time of the operation, and prior to the opening of the bowel.

Cellulitis of the abdominal wall occasionally occurs as a result of imperfect adhesion of the bowel to the abdominal wound. It usually gives rise to troublesome symptoms, amongst which may be mentioned distressing hiccough. A large area of the abdominal wall may be involved which needs to be treated with numerous incisions. Cellulitis is not uncommonly a consequence of secondary interference with the wound; thus in the removal of stitches, or of the means employed for holding up the loop. It should be mentioned that cellulitis is very apt to occur if a Paul's tube be tied in on the second day, in cases where the termination of a two-stage operation has to be decided upon more hastily than was intended. The necessary tension exerted in tying the bowel to the tube loosens its adhesion, and opens the way for infection of the wound in the abdominal parietes.

Failure of the bowel to form proper adhesions and falling back of the loop into the abdominal cavity occasionally occur. Speaking generally, this accident may be said to be most often the result of imperfect fixation at the time of operation, but cases, especially of advanced malignant disease, do occur where not only is the immediate effusion of plastic lymph insufficient, but where the lymph at first effused either fails to develop into proper adhesions, or becomes again absorbed. Failure to obtain sufficiently strong adhesions is also sometimes seen when colostomy is performed in young infants, as for imperforate anus. Escape of the bowel from its new connexions, and even the prolapse of small intestines during expulsive efforts, or during fits of screaming, has in fact occurred sufficiently often to form a definite objection to the performance of inguinal colostomy in the very young. It may be mentioned that even in adults expulsive efforts have been known to cause bursting of the wall of the sigmoid colon itself, with consecutive prolapse of the small intestine. Such a case has been put on record by Barnsley, in which, after replacement of the bowel and repair of the rent, the patient recovered.

Hæmorrhage from a colostomy opening is a rare event except in cases of ulcerative colitis; in this disease it may be alarming, and the writer has also seen hæmorrhage cause death in a patient operated upon for advanced tuberculous ulceration with anal obstruction.

A very embarrassing complication may arise in the occasional *failure of an artificial anus to act.* When it is remembered that in the majority of cases of acute obstruction the immediate cause is a complete loss of tone and contractility of the colic muscle, it is not surprising that this condition should be met with. In some instances the failure of the anus to become functional may be due to the presence of a second source of obstruction, and this question when it arises is one of great anxiety to the surgeon, since such an obstruction, if existent, requires secondary measures, such as an anastomosis, the freeing of adhesions, or a second colostomy, for its relief. The need for such secondary operation is, however, rare, and as a rule sufficiently active purgation will remove the difficulty. The fact that in such cases distension of the cæcum is usually a marked feature often suggests a secondary growth in the neighbourhood of the hepatic flexure. This is, however, seldom the case. An instance of this kind, of an especially striking nature, may be mentioned. The patient, a man of 60, with little previous warning was seized with sudden obstruction, and on the third day of his attack an iliac colostomy was performed. The sigmoid loop was distended, but little beyond gas was immediately evacuated. During the next two days no further action of the bowels occurred, the abdomen was much distended, vomiting was free, and the patient was apparently not in the least relieved. A second colostomy of the ascending colon was performed on the third day, with complete relief of all the symptoms. This man was kept under observation for several months until the time of his death, when a post-mortem examination revealed no trace of obstruction beyond the primary growth of the pelvic colon. Both artificial openings remained patent until death, but the passage of fæces from the iliac anus was fitful and small in quantity, the majority escaping by the upper one.

Later troubles of colostomy lie in *retraction of the spur,* allowing the passage of fæces by the normal route to be resumed; in *contraction* of the artificial anus; in *prolapse* of the mucous membrane or of the bowel itself; and in *extension of the growth* to the mouth of and obstructing the anus.

Retraction of the spur is best guarded against by the formation of a prominent one at the time of the operation, but is sometimes impossible to prevent, particularly in patients with a thick abdominal wall. It is an accident of some importance, since it not only partially destroys the object of the operation by allowing fæces to pass beyond the opening, but it also favours the contraction and spontaneous closure of the anus. Contraction of the opening may be treated by the introduction of tents, followed by the methodical use of a bougie, which often suffice in the earlier periods to sufficiently restore patency. Later it may be necessary to incise the structures of the abdominal wall above and below the artificial anus.

Prolapse—protrusion of the mucous membrane or of the bowel—may prove a serious complication, causing much discomfort to the patient, since it often renders the retentive apparatus inefficient. Again, strangulation of the prolapse occasionally occurs. The prolapse may vary in character; it may affect equally both the proximal and distal limb, the proximal only, or more rarely the distal segment alone. In the slighter cases the condition may be found to vary with the tonicity of the bowel and the consistency of the motions. In more severe cases the redundant mucous membrane may need to be carefully trimmed away with scissors.

When an entire prolapse exists it may be several inches in length, and under these circumstances it is best (after having reduced the prolapse and sewn up the opening as in the procedure for the closure of an artificial anus) to carefully free the bowel, draw a sufficient quantity out of the abdomen, and, after resuturing the bowel to the margins of the wound, to cut off the redundant portion, and to tie a Paul's tube into each segment.

It is not always easy to explain the occurrence of the prolapse, which no doubt depends often on individual peculiarity. In a case in which a colostomy was done in a young girl for a constriction of the rectum secondary to tuberculous disease, the operation of removing prolapsed bowel has had to be repeated twice in the course of four years, as much as 2 feet of bowel requiring to be removed. The claim made in favour of the lumbar operation, that prolapse does not occur, is incorrect, as considerable prolapse from a lumbar anus has been not rarely observed.

Extension of the growth to the mouth of the anus is rare when the latter has been made at a sufficient distance above the obstruction. It does occasionally occur, and under these circumstances the growth may extend into the skin of the abdominal wall, forming more or less warty masses, often retaining an unbroken surface for some time.

Prognosis and results. The operation of colostomy in itself is unattended with any considerable risk of life; thus a preliminary colostomy made with the object of subsequent further procedure seldom gives rise to anxiety or is followed by a bad result. The nature of the indications for the operation—inoperable carcinoma, the last stages of intestinal obstruction, &c.—naturally prepares us for a considerable post-operative mortality. Of sixty-seven cases of simple colostomy for malignant disease performed at St. Thomas's Hospital between the years 1891 and 1907, no less than thirty-four, or 50.7%, died. In Hartmann's practice (*Chir. de l'intestin.*, 1907, p. 386), of sixty-three patients subjected to the operation for relief of the consequences of malignant disease, fourteen, or 22.2%, died.

CHAPTER XI

ENTERECTOMY AND COLECTOMY

GENERAL INDICATIONS FOR ENTERECTOMY

THE main indications for enterectomy may be set forth as follows, details as to the special conditions dependent on the form of disease calling for treatment being considered in the sections devoted to each:—

1. Injuries to the bowel (see Chap. VII).
2. Gangrene in internal or external herniæ.
3. Strictures of the bowel, either congenital or acquired (see Chap. XIII).
4. Fæcal fistulæ, under special conditions (see Chap. XI).
5. Embolism or thrombosis of the mesenteric vessels (see Chap. XIII).
6. Certain intussusceptions (see Chap. XIII).
7. Certain volvuli (see Chap. XIII).
8. Tuberculous disease of the bowel.
9. Certain chronic inflammatory conditions.
10. Morbid growths of the bowel.
11. Growths of neighbouring organs, involving the bowel.

As to the general application of enterectomy, it may be laid down as a rule that the measure is only to be resorted to when absolutely necessary. If a wound or a perforation can be sutured, or the obstruction due to a simple stricture can be satisfactorily overcome by a plastic operation, no doubt can exist as to the superiority of the more conservative method, although at the moment excision and axial union appear a neater and more workmanlike procedure.

Evidence, both clinical and experimental, has shown that in most cases in which a complete axial enterectomy has been employed the segment of bowel proximal to the line of union remains permanently more or less thinned and dilated. These changes have been ascribed to partial obstruction of the lumen due to the presence of an incomplete diaphragm, produced by the inversion of the bowel-wall at the point of union (Ballance and Edmunds, *Med. Chir. Trans.*, 1896, vol. lxxix, p. 300); or to the permanent effects produced by the action of toxines formed in the stagnating contents of the bowel in cases where obstruction has existed (Barker, *Lancet*, 1905, vol. i, p. 1062). A perhaps more plausible explanation may be, that the complete division of the inter-muscular nervous plexus produces a dead point or stop in the wave of peristalsis, with the result that local distension occurs, while a greater strain is thrown on the distal segment of the bowel in the propulsion of the contents forwards. Again, disturbance of the normal trophic influ-ences following section of the plexuses may be concerned in the changes in the intestinal wall.

Putting this objection aside, the significance of which for the well-being of the patient can hardly be determined, it is remarkable how great lengths of the small intestine may be resected without producing any serious signs of interference with the general nutrition of the patient. This observation goes to show that the intestinal tract forms no exception to the rule observed elsewhere in the economy of the body, *i.e.* that the provisions for the performance of the normal functions always afford a wide working margin. It has been pointed out by Schlatter (*Centralb. f. Chir.*, 1906, vol. xxxii, p. 1354) that the length of gut removed is not the sole factor concerned, since 2 yards may be removed from some patients with small effect, while in others the removal of a few inches may be of importance. In two cases recorded by him, 1½ and 2 yards respectively, were removed with no bad result beyond slight loss of strength. In these cases the loss of absorption of albumen and fats was shown to be abnormally great; while the patient from whom 1½ yards were removed needed more food than the one who lost 2 yards, as in the former the case was complicated by the presence of extensive ad-hesions. Care ought to be taken in dieting these patients to compensate for the loss of absorbent surface. Removal of the large intestine is nat-urally of less moment in this particular than is the case with the small gut (see p. 769).

Gangrenous hernia. In gangrenous hernia two classes of cases are met with: (1) Those in which the gangrene is limited to the site of the constriction, or takes the form of a more or less localized patch at the convexity of the strangulated loop corresponding with the area sup-plied by the terminal portion of the circulation. (2) Those in which infective cellulitis exists, either as a cause or a consequence of the strangulation, and extends for a varying distance along the proximal segment of the gut into the peritoneal cavity. In this class some difficulty may be experienced in determining at what level the section of the bowel should be made. The appearance of the gut and its power of con-traction are perhaps the best guides, to which may be added the evi-dence of thrombosis of the mesenteric vessels gathered from their want of pulsation, possible palpability as cords, and the absence of proper bleeding on incision of the bowel.

Tuberculous disease. This may become an indication for enterectomy in three forms: (1) As the hyperplastic, where definite tumours, often of large size, have to be dealt with. (2) As the entero-peritoneal form, in which peritoneal adhesions, surrounding infiltration, and possibly stenosis may one or all be present. (3) As single or multiple stenoses of the intestine, often free from adhesions or surrounding disease, and possibly at the time that operative interference is undertaken offering little evidence, even histologically, of their original nature.

The symptoms demanding enterectomy are in the main those of more or less severe chronic obstruction, interference with the digestive functions, accompanied by progressive weakness and emaciation; or where the disease is active and accompanied by ulceration, those indicating chronic entero-intoxication.

Many of the earlier successful cases of operative treatment were instances in which tuberculous tumours of the hyperplastic variety had been mistaken for malignant growths, and subsequent experience has shown that the discrimination of the two diseases is far from easy clinically, and may necessitate the use of the microscope, if a certain conclusion is to be arrived at. This is happily of comparatively less moment, since extirpation is the method of treatment best suited to either condition. Mayo Robson, in recording some successful cases of intestinal tuberculosis treated by enterectomy, exclusion, or colostomy, compares the results with those obtained by laparotomy in peritoneal tuberculosis, and urges that additional advantage is gained by removing a local infecting centre (*Clin. Soc. Trans.*, 1902, vol. xxxv, p. 58).

In fact, cases of obvious tuberculous disease of the cæcum, of the subserous variety, do appear to have benefited by a simple laparotomy. Thus Hartmann quotes nineteen cases, collected by Campiche (*Deutsch. Zeitschr. f. Chir.*, 1905, vol. lxxx, p. 519), in which 15.7% cures were obtained by this measure. In cases, however, where the disease exceeds in extent the simple subserous form, little is to be hoped for from simple laparotomy, and this opinion is supported by the unsatisfactory results often following appendicectomy for tuberculous disease, if not limited to the part removed.

The conditions to be dealt with differ somewhat in the small and large intestine. In the former, localized strictures, not unfrequently multiple, and adhesions are the conditions most frequently demanding relief. In the latter, tumours of considerable size may require removal, the favourite seat of which is the ileo-cæcal region. Occasionally the disease may assume the hyperplastic form in the small intestine; thus McCosh and Thacker (*Med. and Surg. Rep. of the Presbyterian Hospital, New York*, January, 1902) record the removal of a spindle-shaped tumour of the ileum, 4–5 inches long and 2½ inches in diameter, with several lymphatic glands enlarged to the size of a pigeon's egg in the mesentery, which was probably of this nature.

When the small intestine is the seat of the disease, the most frequent indication for enterectomy is stenosis. Excellent rules for the procedure, in cases either uncomplicated or accompanied by the presence of moderate adhesions and glandular implication, have been laid down by Caird (*Scottish Med. and Surg. Journ.*, 1904, vol. xiv, p. 22):

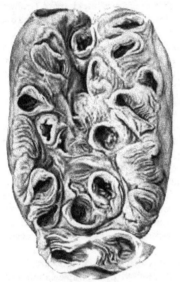

1. 'If the stricture be non-adherent, be localized and solitary, divide well above the proximal dilated portion, since there is a tendency for the development of secondary tubercles and points of erosion and ulceration above the primary lesion. Always search for other strictures. Should there be multiple strictures separated by a lengthy interval of healthy intestine without glandular implication, it is better to deal with each stricture individually, than to excise an undue length of the alimentary canal.'

FIG. 348. ENTERO-PERITONEAL DISEASE OF THE SMALL INTESTINE. The coils are connected by a mass of dense connective tissue. (*St. Thomas's Hospital Museum*, No. 1144.)

2. 'In dealing with an area of coils matted to each other, first ascertain the extent and relation of the parts involved, then identify the free proximal and distal intestine; apply clamps, and proceed to remove the entire mass. The mesentery may be divided close to its origin, as this entails the division of fewer, if larger, vessels, and allows the removal of all the infected lymphatic glands. The latter cannot well be dissected out without damage to the blood-supply of the intestine, hence it may be necessary to remove much bowel in the process of clearing them away. Should the mass be at any point adherent to an adjacent healthy loop, it would appear necessary to excise the implicated wall of that loop, and so avoid the possibility of leaving a future focus of the disease.'

These rules apply equally to the rare instances in which a localized hyperplastic tumour of the small intestine needs removal.   The operative treatment of extensive entero-peritoneal disease is considered under the heading of Exclusion of the bowel.

In a very considerable proportion of cases tuberculous disease of the intestinal tract is limited to the ileo-cæcal region; thus, in 100 cases collected by Fenwick and Dodwell, the cæcum was affected in eighty-five, and in 9.6% of these it was the only part affected.   Ileo-cæcal tuberculosis offers one of the varieties most suitable to surgical treatment, and

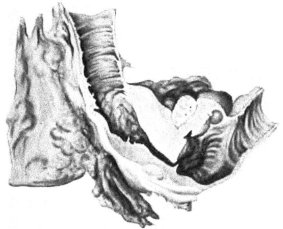

Fig. 349.   Hyperplastic Ileo-cæcal Tuberculosis.   (*Hartmann.*)

the subject has been admirably handled in an address given to the Medical Society of London by Hartmann (*Med. Soc. Trans.,* 1907, vol. xxx, p. 334).

Certain chronic inflammatory conditions.   This indication is founded upon a number of observations made in cases treated by enterectomy, under the false impression that the surgeon was dealing with malignant disease of the bowel.   A small proportion of them are possibly tuberculous in origin, but the large majority probably belong to the category to which practical surgical attention has been particularly drawn by American surgeons, under the somewhat unfortunate designation of diverticulitis.   The association of false diverticula of the intestine with obstruction of its lumen has long been recognized, and a certain number of instances have found their way into modern statistics of the causes of intestinal obstruction, while the condition was described, as early as 1858, by Sydney Jones in the *Transactions of the Pathological Society of*

London, vol. x, p. 13. In recent years a number of observations have been made as a result of operations, in which the symptoms and signs produced by inflammatory conditions have simulated in an extraordinary degree those of malignant disease. Again, the mysterious disappearance of tumours deemed to be malignant and inoperable by surgeons of experience after simple explora-

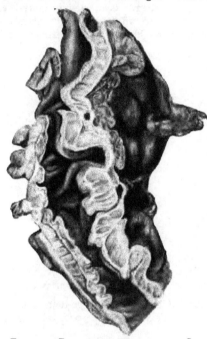

tion, and the surprising results of colostomy under somewhat similar circumstances, all tend to show that inflammatory conditions, especially in the large bowel. giving rise to obstruction and its complications, are far from uncommon (Moynihan, *Trans. Clin. Soc.,* 1907, vol. xl, p. 31).

A certain small proportion of cases of this nature demand an enterectomy. When the inflammatory condition leads to local suppuration, a simple incision may suffice to relieve the patient. but in some instances, where the abscess empties itself into neighbouring viscera, more extensive procedures may need to be undertaken. In an instance reported by Brewer (*Trans. Amer. Surg. Assoc.,* 1907, vol. xxv, p. 258), a perforating ulcer was discovered by abdominal

FIG. 350. PERIDIVERTICULITIS OF THE SIGMOID FLEXURE. Thickening due to chronic inflammation, principally in the muscularis and subserosa. Numerous diverticula. (*Mayo.*)

section, and unsuccessfully treated by suture. When inflammatory tumours lead to the development of acute obstruction, a temporary colostomy may relieve the symptoms and even cure; more commonly the colostomy needs to be followed by a secondary enterectomy. Lastly, where a chronic tumour, accompanied by signs of obstruction, persists, a primary one-stage enterectomy is indicated. In five cases operated upon by W. J. Mayo (*Trans. Amer. Surg. Assoc.,* 1907, vol. xxv, p. 237), the disease was found to be limited to from 4 to 8 inches of the gut.

Malignant disease. The indications for operation in cases of malignant tumour of the bowel are signs of obstruction combined with certain local conditions.

Sarcomatous tumours are of comparatively rare occurrence, forming not more than 2% of all malignant tumours of the bowel. They are met with much more frequently in the small than the large intestine, and are usually only discovered in an advanced stage of growth, since they give rise to little or no narrowing of the lumen of the bowel.

A type axial enterectomy in one stage is the most suitable method of removal in the small intestine. The main difficulty in this procedure may lie in the extirpation of the mesenteric glands, which when involved may far exceed in size the primary growth and necessitate for their removal the resection of an area of mesentery which compromises the vitality of the bowel for a much greater extent than that occupied by the tumour. The occasional existence of multiple tumours must also be borne in mind. In the great majority of instances the growths themselves are free and movable.

Carcinomatous tumours are more common, and of these 95% are situated in some portion of the large intestine. They present themselves in two forms as affecting practical surgery. (1) As a growth of considerable bulk, increasing rapidly in size, accompanied by superficial ulceration towards the lumen of the bowel, and often by considerable surrounding inflammatory infiltration, resulting in the formation of external adhesions both peritoneal and retroperitoneal. Such growths may obstruct the lumen of the bowel but little. (2) As localized annular infiltrations, involving a very limited length of the bowel-wall, unaccompanied by much ulceration, but causing extreme stenosis. A growth of this nature, when viewed from without, may be so limited as to suggest that a ligature with a piece of whipcord has been applied.

In some 40% of all cases a tumour may make the diagnosis comparatively easy; in others the growth may be completely impalpable. When palpable, its presence may only be occasionally demonstrable, and under such circumstances its position may be indicated by local peristaltic waves in the proximal portion of the gut; again, local pain or tenderness may aid in the determination of its site. In many cases the portion of gut above the tumour is thickened and distinctly palpable, but care must be taken not to mistake the cord-like thickening due to enterospasm for the hypertrophy accompanying distal obstruction.

The methods of dealing with colic growths by enterectomy vary with the attendant conditions, but they may be divided into four classes.

1. *The growth is excised, and immediate union, preferably of the lateral type, is effected.* This method constitutes the ideal, and is that

which has been followed by the best results. It is unfortunately restricted in its application, since for its safe performance the general condition of the patient must be good, and no distension of the intestine must be present.

2. *A preliminary anastomosis is effected, to be followed by secondary excision of the growth.* This method, like the first, is only to be undertaken under satisfactory conditions, such as the absence of any considerable chronic distension, or anything approaching acute obstruction. It is founded upon the same principle as a gastro-enterostomy undertaken as a preliminary to the performance of a partial gastrectomy, in cases in which the general condition of the patient is bad, and where temporary relief to the obstruction may be expected to effect improvement both in the general and local conditions. This method possesses the very great advantage over the next of allowing the secondary enterectomy to be performed under normal conditions as far as the risks of operative infection are concerned.

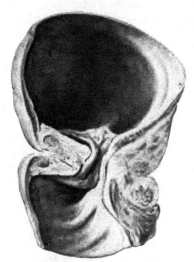

FIG. 351. ANNULAR MALIGNANT STRICTURE OF THE SIGMOID FLEXURE.

3. *Preliminary colostomy, followed by secondary enterectomy and eventual closure of the artificial anus.* This method is that most generally suited for adoption in cases where severe chronic or acute obstruction exists. The establishment of the artificial anus removes immediate risks, allows time for the distension of the bowel to subside, for recovery from atony of the intestinal muscle, and obviates the increased risk dependent on the exceptionally septic state of the contents of the intestine when obstruction has been marked. It has the disadvantages of the discomfort which accrues from the presence of the artificial anus, and the more serious one of prejudicing the chances of the secondary enterectomy by affording an additional source of infection at the time of operation. The desirability of eventual closure of the artificial anus is also a disadvantage, since this step necessitates a considerable prolongation of the time needed for the completion of the treat-

ment. The artificial anus may, however, prove a valuable adjunct, serving as a vent-hole, and preventing distension in cases where the atonic condition of the intestinal muscle is not satisfactorily recovered from. Again, the vent may prove a useful safeguard when the local conditions are such that eventual contraction at the point of union of the bowel may have to be reckoned with later.

4. *Preliminary mobilization and eventration of the growth, combined with colostomy, followed by secondary removal of the tumour, and eventual closure of the artificial anus by an instrument on the principle of the enterotome of Dupuytren.* This method has the disadvantages of requiring a very prolonged period and repeated operations for its completion, but in the hands of von Mikulicz, its chief supporter, it has furnished excellent results both immediate and remote. This is the more striking, in that the possibility of complete extirpation of the lymphatic glands and vessels is less likely than in a one-stage primary enterectomy.

TECHNIQUE OF ENTERECTOMY

Reunion of the intestine after the excision of a portion may be effected by one of three methods:

1. Axial, or end-to-end union.
2. Lateral anastomosis, with closure of the cut ends.
3. Lateral implantation, or end-to-side union.

ENTERECTOMY WITH AXIAL UNION

End-to-end union supplies an ideal result from a cosmetic point of view; one joint only requires to be made, and thus a minimum expenditure of time is ensured, while risk of leakage is limited to a single source.

Certain practical dangers, however, attend the method; thus the necessity of including the 'mesenteric angle' in the line of union in operations involving the small intestine, or the much wider uncovered posterior aspect of the bowel in some parts of the colon. Again, the line of incision crosses the course of the larger branches given off by the vasa recta to the bowel itself, thus tending to endanger the nutrition of the cut margin more than is the case with incisions involving the antemesenteric aspect of the bowel. Further, the main blood-supply to the margins is to some extent compromised by the necessary incision of the mesentery. Likelihood of the formation of a diaphragm as a result of inversion of the united margins may be fairly claimed to have been eliminated by modern methods of suture, although this was a fertile source of trouble in the early history of enterectomy, sometimes giving rise to more or less serious obstruction.

A consideration of the statistics relating to the general results of enterectomy clearly shows that these dangers have exerted an important influence on the success of the operation in the past, and indicate that great care should be exercised in the selection of cases for the axial method, since the numbers undoubtedly prove a greater general mortality to attend it than has been observed after either lateral union or lateral implantation.

The question whether cosmetic reasons, and economy in time of performance, can wholly compensate for the somewhat increased risks of the axial method scarcely allows of an absolute expression of opinion, but is one of those likely always to remain open to argument according to the predilections and specific capability of the surgeon. It must be conceded, however, that axial union is to be regarded as the normal procedure in most cases where the small intestine has to be dealt with, and in many where an operation on the colon is within the limits of the transverse or sigmoid segments.

Operation. The preliminary steps for the exposure and exploration of the portion of the bowel to be removed having been taken, the field of operation is protected by the insertion of gauze plugs. An outer series is first introduced, both to help in the retention of the remaining abdominal contents, and to preserve them from contamination. These will not be removed before the termination of the operation, and should be so arranged that their outer extremities thoroughly protect the tissues of the wound in the abdominal wall. A less bulky series, which can be changed if soiled during the progress of the operation, is then arranged within the protected area.

The portion of bowel to be dealt with, having been previously well drawn forward, is now clamped, the clamps including the corresponding portion of the mesentery. Some stress is laid by Kocher on applying the clamps with a slight obliquity to the transverse axis of the bowel, in order to ensure a slightly more extensive removal of the free margin of the bowel. This ensures a somewhat better blood-supply to the line of union, but care must be exercised not to produce an angle at the point of junction. The proximal clamp should if possible be first applied, the contents of the bowel below gently passed downwards by manipulation with the fingers, and the second clamp placed in position. The bowel is thus rendered as free as possible of contents.

Two inner smaller clamps are applied to control the included segment, enough space being left between them and the retaining clamps to allow a proper length of bowel to project for the purpose of the introduction of the suture.

The bowel is divided at either end about one inch within the retaining clamps, a small plug of gauze having been placed under the point of incision to absorb any leakage, and protect the deeper guards. Each end, as divided, is cleansed by wiping with a dry sponge, and if desired may be treated with an antiseptic—preferably alcohol or solution of biniodide of mercury—prior to wrapping it up in a piece of gauze. Section of the bowel is most simply effected by the use of the knife or scissors. Since, however, this step forms one of the crucial moments in the operation, many devices to lessen the risk of diffusing infection have been employed. Thus a crushing clamp is often applied at the point to be divided, or the section is made with the thermo-cautery.

The ends having been temporarily safely disposed of, the mesentery is divided to the required extent, and removed. There is some practical advantage in commencing the procedure at the proximal point, as by this means the larger vessels are first met with, and the amount of hæmorrhage is minimized. It must be borne in mind that the free escape of blood into the field of operation much increases the risks of diffusing infective matter. The amount of mesentery to be removed varies much, according to the indication for the enterectomy.

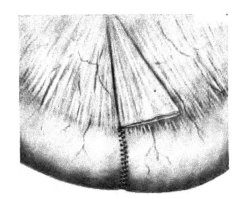

Fig. 352. Plication of the Mesentery. The margin of the mesentery has not yet been sutured.

When the mesentery is healthy, as in cases of wound, and where a small piece of gut only needs removal, the mesentery may be freed from the attached margin, the vessels secured, and the mesentery plicated with sutures (see Fig. 352). In cases where extensive gangrene with thrombosis of the vessels exists or in cases of malignant or tuberculous disease, where it is necessary to extirpate lymphatic glands and vessels, a wedge-shaped area of some size may need removal; in the performance of this step the greatest care must be exercised in dealing with the apex, lest large trunks be unnecessarily wounded, and the blood-supply to the ends of the bowel about to be united seriously endangered.

If the section of the mesentery be made prior to that of the intestine, the amount of hæmorrhage is reduced to a minimum; but this is not always convenient, and hæmorrhage from the cut ends of the bowel may

always be controlled by temporary tightening up of the retaining clamps
to a requisite degree.

The desired area of mesentery and bowel having been removed, the
inner layer of plugs, if soiled, may be changed, and a special narrow plug
folded in narrow layers having been introduced through the gap in the
mesentery and between the ends to be united, these are approximated
(see Fig. 353).

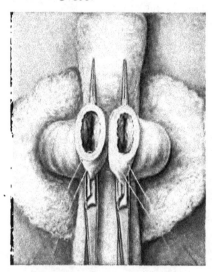

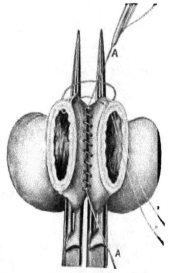

Fig. 353. Clamped Intestine in
Position. The abdominal wound is
protected by plugs, and a longitudinal
plug is in position beneath the line of
suture. Temporary fixation threads are
inserted at the ante-mesenteric margin.

Fig. 354. Enterectomy followed
by End-to-end Union. The first line
of suture A has been inserted. Lee's
stitch * * has been inserted at the
mesenteric margin, but not tied. The
fixation threads have been removed.

The handles of the clamps lying on the abdominal wall serve to
roughly hold the bowel in position, but for the even introduction of the
suture it is convenient to insert temporary fixation threads at the free
margin of the bowel. Fixation of the mesenteric margin is obtained by
utilizing the free end of the first knotted stitch, A, of the sero-muscular
series. The further stitches are introduced one-tenth of an inch from
the cut margin; they include serosa and muscularis, dipping into the submucosa, and are continued as far as the fixation thread at the ante-mesenteric aspect of the bowel. At this point the thread is knotted and left

long to unite with the terminal stitch of the final series to be introduced (see Fig. 358, D).

This first series of stitches having been introduced, the fixation threads may be removed, and attention is turned to the ' mesenteric angle.'

The importance of the mesenteric angle as a source of danger has led to the introduction of numerous devices for its effective closure. One of the most widely employed methods is the ingenious adaptation of a mattress suture of Lee, which pierces all four layers of the mesentery and the intestinal wall, completely obliterating the ' angle ' (see Figs. 354, 361).

The needle is entered from the lumen of the bowel end lying on the operator's right, made to emerge exactly at the point of union of the

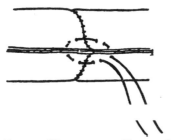 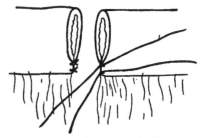

FIG. 355. MITCHELL AND HEAMNER'S MESENTERIC STITCH. (*Senn.*)

FIG. 356. SHOEMAKER'S METHOD OF TREATING THE MESENTERIC ANGLE. Two sutures have been passed through the entire thickness of the wall on either side of the mesentery.

mesentery and bowel-wall externally, and carried across the front of the gap in the mesentery to the opposite side; here it is entered at the junction of the mesentery and bowel-wall, and carried into the lumen of the bowel, whence it is made to emerge again on the posterior aspect of the gap and to enter the opposite end of the gut.   The suture is knotted immediately before commencing the first half of the inner row of sutures, and if passed as above described, its knot lies within the bowel.

The mesenteric stitch lies in the same line as the inner row of sutures, and care should be taken that it does not unnecessarily include any mesenteric vessel near the cut margin.

Two other methods, illustrating the adaptation of a simple suture and a mattress suture respectively, may be mentioned.   It will be noted that Shoemaker's is a preliminary measure; Lee's an intermediate step; and Mitchell and Heamner's a terminal act, in the process of union.

Mitchell and Heamner's stitch is passed at the termination of the union (see Fig. 355). The needle is carried (1) through the mesenteric attachment, dips into the bowel-wall, (2) is thence carried across the line of union, dipping again into (3) the bowel-wall, and emerging to (4) again traverse the mesenteric attachment, thence it crosses the line of union a second time, and a complete circle is established when the ends are knotted.

Shoemaker's method (see Fig. 356) consists in passing two sutures at the mesenteric margin in such a manner as to close the entire lumen of the

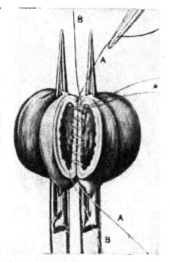

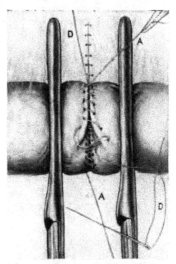

FIG. 357. ENTERECTOMY FOLLOWED BY END-TO-END UNION. The first half of the inner line of suture B has been inserted. Lee's mesenteric stitch * has been knotted, but not cut short.

FIG. 358. ENTERECTOMY. Anterior line of inner stitches completed. First half of final line D inserted. D has been knotted to the free end of A above, and the mesenteric gap has been closed. It only remains to complete D and knot it to the lower free thread of A.

bowel. A complete peritoneal clad ring for apposition is thus obtained, and the mesenteric angle closed. The two threads on one side may be kept long, and employed for the first and second lines of suture.

On the completion of the first line of suture, A, and the tightening of the Lee's mesenteric stitch, the first half of the inner series, B, is inserted, and knotted at the ante-mesenteric margin (see Fig. 357); thence the same line is continued over the anterior aspect, and the bowel lumen closed.

The inner series of sutures, B, is usually made to perforate the whole thickness of the bowel, and thus serves to control all hæmorrhage. If desired, it may be confined to the mucous membrane, under which circumstances it is usually necessary to ligature a few bleeding points. The former procedure is to be generally preferred, as giving more strength of union, and as avoiding the introduction of unnecessary ligatures within the confines of the wound.

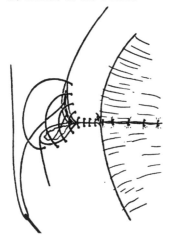

FIG. 359. METHOD OF DEALING WITH INCONGRUENCE IN SIZE.

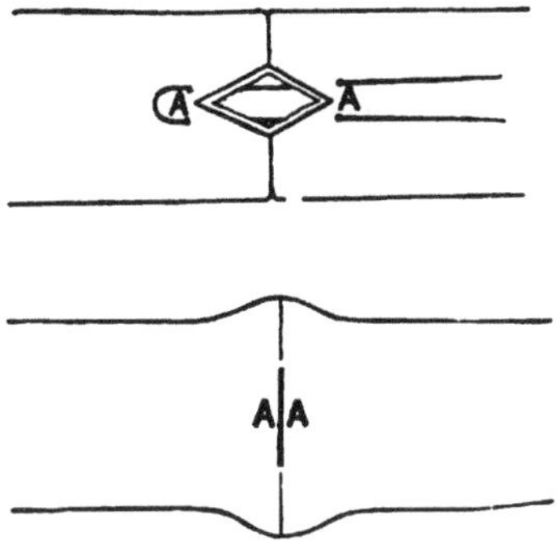

FIG. 360. METHOD OF ENLARGING THE POINTS OF UNION. This is done by a longitudinal incision at the ante-mesenteric margin of both elements of the junction, followed by approximation of the ends of the incisions in the vertical line by a mattress suture. (*Cheatle.*)

The fourth line (see Fig. 358, D), the anterior series of Lembert, is now introduced, the two ends being knotted to those of A, and the union is completed.

It only remains to close the mesenteric gap, if present. This requires a sufficient number of stitches to prevent any chance of leaving a hole which would be capable of giving rise to ulterior trouble as a site of strangulation. Moynihan advises that the procedure should be effected in part by tying the vessels successively on either side of the gap with the same ligature, thus minimizing the number of sutures to be introduced, and avoiding the possible inclusion of uninjured vessels by the stitches.

If preferred, the union of the bowel may be readily effected by the use of two threads of sufficient length, the first stitch being knotted about the centre of the thread, and the long free end left employed for the second half of each line of suture respectively. The two knotted points made in each line prevent any chance of puckering of the union, and consequently of narrowing of the lumen of the bowel.

In some cases considerable *incongruence* exists in the calibre of the two ends of bowel to be united. The difficulty may sometimes be met by the removal of a sufficient portion of the narrow element, but it is seldom that this simple expedient will suffice.

Two simple methods are then at the disposal of the surgeon: (1) The length of the cut margin available for employment may be increased by incising the bowel longitudinally immediately opposite to the mesenteric attachment (see Fig. 359). (2) The narrow element may be cut obliquely (Jeannel), the obliquity being at the expense of the ante-mesenteric aspect.

Of the two methods the former is preferable.

Axial union may also be desired between portions of bowel both of which are considerably narrowed, and for such the method recommended by G. L. Cheatle and resembling that of Chaput may be employed (*Lancet,* 1897, vol. ii, p. 1113).

A similar longitudinal incision, parallel to and opposite the mesenteric attachment, is employed, but in this instance in the case of either end. The whole length of the cut margin thus gained is united transversely, and the lumen of the bowel at the point of union is actually increased (see Fig. 360).

If axial union be for any reason attempted in the continuity of such portions of the bowel as the ascending or descending colons, the problem of obtaining a complete peritoneal ring for apposition is usually insuperable. The difficulty may be lessened by certain methods, but only absolute necessity should allow such unions to be made.

The uncovered aspect of the colon may be to some extent narrowed by care in the division of the parietal peritoneum, and the formation of a small peritoneal flap from it, which flap is stitched to the cut margin of the bowel prior to the commencement the main suture; this method is only practicable when the bowel is somewhat contracted. If the formation of a flap be impracticable, the uncovered portion of the bowel at least should be united by Connell's method, as this affords a firmer immediate union of the opposed parts; the remainder of the line of suture may be completed in the ordinary manner if desired.

Connell's method of union. A single series of completely perforating stitches is employed. The ends of the bowel having been placed in position, a Lee's stitch is introduced at the mesenteric margin, and a series of interrupted mattress sutures are used to unite the applied margins of the bowel (see Fig. 361).

This first half of the suture is passed with ease; the second needs a little practice, and a fully curved needle is required. The needle is introduced from the interior of the right element, and emerging on the peritoneal aspect is carried across the gap to enter the left element from

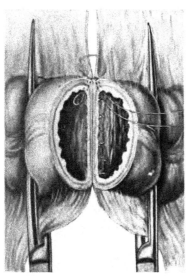 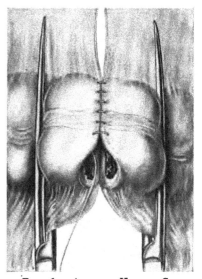

FIG. 361. UNION OF THE TRANS-
VERSE COLON BY CONNELL'S METHOD.
The first series of interrupted sutures
has been inserted and knotted. Lee's
stitch has been inserted at the mesenteric margin, but not tied.

FIG. 362. ANTERIOR HALF OF CON-
NELL'S SUTURE. The stitches are being
inserted with a continuous thread, and
are not drawn tight, in order to show
their direction. Note the necessary inversion of the margin shown at the
lower angle of the union.

the peritoneal aspect and gain the lumen; the needle is then made to again emerge from the lumen ⅛ inch further forwards and is carried across the gap to re-enter the right element ⅛ inch from the point originally pierced (see Fig. 362). The two free ends now hang from the lumen of the right element and are knotted within the bowel. The necessary incurvation of the margin of the bowel may be maintained, if desired, by the application of Poirier's forceps on either side of the gap.

The sutures of the second half are readily tied until the opening is nearly closed.   To allow of the knotting of the last stitches a threaded needle is introduced eye forwards from the deep aspect of the joint between two of the already knotted sutures of the first line.   When the eye of the needle projects, the contained thread is drawn into a loop into which the free ends of the stitch to be knotted are inserted (see Fig. 364). The needle and loop are then withdrawn, bringing the two free ends

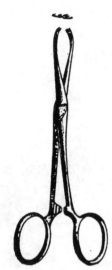

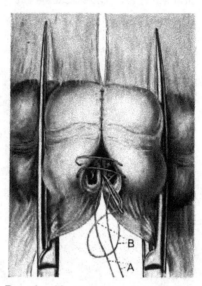

FIG. 363. POIRIER'S FORCEPS. Useful as a substitute   for   controlling threads.

FIG. 364. METHOD OF COMPLETING CONNELL'S SUTURE. B, Loop of thread in the eye of a needle which has been passed between two sutures of the deep line; A, Ends of the superficial stitch passed into the loop preparatory to being drawn through on the deep aspect of the joint and knotted.

with them out of the posterior line of suture.   Traction is now exerted on the ends of the thread in such a manner as to obliterate the lumen of the bowel and bring the two lines of suture at this point into contact: the stitches are then firmly knotted, and cut short, and as the bowel resumes its normal tubular form the free ends are retracted into its cavity.

The method may be varied, if desired, by the employment of a continuous stitch, instead of the interrupted mattress suture (see Fig. 362): but this slightly increases the difficulty, as the thread is not readily held taut during each passage of the needle.   The somewhat troublesome method of inserting the final stitches may be safely avoided by the substitution of two or three deeply passed sutures of the Lembert type to close the last portion of the gap on the anterior surface of the union.

ENTERECTOMY WITH LATERAL UNION

Lateral union is applicable to almost any portion of the bowel, provided only that sufficient length and mobility exist to allow of the desired arrangement of the free ends.   These latter conditions are rarely absent except in the presence of formidable adhesions, or in the case of the lower end of the pelvic colon.   By the lateral method the parts to be approximated may be so arranged as to ensure the contact of plane peritoneal surfaces throughout, without the necessity of any invagination at the point of union.   The incision for the purposes of communication is made in the area of the terminal twigs of the blood-supply, thus reducing interference with the nutrition of the bowel-wall to a minimum, also at a distance from the divided mesenteric trunks.   The opening may be made as extensive as the surgeon may desire, while the tendency to subsequent contraction is slight.   Disparity in the width of lumen of the two portions of bowel is of little importance, and calls for no special procedure. No danger is incurred of either temporary or secondary obstruction of the opening by a diaphragm, and, lastly, experience has abundantly proved the risks from leakage at the line of suture to be far less than in the case of axial unions.   In fact, if the main aperture of communication alone were taken into consideration, the large proportion of competent anastomoses for gastro-enterostomy and ileo-colostomy would show that the risk from this cause is minimal.   In enterectomy with lateral union, however, it must be allowed that the risk of leakage is from the blind terminal ends, which in a lesser degree offer the same conditions which constitute the danger in axial unions; still, even here, the inference cannot be avoided that an axial union might have failed where a closed end has given way.   A full appreciation of this source of danger might perhaps suffice to lessen it, in so far as it is not infrequent for the surgeon unintentionally to employ rather more care and vigilance in the suturing of the actual anastomosis, than in the less exacting closure of the ends of the divided bowel.

Lateral union is the normal method of enterectomy in the large intestine, the transverse colon, the sigmoid flexure, and pelvic colon offering the only debatable exceptions.

Operation.   The preliminary procedures are the same as in preparing for an axial union, with the single exception that a longer length of bowel needs to be exposed for the operation.

The required segment having been excluded by the application of clamps, the bowel is divided, and the portion to be removed is dealt with according to circumstances. As a general rule the ends should be cleansed, wrapped up in gauze, and the removal of the part to be excised proceeded with, since by this means a major source of infection is removed, and the process of suturing is carried out under the best available conditions. In some cases, however, particularly when there is difficulty in effecting a free extrusion of the bowel, it may be safer to sew up each end to be closed as it is divided, and proceed to the removal of the diseased or injured part later.

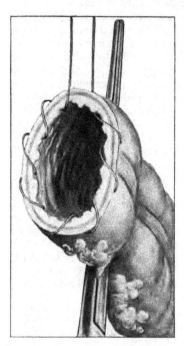

FIG. 365. PURSE-STRING SUTURE PASSED FOR CLOSURE OF THE CUT ENDS.

The removal of the diseased or injured segment in the case of the small bowel offers little difficulty in the absence of adhesions, or extensive infiltration of the mesentery. In the large bowel more difficulty may be experienced, from hæmorrhage during the process, and possibly fixation from infiltration of the retroperitoneal tissue; again, the area involved by the operation is generally appreciably wider. To meet these difficulties, the large vascular trunks should as a rule be first divided and secured, and the existence of extensive infiltration may call for careful dissection. Section of the tissues with the knife is generally preferable to forcible stripping, as the lymphatics are thus more radically removed.

Closure of the cut ends. This is most rapidly effected by the introduction of a purse-string suture at the immediate margin, which perforates all the coats (see Fig. 365); this is tightened and tied. The tied end is inverted (see Fig. 366), a second continuous Lembert's suture involving the serous muscular and submucous coats is superimposed, and the closure is completed (see Fig. 367). If preferred, a crushing clamp may be previously applied at the site of the projected section.

This diminishes the volume of tissue to be surrounded by the purse-string suture, but if the bowel dealt with is wide, the crushed portion is so spread out by the pressure of the clamp, that the extra convenience gained is not great.

In place of the initial purse-string suture, an ordinary continuous suture involving all the coats may be used, and when the end to be

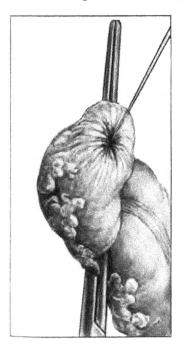 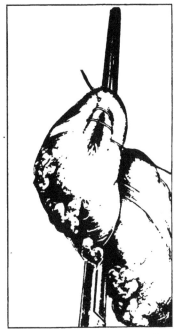

FIG. 366. PURSE-STRING SUTURE INVERTED PRIOR TO INSERTION OF THE SECOND LINE.

FIG. 367. INSERTION OF THE SECOND LINE OF SUTURE OVER THE INVERTED END.

closed is large this method is preferable. In either case the difficulty dependent on the incomplete peritoneal clothing of the ascending and descending colons can be readily dealt with, as a result of the puckering induced by the purse-string suture, and if a simple line has been employed the diminution in extent can be increased by tying the end of the thread left at the commencing knotted stitch to that left at the terminal one.

The closure completed, the ends are carefully cleansed, and some rearrangement may be necessary. The removal and rearrangement of the inner series of pads may suffice to give working room for the establishment of the anastomosis; if not, the ends must be drawn upon, and some readjustment of the retaining plugs may be necessary. Before commencing the anastomosis, it is especially important to fully protect from contamination any surface denuded of peritoneum in the floor of the wound, as such surfaces constitute one of the chief sources of danger in resections of the large intestine.

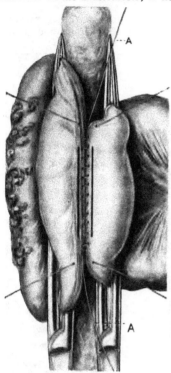

FIG. 368. LATERAL UNION. *First tier of the sero-muscular suture completed.* A, A, Ends left long for future knotting with the superficial tier. The two terminal sutures are inserted opposite either extremity of the line of incision.

Lateral anastomosis. The closed ends are now rendered as far as possible free of contents by gentle manipulation, and clamps are applied distally to the site of the projected anastomosis.

The further steps are identical with those of a simple anastomosis of two loops of bowel.

A continuous line of suture, 2½–3 inches in length, perforating the serous and muscular, and entering the submucous coats, is introduced, each end being knotted, and the projecting portion of the thread placed in artery forceps for union later with the corresponding ends of the final line of suture (see Fig. 368).

Two short threads are introduced in such a manner as to cross the line of the projected incision into the bowel, and are laid aside to be tied as the last step of the procedure. These stitches are intended to thoroughly protect the two extremities of the anastomotic opening.

An incision, corresponding in length to some four-fifths of the extent of the line of suture already introduced, is now carried through the serous and muscular coats, entering the submucosa and exposing the vessels. As the latter are divided it may be necessary to secure some of the larger ones by forceps, as they cannot always be efficiently compressed by the retaining clamps. All hæmorrhage being controlled, a

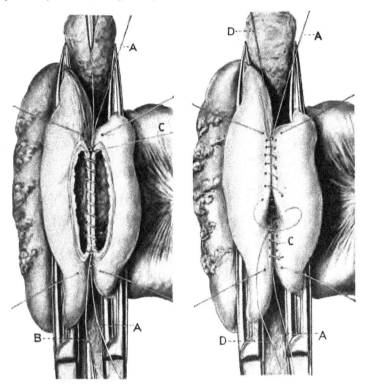

FIG. 369. LATERAL UNION. *The bowel opened.* First half of the inner line of suture B completed. Thread ready for completion of the third line C.

FIG. 370. LATERAL UNION. *Third line of suture* C *complete.* Fourth line, D, half completed, and the terminal sutures still untied.

puncture is made at one end of the exposed mucous membrane, and it is divided in the whole length of the desired opening, any fæcal contents being carefully caught or sponged away. The divided mucous membrane projects from the margin of the wound, and it is desirable to excise an elliptical area ¼–½ inch wide at the centre of the wound, as suggested by Littlewood (*Lancet,* 1901, vol. i, p. 1817), this procedure ensuring a thoroughly patent opening, and obviating any chance of immediate or ulterior obstruction.

For the introduction of the inner line of suture it is convenient to commence by inserting the two threads intended for the deep and superficial segments respectively, knotting one at either extremity of the opening, and leaving a short free end which is secured by a pair of artery forceps. These short ends are useful to steady the bowel, while tension upon them tends to maintain parallelism of the margin of the anastomotic opening. With one long end, continuous through and through stitches are carried along the entire length of the opening, and it is tied to the short end of the second suture thread. A similar line of stitches is carried in the reverse direction through the remaining free margins of the opening with the long end of the second thread; this is knotted with the short end of the first, and the lumen of the bowel is closed (see Fig. 369).

The remaining line of continuous sero-muscular suture is introduced, the free ends being knotted to those of the first, the two short stitches crossing the line of the anastomosis at either end are tied, and the union is completed (see Fig. 370).

The exposed bowel is now carefully wiped over, and if necessary washed with saline solution, and the protecting plugs at the bottom of the wound removed to allow of the repair of the peritoneal defect in the posterior abdominal wall. This latter step is an important one, as the retroperitoneal tissue is liable to exude serum, and infection extends in it with great rapidity. If any extensive area has to be left uncovered, it is advisable to make a puncture in the loin, and introduce a drain prior to closing the abdomen. When a lateral union is made in the small intestine the suture of the mesentery is a comparatively simple matter, as the two segments overlap, but care must be exercised to avoid injury to the blood-vessels in the introduction of the few sutures required.

ENTERECTOMY WITH LATERAL IMPLANTATION—END-TO-SIDE UNION

This method possesses many of the advantages of lateral union, and an individual one, in the reduction of the risk of giving of the blind end to one source instead of two. It has found its chief application in partial gastrectomy by Kocher's method, in ileo-colostomy, and colo-colostomy. The method is most suited to ileo-colostomy. In union of two portions of the colon it has, in the experience of the writer, proved somewhat liable to contract; thus in two instances where the descending colon was implanted into the transverse after removal of the splenic flexure for growth, the establishment of a safety-valve in the transverse colon was necessary some nine months later. This narrowing has also been observed by other surgeons, but the danger of its occurrence may no doubt be lessened by the employment of certain details to be mentioned below. The fact that Kocher, in a series of eighty-four partial gastrec-

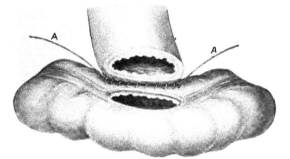

FIG. 371. LATERAL IMPLANTATION. *First stage.*

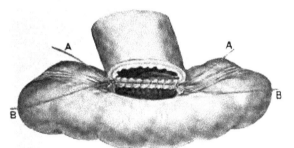

FIG. 372. LATERAL IMPLANTATION. *Second stage.*

tomies, only lost a single patient from leakage at the site of the lateral implantation, speaks strongly for the immediate efficiency of this method, even if the results be discounted by the special advantage offered by the stomach as a basis of support for the union, and the technical ability of the operator concerned.

Operation. The required portion of the intestine having been removed, the cut end of the segment of bowel of larger calibre is closed by one of the methods already described, and the site of the implantation decided upon. The latter should be at least an inch and a half within the closed end, and a longer distance may often be chosen, especially if any doubt exists as to the condition of the intestine at the point of section.

The protecting plugs are arranged beneath the point of union, and the clamped end to be implanted is brought to the side of the part of intestine destined to receive it.

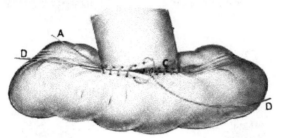

FIG. 373. LATERAL IMPLANTATION. *Third and fourth stages.*

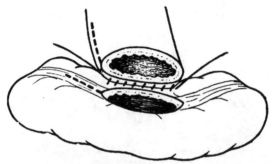

FIG. 374. LATERAL IMPLANTATION. *Method of enlarging a narrow element by incision of the ante-mesenteric margin.* The dotted lines indicate the site of the additional incisions.

The first row of external sutures is inserted in exactly the same manner as in an axial union, and should extend to half the circumference of the portion of bowel to be implanted (see Fig. 371).

When this is completed, the ends of the thread which have been kept long are taken in pairs of artery forceps, for later use as supports, and for knotting with the anterior series at the completion of the union.

An incision of the required length is made in the closed bowel, most conveniently by prior division of the serous muscular and submucous coats, any bleeding points being controlled provisionally by artery forceps. The mucous membrane is incised, and a strip on each side with advantage removed.

A series of through and through continuous stitches is now inserted, closing first the deep, and then the superficial halves of the opening (see Fig. 372).

Finally, the anterior half of the external Lembert's line of suture is completed, the free ends of the threads being knotted to those of the posterior segment which have been used as supports during the later stages of the suture (see Fig. 373).

As already mentioned, the weak point in the method of lateral implantation is the tendency of the opening to contract. As a general rule this is to be combated by the excision of a certain amount of the mucous membrane of the receiving segment at the time of operation. This does not, however, suffice to meet all cases, and when the segment to be implanted is too narrow, the most simple procedure is to make a longitudinal incision at its ante-mesenteric aspect; by this means an opening of at least 2 inches in length is readily procured (see Fig. 374).

Omental flaps and grafts. When there is reason to suspect weakness in the union after a resection, or the inefficient closure of a perforation of the intestine, the omentum may occasionally be employed as a graft or flap sutured over the doubtful spot. Again, the omentum as a whole may be sometimes so affixed to the margins of the abdominal wound as to localize a weak spot, and protect the general peritoneal cavity in case of leakage. With regard to these methods, it may be pointed out that the use of the *omental flap* is only satisfactory in the upper segment of the abdomen, where the risk of leaving a bridge beneath which strangulation can occur may be avoided. Thus the omentum is often useful in gastric or duodenal perforations. In resections of the small intestine, an omental graft is not advisable, and is rarely necessary if sufficient intestine be removed. In resections of the colon, the appendices epiploicæ may often be used, or in the case of the transverse colon the great omentum, since their employment is not accompanied by the risk of giving rise to the development of objectionable adhesions.

Small *omental grafts* may be cut free, and sutured over the required spot. This method again is open to the objection of encouraging the development of adhesions, since the separated graft adheres equally readily to the neighbouring coil of bowel as to that to which it is sutured. As a general rule, therefore, the use of either flaps or grafts is to be deprecated, except in cases the gravity of which renders the development of subsequent adhesions a matter of negligible moment.

ARTIFICIAL AIDS TO ENTERECTOMY

Although the general trend of surgical opinion is strongly towards the view that simple suture is the more desirable method for employment in enterectomy, yet in some positions undoubted convenience is to be obtained by the use of certain mechanical devices, while some operators still employ them habitually by preference.

Two principles are involved in the numerous aids which are at the surgeon's disposal:

1. *The simple provision of a temporary support* to facilitate the ready introduction of the sutures. This is illustrated by the collapsible rubber bag used by Treves and others, while the various bobbins, such as Mayo Robson's, Allingham's, and Stanmore Bishop's, are absorbable, do not need immediate removal, and provide a passage for the intestinal contents during the time they remain in position.

2. *The substitution of a mechanical device for sutures;* such device effecting both the union of the bowel, and the removal, by 'pressure necrosis,' of the redundant tissue grasped by it. In these also a channel is provided for the passage of the intestinal contents during the period that the device remains in position. Such is the 'button' of Murphy, which, it may be well claimed, has exercised a more potent influence in the free application of intestinal surgery than any other individual invention.

The two methods of best proved general utility are those of the decalcified bone bobbin, and Murphy's button, and these will therefore be taken to illustrate the above principles.

Mayo Robson's bobbin. Of the various appliances devised with the object of providing an artificial support, none has proved itself more generally satisfactory than the decalcified bone bobbin. Mayo Robson, writing in 1896 (*Clin. Soc. Trans.,* 1896, vol. xxix, p. 151), after quoting certain statistics, expressed himself as follows: 'I believe artificial aids in enterectomy afford greater safety than the unaided suture; and of the artificial aids a decalcified bone support has shown in the hands of four different surgeons the comparatively low mortality of 8.3%.' The results obtained by Mayo Robson show the success with which the use of the bobbin has been attended in the hands of its designer; none the less he has at the present renounced its routine use in favour of methods of simple suture.

'For the application of the bobbin, two medium-sized sewing needles bent into the shape of the third of a circle are threaded, one with silk and one with catgut, the former for approximating the serous surfaces, the latter the mucous margin. If one suture only be applied, I prefer chromicized catgut.

'A needle-holder is neither necessary nor desirable, since its employment means loss of time.

'After the bowel to be operated upon has been clamped above and below, or if possible isolated by encircling the whole loop with an elastic tourniquet, the affected portion is excised, leaving the open ends to be dealt with. For convenience it is better to apply the serous suture around the distal half first, and to lay aside the threaded needle until the mucous edges have been approximated and the bone bobbin inserted, when the serous circle can be completed.

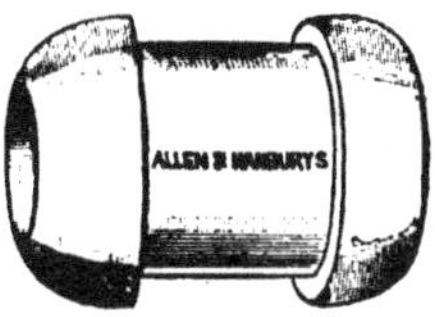

FIG. 375. ROBSON'S BOBBIN.

'The bobbin is not inserted until the marginal suture has been carried around the distal half of the circumference.

'After the insertion of the bobbin, the marginal stitch is continued around the circle, until the loose end of the catgut stitch at the starting-point is reached; the two ends are then drawn on, tied, and cut short.

'The serous suture is now continued around the circle, and when it reaches the starting-point the loose end of the silk stitch is picked up and both are drawn on, tied, and cut off. Both stitches are now buried, and a line only is seen where the union has been effected.

'If on account of want of time one suture only be employed, the marginal stitch, taking up the serous muscular and submucous coats, and avoiding as far as possible the mucous membrane, should be employed.

'The mucous margins will then be approximated though not perforated, and the buried stitch will run little danger of becoming infected.'

Murphy's button. The buttons are at present made in two forms, a circular for end-to-end and end-to-side unions, and an oblong for lateral anastomoses. The buttons are made in two halves, the male half being provided with a spring flange which exercises pressure on the ends of the included gut, while two spiral springs, projecting through openings in the hollow stem, act as the thread of a screw when the male half of the button is telescoped within the female segment (see Figs. 376, 377).

Murphy lays down the following instructions for the use of the button: 'Neither the button, its modifications, nor suture should ever be used in end-to-end anastomosis of the large intestine (except in the rectum and sigmoid), where an end-to-side or a side-to-side anastomosis is possible, as anatomically too large an area of the bowel circumference is uncovered by peritoneum' (Kelly and Noble, *Gynæcology and Abdominal Surgery*, 1908, vol. ii, p. 434).

Axial union. A No. 3 button is most generally applicable.

1. The coil of bowel is freed from contents by careful compression.

2. The retaining clamps are applied to exclude the portion to be excised.

3. An aneurysm needle and thread is passed through the mesentery

of the portion of bowel to be excised, 1½ inches from the intestinal border. A ligature is tied so as to include the vessels only of that portion of the mesentery complementary to the area to be excised.

4. The mesentery is slit centrifugally from the intestine to the ligatured point.

5. A thread, ten inches in length, provided with two needles 2½ inches long, is prepared. The needles are passed as in making a pleat,

 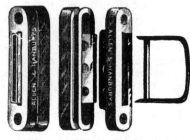

FIG. 376. MURPHY'S CIRCULAR BUTTON FOR END-TO-END OR END-TO-SIDE UNION.

FIG. 377. MURPHY'S OBLONG BUTTON FOR LATERAL ANASTOMOSIS.

one on either side of the gut from the mesenteric to the free margin of the bowel. The threads are not drawn, but the needles are maintained in position to act as splints during the division of the bowel with scissors. By this manœuvre any risk of division of the thread is avoided.

6. The gut divided, the puckering thread is drawn through by the needles, and the button, held by its central hollow stem in a pair of forceps, is placed in position in the end of the bowel. The puckering thread is then drawn tight, knotted, and cut short.

7. The process is repeated at the other end of the bowel. The two halves of the button are now taken up in Hartmann's clamps (see Fig. 378). The necessary amount of mesentery is excised, and, lastly, the two segments are approximated and firmly pressed together. No external supporting sutures are required.

Lateral implantation. The method is the same; a round button is employed, and the segment of the button inserted in the receiving element of the junction is introduced as in a lateral anastomosis.

Lateral anastomosis. For this procedure an oblong button is employed. The site of the incision is encircled with a puckering thread, but here again Murphy passes the needles, and employs them as a splint during the process of incising the bowel. The opening requires to be of a length corresponding with that of the button; the introduction of the latter is effected by introducing the lateral edge first beneath the upper margin of the opening; the button, which is held by its central stem in forceps, is then rotated beneath the lower margin of the opening, which is held up by a pair of forceps. The puckering thread is tightened, and the further details do not differ from those in an axial union.

Murphy lays great stress on the outer margin of the pressure surface of the button being an accurate semicircular curve, and not a rounded

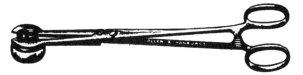

FIG. 378. HARTMANN'S CLAMP FOR HOLDING MURPHY'S BUTTONS.

off angle. He considers this of the utmost importance in the proper limitation of the extent of the ' pressure necrosis,' which he says should have attained its maximum at the expiration of three days.

In spite of the success which has attended the use of the button in the hands of the inventor, and in those of many distinguished operators, its use is best restricted to positions in which methods of suture are difficult or impossible, and to cases in which a minimum of expenditure of time is obligatory. The latter indication is hard on the method, since it relegates its employment for the most part to cases of the most compromising description. The improvement in methods of suture has, however, been so great that most of the early complications and dangers have been removed from their employment, while no doubt can exist as to their greater elasticity of application, and they possess the undoubted advantage of entirely avoiding all the risks which may attend the introduction of a foreign body into the intestinal canal.

A series of entero-enterostomies comprising 750 operations for all causes has been collated from various sources by one of Murphy's assistants. In this series the remarkably low mortality of 19% is shown, or if the cases in which the operations for malignant disease are subtracted, of 14% only (*Philad. Med. Journ.*, 1900, p. 1271).

TECHNIQUE OF COLECTOMY

The removal of portions of the colon involves difficulties not encountered in similar operations on the small intestine. The more important of these depend on the fixation, location, vascular supply, and the arrangement of the lymphatic vessels and glands of the segment of bowel requiring to be resected.

1. *Fixation.* Comparative fixity, whether dependent on anatomical arrangement or on secondary infiltration, has in the past exerted a potent influence on the results of partial colectomy. Extended experience has demonstrated the freedom with which fixed portions of the colon may be mobilized by division of the parietal peritoneum at the outer margin of the bowel, which measure has done much to reduce the importance of this difficulty.

2. *Location.* The depth of the situation occupied by a growth leads to difficulties similar in nature to those of fixation, which are to be met also by free mobilization of the part requiring resection. Further, exposure of the field of operation may be rendered easier by a proper position of the patient during the performance of the operation, and removal of the affected part may be facilitated by the resection of a length of the intestine out of all proportion to that actually diseased. In spite of these aids, certain positions, such as that of growths situated deeply in the pelvis, still retain grave importance from a purely technical aspect.

3. *Vascular supply.* In this respect operations on the colon possess special characteristics, since the effect of obliteration of any main arterial trunk is known to correspond with a loss of vitality in a definite length of the bowel, and hence may determine with some exactitude the extent to be removed.

4. *The arrangement of the lymphatic vessels and glands.*

The subdivision of the system into areas corresponding with the main arterial trunks favours the possibility of dealing with the ' lymphatic area ' in which the growth is situated in a more radical manner than is possible in the case of the small intestine, with its common supply from the large superior mesenteric artery.

Although colectomy may be demanded for the treatment of either simple or malignant conditions, yet the latter form the more frequent and important indication. Until recently no very definite rules have been laid down for the attempt to completely extirpate the lymphatic vessels and glands corresponding to the area occupied by colic tumours, such as have been propounded for the removal of carcinomata in other regions, as the breast and tongue, since the anatomical data on which such rules could be founded cannot be said to have existed. A valuable effort to remedy this deficiency has been made by Jamieson and Dobson in a series of papers dealing with the normal lymphatic system of the colon, in which the course of the lymphatic vessels and the arrangement of the glands are accurately described, and upon the results of these anatomical investigations definite rules for the extirpation of the several lymphatic areas have been laid down.   These investigations are of the greater value, since they correspond in general with the information to be gained by consideration of the numerous isolated pathological observations scattered throughout the extensive literature of the surgery of the colon, and especially with the careful pathological review of 72 cases of colic carcinomata by H. S. Clogg, appended to which are a series of suggested operations differing only slightly from those devised by Jamieson and Dobson on strictly anatomical lines (Jamieson and Dobson, 'Lymphatics of the Cæcum and Appendix,' *Lancet*, 1907, vol. i, p. 1137; Dobson, *Lancet*, 1908, vol. i, p. 149; Jamieson and Dobson, *Proc. Roy. Soc. of Med.*, 1909, vol. ii, Surg. Sect., p. 149; H. S. Clogg, 'Cancer of the Colon,' *Lancet*, 1908, vol. ii, p. 1007).

Jamieson and Dobson's observations were made on a series of specimens prepared by the method of Gerota, and may be shortly summarized as follows :—

It is pointed out that the lymphatics connected with any given segment of the colon correspond in their course and arrangement with the main arterial branches of supply to such segment.   Hence the course and distribution of the latter afford an all-important general indication as to the extent of bowel, parietal peritoneum, retroperitoneal tissue, or mesentery, which requires to be removed in an attempt to completely extirpate the 'lymphatic area' which pertains to a tumour situated in any given position.   Four lymphatic areas are described: (1) ileo-colic, (2) middle colic, (3) left colic, (4) inferior mesenteric.   As an inconstant vessel in origin, with few glands arranged upon it, the right colic is not assigned an individual area.   The lymphatic glands connected with each individual area are divided into four distinct but intercommunicating groups: (1) *Epicolic,* glands contained in the appendices epiploicæ and lying on the wall of the bowel; (2) *paracolic,* glands arranged in a line parallel to the mesenteric margin of the bowel, between the intestine and the arterial arcades and on the arcades; (3) *intermediate,* glands arranged around the trunk of the arteries, about midway between their origin and the gut; (4) *main,* glands arranged around the main trunk of the artery near its origin.

The 'intermediate' groups for the most part receive lymphatic vessels from the epicolic and paracolic groups, but some vessels may pass to them directly from the bowel itself.   The 'main' groups receive chiefly vessels from the three peripheral groups, in certain regions, notably the lower part of the inferior mesenteric system, directly from the intestine itself, and on the other hand are connected centrally with the lumbar and mesenteric glands.   The observations show that the complete removal of any given lymphatic area may be impracticable when infiltration of the 'main' glands has occurred, in consequence of their near connexion with the central system; also, that intercommunication between the colic systems and others, such as the 'splenic, may offer an obstacle to radical extirpation. On the other hand, they clearly indicate the lines on which complete operations should be planned, and are hence of very great value.

It is at the present time hardly possible to lay down definite lines

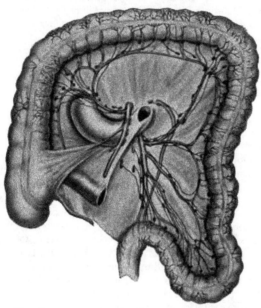

Fig. 379. The Lymphatics of the Colon. The upper part of the pelvic colon, after Gegenbaur, has been added to show the interruption of the arterial arcades below the distribution of the lowest sigmoid artery. (*After Jamieson and Dobson.*)

for the choice of the major or minor operations described below, and in considering the suitability of either to individual cases great discrimination must be exercised. For simple conditions the minor procedures suffice, and even in malignant disease the ulterior results obtained by these cannot be said to have been altogether unsatisfactory. The question, therefore, must arise as to when it is justifiable to submit patients to the increased risks involved by the employment of the more extensive operations designed for the radical removal of the ‘lymphatic area’ concerned, and the points which affect this decision must be shortly considered.

1. *The extent of the local disease.* Surrounding infiltration or the existence of adhesions is as fully opposed to an extensive as a limited operation. Under such conditions, even if adhesions can be dealt with locally by the removal of a portion of adherent bowel, yet it is improbable that the necessary additional removal of the second series of glands could be satisfactorily proceeded with.

2. *The position of the growth with regard to the blood-supply.* It is at once apparent, since the individual lymphatic areas correspond with those of the main arteries supplying any one segment of the colon, that the most extensive resections of intestine will be required when the growth occupies a point corresponding to the anastomosis of any two arterial systems—thus, at the flexures; also that the amount of bowel to be removed bears no sort of proportion to the magnitude of the tumour itself. The fact that these very extensive operations are indicated in situations in which experience appears to have shown the ulterior results of more limited operations to have been comparatively favourable, renders it necessary to exercise some caution before deciding upon their choice.

With regard to the regions in which special care needs to be taken in interfering with the arterial supply, it may be said these are few. Although certain anastomoses, notably that between the middle and left colic arteries, are occasionally absent, yet as a rule the intercommunication between the colic arteries has been shown to be sufficient to maintain the vitality of the bowel in spite of the obliteration of any one main trunk. Certain points are, however, worthy of mention. (*a*) Division of a main trunk is safe only if interference with the system of primary arcades is avoided. (*b*) In removal of the cæcum and ascending colon, division of the lowest ileo-colic branches endangers the vitality of the lower six inches of the ileum. (*c*) The general system of arterial arcades is interrupted between the lowest sigmoid branch and the highest branch of the superior hæmorrhoidal artery. As a consequence the anastomotic circulation in this region can only be maintained by a flow in the reverse direction in the lowest sigmoid artery itself to the superior hæmorrhoidal trunk. Thus Manasse (*Arch. f. klin. Chir.,* 1907, vol. lxxxiii, p. 999) has pointed out that a division of the inferior mesenteric trunk above the origin of this vessel is unattended by danger, while division of the trunk below its origin endangers the vitality of the cut extremity of the lower segment of the bowel.

3. *The extent of glandular infiltration or enlargement.* The date at

which this may commence is incalculable, but it appears probable that it occurs early only in instances of great malignity and rapid growth, such as are occasionally met with in young subjects. Butlin computed that more than 50% of patients affected with colic carcinoma die from obstruction of the lumen of the bowel before glandular metastases have developed, and although this computation of freedom from glandular infiltration is probably too high, yet in Clogg's series (*loc. cit.*), although enlarged glands were found in a much larger proportion of the cases, in a considerable number the enlargement did not depend on cancerous infiltration, and this latter observation is confirmed by those of many other observers. Pathological evidence (Clogg) and clinical observation during the course of operations have shown that in certain positions, *e.g.* transverse colon and sigmoid flexure, and to a lesser degree at the other flexures, the glands affected tend to be those in the immediate vicinity of the growth, and these observations are supported by the normal course taken by the lymphatic vessels in relation to the glands demonstrated by Jamieson and Dobson. The observations of the latter authors of the course taken by the lymphatic vessels in the neighbourhood of the sigmoid and pelvic colons somewhat discounts the importance of this fact in that region, but, generally speaking, clinical evidence of the results of limited resections of the sigmoid flexure shows that it is not to be underrated.

Lastly, it must be remembered that the course of infection is by no means regular, and that glands may often be discovered at a distance from the growth, while those in the immediate proximity of it remain unaffected. Such enlarged glands are not necessarily carcinomatous, but the escape of the proximal glands has been clearly explained by the direct course taken by some of the lymphatic vessels to the intermediate glands by Jamieson and Dobson, and this fact, together with the observation that the intervening vessel is free from growth, moreover, is utilized by them as support for their contention that infection of the glands is embolic in character and not consequent on 'permeation'.

Infection of the 'intermediate' series of glands marks the limit at which a 'radical' operation is worth performance. If the 'main' series be infiltrated, the probability of existing extension to the mesenteric or lumbar glands is opposed to the likelihood of a radical removal being successful.

4. *The actual magnitude of the operation.* This factor is to be discounted, not only by the greater possibilities of permanent cure, but also by the operative advantages gained. Although the free removal of bowel necessitates a somewhat larger incision, and greater exposure of the abdominal cavity, yet, on the other hand, it renders manipulations easier and more rapid, while the risks of infection of the abdominal cavity are

materially reduced. Again, the free removal of intestine in some situations rather facilitates than opposes the union of the divided ends.

Consideration of the above points seems to lead to the somewhat paradoxical conclusion that only the least extensive and apparently favourable cases are those suited to the more extensive methods of operation. Even if this prove to be the case, the results obtained by the more radical methods in other parts of the body indicate that a similar improvement is probable with the application of the same principle to the growths of the colon, and the general trend of surgical opinion is in this direction.

Putting the most extensive operations on one side, it is evident also that advantage may be gained by a systematic search for glands along the line of the vascular trunks in the retroperitoneal tissue, the more so as anatomical knowledge now permits us to determine with some precision the situation in which such glands should and should not exist, and which are of the greater importance. Such knowledge allows of a less extensive removal of the main arterial trunks, and this fact has influenced operators in somewhat limiting the scope of operations, which theoretically should be wider.

REMOVAL OF THE CÆCUM AND ASCENDING COLON

The cæcum shares with the sigmoid flexure certain characteristics; thus, in both portions of the bowel the intestinal contents tend to stagnate, and in both carcinomatous tumours are common. The cæcum differs from the sigmoid flexure in that its contents still retain highly digestive powers; hence perhaps an explanation that in the cæcum the medullary form of carcinoma is more common. The tumours are often large, with a tendency to ulcerate freely, and excite very considerable surrounding tissue reaction, leading to comparatively early fixation, often of a simple inflammatory character. Growths of the cæcum are also occasionally atypical in their structure, conforming rather to the type of an epithelioma than to that of a true columnar carcinoma.

Again, both these segments of the colon are especially liable to become the seats of inflammatory processes, sometimes accompanied by the formation of abscesses and fistulæ, tuberculous infiltration being more common in the cæcum, and simple inflammatory changes in the sigmoid flexure.

The cæcum may need removal not only when the disease is actually located in its walls, but also in many cases where the ascending colon is the part primarily affected, since under the latter circumstances the cæcum is often much dilated, its walls are thickened, and the width of the lumen may render it unsatisfactory either for axial union or closure. Again,

the close connexion of the lymphatic system of the two segments renders
the removal of the cæcum a desirable proceeding, when the ascending
colon is the seat of malignant disease. In some cases, however, where
the growth occupies a high position in the ascending colon, the broad
strong cæcum is well adapted for the lateral approximation of a loose
tranverse colon.

Anatomically these portions of the colon are in some respects favourably situated for operation; the cæcum itself lies ventrally, is surrounded
by peritoneum, and the lower portion of the ascending colon is comparatively movable. In from 26 to 30% a mesocolon is present, but the
ascending colon becomes steadily less movable from commencement to
termination. Occasionally the mesocolon is abnormally long, and then
is continuous with the mesentery of the small intestine, a condition of
much importance for the occurrence of the so-called cæcal volvulus.

Operation. For removal of the cæcum or ascending colon, the
patient should be arranged with the right side of the body raised, and
the pelvis higher than the abdomen, in order that the small intestine shall
fall as far as possible out of the field of operation.

The incision is made in the right semilunar line, and needs to be six
or more inches in length. When the operation is done for malignant
disease, a thorough exposure of the area to be dealt with is of more
importance than the final condition of the abdominal wall; hence no
limitation of the length of the incision is advisable, the more so as free
access to the parts not only renders the subsequent manipulations easier,
but also diminishes the risk of infection.

The portion of bowel requiring removal having been exposed and
defined, the points at which division is to be effected are decided upon,
and plugs are introduced to isolate the area of operation from the general
peritoneal cavity.

If necessary, the bowel is mobilized by division of the parietal peritoneum at its outer margin, the colon being raised together with the
retroperitoneal tissue, and drawn forwards and inwards. This process
involves little hæmorrhage, as the main vessels reach the intestine at its
inner margin and only anastomotic branches are involved.

Clamps are applied on either side of the two points to be divided, and
the removal of the included portion of bowel proceeded with. It is
generally more convenient to first divide the distal end of the colon, and
the cut ends having been carefully cleansed and wrapped in gauze, the
part to be removed is rapidly freed in a downward direction. In this
part of the procedure it is convenient to clamp the large vessels at some
little distance from the margin of the colon before dividing them, as this
measure diminishes the amount of bleeding and facilitates the detection

of any enlarged lymphatic glands lying in their course. The retroperitoneal tissue in the area exposed should be cleanly removed from the posterior abdominal wall, especial care being taken that the ureter is not injured during the process of dissection.

The difficulties that may arise during the procedure of freeing the bowel may depend on inflammatory infiltration of the retroperitoneal tissue, or simple adhesions to neighbouring organs. Peritoneal adhesions are not uncommon when the disease is of an inflammatory or tuberculous nature, or in the florid medullary form of carcinoma; in the annular scirrhus form of growth, fixation due to malignant invasion of the retroperitoneal tissue may be very extensive compared with the small extent of involvement of the bowel itself.

The freed cæcum and colon are delivered from the abdominal cavity, and the uncovered retroperitoneal space carefully protected with gauze plugs prior to section of the small bowel. The ileum having been divided and duly cleansed, two courses are open: either to close both the proximal and distal ends of the bowel, and make a lateral anastomosis, or to close the colic end, and implant the ileum into the side of the colon. Axial union, although it has often been performed, is not to be recommended. Lateral anastomosis is the preferable method, and it is often more conveniently made to the transverse colon than to the more fixed remnant of the ascending colon, should this have been preserved.

When the free ends have been closed, the plugs protecting the retroperitoneal space are removed, and in order to bring the two portions of bowel into position for the anastomosis, it may be necessary to effect some rearrangement of the plugs which have served to retain the general abdominal contents during the operation. When satisfactory adaptation has been secured, the surrounding area is protected in the usual way and the union may be completed.

The last special step in this operation, closure of the defect in the posterior parietal pertioneum, is now proceeded with. When the removal of bowel has been extensive, this may be difficult, but it is rendered somewhat easier by the drawing upward of the mesentery which has accompanied the apposition of the ileum to the colon. The repair of the gap should be as complete as possible, since the opened-up retroperitoneal space is a source of great danger should infection have occurred. If it prove impracticable to entirely close the gap, it is usually advisable to introduce a drain from the loin, which may be removed at the end of from twenty-four to thirty-six hours.

Dobson (*Lancet*, 1908, vol. i, p. 149) gives the following description of an operation performed for the removal of a carcinoma of the ascending colon, together with the corresponding ' lymphatic area ':—

' An incision 7 inches long was made in the right linea semilunar
the tumour in the ascending colon was defined, and the small intesti
was packed off to the left side of the abdomen. The duodenum and t
ileo-colic vessels were then defined, the overlying peritoneum was divide

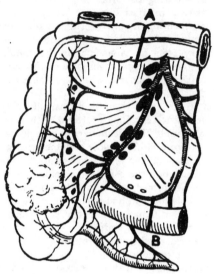

and a fairly large uppe
most gland of the ma
ileo-colic group chain w
pushed downwards. T
artery and vein were th
clamped and ligatured, t
ligature being appli
about ½ inch from t
superior mesenteric artei
At this stage clamps we
applied to the transvei
colon close to the hepa
flexure, and to the ilec
about 6 inches from t
ileo-colic valve.

' The peritoneum
the outer side of the :
cending colon was th
divided, and the whe
mass—ascending colo
cæcum, and terminal pc
tion of the ileum—w
thrown over to the le
the peritoneum, ileo-cc
vessels, and chain
glands being stripped

FIG. 380. ILEO-COLIC LYMPHATIC AREA WITH
A COLIC GROWTH. The division of the colon, A,
is that now recommended, but somewhat wider
than that described in the above operation. B,
Point of section of the ileum. (*Dobson.*)

up to the duodenum; the ureter was seen and avoided and some vess
were tied. The mesocolon was then divided from the duodenum to t
selected point on the colon, some branches of the middle colic artery bei
tied. In the same way the peritoneum of the anterior layer of the mese
tery was divided down to the ileum, and also the posterior layer and t
terminal branch of the mesentery artery were secured. The whole ma
was now easily withdrawn from the abdomen (see Fig. 380), and t
colon and ileum were divided between clamps; both ends were closed
celluloid thread continuous suture, three layers in the colon and two
the ileum. Lateral anastomosis between the two portions of the gut w
effected, thus drawing up the mesentery and covering in the denuded ai
on the posterior abdominal wall. A small tubular drain was insert

through a stab wound in the loin and the anterior wound was closed in the usual way.'

Dobson claims by this operation to ' remove all the primary lymphatic glands receiving direct vessels from the cæcum and ascending colon, the lymphatic vessels, and the tissue in which these vessels run. The blood-supply of the portion of intestine to be removed is effectively controlled and the risk of contamination of the field of operation is minimized by deferring the division of the gut until towards the end of the operation.' The removal of several inches of the ileum enables the small intestine to be brought up to the colon with ease, and allows of a satisfactory anastomosis being performed. Division of the transverse colon at the junction of the middle and right thirds is now recommended.

REMOVAL OF THE TRANSVERSE COLON AND THE FLEXURES

The hepatic flexure is not very commonly (6.4%) the seat of tumours; when present they are comparatively easy to deal with, since the flexure, although fixed, is uncovered and near the anterior abdominal wall. The acuteness of the flexure and the length of the mesenteric attachment fluctuate considerably. A variable fold, corresponding with the costo-colic ligament of the left side, extends from the flexure to the abdominal parietes, and occasionally folds stretch from it to the liver and stomach.

Operation. The incision may be made through the right rectus sheath, or in the semilunar line. The procedure is considerably facilitated by placing an air-cushion or pillow under the back of the level of the lower ribs (as in an operation on the bile passages) ; this manœuvre not only renders the flexure more prominent and easily extruded, but also favours the falling away of the small intestine from the field of operation. Union of the two ends of the colon by lateral anastomosis is the preferable method of junction.

The writer's experience of a limited operation in this region has been a favourable one; thus one patient is alive and well at the end of fifteen years, one survived four years before a recurrence took place, and a third remains well after a short period. But both Jamieson and Dobson, and Clogg, recommend an extensive removal for growths in this situation. They consider it advisable to remove the whole lymphatic area corresponding to the distribution of the middle colic artery. The middle colic artery is isolated and tied at its origin, and the mesocolon incised from this point to the extremities of the parts of the intestine supplied by this vessel. This necessitates the removal of the upper third or half of the ascending colon, and of two-thirds of the transverse colon. The widely separated cut ends are closed, and an ileo-sigmoidostomy per-

formed; or the lower part of the ascending colon, the cæcum, and th
lowest six inches of the ileum are to be removed, and the ileum i
anastomosed with the remaining third of the transverse colon.

The operation is wide, but it is claimed that it permits of free mobil
zation of the growth, complete control of the blood-supply, allows th
intestine to be brought well out of the abdomen with correspondin
diminution in the risk of contamination of the field of operation, an
allows of the anastomosis of movable portions of the gut widely remove
from the seat of disease.

The tranverse colon.   The existence of a long mesocolon muc
simplifies the operation of colectomy in this segment, especially in it
left half.   It is well to bear in mind that the mobility of the bowel a
lows considerable range of position, which may allow a tumour t
descend so low as to be mistaken for one of the sigmoid flexure before
is exposed.   The transverse colon is readily united axially, the usu
precautions being taken with the mesenteric angle.   The glands arrange
along the branches of the middle colic artery are favourably situate
both for detection when enlarged, and for removal; but caution must b
exercised, in dealing with the central parts of the mesentery, that th
superior mesenteric artery be not damaged.   This portion of the bowel i
also especially well situated should it be wished to make use of an oment
flap to cover a union of doubtful stability.

The observations of Jamieson and Dobson go to show that the ir
testinal lymphatic vessels are all intercepted before they have run ver
far by the ' paracolic ' glands, while the ' intermediate and main ' grou
of glands receive no vessels directly from the gut.   Under these circum
stances they only consider it necessary to remove as much colon on eith
side of the growth as to permit of a satisfactory anastomosis, the par
colic glands at some little distance from the growth being secured to
gether with it.

The splenic flexure is deeply situated, and enterectomy in thi
position is more difficult of performance than in any other, except i
that of the pelvic colon.   The flexure is more constant than the hepati
as might be expected from the fact that it perpetuates one of the primar
developmental bends of the alimentary tube.   The bend is usually acut
lies directly upon the left kidney, and is fixed in position by the cost
colic band.   A mesocolon is present in only 5% of all cases.

The deep position, and the fact that this segment of the bowel is par
ticularly often the seat of typical annular growths, render the localizatio
of tumours in this region very difficult, so much so that they have escape
detection, even during an abdominal exploration, when much distensio
existed.

These peculiarities render a vertical incision inconvenient, the flexure being most satisfactorily exposed and mobilized from an incision made obliquely along the left lower costal margin 6 inches in length.

The tumour having been removed, the form of union may be a difficult question to decide. The descending colon lies deeply, and in cases of carcinoma of the splenic flexure is often contracted and small. End-to-end union is dangerous and unsatisfactory; lateral union may be difficult, but if practicable is to be chosen.

The difficulty lies in the fact that while the transverse colon is provided with a mesentery, mobility may be insufficient to allow it to be conveniently placed alongside the fixed descending colon, and the necessary sewing may have to be carried out within the confines of the abdominal cavity. If the descending colon cannot be sufficiently mobilized to facilitate union, the trouble may sometimes be met by closing the cut ends and uniting the transverse colon laterally to the sigmoid flexure. Lateral implantation of the descending colon into the transverse has, in the hands of the writer, proved itself an unsatisfactory method, as in two instances in which it was adopted secondary stenosis occurred, necessitating the formation of a proximal vent.

Madelung (*Archiv f. klin. Chir.*, 1906, vol. lxxxi, Pt. 1, p. 206) has expressed the opinion that the prognosis after removal of growths of the splenic flexure is especially good, even if the disease be advanced, on account of the paucity of the lymph paths, and that metastases are comparatively uncommon. Jamieson and Dobson, on the other hand, express an opinion in favour of a wide removal of this flexure, as in the case of the hepatic. They observed the large majority of the lymphatic vessels to pass into the epicolic and paracolic glands, rarely to the intermediate group, and never directly to the main groups situated on the left colic artery or on the upper part of the inferior mesenteric vein. Some lymphatic vessels were, however, observed to pass to the splenic glands, hence a complete removal of the lymphatic area is impracticable.

Removal of the growth, together with that part of the lymphatic area connected with the branches of the left colic artery, is recommended. The left colic artery and vein are to be defined as they leave the outer margin of the inferior mesenteric vein, and tied. The splenic flexure, together with the left third of the transverse colon, and the greater part of the descending colon are to be mobilized and removed, and an axial union established. This operation, although extensive, has the great advantage of avoiding the difficulties of union above mentioned to a considerable degree.

The descending colon. Tumours in the descending colon are rare (3.1–7.1%), possibly since this portion of the large bowel serves less as a reservoir and there is little tendency of the contents to stagnate. After leaving the splenic flexure the fæces descend rapidly, peristalsis being aided by the force of gravity from the straight vertical course taken by the bowel. In fact, at post-mortem examinations the descending colon is rarely in a state of distension.

The difficulty of a limited colectomy here comes next in order of gravity after the splenic flexure, and, for much the same reasons, depth and fixity. A mesocolon is met with more commonly than in the case of the ascending colon, partly as a result of the lesser degree of distension. The isolated blood-supply, and consequent simple arrangement of the lymphatics, makes the removal of glands less difficult than in the case of the cæcum and ascending colon. According to Jamieson and Dobson, the lymphatic area comprises the epicolic and paracolic glands, and the intermediate glands on the branches of the left colic and first sigmoid arteries; as in the case of the splenic flexure, a communication with the splenic system exists. The operation recommended corresponds with that for removal of the splenic flexure, except that the lower division is of the upper part of the sigmoid flexure instead of the descending colon, and the first sigmoid artery is tied close to its origin.

The sigmoid flexure. This segment of the colon is a more common seat of surgical operation than any other. Malignant growths are frequent, while the function of the loop as a reservoir makes it particularly liable to the occurrence of inflammatory changes. On the whole the arrangement of the sigmoid flexure is singularly constant, although in common with a general transposition of the viscera it may occasionally lie to the right side of the body; and rarely, it may be absent, the descending colon terminating in a direct continuity with the rectum, in which latter case a large cloaca is sometimes developed to take place in the higher reservoir which should normally exist. The loop may vary in width, length, and degree of convolution, but the most important practical variations are dependent on the relative length of the mesentery. Congenital cicatricial bands and lateral adhesions are occasionally met with, while a short mesentery, especially with a distended loop, may equally be a mere individual anatomical arrangement. Either of these conditions may give rise to operative inconvenience, even when the flexure itself is not the actual seat of the disease; but the most frequent source of difficulty lies in the shortening of the mesentery so frequently accompanying the presence of malignant tumours and inflammatory conditions. A long mesentery favours the occurrence of volvulus.

The sigmoid flexure is the seat of malignant disease in from 27 to 38% of all cases of carcinoma of the colon, excluding the rectum, and in this segment the growths show a special disposition to assume the annular form, and to be circumscribed in area. When situated at the distal portion of the loop, they lie within the pelvis and are difficult to palpate, but in such cases help in diagnosis may often be obtained by noting thickening in the proximal portion of the bowel, the collection of considerable masses of scybala, or well-marked local peristalsis. Growths of small size may be visible on exploration with the long proctoscope or sigmoidoscope. Again, growths, impalpable from above, may often be discovered by bi-manual examination *per vaginam* or *per rectum* in the female, or *per rectum* in the male. When the growths are of the pronounced annular form, and situated in the lower part of the loop, an exploratory incision is often the only method of actually palpating them, and in cases where the growth has acquired firm adhesions to the pelvic wall, even if it be of considerable extent, a very moderate amount of distension of the bowel or a thick abdominal wall renders an open exploration the only means of digitally determining its presence.

Operation. The patient should be arranged in the high Trendelenburg position with the left shoulder and side of the pelvis somewhat raised by pillows. The incision is made in the left linea semilunaris, or often better through the left rectus sheath, since the more difficult end of the bowel to manipulate, the distal, lies fairly mesially. Should difficulty arise in dealing with the upper end, the incision may be enlarged towards the left, the line of cleavage of the fibres of the broad muscles of the abdomen being followed when the limits of the rectus sheath are depassed.

The exposure of the tumour is easy if the growth be situated in the central portion and provided with a long mesentery; more difficult, if the part to be removed is at the upper or lower part and the mesentery is short.

The bowel itself along the mesenteric margin and the mesentery in the lines of the arteries are palpated for the detection of enlarged glands, and the amount of bowel to be removed is decided upon. The general abdominal cavity is protected by the insertion of plugs, and the retention clamps are applied to the bowel. If necessary, the bowel is now mobilized by an incision made into the mesentery at its outer line of continuity with the parietal peritoneum, and the excluded loop is drawn forward and removed, together with a portion of the mesentery and such enlarged glands as shall have been discovered. Hæmorrhage may be minimized by securing the large sigmoid branches prior to section of the bowel.

Union may be of the type axial variety, or the ends may be closed and a lateral anastomosis established. The latter method is preferable should any doubt exist as to the healthy condition of the bowel-wall.

When any question arises as to the efficiency of the suture, either from the actual condition of the bowel-wall, the tension existing on the union, or the general state of the patient, it is often possible to make the line of suture extra-peritoneal. In the early days of intestinal surgery this was often done, by retaining the loop of bowel, when long enough, without the limits of the abdominal cavity, and either allowing it to sink, or replacing it at a later date when union had taken place. If the loop was too short to allow of this procedure, the wound was plugged down to the seat of suture and not entirely closed. Both these procedures are open to objection, and have been much improved upon by the method employed by Bloodgood.

' The parietal peritoneum is separated from the margins of the wound for a sufficient distance to allow it to be pushed back and sutured to the mesentery of the bowel on each side of the suture. Above and below, the margins of the peritoneum are brought together as usual, thus securing the line of suture in an extra-peritoneal position at the bottom of the external wound, a gauze drain being inserted down to the bowel. In the case related ' the method protected the peritoneal cavity most effectively, but no leakage from the line of suture occurred; the wound granulated up rapidly ' (*Trans. Amer. Surg. Assoc.*, 1906, vol. xxiv, p. 115).

When the growth occupies the lower extremity of the flexure, or if a considerable length of bowel has needed removal, great technical difficulty may arise in the union of the remaining bowel ends. Under these circumstances two courses are open, the simplest to utilize the upper end for a colostomy, and sew up and sink the lower into the pelvis. When the difficulty depends on fixation of the upper segment this course is the safer and to be preferred.

When the difficulty depends on the shortness of the lower segment, a colostomy may be avoided if desired in the manner suggested in the next operation (see p. 757).

Jamieson and Dobson in dealing with the sigmoid flexure and upper part of the rectum state that the glands implicated are those of the para- and epicolic groups, the intermediate group upon the sigmoid arteries, and the main glands on the inferior mesenteric trunk. They did not observe the passage of any lymphatic vessel *direct* to the glands at a higher point on the inferior mesenteric trunk than that corresponding with the middle and upper thirds, *i.e.* just below the origin of the left colic artery. The proximity of the inferior mesenteric trunk to the bowel in the lower part of its course practically necessitates the removal of some portion of the vessel, but considering the paramount importance of the left colic artery for the anastomotic circulation of the upper

segment of the bowel concerned, they recommend the following operation for growths of the lower part of the sigmoid colon.

The inferior mesenteric artery and vein are exposed and tied immediately *below* the origin of the left colic artery. A long incision is made at the outer side of the mesorectum and mesosigmoid, and the descending colon and sigmoid mobilized by stripping them inwards towards the middle line. In doing this the ureter and spermatic vessels will be encountered and must be avoided. The mesosigmoid is then divided in an oblique line downwards from the point of ligature of the inferior mesenteric to about the middle of the sigmoid flexure, care being taken to preserve as far as possible the secondary arches on the sigmoid arteries. The peritoneum to the inner side of the artery is divided downwards to the inner side of the mesorectum. The mass of tissue to be removed is then stripped forwards from the upper part of the sacral hollow, and the gut clamped and divided at the middle of the sigmoid flexure and at the junction of the first and second parts of the rectum. The part removed will consist of the lower half of the sigmoid flexure and the upper part of the rectum, the greater part of the inferior mesenteric vessels with the accompanying chain of glands and lymphatic vessels, and the surrounding subperitoneal tissue.

The blood-supply of the upper end is assured, owing to the preservation of the left colic artery, that of the lower, which depends on the middle and inferior hæmorrhoidal arteries, suspect (see p. 745); it must be tested by release of the clamp. If no bleeding occurs, one of two courses must be taken: (*a*) to complete the operation by a colostomy; (*b*) to remove more of the lower portion, everting the rectum and drawing the freed sigmoid down through the anus to perform a union by Maunsell's method. If, on the other hand, the lower end bleeds, an immediate suture *in situ* may be performed.

For the middle and upper parts of the sigmoid flexure they point out that an equally severe operation is necessary to secure the ideal, but in view of the fairly satisfactory results obtained in the past by partial operations they recommend a modified operation.

The peritoneum is divided over the inferior mesenteric vessels, and as many of the main glands are stripped off them as is possible without damaging the vessels. This is done from the point of origin of the left colic artery down to the origin of the lowest sigmoid artery. The sigmoid arteries are tied at their origin, the lowest being preserved if its removal be not necessitated by the position of the growth. The descending colon is then mobilized by an incision of the peritoneum at its outer border and the gut divided above at the junction of the descending colon and the flexure, and below in the lower part of the flexure. Almost

the whole of the mesosigmoid will thus be removed, including the intermediate paracolic and epicolic glands, and probably the greater number of the main group corresponding to this part of the sigmoid flexure. If it be found necessary to tie the lowest sigmoid artery at its origin care must be taken to divide the gut below the level of the brim of the pelvis, in order to avoid the ' dead end ' which may be left, as Manasse and Archibald have shown, owing to the non-union of the branches of the lowest sigmoid and superior hæmorrhoidal arteries.

Moynihan (*Surg. Gyn. and Obst.*, 1908, vol. vi, p. 463) gives a full description of similar extensive operations carried out by himself, the main features of which lie in the free mobilization of the bowel which he shows to be practicable, and the free removal of lymphatic glands. An equally extensive operation has been devised by Kümmel (*Arch. f. klin. Chir.*, 1899, vol. lix, p. 555) on the ground of possible inefficiency of the vascular anastomoses when the lower colon is extensively resected.

HIRSCHSPRUNG'S DISEASE

Congenital idiopathic dilatation of the colon involves in more than one-third of the cases the sigmoid flexure, but the whole large intestine may take part in the process, while the rectum and small intestine are practically always spared. The bowel may be greatly dilated, even to a 30-inch circumference, and its walls are thickened by hypertrophy. Most of the cases occur in infants who have suffered emaciation and depletion of strength from their condition, a fact to be borne in mind in selecting an operation.

Enterostomy or colostomy with post-operative lavage by means of a tube in the dilated segment and through the rectum may be done. The colostomy may be followed by a lateral colo-colostomy and resection of the dilated and hypertrophied bowel at the same time or at a third period. In the latter case, the colostomy opening may be closed.

ACCIDENTS SUBSEQUENT TO, AND AFTER-CONSEQUENCES FOLLOWING, ENTERECTOMY

Primary peritoneal infection. This, the most frequent and fatal complication of enterectomy, has become less frequent as one-stage operations have been abandoned in the presence of serious obstruction. It is most commonly the result of infection during the performance of the operation; less often, of a primary incompetence of the suture. Death from this cause is usually rapid, occurring in the course of from two days to a week.

Whatever mode of operation is adopted, the risks of infection during its performance cannot be entirely obviated, but the danger steadily increases with the degree of fixity of the portion of bowel involved, and consequent necessity of performing the section of the lumen within the confines of the peritoneal cavity, also with the relative amount of intestinal contents. Infection is greatly more to be feared during the performance of colectomy than in enterectomy of the small intestine, and the chances of its occurrence increase with the degree of fluidity of the fæces contained in the large bowel. The mechanical difficulty due to fixation must be met as far as possible by free mobilization of the part of the bowel concerned. When circumstances appear to render the occurrence of infection probable, it is to be met by the provision of free primary drainage at the time of operation, and prompt opening up of the wound should the drainage prove insufficient to prevent diffusion.

No extensive experience is forthcoming as to the value of prophylactic injections of anti-colon bacillus serum, but in a few instances administration of the serum on the appearance of signs of serious infection has shown that it may influence the general and local symptoms much as it does in appendical peritonitis.

Thus, a man aged 52, from whom an extensive carcinoma of the ascending colon was removed, and an axial enterectomy performed, passed a sleepless night in spite of morphine, and on the following day the pulse had risen to 130, and the temperature to 103.6° F. The respiratory movement of the abdominal wall was very restricted, local tenderness and some distension developed, and there was great pain. An injection of 25 c.c. of anti-colon bacillus serum was given at the end of twenty hours, followed by a second at the end of a further twelve hours. The first injection was followed by a fall in the pulse to 116, the temperature to 100.4°, relief of the pain, and comfortable sleep. Two injections were given, and after the third day no further alarming symptoms were observed. On the eighth day the temperature rose, and signs of intraperitoneal abscess were discovered. Incision and drainage of the abscess were followed by rapid recovery. This case followed the same course often seen in bacillus coli infections in connexion with acute perforations of the appendix, both as to the relief of general symptoms of septicæmia, and in the occurrence of rapid localization of the area of infection.

When the resistance of the patient is good, or the infection of minor degree, local abscesses may develop. These abscesses usually do well, if early and freely incised and drained, and, except for the possible formation of a fæcal fistula, and the increased risk of the development of permanent local adhesions, may do little harm. Those situated in the

retroperitoneal space are the more difficult to deal with, and give rise
to the more chronic form of fistulæ.

Failure of the suture. Apart from deficiencies in the actual tech
nique, this accident may be the result of several causes, and may also
be followed by general infection of the peritoneal cavity, or the forma
tion of a localized suppuration.

The suture may give way at the point in the line of union in which
the peritoneal investment of the bowel is deficient. This has been most
commonly seen in axial unions of the ascending and descending colons
less frequently in the small intestine, since improved methods of closure
of the 'mesenteric angle' have been devised.

The stitches may cut through the included tissue as a result of de
ficient vitality of the bowel-wall, or as a consequence of the rigidity
of the tissue dependent on inflammatory infiltration. The latter fact
gives a useful warning against drawing the sutures too tight when such
conditions of the bowel exist.

The general condition of the patient may be such that a sufficient
deposit of plastic material for the satisfactory closure of the wound is
not provided, especially where malignant disease is the primary trouble
Again, the plastic material primarily effused may not be converted into
properly organizing tissue, or under these circumstances may become
reabsorbed. The latter process is specially likely to occur in the presence
of peritoneal infection. In this relation the observations of Chlumsky
are of much interest; he has shown that the union of intestinal wounds
is firmer upon the first than upon the three following days, that from
the fifth onwards the strength steadily increases, while at the seventh
it should be thoroughly secure (Kocher, *Chir. Oper.*, p. 937).

Local stitch abscesses may form in the line of union as a result of
infection of the suture thread. Speaking generally, the possibility of
this accident is an argument against the employment of a single tier
of through and through sutures when circumstances do not make it a
necessity.

When lateral unions are made, the closed ends of the bowel may
give way secondarily. Some remarks have been already made on this
subject under the general heading of Enterectomy. The accident ap
pears to have happened much more frequently after the excision of the
bowel tumours than where the ends have been closed in the performance
of unilateral exclusions, a fact probably to be explained by the greater
time needed for the performance of the former operation, and the much
greater amount of interference with the vascular supply of the intestine
involved. This observation serves to impress the necessity of keeping
the possibility of this accident well before us in the performance of

colectomies. The eighth or ninth day is that on which failure is prone to occur, and care must be exercised in the exhibition of purgatives, or still more, the administration of enemata at this period.

The formation of a local abscess in connexion with the suture is not necessarily a serious matter to the patient, either as to danger to life, or great prolongation of the length of treatment, but it is important, as probably leading to the formation of adhesions which may permanently prejudice the viability of the channel in the bowel, interfere with normal peristalsis, and possibly give rise to ulterior obstruction of neighbouring coils of intestine.

The formation of immediate adhesions. Adhesions may develop between the actual seat of union and adjacent coils of small intestine, between the seat of union and the abdominal parietes, or between coils of small intestine in the neighbourhood of the enterectomy. Such adhesions naturally form most frequently in the presence of infection, but more especially when the infection is a slow one, due to leakage from the line of suture from whatever cause. Acute obstruction from kinking of the intestine may result, leading to the necessity of a further laparotomy and possibly to the death of the patient.

Stenosis at the seat of union. As an immediate sequence of enterectomy this complication has practically disappeared with the introduction of improved technical methods. When a later consequence it has more frequently been observed after axial unions and lateral implantation than after lateral junctions of the bowel.

PROGNOSIS AND RESULTS OF ENTERECTOMY

Whatever form of enterectomy be undertaken, the operation must rank as one of the more formidable of surgery. Although isolated small series of cases showing a very low rate of mortality have been published by individual operators, yet if the records of a large number of eminent surgeons be reviewed the death-rate after this operation cannot be placed below 30%. Anatomical conditions render resection of the small intestine a less serious procedure than that of the large, while the nature of the contents of the bowel is more favourable for the safe conduct of the operation; on the other hand, resections of the small intestine often have to be performed under most unsatisfactory conditions.

Two factors mainly influence the prognosis after an enterectomy: (1) the danger of infection during the performance of the operation, (2) the nature of the conditions for which it is undertaken. In the light of present experience it is difficult to see how the risks of immediate infection are to be further greatly diminished, although it is clear that attention to technical details is the predominant factor in obtaining the best results, and that obvious improvement in results has been observed to accompany the more efficient protection of the general peritoneal cavity during the performance of the suture, such precautions as the removal of a sufficient length of the bowel, preliminary mobilization of the large intestine, and perfectionment in the methods of suture itself. As to the second factor, putting aside operations done in the presence of deficient vitality from acute conditions, the nature of the disease is seen to exert a very definite influence on the results attained. Thus while the mortality in malignant disease has not been brought to below one-third of the whole number of cases, the proportion of failures in enterectomies performed for tuberculosis has been materially reduced.

Remarks will be found elsewhere as to the recorded results of enter-ectomy for such conditions as result from strangulation of the bowel but it may be mentioned here that one important factor in the improvement of results has been the removal of sufficient lengths of bowel to ensure the tissues in the line of union being healthy. Thus, of sixteen cases recorded by Roswell Park (*Centralbl. f. Chir.*, 1904, p. 55), in which more than 200 centimetres of gut were removed, only four, or 25%, died.

Enterectomy for inflammatory conditions has been followed by fair results, but even here we find as large a proportion as two deaths among five operations performed on the sigmoid flexure by W. J. Mayo (*Trans. Amer. Surg. Assoc.*, vol. xxv, p. 237).

In Hartmann's collation of enterectomies for tuberculous disease (*Trans. Med. Soc. of Lond.*, vol. xxx, p. 334), he finds that of 75 operations performed before 1900, 22, or 30%, died, while of 58 operations after that date only 7, or 12%, died, a difference no doubt resulting from the more careful choice of cases on the one hand, and improved technique on the other. Caird (*Scot. Med. and Surg. Journ.*, vol. xiv, p. 22) has published a series of 11 operations with 7 recoveries. Nikoljski (*Centralbl. f. Chir.*, 1904, p. 395) has collated 130 cases of operation for tuberculous stenosis, mostly in the cæcal region, in which the mortality after enterectomy was 30% and after anastomosis 17%.

In malignant disease the immediate prognosis is grave, but the ultimate results are fairly satisfactory, since it may be fairly asserted that patients from whom the growth has been removed, even if they only survive a period of months, are in a happier condition than those who have been subjected to colostomy, while a good proportion may remain free from trouble for years.

The late date at which sarcomatous tumours are detected militates against satisfactory results. Lecène (Hartmann, *Chir. de l'intestin,*

p. 433) gives the mortality in 25 cases subjected to enterectomy as 25%
(adults, 18 axial unions with 7 deaths (33.3% mortality); lateral unions,
adults, 4, no death; children, 3 axial unions with no death). Eight of
these patients remained alive and well at 8 years, 4 years, 3½ years,
2 years, 1½ years, 1 year, 10 months, and 8 months respectively.
Moynihan (*Abdominal Operations,* 1st ed., p. 323) in his collation,
which contains several of the same cases, reports similar results. Corner
and Fairbank (*Trans. Path. Soc. of Lond.,* 1905, vol. lvi, p. 20) have
collected 13 cases of sarcoma of the large intestine subjected to enterectomy, with a mortality of 46.1%.

The following table contains the recorded results in 276 enterectomies
for carcinoma. In all 104 died, a mortality of 37.6%.

Collected by Hartmann	.	143	died 48	Mortality 33.5%
St. Thomas's Hospital	.	58	" 23	" 39.5%
Voelcker, Czerny's Klinik	.	58	" 27	" 46.5%
Caird	.	17	" 6	" 35.2%

Without doubt, these statistics contain a large number of patients
operated upon under unsatisfactory conditions, but none the less they
set out the immediate mortality which has been experienced up to the
present time.

Anschütz (*Mittheil. aus. d. Grenzgeb. d. Med. & Chir.,* 1907, 111
Suppl.) in a report from the Klinik of von Mikulicz records 20 one-
stage operations for carcinoma with 11 deaths, while of 30 cases treated
by the several stage operation, only 6 died. He further states that,
including the results of other surgeons, the mortality of the several
stage operation has not risen beyond 12%, while among 139 one-stage
operations collected from the literature the mortality reaches 46%.

In 27 of the above 30 cases which were able to be followed subsequently, 14 patients remained well and free from recurrence at the end
of three years, or 52%.

CHAPTER XII

LATERAL INTESTINAL ANASTOMOSIS AND EXCLUSION

SIMPLE LATERAL ANASTOMOSIS

THIS procedure repeats the natural process observed in the formation of spontaneous communications between neighbouring coils of intestine or other tubes. Originally devised by Maisonneuve in 1845, it resulted in two failures, and probably on this account the operation received no support and little consideration until the question of its utility was raised by Hahn some forty years later. The practical application of the method dates from the publication of the interesting and instructive work of Senn in 1889, and to his able advocacy the now frequent employment of methods of lateral anastomosis is due.

Simple lateral anastomosis has more recently suffered some limitation in its field of application by the introduction of the methods of exclusion. Practical experience has shown that a lateral opening in the delivering segment of the bowel is insufficient to wholly divert the passage of its contents into the distal receiving one. When the operation is designed to overcome the obstruction due to a stenosis this defect may lead to undesirable collections of intestinal contents in the short-circuited portion of the bowel; while, if the anastomosis is made to favour the closure of an intestinal fistula, or with the desire to entirely divert the passage of intestinal contents from the normal channel, it fails in its object. This failure depends in part on the natural tendency of the fluid contents of the various canals in the body to travel in their usual course if possible, in part on the tendency of the anastomotic openings to contract when an alternate route exists.

Indications. 1. Cases of *chronic obstruction* of the bowel by growth, unsuitable for any more extensive or radical measure. If performed for this cause, the undesirable collection of intestinal contents in the short-circuited segment may be met by the establishment of a fistula in this part of the bowel, or, in suitable instances, by the addition of an appendicostomy, to allow a vent for gas and the possibility of flushing out the interior of the excluded portion of the intestine.

2. A lateral anastomosis may be employed *as a preliminary measure to the performance of an enterectomy,* forming a desirable substitute for a preliminary colostomy.

When obstruction is acute it is rare that either of these indications can be safely acted upon, both on account of the danger which depends on the highly septic character of the abundant intestinal contents, and the unsatisfactory conditions offered by the stretched bowel-wall for the purposes of suture. Should the procedure be taken into consideration in dealing with such cases, the amount of distension and the power of contraction still possessed by the intestinal muscle are the two local conditions which, combined with the general state of the patient, must decide the question; but as a rule anastomoses are only desirable when the signs of obstruction are of minor degree or chronic in character.

3. *In cases of tuberculous disease* of the intestine, especially in the entero-peritoneal form and in the small gut, a lateral anastomosis is often preferable to an exclusion in view of the difficulty which may exist in determining the upper and lower ends of the portion of bowel affected in the presence of numerous adhesions. In these cases, moreover, more than one anastomosis may be desirable.

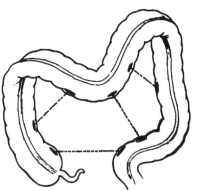

FIG. 381. SOME POSITIONS IN WHICH COLO-COLOSTOMY MAY BE PERFORMED. (*Modified from Hartmann.*)

4. Lateral anastomosis may be employed as *a preliminary to the closure of an artificial anus or fæcal fistula* by suture or enterectomy. On subsequent closure of the ends a lateral enterectomy is obtained.

5. *In cases of gangrenous hernia* a lateral anastomosis is sometimes performed at the base of the loop, the gangrenous apex being drawn out of the wound left for future treatment (Roux's operation).

6. Lateral entero-anastomosis forms a portion of the operation in some forms of gastro-enterostomy and jejunostomy.

In the choice of the most suitable situation for the establishment of an intestinal anastomosis, certain points are open to consideration. When possible a spot should be selected at which the bowel-wall is as far as possible in a normal condition; while, when the disease for which the operation is performed is malignant in character, the new communication should be sufficiently widely removed from the primary dis-

ease to render secondary invasion of the opening improbable. T!
situation of the anastomosis should be so chosen as to avoid the produ
tion ·of any undesirable degree of tension on the joint. Thus, an ile
colostomy or ileo-sigmoidostomy is as a rule superior to any form ·
colo-colostomy, because the comparative mobility of the small intesti·
allows it to be placed practically in almost any position without strai
Colo-colostomy may be said to be generally undesirable if it can
avoided, for in addition to the question of fixation of the colon it is
be remembered that the peristalsis is comparatively weak in this porti(
of the bowel, and hence the chances of an efficient anastomosis are (
minished (see Fig. 381). Published results show that a greater propc
tion of failures have attended the establishment of colo-colostomies th:
of anastomoses between the small and large bowel.

Operation. The technique of uniting the bowel in lateral anast
moses differs in no way from that already described on p. 732, under tl
heading of Lateral union in enterectomy (see Figs. 368–70). The il
portance of ensuring an iso-peristaltic union should be borne in mind.

METHODS OF EXCLUSION

Since the advocacy of total exclusion by Salzer in 1889 (*Verhan*
der Deutsch. Gesellsch. f. Chir., 1891, vol. xx, p. 305) these metho
have undergone numerous modifications, and several are employed ·
the present time. All, however, are variants of the two main types: (1
Unilateral exclusion, in which the delivering segment is interrupted ·
its continuity immediately beyond the seat of the anastomosis: (:
Bilateral exclusion, the original method of Salzer, in which the bowel
divided a second time at the distal extremity of the excluded segmen

Pure bilateral exclusion has been shown to be an undesirable pr(
cedure, since the collection of intestinal secretions, of gas, and in son
cases the accumulation of the products of ulceration of the wall of tl
excluded segment of bowel, give rise to the formation of a sac from tl
interior of which systemic auto-intoxication and infection take place, an
which, by bursting, may give rise to local disaster.

To obviate these defects various methods have been devised: (1) .
unilateral exclusion is performed, and the proximal end of the exclude
segment is drained by its implantation into the colon beyond the poi
at which the anastomosis has been established (Monprofit) (see Fi|
382). (2) The distal end of the excluded segment may be brought t
to a special opening in the abdominal wall. (3) To the last arrang(
ment may be added the establishment of a small safety vent near tl
proximal end of the excluded segment. (4) In a cruder method, that (
Hochenegg, the two open ends of the excluded segment are brought t

the surface at special openings made in the abdominal wall for their reception away from the original operation wound (see Fig. 383). This method is convenient in cases in which it is desired to treat the interior of the excluded segment with medicaments, and it has been found by experience that only the distal opening remains of any material size, the normal peristalsis directing the discharge of contained matter in the habitual direction.

The method of unilateral exclusion is more widely employed, although it is not altogether free from the objections that have been raised against simple anastomosis. A tendency still exists for the accumulation of intestinal contents, especially gas, which enter the excluded portion of

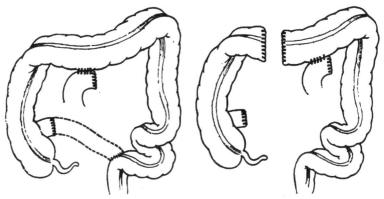

FIG. 382. METHOD OF MONPROFIT. The proximal end of the ileum has been anastomosed to the transverse colon. The dotted line shows the distal end of the ileum implanted at the upper end of the pelvic colon. (*Modified from Hartmann.*)

FIG. 383. BILATERAL EXCLUSION. Ends of the excluded segment closed. The ends may be treated in other manners. (1) They may be brought up and sutured into separate special openings made in the abdominal wall. (2) A vent may be established in the cæcum, or by an appendicostomy, and the distal end of the excluded segment brought to the surface. (*Modified from Hartmann.*)

bowel by reflux from the point of anastomosis. This occurrence has been denied by Roux, who states that it occurs only when an intestinal fistula exists in the excluded portion, and interferes with the normal peristaltic action. Roux's theory has not, however, been substantiated by other observers, hence the temporizing expedient of establishing a vent at the proximal end of the excluded segment from which the bowel can be periodically flushed out has been introduced. In other instances the difficulty has been met by excising the whole portion of bowel excluded, the parts in some instances amounting to almost the entire length of the colon.

Indications for unilateral exclusion. The operation may take the place of simple lateral anastomosis in chronic obstructions of the bowel unsuitable for radical measures. In the case of malignant growths, however, experience has not shown that any better results are attained (Hartmann, *loc. cit.,* p. 88), while it is probable that the products of degeneration, should the growth be breaking down, are the more likely to be passed steadily onwards the less the peristalsis is interfered with. As far as the other indications set forth for simple lateral anastomosis are concerned, it is evident that unilateral exclusion should not be performed when the result required is only a temporary one.

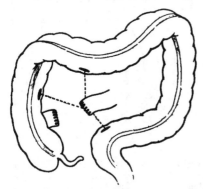

Fig. 384. Unilateral Exclusion. Ileum divided. Both ends closed. The dotted lines indicate some of the positions in which an anastomosis may be established. A proximal vent may be established in the cæcum or by appendicostomy if desired.

The operation is more frequently indicated in the following conditions:—

1. *Pyo-stercoral fistula,* such as may be met with after attacks of gangrenous appendicitis. In these cases local operations generally fail from the same cause that has prevented the closure of the fistula, namely, the presence of continued suppuration. The plastic closure of the opening in the bowel nearly certainly gives way with the advent of suppuration in the abdominal wall, while the necessity of providing drainage in such cases still further prejudices the probability of success. On the other hand, a simple lateral anastomosis is insufficient to completely divert the passage of the fæces from their normal course.

2. *Pyo-stercoral fistulæ consequent on tuberculous disease,* unsuitable for treatment by more radical measures. In tuberculous disease beyond the question of removing the inconvenience of the fistula; the diversion of the fæces from the diseased portion of the bowel, and the possibility of the local application of medicaments by means of either

the fistulous opening itself, or a more efficient supplemental vent, may allow a rapid improvement in the primary diseased area.

3. *Fistulous communications* between the bowel and other abdominal or pelvic viscera. Hartmann has successfully treated a vagino-intestinal fistula by bilateral exclusion of the affected segment of small bowel. The two ends of the excluded portion were sunk, since a vent for their contents existed in the presence of the vaginal fistulæ, and it was observed that the vaginal discharge rapidly diminished in amount, and eventually ceased, the unused intestine no doubt rapidly contracting and atrophying.

4. The method has been employed in various forms of colitis *as a substitute for colostomy*. Its application for such cases can only be a very limited one, since for the slighter cases of membranous colitis or dysenteric ulceration the measure is too grave, while in the presence of severe ulceration the possibility of reflux into the excluded portion of the bowel contra-indicates its use; again, the lower portion of the large intestine is rarely itself free from ulceration. Moreover, if employed, a vent (possibly an appendicostomy, which it must be allowed is a far less serious inconvenience than a colostomy) is necessary in order to prevent accumulation of gas and fæces, and to allow of local applications being made.

5. Unilateral exclusion has been somewhat largely resorted to in cases of chronic constipation, especially by Arbuthnot Lane (*Brit. Med. Journ.*, 1908, vol. i, p. 126). The experience gained by this operation has been to emphasize the occurrence of distension in the excluded segment, and although troublesome symptoms from this cause are not constant, they have been sufficiently frequent to lead Lane to recommend a secondary removal of the excluded colon in a large majority of cases.

That the exclusion of the colon by an ileo-sigmoidostomy is not incompatible with fair body nutrition, and may even result in a large gain in subjects who have long suffered from the effects of auto-intoxication from the colon, has been abundantly proved by the operation of Arbuthnot Lane, and in a lesser degree by the observation of patients in whom the same operation has been performed for the relief of obstruction from malignant disease. Moreover, it has been proved that trouble arising from the fluid nature of the intestinal contents delivered into the sigmoid flexure of the rectum is very shortly got over. That the latter should be the case is no cause for surprise, when the experience of a similar solidification of the fæces is observed in colostomies performed in the cæcum, even if the conditions for the absorption of fluid are not equally good. In this relation the free absorption of saline fluid introduced into the lower bowel, and the rapid gain in consistency of a diarrhœic motion, if retained for a time in the rectum, may be instanced to show that the reputed special capability of the cæcum to absorb the unnecessary fluid component of the fæces may be more an accident of position than due to any special character possessed by that portion of the colon.

E. W. Hey Groves and J. Walker Hall have reported on the analysis of the excreta in two cases in which portions of the colon had been excluded by operation (*Lancet,* 1909, vol. i, p. 236).

The results in the first case showed: (1) 'that the amount of absorption of water was abundant, the diarrhœa being due simply to the discharge of mucus; (2) that the amount of nitrogen and fat in the fæces, although high in proportion to the intake, represented the almost irreducible minimum that was always present in the fæces.'

In the second case, an ileo-sigmoidostomy in a youth of nineteen, where the bowels acted regularly once daily, 'that water absorption was amply carried on by the pelvic colon and rectum, and that while the absorption was not quite so good after the colon had been removed, it was quite sufficient for the nutritive economy.'

When, however, these points are conceded, it appears doubtful whether the operation should be often performed for simple constipation, in view of the facts that a secondary removal of the colon is often required, and that, in spite even of these radical procedures, purgative medicines may still be necessary to ensure the action of the bowels. The results of ileo-sigmoidostomy have indeed only afforded another illustration of the difficulty of dealing with chronic constipation due to inefficient action of the intestinal muscle by any surgical method.

6. In some instances, where an enterectomy has been performed, approximation of the remaining bowel ends may be extremely difficult or impossible. Under these circumstances it may be desirable to perform an ileo-sigmoidostomy, and fix either the distal end of the excluded segment into an opening in the abdominal wall, or the two ends of the bowel may be brought up to the surface at separate openings by Hochenegg's method.

Operation. The first stages in the performance of a unilateral exclusion differ in no way from those necessary for the establishment of a lateral anastomosis, the only addition consisting of the division of the proximal element of the junction immediately beyond the anastomotic opening.

The division may be accomplished by simple section of the bowel and closure of the ends by suture as already described on pp. 731–4. In this operation, however, the additional security obtained by the use of a crushing clamp, as advised by Kocher, Doyen, and others, is very great, since any actual opening of a patent intestinal lumen is avoided. The clamp may be applied prior to the establishment of the anastomosis, and left in position until the suturing of the junction is complete, by which method the complete adhesion of the compressed intestinal mucous membrane is assured; but really only a few minutes are necessary to attain this end.

Some of the various methods of intestinal exclusion are indicated in

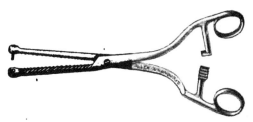

FIG. 385. KOCHER'S CRUSHING CLAMP.

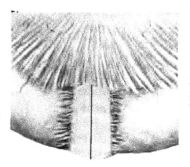
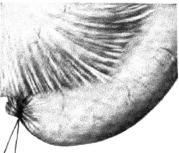
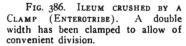

FIG. 386. ILEUM CRUSHED BY A CLAMP (ENTEROTRIBE). A double width has been clamped to allow of convenient division.

FIG. 387. END OF ILEUM CRUSHED AND LIGATURED PRIOR TO ITS INVERSION BY A LINE OF SUTURE.

Figs. 381–4, and no further description of detail seems necessary for their comprehension.

Prognosis and results. The establishment of an intestinal anastomosis is an operation in itself so simple, and it is so frequently performed on the bowel in a comparatively normal condition, that the results obtained might be expected to surpass those of most other operations on the intestinal canal. The rare occurrence of failure in obtaining good local union in gastro-intestinal anastomoses also supports this expectation. Lateral anastomoses and partial exclusion are, however, methods so commonly employed in patients whose general and local condition is in the last degree unsatisfactory, that we find the published statistics of the results of the operations far from good. The operations are naturally most successful when performed for non-malignant conditions, as in intestinal fistulæ, for some forms of intestinal obstruction, or somewhat less so in cases of tuberculous disease.

Of 21 anastomoses established in cases of carcinoma of the colon in St. Thomas's Hospital 7 (or 33.3%) died, the average result approximating itself closely to that obtained after partial colectomy. Hartmann quotes 37 cases collected by De Bovis, with 9 deaths; 11 by Terrier, with 3 deaths; and 14 by himself, with 4 deaths (all colo-colostomies). Thus, 62 cases in all, with 16 deaths, a mortality of 25.9%. Of 10 cases of ileo-sigmoidostomy for chronic constipation published by Arbuthnot Lane, in which further interference with the colon was not undertaken on account of the bad general condition of the patient, 2, or 20%, died.

CHAPTER XIII

OPERATIONS FOR FÆCAL FISTULÆ AND ARTIFICIAL ANUS

FÆCAL fistulæ may be congenital, and then usually consist in the external orifice of a patent vestigial vitello-intestinal duct. The operative treatment under these circumstances does not differ from that described in the section relating to Meckel's diverticulum, except in so far as a preliminary closure of the opening by suture is needed prior to the removal of the diverticulum. This operation should not be undertaken at too tender an age.

Acquired fæcal fistulæ may result from injury, the sloughing of strangulated portions of the bowel, sloughing of the bowel-wall due to gangrenous cellulitis, or the perforation of simple stercoral ulcers. Certain diseases of the intestine, such as tubercle, actinomycosis, and carcinoma, may also be accompanied by the formation of fæcal fistulæ, usually secondarily to the development of an abscess. More rarely, disease of neighbouring structures, e.g. tuberculous disease of the bone or disease of other abdominal viscera, may give rise to the formation of an abscess, which by opening spontaneously both into the bowel and on to the surface of the body, results in the development of a fæcal fistula.

For purposes of treatment fæcal fistulæ must be divided into two classes: (1) the purely stercoral, and (2) the pyo-stercoral.

OPERATIONS FOR STERCORAL FISTULÆ

In the least important variety, such as is seen after appendicitis operations or suppurations, and sometimes in herniæ where the gangrene has been of a limited character, the track of the fistula is of some length, and no fusion of the skin and mucous membrane takes place. The track of the fistula is then lined by ordinary granulation-tissue, and spontaneous closure is the rule if sufficient patience be exhibited in the treatment.

Operation. When such fistulæ are short, and open directly upon the surface, healing may sometimes be aided by the formation of a small skin flap which is slid over the opening and fastened in such a manner as to allow free vent to the discharge at the margins. The valvular exit and obliquity in the course of the track thus attained will aid spontaneous closure.   This method is well worthy of trial in small fistulæ with slight amount of discharge, when a more extensive procedure is not advisable.

When the fistula is of more important dimensions and fusion of skin and mucous membrane has taken place at its mouth, a more thorough operation is required.

The preliminary preparation of the patient for any of these procedures is of the first importance for their success.   Care should be taken, by the previous administration for some days of intestinal antiseptics such as salol (gr. 5–10 t. d. s.), or a culture of lactic acid producing organisms, that the intestinal canal be as aseptic as practicable; a purgative should be administered thirty-six hours previous to the time of operation, and the bowel should be well washed out locally some five hours before the patient comes to the table.

If the small intestine is to be dealt with, and there is reason to suppose that the distal segment of the bowel is contracted, it is well to attempt to dilate this by the passage of bougies for a few days.   In the case of the large intestine, a Mitchell Banks's tube may be inserted with the same object.   If an ascending or transverse colostomy opening is to be closed, the administration of large enemata by the natural anus, to dilate the lower colon, may help to increase the calibre of the contracted bowel and prepare it for the resumption of its normal function.

Lastly, the preparation of the skin of the field of operation is a matter of much importance and difficulty.   When the fistula is connected with the small intestine, or the cæcum, the power of digestion possessed by the fluid intestinal contents needs to be combated.   This may be attempted mechanically by the application of a fenestrated rubber apron, fixed at the margin of the opening by rubber solution.   Again, the introduction of a tube may allow the greater portion of the escaping fluid to be diverted from contact with the surface.   The other mode of protection is by the application of ointments.   Hard paraffin ointment, which is liquefied by heat and applied with a brush, sometimes serves well, but it has a tendency to crack off and expose the skin in lines.   If this be so, a softer ointment must be thickly applied.   In spite of all endeavours, however, the operation has often to be performed in the presence of an unsatisfactory condition of the skin, and in this case the employment of an apron fixed to the margin of the incision is desirable during the performance of the operation.

The first step, after a thorough cleansing of the surrounding integument and the bowel in the immediate neighbourhood, is to make an encircling incision of the skin about a tenth of an inch from the margin of the fistula.   The opening is then closed by a continuous suture, the ends of which are left long to give the surgeon control of the bowel.

A longitudinal incision is carried from either end of the oval defect, and by means of this the tissues of the abdominal wall are carefully dissected away from the central neck enclosing the fistula.   For this purpose the incision is first deepened from either end, until the parietal peritoneum is reached, and the dissection is then carried up to the neck of the fistula.

The further procedure varies with the size of the opening, and the amount of tissue enclosed in the neck.   If these be small, a purse-string suture may be passed around them, tied, and the projecting neck cut away.   If large, a controlling suture should be passed at either extremity of the closed opening in the bowel, the bowel and peritoneum are drawn forward, and the wound is protected by gauze.   The projecting neck is then cut away, and a continuous through and through suture is rapidly passed to close the defect in the bowel-wall.

The closed opening is now sunk by a second line of suture passed through both parietal peritoneum and the bowel-wall itself.   In the small bowel the line of suture should be transverse to the long axis of the bowel; in the large intestine the direction of the line of suture is a matter of little moment.

The above operation (Grieg Smith) aims at not opening the peritoneal cavity.   In many cases, however, this aim is frustrated by accidental injury to the peritoneum during the process of freeing the neck, and generally the introduction of the second line of suture may be much more efficiently performed if the peritoneal coat of the bowel is exposed. If therefore the earlier stages of the operation have been carried out without the escape of fæcal matter, it is preferable, after the first line of suture has closed the opening, to bring the bowel forward from the peritoneal cavity, if necessary freeing adhesions, insert some protecting gauze, and complete the suture with the bowel freely exposed.   Not only does this plan allow of more satisfactory stitching, but it also avoids the necessity of leaving the bowel firmly anchored to the abdominal wall.

The opening in the bowel having been closed, the defect in the peritoneum is repaired, the muscular layers of the abdominal wall are reunited by means of catgut sutures, and the skin wound is sutured with silkworm-gut.

OPERATIONS FOR PYO-STERCORAL FISTULÆ

These fistulæ are unsuitable to the mode of treatment last described, since the presence of suppuration introduces a new and greater element of risk to the peritoneal cavity; while union of the external wound cannot be hoped for unless drainage is provided, which latter seriously prejudices the success of the whole undertaking. Such fistulæ, moreover, are often multiple, and the result of tuberculous or other forms of disease, in which more radical treatment is desirable.

As a rule, then, in pyo-stercoral fistulæ one of the forms of exclusion is indicated (see p. 768), and this may require to be supplemented by local treatment of the original focus of disease.

Of a somewhat similar character are the long tortuous fistulæ travelling between coils of intestine, such as may pass from the surface deeply into the pelvis in cases of tubal or ovarian suppuration, in which the intestine has been implicated. The greatest patience is necessary in dealing with these. The exposure of the opening in the bowel is difficult, and entails great risk of the diffusion of infection with whatever care the general abdominal contents are plugged away, while when exposed, the opening may be in a part of the bowel so fixed by adhesion to surrounding parts and so deeply placed, that suture is impracticable. As a general rule, therefore, the treatment of such fistulæ should be confined to providing a free passage for escape of the intestinal contents and promoting the formation of granulations.

OPERATIONS FOR ARTIFICIAL ANUS

This condition, in which the great majority of the entire mass of fæces is passed by the adventitious opening, is usually the result of surgical procedures, although it occasionally follows extensive sloughing of the bowel in herniæ, or as a result of gangrenous cellulitis.

Operation. The methods available for the closure of an enterostomy opening differ with the form of operation which has been primarily employed. In many cases in which a temporary vent only has been required, the lateral wall alone has been involved. Such openings possess rather the character of a fæcal fistula, than those of an artificial anus, and the treatment of them differs merely in degree from that already described.

When the whole calibre of the bowel has been involved, either by excision or loss of substance from sloughing, an additional obstacle to closure is offered by the ' spur ' furnished by the projection of the mesenteric border. When the spur is of moderate dimensions, especially in the large intestine, its prominence may be gradually lessened by the method of Mitchell Banks. To the centre of a piece of large rubber tubing some 4 inches in length a strong string is attached. The tube thus provided is inserted into the distal segment of the bowel through the artificial anus, and passed downwards until entirely within the external opening.

By means of forceps and the controlling string the tube is now drawn upwards into the proximal limb of the bowel until the string is in the centre of the opening. Lastly, the string is tied around a pad, or a second piece of tubing laid on the abdominal wall across the anus, and parallel with the course of the bowel beneath. In some cases the tube is with difficulty retained; in others it may be kept in position for days and the whole intestinal contents diverted into their proper channel. This method is extremely useful as a test of the capability of the bowel to resume its function, when the closure of a temporary artificial anus for such diseases as ulcerative colitis is contemplated.

Should this preliminary measure prove successful, not only will the projection of the spur be lessened, but the adventitious anus will also decrease in size, and a simple plastic operation may suffice.

FIG. 388.   VON MIKULICZ'S KENTOTRIBE.

In more complete cases the method of closure differs in the case of the small and large intestine.

In the small intestine, if the diversion has been complete, and any considerable time has elapsed since the anus was established, a great incongruence usually develops between the upper and lower limbs of the bowel. Hence, not only is an enterectomy needed, but a considerable portion of the lower segment may require to be resected. (For methods of meeting the difficulties of incongruence in size, see p. 724.) Resection of the ends and a typical axial union is the preferable method in all such cases.

A type enterectomy is less often desirable in the large intestine, since the dangers of the procedure from the possibilities of operative infection are greater, while the persistence of a fæcal fistula in the event of incomplete success is a matter of far less importance.

Two methods of overcoming the difficulty dependent upon the existence of the ' spur ' are available: (1) destruction of the spur by pressure with an instrument of the nature of Dupuytren's enterotome, or von Mikulicz's kentotribe; (2) the establishment of a lateral anastomosis at a distance from the artificial anus, which latter is closed by one of the plastic methods employed in fæcal fistulæ.

Of these methods the latter is the more rapid, and on that account often preferable. The former involves a considerable expenditure of time, but in the hands of von Mikulicz has proved itself remarkably safe.

When it is desired to establish a lateral anastomosis as a preliminary to a plastic operation for the closure of the artificial anus, the only special details to be taken into account are the cleansing of the skin and the exclusion of the anus from the field of operation by plugging both limbs of the bowel, and by careful sealing with collodion during the perform-ance of the operation.

When it is intended to employ an enterotome, the method of von Mikulicz is the best. At the time of the primary operation the two limbs of the bowel are sutured side by side for some 3 or 4 inches, in order to ensure their parallel arrangement and a certain degree of adhesion prior to the application of the enterotome. The enterotome (kentotribe) exerts its pressure by means of an elastic band applied round the handles. The pressure is moderate, thus 6–8 days elapse before the instrument separates, instead of the 3–4 necessary when the enterotome of Dupuy-tren is employed. Only ¾–1 inch of the tissues are included at a time,

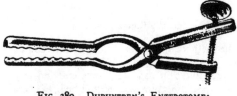

FIG. 389. DUPUYTREN'S ENTEROTOME.

and the projecting margin of the spur is left to the last and then destroyed by the appli-cation of an elastic ligature. The deter-mination of when a sufficient amount of spur has been de-stroyed to ensure a free passage is made by digital examination, and when this has been effected the anus is closed by a plastic operation.

F. Krauss has modified the kentotribe of Mikulicz, in such a manner that only the deeper part of the spur is perforated. Thus, a lateral anas-tomosis is established from within the bowel, and the external opening is then closed as in the other procedures.

The treatment of the intestino-vesical and intestino-vaginal fistulæ is referred to under the headings of colostomy (p. 696) and lateral anas-tomosis and exclusion (p. 768). It is rare that such conditions are suitable for direct treatment unless due to simple inflammatory disease. Fistulous communications between neighbouring coils of intestine, as for instance between jejunum and rectum, may occasionally demand treat-ment, and for such an abdominal exploration is the only resort. The adhering portions of intestine may be able to be separated and the open-ings closed by suture. If this prove impossible, as in the case of disease of the intestine, the small bowel must be clamped and divided above and below the opening, and an axial union effected between the extremities. The two ends of the portion of small bowel communicating with the large are then closed, and a total exclusion is made.

Prognosis and results. The minor operations for the closure of fæcal fistulæ entail little danger when carefully performed. The operations for the closure of an artificial anus are more serious, but the gravity in great part depends upon the nature of the cases for which they are needed.

Resection of the small bowel for artificial anus has been followed by good results. As long ago as 1885, when the writer, on the occasion of performing the first successful resection of the small intestine in this country, collected some Continental results (*St. Thomas's Hosp. Rep.,* vol. xiii, p. 181), the mortality was shown to be 38.4%, but it is now far lower.

Resections of the large intestine have been less favourable, but the results of short-circuiting and the use of the enterotome have been good. The closure of an artificial anus made for the treatment of ulcerative colitis is especially attended with risk (see p. 695).

CHAPTER XIV

OPERATIONS UPON THE VERMIFORM APPENDIX

APPENDICECTOMY

INDICATIONS FOR THE OPERATION

(i) **Acute appendicitis.** Acute inflammation of the appendix, the most important indication, is often the most difficult to insist upon, since the surgeon has not always a free hand. It is necessary, therefore, to discriminate between cases in which an operation is indispensable and those in which it is merely expedient or justifiable. Thus, while the removal of an appendix in a condition of acute catarrhal inflammation may be fully justified, yet in the large majority of instances it cannot be said to be absolutely necessary; while, on the other hand, certain conditions, such as acute gangrene or gross perforation, demand immediate operation if a fatal issue, widespread infection, or the undesirable complication of an abscess is to be avoided. The judgment of the majority of American surgeons is that immediate operation at whatever time the inflammation of the appendix is recognized is not only justifiable but will conserve the best interests of the patient.

Time at which to operate. Operations for acute appendicitis may require to be undertaken in three definite stages of the disease.

1. *Early.* These operations are performed during the first twenty-four to forty-eight hours after the commencement of the disease. In such the formidable complications due to severe or extensive peritoneal infection are rarely met with, and the 'early operation' is one of the most successful and satisfactory in abdominal surgery.

2. *Intermediate.* Operations in this stage are designated 'operations of necessity'. They are performed on from the third to the sixth day, and form the most dangerous and least satisfactory class of the whole series. General or very extensive peritoneal infection or severe local spreading infection is the condition which commonly needs to be dealt with. The indications for operation have often supervened upon the so-called 'latent period', and the experience of such cases has done more to popularize the 'early operation' than any records of success in the performance of the early operation itself.

3. *Late.* Operations performed from the sixth day onwards. These

are usually demanded by the occurrence of symptoms indicating a slow spreading infection, or when severe symptoms indicate that a secondary extension has spread from a previously localized infection. This seriousness places them between the early and intermediate operations in gravity.

(ii) **Recurring appendicitis.** Since the early advocacy of appendicectomy for this condition by Treves, this indication has been the one most commonly acted upon. Such operations, commonly spoken of as 'interval operations,' can be performed with little risk to the patient, are often very easy of accomplishment, and, it must be owned, have been practised with a greater degree of frequency than necessity warrants. It is of much importance that the operation should not be performed in cases of uncomplicated mucous colitis or enterospasm, since such operations are responsible for the greater number of the failures to relieve existing symptoms, and bring the procedure into discredit.

Indications. Certain questions need to be considered. First, is a single attack allowed to pass from the acute stage to be recognized as an indication? The majority of surgeons feel that an appendix that has once shown evidence of infection should be removed, although this is not so imperative if the attack has been one without fever and without definite evidence of peritoneal irritation.

If a second attack occurs, even if slight, no doubt exists as to the advisability of an operation. The risks of any subsequent seizure are quite incalculable; thus, after numerous insignificant attacks, which have not necessitated more than a day's rest in bed, a seizure of the most severe grade may ensue, and place the life of the patient in imminent risk. Again, the mere inconvenience attending the recurrent interruptions to health and occupation is in itself a strong indication for removal of the cause of the attacks, when the small risk to life or health involved in the operation is considered.

(iii) **Chronic appendicitis.** This is an important indication, only separable from the last on the ground that the symptoms of the disease, particularly those dependent on auto-intoxication, are more or less constant. In this condition, as in that of rapidly recurring attacks, the good effect of removal of the appendix is most striking.

(iv) **The previous occurrence of a local abscess.** In every instance where possible without too great danger to the patient the appendix should be removed, even in the presence of a local abscess. If, however, owing to the inexperience of the operator, to the gravity of the patient's general condition, or to difficulty in finding the appendix, this is not possible, it is advisable at a subsequent operation to remove the appendix or what part of it remains. This should be done if possible before the patient leaves the hospital, since he may not return if he is discharged. In such a condition after the infection has subsided in three to four weeks, an incision is made directly down upon the site of the appendix and its remains sought for. In the majority of instances it will be found that a considerable part òf the appendix remains, although at times cicatrization or destruction or atrophy of the organ may have obliterated it.

With regard to the difficulty of such operations it is remarkable, if some eight or ten weeks are allowed to elapse before proceeding to remove the appendix, how more or less completely peritoneal adhesions may have disappeared. The most frequent exception to this last statement is found with a retrocæcal position of the appendix; it must be allowed that in this instance very formidable difficulties may be met with, and for this reason the rectus-sheath incision (see p. 785) is to be preferred in dealing with such cases as affording greater possibilities of easy extension of the wound.

(v) **Abnormal conditions of the mesentery of the appendix.** The most common of these is the sharp bend in the appendix due either to a congenital peculiarity, or more frequently to mesenteritis, the result of an intramesenteric perforation. In either case attacks of colic are common, and more serious inflammatory attacks due to retention of fæcal matter in the distal part of the organ are to be feared.

Occasionally an abnormally long mesentery allows a torsion or volvulus; this has been known to give rise to gangrene of the appendix, also to well-marked recurrent attacks of appendicitis. It is a definite indication for appendicectomy, but more often discovered by operation than diagnosed beforehand.

(vi) **The presence of a stercolith or foreign body in the appendix.**

(vii) **Appendicitis accompanying or complicating mucous colitis.** This indication is one of the most difficult to lay down with precision.

In some instances mucous colitis is undoubtedly secondary to appendicitis, and in such appendicectomy suffices to bring about a cure, especially if followed by careful after-supervision as to diet and regulation of the bowels.

In others the signs of appendicitis are only a part of those of a general colitis, and removal of the appendix at the most affords but a temporary relief from the symptoms.

The discrimination of the two conditions is one of great difficulty, while the discredit which obtains to errors in the choice of cases for operation renders the greatest care necessary.

Speaking generally, the free passage of mucus in the stools is a definite contra-indication to the performance of appendicectomy, except in the presence of gross local signs of disease of the organ.

(viii) **Malignant disease of the appendix.** The actual frequency of this condition is a matter of some uncertainty, since it has been discovered only as a result of operation or post-mortem examination. Rolleston and Jones (*Trans. Med. & Chir. Soc.*, 1906, vol. lxxxix, p. 125) have collected 33 instances in which primary malignant disease was found in appendices removed during life; 4 of these operations were undertaken for the relief of symptoms referable to the female pelvic viscera, 2 in consequence of the existence of fistulæ, and 27 for symptoms pointing to appendicitis in one form or another. As an indication for operation, the uncertainty or impossibility of diagnosis robs the condition of much importance. The growths are usually carcinomata, but cases of sarcoma and endothelioma have been reported.

(ix) **Tuberculous disease.** This is not often localized to the appendix, and removal of the latter has not been attended by very gratifying results. In connexion with the operation the beneficial effect of the mere opening of the abdomen for tuberculous conditions is to be borne in mind. Should advanced tuberculous disease of other organs exist, the operation of appendicectomy is contra-indicated, since tuberculous disease of the appendix is rarely followed by the acute complications common in the pyogenic infections.

(x) **Actinomycosis.** It is uncommon for actinomycotic infections to be discovered until the cæcum or surrounding parts have become invaded by the disease; hence the disease is rarely to be regarded as an indication for a simple appendicectomy.

METHODS OF OPERATION

The incision. One of two methods of incision of the abdominal wall suffices for the removal of the appendix in most cases.

McBurney's incision. This method is the most suitable for interval operations where there is no reason to suspect any unusual difficulty in the removal of the appendix. The incision gives good access to the field of operation, hence is greatly superior to the small opening by division of muscle where the whole process of detection and separation of the appendix needs to be accomplished by aid of the sense of touch and out of the sight of the surgeon. The resulting cicatrix is also stronger and less likely to form the seat of a ventral hernia.

An oblique incision about 3 inches in length, but varying with the size or degree of obesity of the patient, is made, commencing about 1 inch above a line drawn from the umbilicus to the anterior superior iliac spine, and crossing the line about 1½ inches from the latter process, and is carried through the skin and subcutaneous fat. A small vessel usually needs to be secured at the upper angle of the wound, and at the lower end of the superficial epigastric vessels may be divided (see Fig. 390).

The fibres of the aponeurosis of the exposed external oblique muscle are separated by an incision running parallel to their course, and the

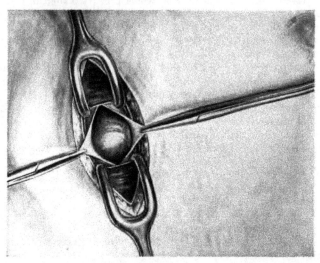

FIG. 390. McBURNEY'S INCISION. The divided aponeurosis of the external oblique muscle is indicated by the white line. Retractors control the separated margins of the internal oblique and transversalis muscles. The peritoneal margins are held in forceps.

fibres of the internal oblique muscle are exposed, running in a direction at right angles with those of the overlying aponeurosis. By the aid of a retractor and blunt dissector the fibres of the muscle at one of the more obvious intersections are separated (that containing the cutaneous branch of the ilio-inguinal should be avoided) and drawn apart, exposing those of the transversalis and a portion of the anterior aponeurosis of that muscle. The fibres of the transversalis are similarly drawn apart, and the transversalis fascia exposed. Traction by a pair of retractors may now be employed to obtain a sufficiently wide opening. Some small branches of the deep circumflex iliac artery may be torn and need to be secured, but hæmorrhage is minimal.

If a pair of slightly hooked retractors be employed, as in Fig. 390.

the floor of the wound may be raised by an assistant, the transversalis fascia divided in the line of the external incision, and the peritoneum carefully opened and incised to a corresponding extent. The two edges of the cut peritoneum being secured with pairs of artery forceps, the field of operation is now freely exposed.

If during the subsequent stages of the operation the space provided by McBurney's incision should prove insufficient, it may be increased by division of the anterior aponeurosis of the transversalis carried onwards into the sheath of the rectus muscle. In prolonging the incision the fibres of the rectus may be displaced inwards, and the opening continued nearly to the middle line, care being taken to spare the deep epigastric vessels, if possible, by displacing them with the muscle.

The rectus-sheath incision. This incision is suited to all appendicectomy operations.

While drainage is more easily secured through this incision, the

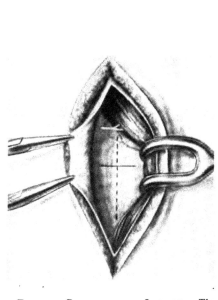

Fig. 391. Rectus-sheath Incision. The rectus sheath has been opened, and the muscle and epigastric vessels retracted inwards. The posterior layer of the rectus sheath remains undivided. The dotted line indicates the ordinary incision, the firm line the direction of the transverse.

danger of secondary hæmorrhage from the deep epigastric is such that many surgeons prefer drainage through McBurney's incision rather than through the right rectus. The right rectus incision does permit one to explore more widely in case of doubt as to the origin of the disease, but where suppuration is distinctly recognized in the region of the appendix before operation, the McBurney incision is used by the majority of surgeons. It should be borne in mind, however, that if the

right rectus incision is used and secondary hæmorrhage does ensue after some days, immediately after the patient has recovered from the shock of the hæmorrhage, the wound having been packed temporarily to control it, the surgeon should proceed to a ligation of the deep epigastric artery and not await further hæmorrhage in these wounds.

The rectus-sheath incision has the disadvantages of not being so directly situated over the root of the appendix, hence some greater degree of traction on the outer margin of the wound may be needed, the area of the abdomen occupied by the small intestine is more widely encroached upon, and a part of the nerve-supply of the rectus is endangered. These minor defects are, however, to be met by care, and are more than fully counterbalanced in suitable cases by the advantages of the incision set forth above.

As originally devised by Battle, the incision through the skin and subcutaneous tissue is an oblique one, about 4 inches in length. The centre of the incision bisects at right angles the line from the umbilicus to the anterior superior iliac spine at its mid-point, and it lies within the right linea semilunaris.

A vertical incision over the outer third of the rectus of the same length, and commencing below the level of the umbilicus, serves equally well. Some small subcutaneous vessels only need to be taken up with artery forceps (see Fig. 391).

The sheath of the rectus is divided for the whole length of the wound, this structure being arranged in two distinct layers in at least the lower two-thirds of the wound. The outer margin of the rectus muscle is exposed by a few touches of the knife, the open sheath drawn outwards, the margin of the muscle freed and drawn inwards, the deep epigastric artery being freed if necessary and retracted together with the muscle. One transverse arterial branch usually needs division, and two branches of the twelfth intercostal nerve are met with. The lower nerve, a small one, is usually divided; the upper large branch must be preserved if possible.

The exposed posterior layer of the sheath, the fascia transversalis, and the peritoneum are successively incised vertically, and the abdomen opened.

The outer margin of the wound is now freely retracted, and, after necessary exploration, the area of operation is limited by the introduction of protecting plugs as in the other incision.

When no great amount of space is required the incision of the posterior layer of the rectus sheath may be made transversely so as to avoid risk to the nerves to the rectus muscle, but this method compromises one of the chief merits of the incision, *viz.* the capacity for prolongation and consequent free access to the abdominal cavity.

THE OPERATION IN QUIESCENT INTERVALS

McBurney's incision is generally preferable. The abdomen being opened, search for the appendix is made. The portion of bowel exposed by the incision is usually the ascending colon, 2 or 3 inches above the cæcum. When previous attacks of appendicitis have been accompanied by peritoneal inflammation, adhesions often exist between this portion of the colon and the anterior abdominal wall. Due care must be observed in the separation of these, and the possibility of their existence must be borne in mind in the preliminary incision of the peritoneum. The existence of permanent adhesions in this position is of interest as indicating the increased disposition to their formation when a fixed portion of bowel is concerned, since the more mobile cæcum is rarely adherent anteriorly, although often fixed deeply by occlusion of the fold of peritoneum passing from its deep aspect to the iliac fossa.

The appendix when enlarged, or if free, is generally readily detected on palpation; if free, it may be at once drawn up into the wound; if adherent, it may often be easily freed by careful manipulation with the finger; when this is not the case, dissection may be needed.

The appendix discovered, and if possible delivered together with the free end of the cæcum, plugs are introduced downwards to the entry into the pelvis, inwards to protect the small intestine, upwards on the surface of the colon, and into the groove between the outer wall of the colon and the abdominal wall. The ends of these plugs, where brought out, protect the external wound. In this way all chance of internal dissemination of infection is avoided; a piece of gauze is placed over the exposed cæcum, and the removal of the appendix is proceeded with.

When difficulty arises in the detection of the appendix, search is made on the following lines. The anterior longitudinal band on the surface of the cæcum is followed to its commencement, which procedure gives a rough indication of the position of the base.

Attention is then given to the more common positions.

1. *The appendix may project forwards.* In these instances the distal portion is usually sharply bent, and this and the tip are often surrounded by adherent omentum. The combined mass is usually readily detected on digital exploration (indeed a previous conclusion as to this position may have been made from external examination), but the mass is usually held out of sight to the inner side of the wound by adhesions to the anterior abdominal wall which require to be separated.

2. *The appendix may lie at the pelvic brim*, often then closely asso-

ciated with the under surface of the mesentery; or it may lie deeply in the pelvis, commonly adherent to the pelvic wall, less frequently to the bladder in either sex, while in the female it may be intimately connected with the uterine appendages.

3. *The appendix may be retrocæcal.* In this case it may possibly be palpable through the walls of the cæcum. The retrocæcal appendix is one of the most troublesome to remove, as very firm adhesions often exist between the posterior wall of the cæcum and the iliac fossa. When the latter are separated the base of the reflection of the peritoneum is generally broken, and the rectrocolic subperitoneal space is opened up, and this may need to be extensively disturbed in the removal of the appendix if long. In such instances especial care is needed to avoid infection, and if there is reason to think this has occurred it is wise to provide drainage.

When the appendix lies to the outer side of the cæcum, trouble may also be met with. The position in itself is apt to indicate a long appendix, and in fact such is often found, the tip of the organ even extending as far upwards as the under surface of the liver. It is in these cases that the McBurney incision is least convenient, and may require considerable extension to allow of the necessary manipulations.

The freeing of an adherent appendix is usually much facilitated by delivery of the cæcum from the wound, and entrusting it to the hands of an assistant to be held up after carefully wrapping it in gauze.

Other difficulties in tracing the appendix. Other difficulties may arise from the condition of the tube itself. The ordinary bulbous appendix resulting from the retention of secretion or muco-pus beyond a stricture gives little trouble, except that needed to avoid the bursting of the structure during removal. In some instances the appendix may be practically divided, the distal portion having become atrophic instead of dilated, and this portion may be easily overlooked. In extreme instances of the latter condition the organ may be represented by its base and extreme tip only, the central portion forming a more or less tenuous cord. This cord, although with difficulty palpated by pressure against the abdominal wall, is generally to be traced as a band by traction on the cæcum. Such appendices are usually produced by repeated attacks of inflammation unaccompanied by suppuration. When the tip is attached to a neighbouring free viscus the band is a source of possible future intestinal obstruction; hence this reason for complete removal is to be remembered in addition to the possibility of the retention of secretion in the separated tip (see p. 827).

Difficulty in delivering the appendix more frequently depends on shortening and distortion of the meso-appendix than on surrounding adhesions. This condition is most common subsequently to attacks of appendicitis in the course of which perforation has occurred between the layers of the mesentery. In such cases a firm band of hard tissue usually gives rise to very firm fixation, and it must be remembered that the division of this tissue after at all recent attacks involves the laying open of infected tissues, and is consequently a cause of risk which may raise the question of the necessity of drainage. When the characteristic yellow areas of infected tissue in a state of coagulation necrosis are met with, it is advisable to snip them carefully away, and possibly to apply an antiseptic to the area under supervision.

Surrounding adhesions having been separated, the mesentery of the appendix is divided. If the mesentery be of sufficient length a single ligature is drawn by an aneurysm needle or pair of artery forceps through an opening in the bloodless area found near the base of the appendix and tied. A small vessel at the junction of the cæcum, which is not included, may generally be clamped for the moment, and is eventually controlled by the purse-string suture employed in sinking the appendix. When the mesentery is short and rigid it is better divided in sections after the previous application of artery forceps, and two or three ligatures may be required. It is convenient to keep the ligatures long until all have been tied, as control is thus retained should the hæmorrhage be not completely stopped.

Although the usual and most satisfactory procedure is to free the appendix prior to its removal, yet in some instances the density and extent of the adhesions present render this difficult or impossible. Again, the process may demand so free interference with the cæcum as to involve much risk of damage to the integrity or vitality of the organ, as well as opportunity for the spread of infection. Under these circumstances it is often preferable to define the base of the appendix, and after dividing it, to dissect or strip out the organ from its base. If this method be decided upon, it is convenient to insert two mattress sutures into the cæcal wall on either side of the base of the appendix, prior to its division and ligature. In this way a safe command of the divided base is retained when that depending on traction of the appendix itself is removed, and no difficulty occurs in drawing over a proper covering of cæcal wall to sink the stump. The separated appendix, the base of which has been secured by a clamp or a provisional ligature, is now held up and the dissection or separation commenced from the proximal end.

When the appendix is embedded in adhesions of such density and extent that its safe separation appears impracticable, Kelly's method may be employed. The appendix is freed at its base, a longitudinal incision down to the internal muscular coat or submucosa is made over it, and the tube is stripped out of its bed by gentle traction and blunt dissection.

Removal of the appendix. Previous to this step, the cæcum, or exposed bowel, is covered with some layers of gauze. Much ingenuity has been expended on devices for the actual separation of the appendix from the cæcum, the main objects of all being the avoidance of immediate infection from the stump, and the provision of a firm cicatrix to cover it in.

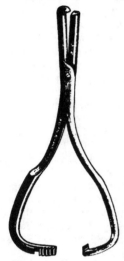

The most satisfactory methods are those in which the lumen is obliterated previously to section of the appendix. This end may be obtained by employing a special crushing clamp such as Kocher's (see Fig. 392). If the clamp be used an artery forceps is applied to the distal part of the appendix to prevent any escape of contents when it is divided. The edge of the thin ribbon-like crushed portion exposed on the upper surface of the instrument is rubbed over with a probe dipped in pure carbolic acid, the excess removed with a dry sponge, the clamp removed, and the base of the crushed portion is ligatured.

FIG. 392. KOCHER'S AP-PENDIX CLAMP. *Corner's modification.*

A purse-string suture is inserted around the stump, and the latter sunk. When there is any difficulty in raising the cæcum, or if it be held forward with tension, it is desirable to insert either the purse-string or two mattress sutures prior to the separation of the appendix, and in this way trouble in introducing the sutures in the depth of the wound is avoided.

When the clamp is not preferred the same crushing method can be attained by the use of an ordinary pair of artery forceps. The best method consists in the application of three pairs side by side (Halsted). The middle pair is first removed, and the appendix divided in the groove between the two remaining ones. The distal clamp serves to prevent the escape of contents from the distal portion of the appendix.

When the base of the appendix is inflamed and thickened by either acute or chronic disease, the crushing method is inapplicable, since the clamp is apt to cut through the tissues entirely, the infiltrated and brittle mucous membrane giving way together with the serous and muscular coats.

A flap method is then desirable, and the coat-sleeve circular amputa-

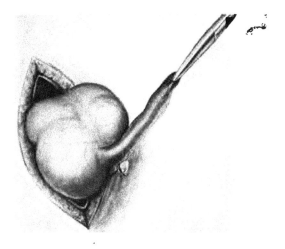

FIG. 393. THE CÆCUM DELIVERED. The appendix has been freed from its mesentery, which has been tied.

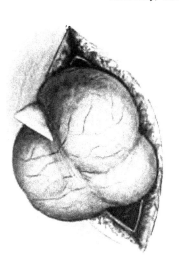

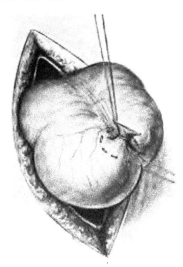

FIG. 394. THE APPENDIX REMOVED. The stump has been freed from the clamp.

FIG. 395. THE APPENDIX STUMP LIGATURED, AND A PURSE-STRING SUTURE INTRODUCED.

tion of Barker may be employed. The knife is carried by a series of light sweeps through the serous and muscular coats until the pale mucous membrane is exposed; with a blunt dissector, the cuff is separated and turned upwards, a ligature is applied to the mucous membrane, and, after the application of a retaining forceps on the distal side of the ligature, the appendix is removed.

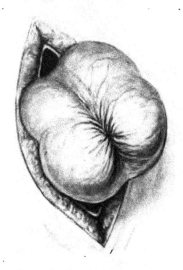

Some risk may arise in the removal of a so-called hydro-appendix, which may be a tightly distended sac, from the possible escape of fluid. Under these circumstances it is often better, after thoroughly protecting the subjacent area, to puncture the appendix and remove the fluid, when the remaining steps can be completed as before.

When the suturing of the stump is completed, the protecting plugs are removed and the closure of the wound is proceeded with. The peritoneum is closed with interrupted silk stitches. The

Fig. 396. The Appendix sunk, and the Purse-string Suture tightened and knotted.

separated muscle fibres are brought into position, and if necessary, which is rarely the case, unless the type wound has been extended, secured by one or more loosely drawn catgut sutures. The external oblique aponeurosis needs three catgut sutures; these should be so passed as to draw the upper margin slightly over the anterior surface of the lower in order to ensure a firm union. With this object the needle, after piercing the upper segment, is entered on the surface of the lower segment and brought out in the same manner as in introducing a Lembert's suture in the intestine. The closure of the wound is now completed by the introduction of a sufficient number of cutaneous stitches.

THE OPERATION IN ACUTE APPENDICITIS

In really ‘early’ intervention this procedure is not usually accompanied by the serious difficulties which may attend ‘interval’ operations, but the conditions met with in the intermediate and late stages vary consirerably and great judgment is required in the treatment of individual cases.

On opening the abdomen free fluid may at once escape, rarely clear, more often of a gruel-like character, or so-called sero-pus. This should be at once absorbed by dry gauze plugs, care being taken not to unnecessarily disturb the immediate region of the appendix, especially if the effusion is not offensive in odour, since during the first forty-eight hours this fluid may be mainly reactionary effusion, and not necessarily highly infective. Plugs to protect the main abdominal cavity are introduced, and the search for the appendix carried out on the same lines as has been described in the previous operation.

If no gross perforation has occurred, the appendix is usually readily brought to the surface, exhibiting signs of acute inflammation, sometimes covered with lymph.

Under these circumstances it is removed and dealt with as in the interval operation, but it is important to bear in mind that the walls of the appendix are often in such a condition as to render the use of the crushing clamp dangerous.

If a gross perforation has occurred the immediate neighbourhood is occupied by stinking pus, sometimes mingled with fæces or escaped stercoliths, and to a certain extent localized. Perforations vary in position. A frequent and happy direction is into the meso-appendix. Under these circumstances peritoneal infection is often very limited in extent. If the perforation be in a free portion, the tip or a bend in the organ is a common site. If the appendix be pelvic in position, widespread pelvic peritonitis is usually present; if retrocæcal or at the outer border of the cæcum, infection is less extensive, but more difficult to deal with. The pus is to be carefully sponged away, and then the appendix is sought for and freed. This stage of the procedure may be fraught with much difficulty; the appendix may be very adherent, possibly as the result of both old and recent adhesions, while the organ itself is softened and frequently more or less broken at the site of the perforation. The separation must be accompanied with all due care, but it is often necessary to carry it out quickly, and the elaborate precautions employed in interval operations to avoid infection are unnecessary under the circumstances. If the cæcum be very adherent it is not advisable to try and fully deliver it, since this step entails risk to the bowel itself, and also that of opening up and infecting the loose tissue of the retrocolic space. If the base of the appendix cannot be readily brought up, controlling sutures should be passed into the cæcal wall, an attempt made to fashion a peritoneal flap from the peritoneal and muscular coats, the mucous coat ligatured, and the organ removed. The controlling sutures previously introduced into the cæcal wall may now be employed to sink the stump.

In some cases the condition of the appendix, or its situation, may be such that a simple ligature of its base *en masse* is the only practical alternative.

When the appendix is in a state of general necrosis from gangrenous cellulitis, its removal is often easy, since adhesions are slight or absent: the danger in such cases is the extension of the infective process to the wall of the cæcum, or even to the ileum.

The appendix having been removed, the area of operation is carefully cleansed; if bowel has been delivered this may be washed over with normal saline, but the interior of the abdomen is better treated with dry gauze plugs only. The difficulty at this stage of the operation increases with the area of the peritoneal cavity involved; when not more than a quarter is invaded, the whole manipulations are carried out from the primary incision; if the condition be one of widespread diffuse peritoneal infection, secondary incision of the left side of the abdomen is sometimes advisable, both for immediate convenience and for the purpose of future drainage.

The question of drainage must be decided on the conditions present. When the appendicitis is of the acute catarrhal type and the effusion sweet, no drainage is required. The same may be the case even in acute gangrene, if no gross perforation has occurred, and the operation is performed during the first twenty-four or thirty-six hours. More frequently wide infection has occurred, and then drainage must be provided by the introduction of tubes and plugs. It is generally advisable to introduce two tubes, one into the pelvis, and the second into the iliac fossa in the neighbourhood of the base of the appendix, a long plug being introduced around and between the two tubes. Drainage by plugs alone is unsatisfactory, since when once removed they cannot be satisfactorily replaced. The removal of the plug should be commenced on the third day, or the whole may be drawn out at the same time, a smaller plug being reintroduced to ensure sufficient gaping of the external wound.

The arrangements for drainage having been completed, the external wound is closed to a sufficient degree not to interfere with the outlet of discharge, or if drainage has been unnecessary, the wound is closed in layers in the ordinary way, silk stitches being used for the peritoneum, catgut for the rectus sheath, and silkworm-gut for the skin.

COMPLICATIONS AND SEQUELÆ OF APPENDICECTOMY

The frequency of occurrence of complications after the operation of appendicectomy varies in accordance with the stage of the disease in which it has been undertaken. Thus, complications are rare after operations performed during the first forty-eight hours, and in those undertaken during a quiescent interval. They are numerous and serious in operations performed in the intermediate period, in consequence of the more serious conditions induced by the progress of the disease.

The operation may fail to give relief from the symptoms of general infection. This is usually the result of too late interference and offers little scope for further measures. The special want of resistance exhibited by some patients must also be credited to the operation in some cases.

If the abdomen has been closed, the wound must be reopened and free drainage established. Other measures to be considered are continuous rectal injections of saline; or when collapse occurs, intravenous infusion, as much as 2 or 3 pints being introduced.

(A discussion of the treatment of general peritonitis will be found under that head in later chapters.)

Subcutaneous injection in the flanks of anti-colon bacillus serum may be tried. 30 cubic centimetres should be given as a first dose, followed by 20 cubic centimetres at the end of the first twenty-four hours. The writer believes that great benefit results from this method of treatment. In any case the injections are followed by fall in temperature, decrease of pulse rate, easier respiration, greater ease, and frequently sleep. Injections of 10 to 20 cubic centimetres may be given every other day. Observation has shown that the use of the serum appears to further the process of localization in addition to its effect on the general condition, and even in cases which do not recover it definitely retards the progress of the disease (Makins and Sargent, *Trans. Clin. Soc.,* 1907, vol. xl, p. 146).

Spreading suppuration. The operation may fail to arrest the tendency of the process to extend. In some instances the extension may lead to a rapidly fatal issue; in others the patient may only succumb at the end of weeks, more rarely even months, after the operation. The treatment of this condition is identical with that of the last, the provision of secondary outlets for the suppuration being the main distinctive feature.

Infection and progressive suppuration and sloughing of the muscles of the abdominal wall. This distressing complication of operation in the acute stages is fortunately rare, but it may necessitate numerous incisions, and only terminate favourably after the destruction of large areas, even nearly half of the entire muscular element of the abdominal wall.

The formation of secondary abscesses after operations in the acute stages. The abscesses vary in degree of contiguity, the most common being, in relative order of frequency, pelvic, left iliac, right lumbar, subdiaphragmatic, subhepatic, and perisplenic. The position in each case is likely to be dependent on the original localization of the appendix. Early incision is indicated in either position.

More rarely, suppurations may be more distant; thus in the pleura or lung. Such may occur independently of subdiaphragmatic abscesses, and may be remote complications occurring weeks or months after the original operation.

In operations performed during quiescent intervals secondary suppuration is rare, the most important forms being the stitch abscess and suppuration of blood-clot in the abdominal wall.

In a small proportion of interval operations abscesses may form at the end of the first week in connexion with the appendix stump, the area of operation, or in connexion with a small residual abscess cavity which was disturbed during the operation. Such abscesses require the provision of a free outlet and the maintenance of a short period of drainage. Many so-called stitch suppurations are really of this nature.

Pylephlebitis and pyæmia.

Fæcal fistula. This sequela may result from various causes. (*a*) Insufficient closure of the appendix stump, often unavoidable where the latter is much thickened and inflamed, and the cæcum fixed. (*b*) Spread of gangrenous cellulitis to the bowel-wall after the removal of the appendix. (*c*) Damage to the bowel during the performance of the operation, either in the separation of the adhesions, or from the softened condition of the bowel-wall. In either of the latter circumstances the ileum may be the seat of the fistula. The strong tendency to rapid spontaneous closure of these fistulæ, even when a very large proportion of the contents of the small intestine escapes, must be borne in mind, and as a rule many weeks or even months should be allowed to elapse before any operation for their closure is undertaken (see p. 773).

Fistulous communications between the abscess cavity and the bladder, sloughing of the right ureter, or openings into the rectum or vagina.

All of these, except the ureteral complications, are unlikely to need special treatment, since they heal spontaneously. The unimportance of the bladder complication is very striking, the amount of cystitis produced being slight, in some cases *nil;* and spontaneous closure is the rule. Injury to the ureter may demand a plastic operation, or possibly the removal of the kidney.

Intestinal obstruction. This complication is most common in connexion with localized appendical abscesses, but may occur after appendicectomy operations where suppuration has occurred. It is most frequently due to kinking of adherent small bowel, and is readily relieved by operation. Rarely, large inflammatory masses may form in the pelvis, and give rise to obstruction of the large intestine. In such a case a temporary colostomy has even been needed.

Permanent adhesions may give rise to incomplete obstruction as a remote sequela, such obstruction occasionally needing relief by abdominal section and freeing of the implicated bowel.

Pulmonary complications. These form a considerable proportion of those observed after either operations in the acute, intermediate, or quiescent periods. The part played by the anæsthetic in their production is difficult to determine, but there is no doubt that a considerable proportion of the cases of bronchitis and pneumonia are to be ascribed to this cause. Pleurisy is more commonly the result of direct extension of the inflammation, while pulmonary embolism must be directly connected with thrombosis of the veins of the area of the operation itself.

Femoral thrombosis, more commonly of the left limb, has been observed with some frequency, and has been explained as due to an extension from the branches of the deep epigastric vein (Witzel), or to a too prolonged period of absolute rest in bed.

Contraction of the right psoas muscle; producing flexion of the corresponding hip. This only occurs in the comparatively rare instances of extension of serious inflammation to the muscle.

Catarrhal jaundice. As in cases untreated by operation, this complication is sometimes observed, more frequently after operations in the acuter stages.

Ventral hernia. This should never occur in cases in which either of the incisions recommended are employed, except when drainage has had to be maintained for a considerable period. When muscle is divided, however small the incision, ventral hernia occurs in a much larger proportion as a post-operative sequela.

OPERATIONS FOR PERI-APPENDICAL ABSCESSES

The choice of an incision for the drainage of an appendical abscess is primarily determined by the position of the abscess, but in certain cases it may also be influenced by the wish to utilize the resulting cicatrix for subsequent removal of the appendix.

For purposes of operation the abscesses may be considered under two headings. First, those which are thoroughly localized and connected by adhesion with the anterior or lateral abdominal wall; secondly, those which, although sharply localized, cannot readily be reached except by a route crossing the free peritoneal cavity.

The drainage of the first class offers little difficulty, the main points in the treatment being the exercise of care in planning the incision so as to cross the area in which the abscess is adherent to the abdominal wall, and the provision of an adequate opening for future escape of the pus. In order to meet the first point, a reliable sign of adhesion during the operation is usually offered by evidence of inflammatory infiltration of the deeper layers of the abdominal wall, and if this be absent the opening of the peritoneum should not be proceeded with before the margins of the wound have been laterally retracted, in the hope of finding a more suitable spot in the near neighbourhood. If the peritoneum be found free throughout the floor of the wound the further procedure must be as described below. To provide a sufficiently free exit opening it is often advisable to divide the muscle fibres rather than to separate and span them.

In the drainage of appendical abscesses across uninfected areas of the peritoneal cavity, the risk of diffusion of infection and setting up widespread or general peritonitis has been much lessened by the adoption of precautions suggested by the experience gained in operations for acute appendicitis. Indeed, the danger has been so nearly extinguished as to render the necessity of employing any of the special incisions mentioned below rare.

When the incision made to evacuate the abscess impinges on the free peritoneal cavity, the first step consists in careful displacement of the free intestine, until the inflamed area is reached. Gauze plugs are now introduced so as to hold back the normal bowel and to thoroughly protect the main cavity of the peritoneum. This ensured, the adhesions are carefully broken down at one point, and the pus rapidly absorbed as it escapes. When free flow has ceased, the abscess cavity is more widely opened up and its interior carefully wiped out with dry gauze. A large drainage tube and a surrounding gauze plug are introduced to the bottom of the cavity, the soiled retaining plugs being carefully withdrawn and replaced by a smaller plug if necessary. The plug and tube having been arranged in the most convenient position in the opening of the abdominal wall, the tube is fixed by a stitch, and the wound may, if required, be reduced in size by the insertion of sutures.

If it should prove that the primary incision, although carefully planned, is in an inconvenient position both for immediate evacuation and subsequent drainage, two courses are open: (1) The abscess being now accurately localized, a second incision may be made directly over the adherent area, and the exploratory incision closed; the primary incision being sutured and protected prior to the escape of pus; or (2) the adhesions may be broken down with the finger, and the abscess cavity entered; the finger is then cut down upon from without, and the counter-opening is used for the permanent drainage of the cavity, a temporary drain being inserted by the primary incision.

The large majority of primary appendical abscesses are met with in the *right iliac* region, and here one of the type incisions for appendicectomy already described may be utilized. One or other can usually be made to cross the point at which the abscess cavity is nearest to, or has already reached, the anterior abdominal wall. In the greater number of cases McBurney's incision is the better situated, but some limitation must be placed on its general adoption, since the disturbance of the muscular layers favours the spread of infection in the abdominal wall, and the opening, from its tendency to rapidly contract, may provide only inadequate space for drainage. When the abscess is large, and especially when the bounding wall is very irregular, spanning of the muscle fibres is better replaced by incision, and indeed this rule obtains equally in incisions made in any other position.

When the abscess is situated near the median line, the rectus-sheath incision may always be employed, and is exempt from the disadvantages which pertain to the gridiron method. This incision is also generally preferable for pelvic suppuration.

Abscesses in the right lumbar region, or the left iliac region, are best opened over the point of greatest prominence, and this principle holds good in most of the other positions in which either primary or secondary abscesses may form.

Certain regions may be occasionally approached by special routes, such as the retrocæcal and pelvic.

Retrocæcal abscesses frequently attain large dimensions, even sufficient to obviously raise the abdominal wall in the line of the ascending colon without acquiring any anterior or wide lateral adhesion. Due regard being had to the remarks made below on the question of evacuating and draining appendical abscesses across uninfected portions of the peritoneal cavity, yet it is clearly preferable to avoid this complication if it can be readily done. Two methods are at the disposition of the surgeon. When the abscess is low in the iliac fossa, the classical incision, one finger's breadth above Poupart's ligament, may be made, the muscles divided, and the extra-peritoneal cellular tissue exposed. The peritoneum is then carefully separated from the iliac fossa, and the cæcum lifted until the abscess cavity is reached. The second alternative is to approach the abscess from the loin. This method is more suitable to retrocæcal abscesses situated at a higher level.

Operations upon pelvic abscesses. Abscesses in the pelvis frequently require evacuation and drainage long before they reach the anterior abdominal wall. In such instances the small intestines are usually more or less distended and raised from their normal position; hence, if reached by an abdominal incision, a non-infected area of some extent frequently needs to be traversed. Under these circumstances some risk may be avoided by opening the abscesses from below, by an incision through the rectum or vagina into the pouch of Douglas. This method has the disadvantage of partaking of the character of a stab in the dark, but it is somewhat widely employed, although much less so since experience has shown that, with proper precautions, drainage may be safely established across an uninfected portion of the peritoneal cavity.

If the rectal route be chosen, the anus is first fully dilated, both for purposes of immediate convenience and to facilitate the later escape of pus. The rectal mucous membrane is then incised, and the further perforation effected by means of a blunt dissector or a pair of forceps. When the pus is reached, the opening is sufficiently dilated. The retention of a drainage tube is not practicable or advisable, since it opens the way not only for the escape of pus, but also for the entrance of fæcal matter into the abscess cavity.

When the vaginal route is preferred the procedure is similar, the primary incision being made in the posterior fornix, and the opening is again completed by a blunt instrument. Vaginal drainage is more commonly employed in the form of a counter-opening, the pelvic abscess having been previously opened from above. The risk of injuring adherent coils of intestine by either route of incision goes far to counterbalance the advantage of avoiding the free peritoneal cavity; hence, the use of these methods should be restricted to cases in which the general condition of the patient renders the risk of an abdominal incision unusually great.

Operations for abscesses in the upper regions of the abdomen due to extension. Appendical abscesses as the result of extension are frequently far distant from the original focus of disease. The extension is usually of a direct character, but rarely it may be the result of a spreading lymphangitis, or an accompaniment of local septic phlebitis, or pylephlebitis and portal pyæmia.

The routes by which extension to the upper abdomen may travel are shown in Fig. 397.

Abscesses ascending by the *right lumbar fossa* usually originate in connexion with an appendix lying to the outer side of the cæcum. They may extend inwards at the level of the hepatic flexure of the colon and occupy the hepato-renal pouch, forming the subhepatic variety, and from this position the pus very occasionally enters the foramen of Winslow and may travel across behind the stomach to the left half of the abdomen.

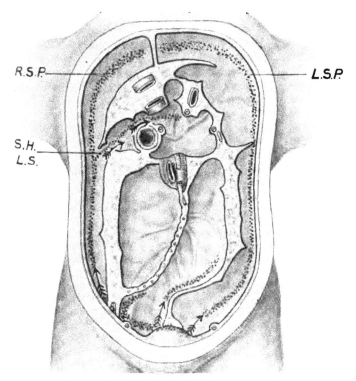

R.S.P.   L.S.P.

S.H.
L.S.

FIG. 397. ROUTES BY WHICH SUPPURATION MAY TRAVEL FROM THE RIGHT ILIAC FOSSA. Modification of Cunningham's diagram of the mesenteric attachment. R.S.P., right subphrenic; L.S.P., left subphrenic; S.H., subhepatic; L.S., route to lesser sac.

Subhepatic abscesses. These are most conveniently opened by an incision in the right loin below and corresponding in direction with the last rib. The condition of the peritoneum should be carefully observed when it is reached, and it may be possible to evacuate the pus without opening the general peritoneal cavity. If this be not the case, the peritoneal cavity should be plugged before the pus is evacuated by the finger. In early cases the condition may more nearly approximate itself to a localized peritoneal infection than a true abscess, only highly stinking turbid fluid being evacuated. The character of the effusion may also depend on the resistance shown to a bacillus coli infection by the individual, and possibly on the particular virulence possessed by the organism concerned.

Subhepatic abscesses may exist in connexion with an extension to the upper surface of the diaphragm; if this be so the two cavities may be drained by the same incision, tubes being passed over the upper and under surfaces of the liver. In a case of the writer's, a collection in the lesser sac of the peritoneum was successfully drained by the lower tube, without the necessity of any further incision.

When the abscess is truly *subphrenic* and limited to the intraperitoneal space between the upper surface of the liver and the diaphragm, a posterior transpleural incision is the best method of treatment.

The patient is placed on the left side, and the trunk rotated to the three-quarters prone position.

The diagnosis is first confirmed by preliminary puncture with a full-sized aspirating needle, passed to the depth of 3 inches through the lower intercostal spaces in the line of the angle of the scapula. The three or four lower spaces may need to be searched, and a second series of punctures may be necessary in the mid-axillary line. These abscesses are, however, more commonly situated in the posterior part of the space, and limited anteriorly by adhesion between the liver and the diaphragm.

It must be borne in mind that two sources of fluid may exist, *e.g.* the pleura and the subphrenic space. The pleural collection only may be reached; if this forms the primary escape the pleural effusion is abundant, or if the fluid only escapes with the withdrawal of the needle it may be small in amount. If clear or turbid fluid only be evacuated, no further interference with the pleural sac is indicated; if it be purulent, an empyema has to be dealt with.

When pus is found beneath the diaphragm, 3 inches of the most suitable rib is excised. This should be one of the lower five; above the seventh rib the diaphragm cannot be approximated to the intercostal muscles to close the pleural space. If the pleural space proves to be unobliterated by adhesions, the margins of the opening must be stitched to the surface of the diaphragm, and the abscess is incised. Barnard (*Brit. Med. Journ.*, 1908, vol. i, p. 371) has laid stress on the importance of suturing the diaphragm to the intercostal wall in all cases, since with the evacuation of the contents of the abscess the diaphragm descends and recent adhesions become torn, opening up the pleural space secondarily. If adhesions be present, however, the suturing of the diaphragmatic opening to the thoracic wall is more easily and satisfactorily performed after the incision has been made   A large drainage tube, penetrating to the whole depth of the cavity, should be inserted.

Retrocolic suppurations may extend upwards in the retroperitoneal tissue in the line of the colon, and reach the posterior surface of the liver, forming extra-peritoneal subphrenic abscesses.   In the earlier stages they may be reached by a right loin incision; the writer has successfully opened one by an anterior incision.   This abscess formed a prominence below the liver, while there was no fullness in the right iliac region.   The incision into the abdomen revealed a free peritoneal cavity, the abscess bulging the upper layer of the transverse mesocolon.   After plugging off the surrounding area the abscess was opened and drained. The appendix (retrocæcal in position) was removed three months later.

When subphrenic, these abscesses are best reached by the posterior transpleural route.

Perisplenic abscesses are generally secondary to pelvic suppuration. They travel by the left lumbar fossa at the outer margin of the descending colon.   They usually demand a posterior transpleural incision, occasionally they may be reached by a left loin incision.   The latter is preferable in view of the direction from which the extension has come.

Barnard (*loc. cit.,* p. 376) has drawn attention to the advantages gained by delaying operation on subphrenic collections for a few days when the local signs are not extensive.   He points out that a wait of three or four days allows the abscess to enlarge, which it does by pressing down the abdominal viscera; this permits the operation to be done at a lower and more satisfactory level, and also renders the probability of pleural adhesion much greater.   In some cases it may even allow a subcostal incision,—an undoubted advantage.

PROGNOSIS AND RESULTS

The general mortality after operations for diseases of the appendix may be said to vary from 2% (Murphy, *Keen's Surgery,* vol. iv, p. 778) to 12%, if the results of a large number of operators under varying conditions are reviewed.   The mortality rises and falls with the relative number of acute and complicated and quiescent cases included in any given set of statistics; it depends, in fact, upon whether the primary disease or its secondary consequences assume the place of first importance in the cases operated upon.

To obtain a fair view of the actual operative mortality it is necessary to divide the operations into two classes: (1) those performed during quiescent intervals of the disease, (2) those performed in the presence of acute conditions.

Mortality after interval operations. Little requires to be said with regard to appendicectomy during a quiescent period. It has been fully proved that the mortality attending this procedure is under 1%, in spite of the fact that many of the operations are of considerable severity. The main factor in ensuring success lies in the choice of a moment for the operation in which not only all acute or slighter symptoms have subsided, but also when it may be assumed that all traces of infective material in the neighbourhood of the appendix have disappeared. Such accidents as occur, apart from those attributable to actual faults in operative technique, are usually due either to the disturbance of small localized infective areas which escape notice during the operation, or to the diffusion of infective material from the interior of the appendix during the process of its sequestration and removal.

Many individual operators have published series of 100 to 200 operations without the occurrence of a single fatality, while such large numbers as 2,000 with one death (0.005%, Murphy), 702 with two deaths (0.28%, Roux), or 695 with four deaths (0.51%, Kümmell) have been reported.

·**Mortality after operations for acute appendicitis.** More detailed consideration becomes necessary in dealing with the results of removal of the appendix in the presence of acute conditions, in consequence of the frequency with which serious complications have already developed when the patient comes into the hands of the surgeon.

It may be said that this contingency should not have to be taken into account, but unless the conclusion that all cases of appendicitis are to be dealt with by immediate operation is generally arrived at, which opinion is far from universally held in this country, the treatment of complicated cases will remain one of the serious problems of surgery. Under existing conditions of professional opinion, the hospital surgeon or the consultant frequently sees cases of appendicitis under one of two conditions, either to confirm a diagnosis in view of the ulterior procedure of an ' interval ' operation, or because the attack is of unusual severity and has developed serious peritoneal complications. Hence the surgeon first comes into contact with patients at the termination of the second or the commencement of the fatal third day, far more commonly than on the first or second days, when a really ' early ' operation can be taken into consideration.

For a satisfactory estimation of the results of operations during the acute stages, the classification adopted by Sprengel (*Deutsche Chirurgie,* Appendicitis, 1906, p. 569) is the most convenient. Thus, ' early operations,' those undertaken during the first 48 hours, ' intermediate operations,' those performed on from the second to the sixth day inclusive, and 'late operations,' those performed from the sixth day onwards.

Mortality after early operations. In this category are included two very different sets of cases from a prognostic point of view: (1) those in which the inflammation of the appendix is accompanied by no more than simple reactionary changes in the peritoneum, (2) those in which definite peritoneal infection has already occurred.

The former class includes cases of simple catarrhal appendicitis, and also a considerable number of instances of acute general gangrene of the appendix. The results of appendicectomy for either of these conditions are almost as good as those of the interval operation, and their inclusion in the general results of early operations is the main factor in the attainment of the low mortality experienced by surgeons who most strongly support an active attitude in the treatment of appendicitis in its acute stage.

In the early operation, peritoneal infection does not acquire the enormous importance it possesses for operations in the intermediate stage. If, however, nearly the whole of the first 48 hours have been allowed to elapse, the area of peritoneum infected may be considerable and the consequent systemic infection severe, especially in children, with a corresponding grave prognosis.

Mortality after intermediate operations. Appendicectomies performed between the second and seventh days of the disease afford the worst results. When peritoneal infection is diffuse, the prognosis is affected both by the duration of the condition and the area of the peritoneal cavity implicated.

Duration is of importance as denoting the degree of systemic infection reached, and it should be borne in mind that the general appearance of patients in whom infection has been in existence for some days by no means always corresponds with the actual gravity of their condition. The subjects may be bright-eyed and cheerful and yet prove quite unequal to resist the sudden increase in toxæmia which results from absorption by the freshly cut surface of the operation wound, and rapidly succumb after an appendicectomy.

The extent of the peritoneal cavity implicated is of little less prognostic significance than the duration of the infection. Amongst my own cases I have separated those in which the process had not extended beyond the right half of the abdominal cavity, from those in which the affection had spread to the left half, and the percentage mortality for the former is 22 against 77 for the latter.

The mortality in such cases necessarily varies with the ability of the surgeon, some being as low as 2–3% and others running as high as

12–15%, of course much higher in the hands of inexperienced surgeons.

Mortality after late operations. Appendicectomies performed after the sixth day have a relatively favourable prognosis. This is dependent on the facts either that a localized infection has to be dealt with, or that if diffuse infection is present, it is commonly the result of extension from a previously localized centre, and is attacked early as far as the general infection is concerned. With regard to the latter point, however, the local condition may severely compromise the possibility of dealing satisfactorily with the recent diffuse infection, and, moreover, it is in cases of this class that subsequent creeping extension of the infection is particularly to be feared.

Mortality after operations for local abscess. The prognosis of well localized suppurations acquires especial interest from the claim which has been made of their occurrence terminating the liability to further attacks of appendicitis, even when treated by simple incision and drainage.

The condition is liable to be accompanied by many of the complications of the disease in general; thus of 59 cases serious complications were met with in 22 (intestinal obstruction 5, fæcal fistula 6, spontaneous opening into the bladder 2, and into ureter 1, subdiaphragmatic abscess 3, empyema 3, cerebral abscess 1, pulmonary abscess 1), and 7 of the patients (13.4%) died.

Of the cases in which the future course has been able to be followed, 23, or 39.9%, are known to have suffered from recurrences, and in 17 of these the recurrence was accompanied by suppuration. All the patients were recommended to undergo an ‘ interval ’ operation, with the single exception of one case in which the gangrenous appendix was found floating free in the cavity of the abscess. In 18 a subsequent interval operation was actually performed, and in all an appendix was found capable of giving rise to further attacks; all recovered.

Finally, it may be stated that a general review of the published results of appendicectomy appears to show clearly that the ‘ early operation,’ if performed as a routine procedure, would lead to the disappearance of practically the whole of the complications which at the present time account for the fatalities which occur; further, that the ‘ early operation ’ may be fairly placed in almost the same category as regards mortality with that performed during a quiescent interval.

CHAPTER XV

OPERATIONS FOR INTESTINAL OBSTRUCTION

GENERAL CONSIDERATIONS

OPERATIONS for the relief of intestinal obstruction are so varied in detail as to be most conveniently considered under the special headings corresponding to their nature.

Indications. Certain broad indications for operation are common to all varieties, such as pain, vomiting, and complete or incomplete obstruction to the passage of flatus or fæces, these symptoms being followed by those of intestinal toxæmia, often by peritonitis, and, if the condition remains unrelieved, by death.

Preparations for operation. The condition of the patient is often bad, and in cases of acute obstruction especially the operations are of an 'urgent' nature. The first precaution should be directed to the temperature of the room in which the operation is to be performed, which should not be below 68° F. Next, care should be taken to see that the patient is well clad; for this object the limbs may be encased in cotton-wool and flannel bandages, and the table should be kept warm by hot bottles so arranged as to run no risk of burning the patient.

Cleansing of the abdominal wall should be carried out with as little expenditure of time and exposure of the patient as possible, and due precautions should be taken during the washing that the table on which the patient lies is not soaked. An abdominal apron, provided with an opening opposite the site of the wound, is an advantage in view of the hasty preparation of the skin which has been possible.

When vomiting is a prominent symptom, the stomach should be washed out. This procedure avoids the risks attendant on aspiration of vomit which may be imperfectly ejected during the operation, and relieves a stomach often objectionably dilated; it is preferably carried out prior to the administration of the anæsthetic. When the general condition of the patient is bad, especially if attended by great abdominal distension, a hypodermic injection of a thirtieth of a grain of strychnine may be administered with benefit.

The most satisfactory anæsthetic is chloroform, or a mixture of chloroform and ether. When the condition is such as to warrant at the most the performance of an enterostomy, local infiltration anæsthesia may be employed, but this method is not convenient or advisable if more extensive measures are contemplated.

Operation. The foot of the table should be raised, or a modified Trendelenburg position arranged which helps to counteract the tendency of the loaded bowel to protrude. When the seat and nature of the obstruction are undetermined, a paramedian incision commencing just above the level of the umbilicus, with displacement of the rectus, provides the most convenient route of access, and allows of ready extension if needed.

When the abdomen is opened, distended coils of intestine are exposed and tend to prolapse, and it is at this period of the operation that the anæsthetization needs to be deepest. Care should be taken to prevent the escape of intestine at this stage, since its exposure favours further distension and an increase in general shock.

It is most important that the search for the seat of obstruction should be made systematically, otherwise much valuable time may be lost. Points in the history or local signs may indicate the advisability of searching certain regions first, but in the absence of these the condition of the cæcum may be best at once determined, as distension or a contracted state of this localizes the obstruction in the large or small bowel respectively. If the cæcum be contracted and empty, an attempt should be made to find a collapsed portion of the small intestine in the pelvis, and in the course of this attempt the various ' hernial openings ' may be rapidly passed in review. If collapsed intestine be discovered, the gut should be as rapidly as possible passed through the hands, an assistant replacing each length of bowel as it is drawn out by the surgeon. The degree of distension of the intestine may render this mode of procedure impossible, in which case either a considerable extent of the small intestine must be allowed to escape into warm towels, or the intestine may be unloaded by an enterotomy (see p. 686). The latter procedure is preferable, especially in the presence of signs of intestinal toxæmia.

If the cæcum be loaded, the sigmoid flexure must next be examined, and then the remainder of the colon. In searching the large intestine it is important to bear in mind that the gut on the distal side of the obstruction is occasionally ' ballooned,' hence every effort must be made to localize the actual point of obstruction; want of attention to this rule has occasionally led to the performance of a colostomy on the distal side. It is in cases of obstruction due to malignant growths that this phenomenon is most commonly met with; it resembles in nature the corresponding condition of the rectum when malignant disease affects that portion of the bowel.

If a considerable degree of escape of distended bowel has been inevitable, its replacement may be a matter of great difficulty. This may be facilitated by evacuation of the contents of the bowel, or more rapidly by the ' towel method ' of Murphy. The exposed intestine is covered by a towel, the margins of which are tucked in to the abdominal cavity around. The abdominal wall is now lifted on either side alternately by an assistant, and by means of pressure and manipulation the intestines are made to re-enter the abdominal cavity. The towel is withdrawn gradually during the progress of suture of the abdominal wound. In less difficult cases an excellent broad metal retainer to insert during the introduction of the sutures has been devised by P. W. G. Sargent (see Fig. 398).

After-treatment. Post-operative vomiting may at first be due to the anæstletic, and then is to be treated if it continues by free draughts of warm water, or a tumbler of water containing a drachm of sodium bicarbonate. The occurrence of vomiting of this class may often be prevented by allowing the patient to inhale a small amount of oxygen until the effects of the anæsthetic have passed off.

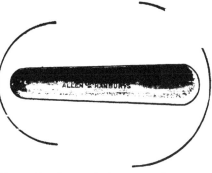

FIG. 398. SARGENT'S INTESTINE RETAINER.

More persistent vomiting may be checked by the administration of half a grain of cocaine, or five minims of tinct. iodi in a tumbler of water. When the vomit continues to be of the offensive character existent before the operation, washing out of the stomach with warm water is advisable.

Hypodermic injections of one-sixtieth of a grain of strychnine may be given to counteract shock, and these are also useful when there is much abdominal distension. Shock and thirst are to be combated by the administration of enemata of normal saline solution, one pint every four or six hours; in bad cases, especially those in which intestinal toxæmia is marked, continuous proctoclysis after the method of Murphy is desirable, 1½ pints being introduced during each two hours (see p. 848).

Peristalsis is to be encouraged by the administration of repeated small doses of calomel, a grain every two hours until five grains have been taken. Turpentine enemata may be useful to relieve distension and encourage the passage of flatus; hypodermic injections of eserine salycilate gr. 1/100 may be given with the same object in conjunction with a dose of magnesium sulphate. On the third day a purgative is generally desirable, and in cases of intestinal toxæmia purgation may often be commenced earlier.

General results for operations for intestinal obstruction.
The results obtained by these operations up till the present leave much
to be desired, although a more general appreciation of the necessity
of early operation, and of the ill-effect of delay, has been followed by a
certain amount of improvement.

The following tables give the results of 400 operations performed
for obstruction due to simple causes, and of 143 performed to relieve
obstruction occasioned by malignant disease.

The operations represent the entire consecutive series performed in
a large London hospital during the twenty years ending with December,
1907, and possess the great advantage over any collection of cases from
outside sources of including every patient operated upon, while the
operations have been performed by a number of different surgeons.

Of 400 patients operated upon for obstruction from simple causes
(excluding external herniæ), 227 died, or 56.7%. Of 143 patients suffering from obstruction from malignant disease, 92 died, or 64.3%.

If the cases operated upon during the last five years of the period are
separated, some improvement in the results is shown.

Thus, simple cases, 155; died, 70, or 45.1%. Malignant cases, 79;
died, 48, or 60.7%.

FOUR HUNDRED CASES OF INTESTINAL OBSTRUCTION FROM SIMPLE CAUSES,
ST. THOMAS'S HOSPITAL, 1888-1907.

Nature.	Total.	Recovered.	Died.	Percentage mortality.
Intussusception	202	109	93	46.3
Volvulus	29	10	19	65.5
Broad Peritoneal Adhesions	60	24	36	60.0
Cicatricial Bands	42	11	31	73.8
Mesenteric Holes	5		5	100.0
Meckel's Diverticulum	22	8	14	63.6
Adherent Appendix	1		1	100.0
Opening in Mesocolon	1		1	100.0
Opening in Omentum	1	1		
Strangulation in Retroperitoneal Fossa.	1		1	100.0
Properitoneal Hernia	1		1	100.0
Retroperitoneal Hernia	1	1		
Diaphragmatic Hernia	1		1	100.0
Cicatricial Stricture	9	1	8	88.8
Impacted Gall-stone	5	1	4	80.0
Fæcal Impaction	1	1		
Angulation of Sigmoid	1		1	100.0
Idiopathic Dilatation of Colon	3	2	1	33.3
Gangrenous Ileum, ? cause	1		1	100.0
Acute Obstruction, ? cause	9	3	6	66.6
Uterine Fibroids	3		3	100.0
Lipoma of Sigmoid	1	1		
	400	173	227	56.7

Situation.	Total.	Recovered.	Died.
Ileum	2		2
Cæcum	7	1	6
Ascending colon	2		2
Hepatic flexure	7		7
Transverse colon	4	1	3
Splenic flexure	12	7	5
Descending colon	6	1	5
Sigmoid flexure	67	22	45
Rectum	28	15	13
Colon, ? site	2	1	1
Stomach	1		1
Ovary	2	1	1
Cervix Uteri	1	1	
Uterus	1	1	
Pelvic Tumour	1		1
	143	51	92

Percentage mortality, 64.3.

OPERATIONS UPON SPECIAL FORMS OF OBSTRUCTION

SYMPTOMATIC OBSTRUCTION

Indications. The commonest form is that accompanying peritonitis consequent on infection. Organic obstruction may also be simulated in cases of injury to, or disease of, the abdominal viscera. Thus, signs of obstruction may follow severe blows. retroperitoneal hæmorrhage resulting from injury, fractures of the spine; the passage of biliary or renal calculi; torsion of the testis, the pedicle of an ovarian cyst tumour, or a floating kidney; and acute pancreatitis.

Symptomatic obstruction characterized by great distension, sometimes persisting for weeks, may be due to hysteria, comparable in its nature to the pseudo-paralysis often noted in the limbs. Of a similar nature is the opposed condition of enterospasm, especially liable to occur in the large intestine.

Of these forms of symptomatic obstruction operation on the intestine is sometimes indicated in the case of peritoneal infection (see p. 847). Certain forms of symptomatic obstruction are of more importance from the point of view of operation, such as those accompanying torsion of the omentum, and embolism or thrombosis of the mesenteric vessels.

Torsion of the omentum may occur within the abdominal cavity, or in a hernial sac. in this respect closely resembling the allied condition of volvulus of the intestine. The symptoms vary; in some cases the bowels act, or even diarrhœa may be present; in others flatus only is passed, or obstruction may be absolute. *The indications for operation* consist in pain, the presence of a tumour in the abdomen, or signs of strangulation or incarceration in a hernial sac. A rise in the temperature and pulse rate of moderate degree accompanies these signs. Cases have been operated upon usually on a false diagnosis.

The operation consists in the removal of the twisted portion of the omentum, the point which needs division being frequently a more or less atrophied pedicle. When the twisted portion is within a hernial sac the omentum can be readily drawn down. In instances of torsion within the abdomen, the paramedian subumbilical rectus-sheath incision is the best. In the six cases of pure abdominal torsion collected by Corner and Pinches (*Trans. Med. and Chir. Soc.*, 1905, vol. lxxxviii, p. 611), the tumour was situated in the right half of the abdomen, which fact would clearly indicate the most suitable site of incision to the operator.

OBSTRUCTION DUE TO ARTERIAL EMBOLISM AND VENOUS THROMBOSIS

Indications. The arrest of the embolus is followed by a short stage of irritation evidenced by increased peristaltic activity, bloody diarrhœa (in 34.7% of 46 cases, Wilms, *Path. und Klinik des Darmverschlusses,* 1906, p. 116), vomiting, which in a few instances has been noticed to be sanious, and distension of the abdomen. These preliminary symptoms are followed by those of absolute obstruction. When the obstructed arterial branch is small and a limited area of the small intestine is affected only, distension of the affected coil and hardening of its wall may give rise to a localized elongated tumour which simulates an intussusception. When the embolus lodges in a branch of the inferior mesenteric artery, in addition to bloody diarrhœa, tenesmus and a patent anus have been observed.

Signs of obstruction of a similar character less frequently develop as a result of thrombosis of the mesenteric veins. The symptoms may be somewhat less acute, while the history often indicates the origin and nature of the lesion. Thus, ascending thrombosis may follow inflammation about the anus, pelvic organs, or the appendix; descending thrombosis has been observed in connexion with syphilitic disease or cirrhosis of the liver, pylephlebitis, or operations on the gall-bladder, bile ducts, duodenum, or pancreas. In Bradford's case (*Trans. Clin. Soc.*, 1898, vol. xxxi, p. 203), the thrombosis was apparently secondary to suppuration of the mesenteric glands.

The occurrence of the above train of symptoms, whether due to embolism or to thrombosis, indicates the necessity of an abdominal exploration, provided the general condition of the patient warrants the procedure.

Operation. The ideal procedure is an enterectomy, in the performance of which the following points are to be borne in mind:—

When a definite tumour has been previously located, its position determines the most suitable level for the incision. In the absence of this indication a paramedian incision with outward displacement of the rectus, starting from the level of the umbilicus, is the most suitable, since in the great majority of instances the small intestine needs to be dealt with.

On opening the peritoneal cavity, blood-stained fluid will probably escape in early operations; in later ones inflammatory exudation and the presence of lymph on the intestines are more likely. The affected portion of bowel may be bright red, ecchymosed, blue and stiff, or possibly gangrenous, and is usually readily palpable. The corresponding mesentery is also stiff and ecchymosed, or the thrombosed vessels may be felt.

Distension of the bowel is commonly a prominent feature, a matter of great moment, since fouling of the peritoneal cavity by intestinal contents has occurred in a considerable proportion of the cases operated upon. A preliminary enterotomy and evacuation of the contents of the bowel should therefore precede the performance of the enterectomy if much distension exists.

Sufficient bowel should be removed to ensure that the parts to be united receive a direct blood-supply. In five successful operations for thrombosis the length needing removal varied from 3½ to 48 inches, and on two occasions a Murphy's button was employed as the means of union.

In the small intestine an axial union is generally preferable. In the colon it may be better to unite the bowel by the lateral method, or to make a primary lateral anastomosis, and then resect the portion of damaged colon.

The patient's condition may render it necessary to rapidly resect the affected portion of intestine, and establish a temporary enterostomy with the aid of Paul's tubes. In the small intestine this plan is naturally undesirable, but it may give time, and tide the patient over the immediate risk.

Prognosis and results. The prognosis depends primarily on the length of the gut implicated; secondarily, on the general condition of the patient, and the time which is allowed to elapse prior to the performance of the operation. Haagn (*Deutsche Zeitschr. f. Chir.*, 1908, vol. xcii, p. 79) points out that the most satisfactory cases for operation are those in which acute symptoms of obstruction are marked, and it is in such that the indications for exploration are clearest.

Brunner (*Deutsche Zeitsch. f. Chir.*, 1907, vol. lxxxix, p. 624) has collected 125 cases of arterial thrombosis, of which 26 underwent operative treatment, and 2 only recovered (mortality 92.3%). In the same paper 89 cases of venous thrombosis are collected, of which 31 underwent operation, and 4 recovered. To these 31 cases may be added the 2 successful ones recorded by Brunner and Haagn, which reduce the mortality to 81.8%.

INTUSSUSCEPTION

Indications. Symptoms of acute obstruction, or, more rarely, of intermittent or incomplete obstruction in subacute or chronic cases. The following features point to the special nature of the condition present :—

Sudden pain, which may be persistent, but is more commonly intermittent, and of a colicky character. Vomiting, at first reflex, which later may become continuous. Even in untreated cases it rarely acquires fæcal characters (25%). When active, vomiting tends to prevent the development of distension and is to some extent a favourable moment both as regards diagnosis and treatment. The passage of blood-stained mucus or blood and mucus in the stools. This sign is less constant in enteric intussusceptions, and is more frequently observed in adults than in children. Chronic intussusceptions are often accompanied by diarrhœa.

Examination of the rectum may allow the apex of the intussusception to be felt. In such cases especially there may be tenesmus. On palpation, an elongated tumour may be felt in the abdomen; this sign is fairly constant, but it must be remembered that the tumour is often palpable only during an attack of enterospasm and pain, when it may be felt to harden under the hand; again, that the position of the tumour shifts with the advance of the invagination. This latter fact sometimes allows a definite want of resistance in the right iliac fossa to be determined (signe de Dance). Enteric intussusceptions are generally palpable in the neighbourhood of the umbilicus; the other varieties in the course of the colon.

It is important to bear in mind that infants and children, the subjects of intussusception, are often particularly strong and healthy, and during the first twenty-four hours they may look remarkably well, suffering from pain only at intervals, while the pulse rate is little quickened.

An intussusception of any form or variety demands an abdominal section at the earliest possible moment after its detection. Treatment by inflation or injection is always untrustworthy and generally useless.

Operation. The most suitable site for the abdominal incision is subumbilical and through the sheath of the right rectus muscle. The muscle may be displaced either inwards or outwards; if the intussusception be extensive the latter direction is preferable, since it facilitates access to the left half of the abdomen.

Prior examination may have determined the position of the apex of the intussusception, and in this case it may be dealt with at once. If the position of the intussusception has not been able to be defined, the cæcum should be first sought; if this be absent from the right iliac fossa, the colon must be traced, preferably from below upwards.

The apex of the intussusception having been discovered, it is steadily passed backward by pressure exercised by the finger and thumb on the containing bowel from below. The early part of this procedure is easy, but gradually becomes less so as the neck of the intussusception is reached. When the difficulty becomes pronounced, the intussusception should be brought into view, the wound, if necessary, being elongated for this purpose, and the final manipulation should be concluded by the employment of sight as well as touch. This part of the procedure is much facilitated by the envelopment of the compressing digits in a layer of gauze, and the addition of gentle traction on the intussuscepted part. It is at this stage of the operation that rents in the softened peritoneal covering of the bowel are in greatest risk of being produced, both by the resulting distension of the intussuscipiens, and the traction on the fixed point at the neck. Such rents are dangerous, as liable to lead to subsequent auto-infection, and they also favour the ulterior formation of adhesions. Every effort must therefore be made to avoid their production, and should they occur, the rents must be repaired by the introduction of fine sutures.

When reduction is complete, the swollen and œdematous mucous membrane, particularly the segments of the ileo-cæcal valve, may suggest the presence of a polyp in the interior of the cæcum. The explanation of this condition must be borne in mind, since the false impression produced by it has sometimes led to an unnecessary exploration of the interior of the cæcum.

Exploration of the abdomen and the necessary manipulation for reduction are to be as far as possible carried out without unnecessary exposure of the intestine—an important prognostic precaution—but in cases of difficulty it is preferable to allow some of the abdominal contents to escape into warm towels, rather than to expend valuable time and carry out the manipulation under manifest disadvantage.

Moynihan recommends that a few sutures should be finally inserted to fix the cæcum in position, on the ground that an abnormal mobility of the cæcum is responsible for the possibility of occurrence of extensive ileo-cæcal intussusception. It may be remarked that recurrence of an intussusception after operative reduction is a rare event, possibly in part because the strain to which the bowel has been exposed does not permit the resumption of over-active peristalsis for some time.

The last portion of the intussusception having been douched with saline solution, the bowel is replaced and the abdomen closed. Rapidity of execution in the case of this operation is specially to be desired.

Difficulties. 1. Enteric intussusceptions, especially of more than twenty-four hours' standing, are less easy of reduction than the other varieties; the adhesion of the layers is m o r e pronounced, probably on account of the favourable conditions offered by the smooth even wall of the small intestine for cohesion.

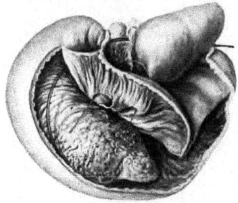

2. Reduction o f the invagination may prove impracticable, or the involved bowel may b e hopelessly damaged by the manipulations exercised.

3. Gangrene o f t h e intussusception may have already occurred.

FIG. 399. ENTERIC INTUSSUSCEPTION OF EIGHT DAYS' STANDING. Gangrene at both the neck and apex of the intussusception. Separation of the neck has occurred. (*St. Thomas's Hospital Museum*, No. 1203 A.)

In either of the two latter events recourse must be had to enterostomy or enterectomy. Enterostomy is a highly undesirable alternative, and is to be reserved for cases in which the general condition of the patient forbids any but the most rapid procedure. If performed, a Paul's tube should be tied into either end of the intestine, and secondary closure should be attempted as soon as practicable. Very few patients survive in whom this course has to be taken.

In rare cases a substitute for enterostomy is to be found in a lateral anastomosis. This can seldom be the case in infants or children suffering with an acute intussusception, since the time needed for the operation is little less than that needed for the form of enterectomy to be below described; moreover, if an anastomosis be established it runs the risk of secondary occlusion by further descent of the intussusception. Lateral anastomosis may, however, rarely be indicated in cases of chronic intussusception, in which the state of the patient renders an enterectomy too dangerous, and here the objection depending on possible secondary occlusion is less strong. In such cases an expectant attitude has been recommended, in order to allow the possibility of spontaneous separa-

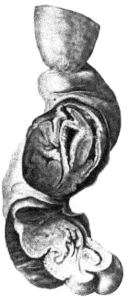

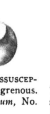

FIG. 400. ILEO-CÆCAL INTUSSUSCEP-TION. Intussusceptum gangrenous. (*St. Thomas's Hospital Museum*, No. 1198.)

FIG. 401. DIAGRAM ILLUSTRATING TREATMENT OF THE INTUSSUSCEPTION SHOWN IN FIG. 400 BY THE JESSETT-BARKER METHOD.

tion of the intussusception; a safer course is to await a general improvement in the condition of the patient, and then proceed to its removal.

Where the reduction of the bowel has been practically completed, and enterectomy appears a necessity, or if the tissues of bowel beyond the intussusception itself have become infected by extension, a resection of the usual type must be performed, with the ordinary treatment of the mesentery. An axial union should be performed in the case of the small intestine, or a lateral union with closure of the free ends where small and large intestine are concerned.

Where removal of the intussusception is decided upon at once, either on account of the initial difficulty experienced in its reduction, or on account of the doubtful state of vitality of the bowel, the operation conceived by Jessett, and carried out and perfected by Barker, Rydigier, and others, is preferable. The principle of the operation is founded on the observation that in some cases of subacute or chronic intussusception adhesion takes place at the neck, and the intussusception perishes and is passed spontaneously *per anum.* The result attained by the operation closely resembles that following an enterectomy by Maunsell's method.

For the performance of this operation the neck of the intussusception is drawn well forwards, and the normal gut clamped above, and if possible below. If the latter procedure be impracticable, by reason of the extent of the intussusception, the clamp must be placed on the whole mass and provisionally removed during the later withdrawal of the intussusception. The abdominal cavity and wound are protected by gauze plugs.

The entering gut is sutured to the prominent neck of the ensheathing segment, the line of suture being carried on to the mesentery in such a manner as to preserve the folds produced jn it by the descent of the intussusception.

A longitudinal incision, 1 or 1½ inches in length, is made into the intussuscipiens ¾ inch below the neck, and from the opening thus obtained the intussusceptum is delivered, the lower clamp being provisionally removed if required.

The intussusceptum is now drawn forward, and its base is divided in segments, stitches through the whole thickness of the wall of the two elements being introduced as the division proceeds. Special care is to be exercised in dealing with the mesenteric margin, in order to prevent any risk of hæmorrhage from this part.

Lastly, the longitudinal incision in the bowel-wall is repaired by the introduction of two tiers of sutures, one perforating all the coats, and the superficial one of the Lembert type. Care should be taken not to include too great an extent of the bowel-wall, since a transverse closure of the wound is not advisable in these cases, in consequence of the near proximity of the other line of suture.

4. Other complications may be met with occasionally. The simplest is the discovery of an intestinal polyp as the original cause of the condition; much more rarely a simple tumour, such as a lipoma of the bowel-wall. In either case the removal of the tumour is indicated, a polyp being cut off at its base and the gap in the mucous membrane repaired over the resulting gap. For this procedure a simple longitudinal incision of the bowel-wall suffices. For a tumour of any size,

either simple or of sarcomatous nature, a type resection of the affected portion of intestine is required. A rare complication may be the discovery of the cause as a Meckel's diverticulum, when the removal of the latter will be indicated after the reduction of the intussusception.

5. Malignant growths of the large bowel of the annular variety not very infrequently become invaginated. When this occurs within the abdominal cavity, the case is to be treated on the lines which govern the surgeon in dealing with such growths in general. Occasionally, however, tumours of the pelvic or sigmoid colon descend to the anus, or even prolapse. This accident may be regarded as a happy one, since the operation for the relief of the condition is one of the easiest in connexion with the intestines. The growth is well drawn down, and then the base of the two thicknesses of bowel-wall is divided in segments, through and through stitches being introduced as the division is proceeded with. When released the line of suture either re-enters the anus spontaneously, or may be readily replaced. In fact, the line of suture may at once rise far out of the reach of the finger.

These operations have been followed by surprisingly good results, both immediate and remote, in spite of the fact that any interference with the lymphatic glands far from the margin of the bowel is impracticable. The mere fact of the possibility of such free prolapse indicates a condition of the mesentery which renders it improbable that extensive lymphatic infiltration has occurred.

Prognosis and results. Experience in operations for intussusception has clearly demonstrated the importance of early interference, and recorded statistics show that in operations performed during the first twenty-four hours, the results obtained compare favourably with those of all other forms of obstruction. Early operation excludes the probability of all the serious complications alluded to above, while the patients themselves usually offer the real advantage as subjects of being perfectly healthy up to the immediate occurrence of the accident. The second element of importance in the prognosis is the relative time spent in the reduction of the intussusception. There is no doubt that, especially in infants, a rapid operation is of the first moment, hence the operator should be careful to choose that method which ensures to him the greatest rapidity and involves the least amount of intra-abdominal manipulation and exposure of the intestines.

The general results of operations are in fact good, and the mortality which exists is in great measure to be ascribed to cases already complicated by the existence of gangrene, the supervention of peritonitis, or general toxæmia.

That even the formidable operation of complete resection is not in itself to be unduly feared, is shown by the results obtained by von Eiselsberg (*Arch. f. klin. Chir.*, 1903, vol. lxix, p. 26), who records nine recoveries in twelve cases of ordinary intussusceptions treated by excision; mortality 25%. These results are of course not comparable with those of resections performed for gangrene, or in toxæmic patients. The latter class of case unfortunately still depresses the percentage of recoveries obtained in General Hospitals, and in consequence of the rarity of this condition amongst the children of the better classes it is to hospital records alone that we can look for information.

During the years 1888–1908 inclusive, 202 patients were consecutively submitted to operation of various forms at St. Thomas's Hospital; of these ninety-three died, a mortality of 46.3%. Of these operations twelve consisted in resection with immediate union, of which number only two adults recovered; and fifteen of enterostomy alone, or enterostomy combined with excision, of which number all succumbed. If the latter twenty-seven cases be subtracted, the mortality for abdominal section combined with reduction is reduced to 38.8%.

If the cases occurring during the last five years of the period are considered alone, the numbers are slightly better. Thus, of sixty-five cases, twenty-three died, a mortality of 35.3%. In this series nine cases of enterostomy, or resection, are included, with only one recovery (an adult); if these be subtracted we have fifty-six cases with fifteen deaths, a mortality for cœliotomy and reduction of 26.7%.

Clubbe (*Brit. Med. Journ.*, 1905, vol. i, p. 1327) records 100 consecutive operations with a mortality of 37%. He further divides these cases into two successive periods, each including fifty, and finds that while in the years 1893–1901 the mortality was 50%, in the years 1901–4 the mortality was reduced to 24%. Clubbe ascribes the improvement in the later results to the fact that the patients came earlier under observation. Cuthbert Wallace (*Clin. Soc. Trans.*, 1905, vol. xxxviii. p. 55) has recorded twenty consecutive operations with a mortality of 20%. Excluding cases in which resection was necessary, Wallace's mortality is decreased to 11.11%.

VOLVULUS

Indications. The indication for operation is usually acute intestinal obstruction of undetermined nature, except in the case of sigmoid or cæcal volvulus, where isolated distension of the loop is often sufficiently well marked to allow a distinctive diagnosis being made. The latter cases also frequently give a history of previous attacks of temporary obstruction of a similar character.

Operation. The primary incision should be subumbilical, this being the most suitable for dealing with either cæcal or sigmoid volvuli or the exploration of the small intestine. If the signs indicate a cæcal or sigmoid volvulus the incision may be over the outer part of the rectus sheath, and the muscle is displaced inwards; for cases of indeterminate cause the paramedian position with displacement of the muscle outwards is preferable.

The abdominal cavity having been opened, the volvulus may present itself in several forms.

Volvulus of the small intestine. 1. In young patients, practically the whole small intestine may be implicated, appearing black and even gangrenous. This condition has most frequently been observed in young infants, and is accompanied by very acute symptoms. In such cases the ileal mesentery may be so deficient as to give rise to a much narrowed line of attachment to the posterior abdominal wall; or the cæcum having failed to descend and travel to the right, a similar narrowed area of fixation is present in spite of the possible existence of a common mesentery.

2. A local coil, or coils, only may be implicated. In this case adhesions may be present, either fixing the coil of intestine itself, or crossing the attachment of the mesentery in such a manner as to narrow its width. In other instances no definite cause for the torsion can be discovered. Volvulus of local coils is naturally the most common variety met with in connexion with herniæ.

When the volvulus is extensive, the ileum is always involved, sometimes the whole ileum and jejunum, but never the jejunum alone. Such cases are frequently hopeless, but the treatment consists in the untwisting of the intestine from right to left, and an attempt to fix the upper and lower extremities of the mesentery in such a manner as to render a second torsion impracticable. Five cases in which operation was successfully performed have been collected by G. Serda (*La Riforma Med.*, 1908, No. vii, p. 177).

When a volvulus affects a single loop of small intestine the treatment depends upon the variety; if the torsion has occurred as a result of rotation around an abnormal adhesion, or as a result of plication of the mesentery by a band, simple division of the latter is sufficient. Again, when a volvulus develops in, or in connexion with, a hernial sac, liberation of the loop and extirpation of the sac is alone indicated. If, on the other hand, no explanation of the twist is to be found in acquired conditions, the affected loop should be resected, and an axial union established if the state of the patient and the local condition of the bowel permit this step.

Volvulus of the large intestine. In the large majority of cases, either the cæcum or the sigmoid flexure is the segment implicated. More rarely, the ascending or transverse colon. The writer has had to deal with the latter condition by resection in an umbilical hernia.

Cæcal volvulus. The cæcum is absent from its normal position; in more than half the cases it lies in the lower abdomen, but it has been met with beneath the mesentery, in the left flank, or in contact with the hepatic or splenic flexures of the colon. A long free mesentery to the cæcum, or cæcum and ascending colon, usually exists; in other cases the rotation appears to have been due to the overloading of acquired lateral pouches of the cæcum. Considerable distension of the cæcum is common, the contents being in great part gaseous. A preliminary temporary colotomy and evacuation of the contents allows the distended loop to be delivered more easily, and much facilitates the untwisting of the mesentery in a direction from left to right. In one case the writer was, in fact, unable to deliver the cæcum, which was impacted in the pelvis, until this measure had been undertaken. A firm palpable band is frequent, passing from below to the point in the ascending colon marking the distal extremity of the loop; this is formed by the mesocolon.

The rotation having been corrected, the cæcum should be fixed as nearly in its normal position as possible. In some instances this may be high, as the cæcum has never descended to its proper level, although provided with an abnormally long mesentery.

Fixation may be by a few sutures passing from the bowel itself to the abdominal wall, but if the mesentery is very long it is better to plicate this on its right aspect, or to stitch the mesentery to the parietal peritoneum. Corner and Sargent recommend plication of the cæcum itself in some cases.

Sigmoid volvulus. The distended coil may lie in any part of the abdomen, but most commonly it passes obliquely upwards and to the right. Its dimensions may be enormous. As in cæcal volvuli, evacuation of the contents is advisable prior to making an attempt to untwist the loop. When the bowel has been emptied the rotation necessary is easily effected, and the question arises as to what measures must be taken to prevent a recurrence.

Sigmoid volvulus is particularly the form in which chronic distension of the bowel and consequent great elongation of the loop take the main causative position. This chronic distension may depend on simple constipation; it may be a part of a general neurosis, as in hysterical subjects; or of a local condition due to some imperfection in the nerve-supply, as in the congenital dilatation of the colon. The chief measures which have been employed to prevent recurrence are fixation of the loop, lateral anastomosis at the base of the loop, and removal of the loop. Each and all have proved themselves unsatisfactory.

Fixation of the loop may be to the abdominal wall in the iliac region, or an attempt to limit its mobility may be made by suturing the left aspect of the mesentery to the parietal peritoneum. Fixation of the loop to the abdominal wall does not suffice to prevent future distension; in one case of the writer's, a woman of fifty, in spite of this measure, the sigmoid flexure a year later was sufficiently distended to reach the liver, and obstruction again developed.

Lateral anastomosis at the base of the loop is dangerous; in two cases of the writer's this was followed by recurrent torsion, once within a week, and once at the end of twelve months. In a third case, of megacolon in a boy of five, the anastomosis has been a success, the patient remaining well at the end of five years. Lastly, as to removal of the loop, the writer has twice performed this, once with success; in the second case dilatation of the distal segment slowly developed, a large sac being formed by the pelvic colon, which again gave rise to obstruction (see Fig. 402).

This experience shows that except in cases of recent sigmoid volvulus

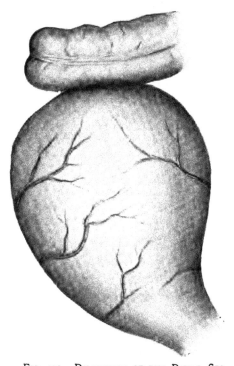

FIG. 402. DILATATION OF THE DISTAL SEGMENT OF THE PELVIC COLON, SUBSEQUENT TO THE REMOVAL OF THE SIGMOID FLEXURE AND UNION BY LATERAL APPROXIMATION. The proximal segment retains its normal size, and the projecting closed end is unaltered.

with a single loop, all existing modes of treatment are unsatisfactory. In fact, a simple colostomy and drainage of the dilated loop may be as satisfactory as any of the more radical methods when a large loop exists.

In cases of volvulus, whether of the large or small intestine, in which the general state of the patient or the local conditions are bad, resection of the loop combined with an enterostomy is indicated.

In connexion with sigmoid volvulus may be mentioned the condition in which a long sigmoid loop rises into the abdomen and the upper part again falls, compressing in the angle a coil, or coils, of small intestine. When possible, the loop should in such cases be resected.

What has been said above as to sigmoid volvulus applies with equal force to the treatment of obstruction due to congenital hypertrophic dilatation of the colon, but in these cases it must be borne in mind that a simple colostomy opening in the sigmoid colon may fail to act if the entire colon be involved in the condition.

Prognosis and results. The mortality after operations for volvulus is high, and highest in cases of volvulus of the small intestine. Of the 29 cases contained in the St. Thomas's series 19 died, a mortality of 65.5%. The cases were distributed as follows: sigmoid flexure 9, cæcum 8, ascending colon 5, small intestine 7. The operations performed were—untwisting and fixation: sigmoid 7 with 2 deaths, cæcal 4 with 3 deaths, ascending colon 2 with 2 deaths, small intestine 5 with 5 deaths. Untwisting alone: cæcal 1, fatal; cæcoplication 1, recovery. Primary resection and reunion of bowel: sigmoid 1, small intestine 1; both recovered. Resection and enterostomy: cæcal 3, small intestine 1; all four fatal.

Corner and Sargent (*St. Thomas's Hospital Rep.*, 1903, vol. xxxii, p. 413) state that of 40 cases of cæcal volvulus collected by them, and in which operations were performed, 21 died, a mortality of 52.5%.

OBSTRUCTION PRODUCED BY INTRAPERITONEAL ADHESIONS

Indications. Obstruction by the action of adhesions may be of the most acute form, especially when of the nature of a strangulation beneath a band. When the adhesions are of the broad form, or multiple, complete obstruction may only follow a period of variable length during which signs of chronic obstruction have been noticed.

A history of previous peritonitis, accompanying inflammation of the gall-bladder, vermiform appendix, or the female generative organs; a history of tuberculous peritonitis, a severe attack of enteric fever, or the presence of an old hernial sac may aid in indicating the existence and also the locality of adhesions. In other cases similar information may be afforded by the presence of a scar in the abdominal wall, the result either of injury or a previous surgical operation.

The site of the adhesions may further be indicated in the early stages of obstruction by the position of the initial pain, the existence of localized tenderness and rigidity, and in conjunction with these signs evidence of distension of a circumscribed length of bowel and increased local peristalsis.

Operation. The site of the incision in the abdominal wall is frequently indicated by the history, or local signs; in the absence of reliable evidence of this character, the paramedian subumbilical incision with displacement of the rectus muscle outwards should be chosen.

When the abdomen has been opened the search for the point of obstruction is governed by definite lines: (1) If the history or the local signs have indicated a special region this should be first explored. (2) If this be not the case, the pelvis should first be investigated in the hope of discovering a collapsed portion of the small bowel. If this be found, the gut is rapidly passed through the fingers, each length being replaced as a further is brought out until the source of obstruction is reached. (3) If the cæcum be distended, the sigmoid flexure is first sought, and should the latter prove collapsed, the incision must be prolonged somewhat, to give ample space for the introduction of the hand for exploration of the upper half of the abdomen and remaining segments of the colon.

The obstructing adhesion discovered, it is dealt with according to necessity.

Cord adhesions may pass between neighbouring coils, between coils and the solid viscera, between the gut and the mesentery, or between the intestine and the parietal peritoneum. They should be divided between two pairs of artery forceps, and then ligatured at the base, and any projecting free portion removed.

Broad adhesions are dealt with somewhat differently; if recent they are most suitably separated by gentle pressure with the fingers covered with a piece of gauze, and if there appears to be a chance of reabsorption it is well to separate any adhesions which come into view. When the adhesions are old and of firm cicatricial tissue, it is not advisable to separate more than appear to be necessary to relieve the obstruction The actual process of separation involves risk to the integrity of the intestine, the knife or scissors often needing to be employed, and the bleeding from the torn surface may be difficult to control. Lastly, the raw surfaces are practically certain to acquire new connexions, probably with the development of two adhesions in the place of the one temporarily separated.

Difficulty in dealing with the adhesions may arise from the degree of distension of the bowels present. Under these circumstances the contents of the bowel should be evacuated by enterotomy (see p. 687). This procedure renders extensive evisceration unnecessary, and much diminishes the immediate risk of the operation. Pelvic adhesions often give rise to the greatest manipulative trouble; considerable advantage in dealing with these may be gained by placing the patient in the Trendelenburg position.

In cases of very acute strangulation, or when the patient comes to the operating table at a late date, simple freeing of the adhesions may not suffice, since the bowel may already be gangrenous, under which circumstance an enterectomy may be necessary.

In other cases the condition may be too bad to allow of an enterectomy being undertaken, and an enterostomy must be performed. The artificial anus will usually be made at the seat of obstruction, but if there is reason to believe that the obstruction is not due to strangulation, and this is especially likely to be the case with recent inflammations. a temporary enterostomy above the seat of obstruction may be the safest procedure. An enterostomy serves to tide the patient over until the toxæmia secondary to the obstruction has been sufficiently removed to allow a more extensive procedure being performed with safety, and minimizes the risks of the immediate operation.

Multiple adhesions, especially such as are met with in tuberculous peritonitis, are often too extensive to be dealt with by separation, and the arrangements of the matted coils too intricate to allow a resection to be performed with safety. In such cases lateral entero-anastomosis is the most suitable method, and more than one intercommunication may be desirable. Entero-anastomosis is also the only resource in cases of adhesion of the intestine to inoperable morbid growths. A single knotted mass formed by intestine which has lain in an old hernial sac may, on the other hand, be resected with advantage.

Prognosis and results. In spite of the comparative simplicity of the operations for separation of adhesions, the form of obstruction due to this cause is a remarkably fatal one. That this in considerable measure depends on too tardy interference cannot be denied, but in many instances, particularly those dependent on internal strangulation, the degree of early toxæmia is striking. Of 102 cases of obstruction from adhesions treated by operation at St. Thomas's Hospital between 1888 and 1907, 64 died, a mortality of 62.7%. In 60 of the cases broad adhesions were the cause, with a mortality of 60%; in 42 band adhesions. with a mortality of 73.8%. The best results are obtained in internal strangulations attacked early, and in recent broad adhesions such as follow on operations, or develop in connexion with appendical abscesses. In the latter form early recurrence sometimes takes place. In any case in which numerous old adhesions exist, recurrence of the trouble at some future date is not uncommon, and such attacks of obstruction may be many times repeated.

OBSTRUCTION BY ADHERENT VERMIFORM APPENDIX

This is not very uncommon; it partakes in one character with the form next to be described, *viz.* that a double source of danger may exist in gangrene of the constricting tube as well as of the constricted portion of intestine. This danger is, however, in some cases eliminated by the fact that the constricting appendix has previously undergone a process

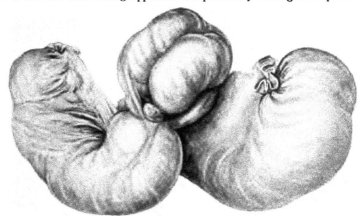

FIG. 403. STRANGULATION OF A LOOP OF INTESTINE BY A VERMIFORM APPENDIX. The tip of the appendix is adherent to the mesentery at the site of a softened mesenteric gland. H. B. Robinson's case. (*St. Thomas's Hospital Museum*, No. 1287 A).

of obliteration; while in others, either only a cicatricial band passing from the tip of the appendix is concerned in the strangulation, or the band causes obstruction by tension and kinking, and not by encircling the affected portion of intestine.

Operation. The operative treatment differs from that of cicatricial bands only in the fact that removal of the appendix by the ordinary method should form a part of the operation for the relief of the obstruction.

OBSTRUCTION BY AN ADHERENT MECKEL'S DIVERTICULUM

This persistent remnant of the omphalo-mesenteric duct is found in some 2% of all subjects, but much more frequently in male subjects (86–14, Hilgenreiner).

Indications. Half the patients are children or young adults under twenty years of age, but obstruction from this cause is met with much later. A history of previous temporary attacks of obstruction often exists; this is probably particularly the case when the diverticulum itself is the strangulating agent and not a band passing from it, since the diverticulum forms a comparatively soft and broad constricting ring, and the engaged intestine may escape with changes in the position of the patient and of the abdominal contents. For the same reason the symp-

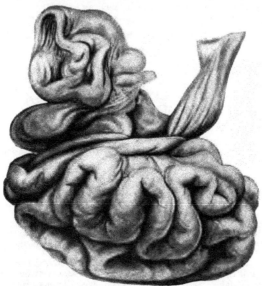

Fig. 404. Strangulation by a Meckel's Diverticulum. A group of coils of small intestine encircled and strangulated by a Meckel's diverticulum, the distal end of which is attached to the mesentery. (*St. Thomas's Hospital Museum*, No. 1282.)

toms of obstruction may be comparatively mild. When the patient is seen early local distension and peristalsis may be detected, and local tenderness just above McBurney's point may be elicited. In a considerable number of instances an abnormal degree of scarring at the umbilicus exists.

Operation. A paramedian subumbilical incision, with outward displacement of the rectus, is the best, since the point of origin of the diverticulum from the ileum is usually within thirty inches of the ileocolic valve.

In carrying out the exploration several points should be kept in mind. (1) The probable seat of origin of the diverticulum. (2) The position of its distal attachment. This is most frequently to the mesentery, somewhat less so to the umbilical cicatrix, and rarely to the intestine. With a mesenteric attachment the strangulated coil may lie deeply; when the attachment is to the intestine the obstruction may be due to kinking. (3) The varieties of arrangement which may be present. Thus, the tube varies in length from 2 to 4 to 8 inches; its calibre may equal that of the ileum itself, or be small or irregular. A mesentery may be present; this may be complete with a thick fibrous margin, representing the original omphalo-mesenteric artery. In other instances the mesenteric fold atrophies and disappears, leaving the fibrous cord unattached to the diverticulum, but retaining its original position; or both mesentery and tube may have disappeared, leaving the vestigial fibrous cord alone. (4) The nature of the obstruction is not in all cases a strangulation; in a minor proportion of instances tension by the diverticulum may produce kinking and valvular obstruction of the bowel, while tension, invagination, prolapse, and secondary stenosis of the intestine have all been observed. (5) In some instances signs of obstruction appear to develop secondarily to an acute inflammation of the diverticulum resembling the corresponding condition of appendicitis.

Examination of the lower end of the ileum and the umbilical region of the anterior abdominal wall is the first step in the exploration; if the search here proves unsatisfactory, a certain degree of evisceration may be necessary to expose the seat of obstruction. When the diverticulum has been localized it is usually necessary to separate one extremity, preferably the distal, in order to free the strangulated bowel. If this attachment be to the umbilicus, the same precautions must be taken as if the bowel required to be opened, since a lumen may exist up to the actual point of termination. When the obstructing agent is formed by the band already alluded to, simple division between clamp forceps suffices.

The distal attachment freed, the engaged bowel is examined, and if in good condition replaced. The coil of intestine from which the diverticulum springs is then drawn out of the belly and clamps are applied, either a proximal and distal one, or, where a long mesentery exists, one long clamp may be applied across the base of the loop. The cavity and margins of the abdominal wound are protected by plugs and the diverticulum removed.

Removal is best effected by the application of Kocher's crushing clamp to the base, as in removing an appendix. The resulting stump is ligatured, and sunk by the introduction of a continuous Lembert's or mattress suture, passed in the transverse axis of the bowel. If the clamp be not to hand, the base, if small, may be crushed with an artery forceps and similarly treated.

When the diverticulum is inflamed and stiffened, the clamp method is inapplicable, and it is preferable to incise the serous and muscular coats and raise them either as a circular cuff or in two flaps. The mucous membrane is then ligatured, and the defect sutured as above described. Should the condition of the mucous membrane, or the width of the base of the diverticulum, preclude the use of the ligature, the opening must be closed by two tiers of sutures passed in the transverse axis of the bowel.

Complications in the performance of the operation may depend either on the condition of the bowel or of the diverticulum itself. Strangulation may have resulted in gangrene of the included loop; in this case an enterectomy will be indicated, unless the general condition of the patient should be such that the performance of a temporary enterostomy alone can be entertained. If the condition has commenced with, or resulted in, inflammation of the diverticulum itself, the latter may readily tear and give exit to highly infective material, or a condition of gangrenous cellulitis may have extended to the ileum. The latter condition may demand an extensive resection such as is occasionally required in cases of gangrenous hernia.

Prognosis and results. The prognosis depends upon the date at which the operation is undertaken, and upon the nature of the obstruction. The chief cause of mortality is peritoneal infection, which in cases of strangulation or inflammatory conditions may have already developed on the second or third day. The local complications already alluded to also obviously depend on the flux of time, and operation is not to be held responsible for deaths from such causes. Of twenty-two operations performed at St. Thomas's Hospital between 1887 and 1908, eight were successful, a mortality of 63.6% occurring, which is 1% higher than that observed in all the cases of obstruction, excluding malignant cases and external hernia. In Hilgenreiner's (*Beit. z. klin. Chir.,* 1902, vol. xxxiii, p. 177; also vol. xl, p. 69) 102 collected cases the mortality amounted to 71.5%.

Strangulation by the Fallopian tube, or by a long pedicle of an ovarian cyst, has been occasionally observed. The portion of intestine included may be small gut, as in Fagge's cases, or the sigmoid flexure. In the latter instance isolated distension of the loop may give rise to a diagnosis of sigmoid volvulus. In such a case of the author's the cyst, having risen into the abdomen from the left ovary, crossed the base of the sigmoid flexure from right to left, and descended into the pelvis, where it became impacted. The first step consisted in enterotomy for evacuation of the contents of the sigmoid, followed by puncture of the cyst; the latter was readily lifted from the pelvis, the intestine freed, and the emptied cyst was then removed.

Intestinal obstruction due to the presence of ovarian tumours is much more commonly the result of intestinal adhesion to cysts which have become inflamed or of which the pedicle has undergone torsion.

OBSTRUCTION DUE TO STRANGULATION IN ABNORMAL OPENINGS IN THE MESENTERY, OMENTUM, AND BROAD LIGAMENTS

Indications. These forms of obstruction are rare, and the indications for operative treatment are usually signs of an acute nature calling for abdominal exploration.

Operation. *Apertures in the mesentery* are discovered by abdominal exploration, and the treatment consists in delivering the bowel and closing the adventitious opening. Should the constricting margin require incision, the latter should be radial in the course of the main vessels. Experience has shown that the constriction in these cases is usually not very severe in character. Thus, in Stabb's case (*St. Thomas's Hospital Reports,* 1891, vol. xxi, p. 174) two separate loops of intestine, one 5 inches long, and a second 10 inches long, situated 30 and 64 inches from the ileo-colic valve respectively, were readily withdrawn from the circular opening in the mesentery. The strangulated bowel and corresponding mesentery were only slightly nipped, in spite of the fact that the symptoms had been very acute. In Howard Marsh's case (*Brit. Med. Journ.,* 1888, vol. i, p. 1157) again, the intestine was released after stretching the yielding margin of the ring with the finger-nail.

Apertures in the omentum, either traumatic or developed in connexion with disease of the omentum, may give rise to strangulation, but their treatment calls for no special attention.

Apertures in the broad ligament are rare sites of strangulation. In the cases described, a similar slight degree of constriction to that observed with mesenteric apertures has been noted.

Prognosis and results. During the twenty years ending with 1907 5 cases of strangulation in mesenteric apertures, 4 in the classic situation near the ileo-colic junction, and 1 secondary to tuberculous disease in the transverse mesocolon, were admitted into St. Thomas's Hospital. Of these 1 died before operation could be undertaken; the other 4 succumbed after operation, 1 needing resection of gangrenous gut. Prutz (' Die angebornen Lücken und Spalten des Mesenteriums,' *Deutsche Zeitsch. f. Chir.,* 1907, vol. lxxxvi, p. 399) has collected 18 cases treated by operation, of which 13 died (72.2%). Of 6 cases of strangulation in broad-ligament gaps collected by Wilms (*loc. cit.*, p. 362) 1 only recovered.

HERNIA INTO THE RETROPERITONEAL POUCHES

From an operative point of view these herniæ may be divided into two series, an upper and a lower. The first group includes hernia through the foramen of Winslow and the various fossæ in the region of the duodenum and root of the mesentery; the second group, those into the fossæ around the cæcum, the intersigmoid, and the rare hernia into Douglas's pouch.

Upper series. These herniæ possess some special features in common: they are commonly large; they belong to the category in which recurring temporary attacks of obstruction are not rare; they give rise to somewhat characteristic localized distensions of the abdomen in the upper and central areas, and they are to be explored when diagnosed or suspected by an incision giving access to the epigastric and umbilical regions.

The indications for operation are those of acute obstruction of the small intestine, although in the herniæ into the foramen of Winslow the colon may be affected.

Herniæ into the lesser sac of the peritoneum. The most common form is that in which the neck of the sac is formed by the foramen of Winslow. The contents consist most frequently of coils of small intestine, but both small and large intestine have been included, also large intestine alone. The contents of the hernia may be confined to the normal limits of the sac, or they may extend into unobliterated portions of the spaces between the layers of the gastro-hepatic or gastro-colic omenta, or even secondarily penetrate one of these layers from within to re-enter the main peritoneal cavity.

Operation. In the exploration of a hernia through the foramen of Winslow, if the nature of the case be suspected, a paramedian supra-umbilical incision through the right rectus sheath with displacement of the muscle upwards will be the most suitable.

The points which will need consideration during the prosecution of the operation are the following:—

1. The neck of the hernia is first to be explored; this is at the right extremity of the sac, and the distension present will mainly affect the part of the intestine contained within the sac. It may be found that the contained intestine can be withdrawn without much difficulty; in this case the obstruction may have depended on twisting of some of the coils within the sac, or it may be found to depend on a second constriction at

a point in the walls of the omental sac where the contents have made a secondary exit.

2. When the large intestine is included, it has been pointed out by Moynihan that this depends on abnormal mobility of the cæcum, and possibly of the ascending colon due to the presence of a ' common mesentery.' Under these circumstances it may be well to attempt to try and limit this mobility by fixing the cæcum into its proper position by the introduction of sutures between its base and the abdominal wall, or by pleating its mesentery, since an effectual closure of the peritoneal clad ring cannot be made.

3. When difficulty arises in the extraction of the contained bowel, the first step should be the evacuation by enterotomy of its contents, since the strangulated intestine can be readily reached by tearing through the thin omental wall in a convenient position. This will much facilitate subsequent procedures. In Delkeskamp's case the evacuation was effected by merely pressing the contents of the incarcerated cæcum and ascending colon onwards through the hepatic flexure, when the bowel was readily drawn out of the foramen.

The extraction of the bowel has, however, proved impossible, as in the classical case of Treves, where even after death the bowel could not be drawn out until the portal vein, hepatic artery, and the bile duct had been divided. It has been suggested by Moynihan and Wilms (*loc. cit.,* p. 384) that the constricting neck may be enlarged by division of the peritoneum as it passes from the duodenum to the posterior abdominal wall, the incision being carried up to the lower margin of the foramen. This mobilizes the duodenum, and allows of its displacement downwards with some enlargement of the ring.

4. Other forms of hernia into the omental sac need no special measures, the constricting ring formed by the omentum being thin and easily stretched or divided without danger of injury to any important structures.

Hernia of the duodeno-jejunal, parajejunal, and retromesenteric varieties. The most important forms are those which have been conveniently classed by Moynihan under the names of right and left duodenal hernia. For these, a sufficient number of observations have been collected by Moynihan to allow of some definite lines being laid down for operative treatment; the rarer varieties need to be dealt with as the conditions discovered at the moment may suggest.

Left duodenal hernia (hernia into the duodeno-jejunal fossa). A correct diagnosis of the nature of the obstruction in strangulations in the duodeno-jejunal fossa is sometimes possible if the indications first laid down by Leichtenstern be borne in mind. Thus, the presence of a globular swelling in the mesogastrium; hollowness in the colic area; in thin patients, the detection on palpation of a circumscribed elastic tense globular tumour resembling a large slightly movable cyst extending from the mesogastrium to the left; a sonorous percussion note over the tumour; and possibly the presence of hæmorrhoids, and the passage of blood *per anum;* the last symptoms resulting from obstruction and pressure at the neck of the hernia on the inferior mesenteric vein.

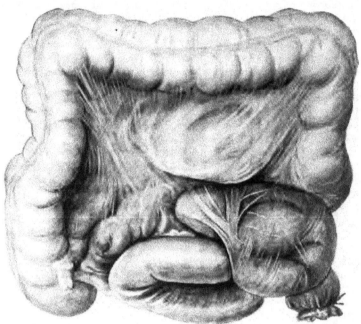

Fig. 405. Small Left Duodenal Hernia. The highest coils of the jejunum are in the sac. The vessels are seen in the neck of the latter. Shattock's case. (*St. Thomas's Hospital Museum*, No. 1279.)

If the hernia be suspected to be into one of the duodenal pouches a paramedian incision is that most likely to be convenient, and as left duodenal hernia is the most common variety, the incision should be as a rule made through the left rectus sheath.

The size of such herniæ varies enormously; the contents may consist in a single short coil of intestine, or nearly the whole small intestine may be included. As a rule the cases subjected to operation have been of the larger class, and these are perhaps prognostically the relatively favourable, since in small herniæ the strangulation is apt to be the more acute (see Fig. 405). In the large herniæ the appearance on exploring the abdomen is very striking, since nearly the whole small intestine may be hidden from view. In extreme cases the peritoneum of the mesenteries of the descending and transverse portions of the colon may have been so drawn upon in the development of the sac, that these portions of the large bowel are as it were spread out upon its surface.

In left duodenal hernia the neck lies to the right of the sac, and is situated to the left of the third lumbar vertebra. If the hernia be small the opening retains the normal direction of the mouth of the fossa, looking forwards and to the right. As the hernia increases in size the opening tends to rotate backwards, looking first directly to the right, then directly backwards. In this case it will be necessary for exposure of the neck to drag the sac over towards the left.

The size of the opening does not always correspond with that of the hernia, and may in fact vary inversely, being large with a small sac. The neck is bounded anteriorly by the fold containing the inferior mesenteric vein, and possibly the left colic artery; the posterior boundary is formed by the posterior parietal peritoneum.

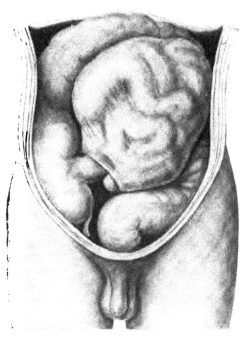

FIG. 406. LARGE DUODENAL HERNIA. Escape of a single limb of the bowel. (*Aschoff.*)

Certain peculiarities of this hernia are to be borne in mind: (1) as a result of the mode of the formation of the neck, the duodeno-jejunal junction may be enclosed within the sac, so that the emerging intestine only is seen (see Fig. 406); (2) the upper portion of the contents may have escaped, leaving perhaps only ileum in the sac, in which event both the entering and emerging limbs will be seen; (3) in large herniæ one or more individual coils may escape from the sac, and again enter the peritoneal cavity. The strangulation may then involve one of such coils and not the main contents of the sac.

In many cases reduction is easy; if this be not the case, the neck of the sac must be cautiously divided at its lower margin, care being exercised to avoid injury to the inferior mesenteric vein or left colic artery. When difficulty is met with, the parietal peritoneum and the anterior wall of the sac itself should be incised, and the intestine drawn forward and emptied. Removal of the sac is usually impracticable, but an attempt to close the neck by suture should be made. Bearing in mind the mode of development of these herniæ, any possibility of re-formation would probably be prevented by a limited fixation of the jejunum to the wall of the abdomen, to the left of the inferior mesenteric vein. Sherren (*Clin. Soc. Trans.,* 1906, vol. xxxix, p. 99) reports a successful case of operation. The vessels occupied the upper and left border of the neck for a short distance only. He divided the neck downwards, removed as much as possible of the peritoneal reduplication, and sutured the edges with catgut.

Right duodenal hernia. In general characteristics this hernia closely resembles the last, except in the fact that the body of the sac and its neck occupy the right half of the abdominal cavity, the sac only spreading to the left when it assumes large proportions. The right variety has not been so often observed; thus Moynihan was only able to collect 17 cases, against 57 of left duodenal hernia.

Operations for the relief of strangulation are to be conducted on the same lines as in left duodenal hernia, but it must be remembered that the sac itself often occupies a lower position in the abdomen, that the neck is at the left end of the sac, but situated to the right of the vertebral column, and that the superior mesenteric artery takes the place of the inferior mesenteric vein in the anterior boundary of the neck. The wandering of the neck of these herniæ appears to be responsible for some of the rare varieties of retromesenteric hernia which have been observed.

Lower series. The herniæ of this series, when strangulated, are commonly to be diagnosed only by abdominal exploration, the indications for operation being symptoms of acute obstruction of unknown cause. The most convenient site for the exploratory incision is subumbilical through the right rectus sheath, since an opening in this position gives access to all the varieties.

The cæcal region is first to be explored, as the very large majority of the herniæ are to be found here (see Fig. 407). Intersigmoid hernia has only been certainly observed on two occasions (Eve, McAdam Eccles), and the hernia through a diaphragm occupying the entry to Douglas's pouch once (Saniter).

Release of the strangulated portion of bowel is usually easy, and the neck of the sac should be obliterated by suture, if practicable. In herniæ into the ileo-appendicular fossa (the hollow between the ileo-appendicular fold and the mesentery of the vermiform appendix), removal of the appendix serves to completely remove the fossa (Moynihan).

Prognosis and results. Operations in these forms of obstruction are rare. Moynihan mentions five operations for herniæ through the foramen of Winslow with two recoveries. In one fatal (Treves), and in one successful case (Neve), reduction proved impossible. Eight cases of herniæ in the fossa in the neighbourhood of the cæcum with four recoveries, and one successful operation on an intersigmoid hernia (McAdam Eccles), are also recorded by him.

A wealth of information on the subject of these herniæ is contained in Moynihan's work (*On Retroperitoneal Herniæ*, Second Edition, 1906) on the subject, to which the writer has been mainly indebted in the compilation of this short section.

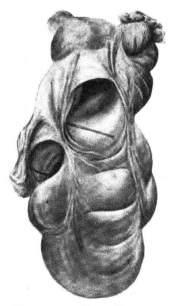

FIG. 407. TWO RETROCÆCAL POUCHES ASCENDING BEHIND THE COLON. The vermiform appendix lies in the lower pouch. (*St. Thomas's Hospital Museum*, No. 1281.)

STRICTURES OF THE INTESTINES

Strictures of the intestine may be congenital or acquired, and are met with in all parts of the intestinal canal.

Congenital stenoses. Of 89 cases collated by Schlegel (Wilms, *loc. cit.*, p. 140), 29 or 32.5% were duodenal, 54 or 60.6% jejuno-ileal, and 6 or 6.6% colic.

Duodenal stenoses are more common above the level of the papilla of Vater; the signs then resemble those of pyloric obstruction; when the stricture is situated below the papilla the vomit contains bile and pancreatic ferments.

Strictures of the jejunum and ileum may be situated in any part and are sometimes multiple. Ileal strictures may be associated with a persistent Meckel's diverticulum. In the large intestine the ascending colon and the sigmoid flexure are the most common seats.

The condition to be dealt with varies. In the small intestine there may be a complete absence of continuity, the proximal and distal segments may be connected by a fibrous cord, the connecting cord may possess a minute lumen, or the gut may be completely occluded by annular constrictions. In the colon either a thin septum or a complete interruption of continuity is the more common form.

Operation. The possibility of an enterectomy seldom exists, not only on account of the tender age and general condition of the infants, but also on account of the disparity in size between the upper and lower segments of the bowel.

For the high duodenal stenoses a gastro-enterostomy is indicated. In the low duodenal stenoses the dilated duodenum may be connected with the jejunum, the latter being brought through the transverse mesocolon. Murphy advises that the jejunum be divided for this purpose, the free end closed, and a lateral anastomosis made.

For most strictures in a lower position an enterostomy is the only immediate resource, the opening being utilized for purposes of nourishment pending the later establishment of an anastomosis.

Results. The recorded results have not been of an encouraging nature; thus of 25 infants on whom operations have been performed (19 enterostomies, 4 anastomoses) not one recovered (Braun, *Beitr. z. klin. Chir.*, 1902, vol. xxxiv, p. 993).

Acquired stenoses. These may be the consequence of injury, and are then commonly complicated by the coexistence of adhesions. Circular stenoses may develop at the site of a hernial constriction of the gut, at the neck of an intussusception which has sloughed away, or follow an axial enterectomy. In other instances the stricture may follow disease of the wall of the bowel; thus, the cicatrization of stercoral ulcers, the ulceration of enteric fever or dysentery, or tuberculous or gummatous infiltration. Strictures resulting from tuberculous or enteric ulceration are usually situated in the ileum.

Operation. The ideal treatment in cases of stricture consists in some form of enteroplasty, but this is only applicable to cases in which at least a half of the natural lumen persists, and in the localized annular forms.

The simplest and most satisfactory procedure consists in making an incision in the long axis of the bowel at the antemesenteric margin, 1 to 1½ inches in length.

A single mattress suture is passed through the bowel-wall in such a manner as to include the two ends of the incision. Traction on this stitch allows the two angles to be approximated at a point which corresponds with the centre of the subsequent transverse line of suture. The coaptation stitch may be tied loosely with a surgical knot, and the transverse suture is commenced from above downwards. The latter should be continuous, and carried through all the coats of the intestine; when complete the coaptation stitch may be removed, and the whole line of suture sunk by the introduction of a second tier of continuous Lembert's stitches (see Fig. 408).

Conditions such as the presence of external adhesions, neighbouring diseased tissue, the implication of a considerable length of the bowel-wall, or the presence of multiple stenoses, frequently contra-indicate a simple enteroplasty. Under these circumstances, resort must be had either to lateral anastomosis or enterectomy. When the stricture is single, an enterectomy is preferable; when the stenoses are multiple, the obstruction is best relieved by the establishment of a lateral anastomosis. In such cases as those due to tuberculous disease, more than one anastomosis may be required (see p. 765).

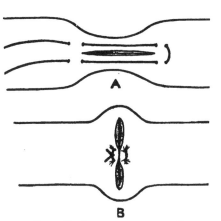

FIG. 408. INTRODUCTION OF A COAPTATION MATTRESS STITCH IN SIMPLE ENTEROPLASTY.

Enterostomy comes under consideration as a temporary measure only in those instances in which the general state of the patient is bad, or the local condition of the intestine forbids for the moment any more satisfactory procedure.

Prognosis and results. The prognosis in cases subjected to either enteroplasty, enterectomy, or anastomosis should be good, but many patients come into the hands of the surgeon having already developed serious complications. This is well illustrated by the series of 9 cases included in the St. Thomas's table, of which only 1 recovered. Five were strictures of the small intestine, of which all died. In 3 of the fatal cases the operation was indicated by peritoneal infection resulting from spontaneous perforation. The remaining 4 cases were situated, 1 in the ascending colon, 2 in the sigmoid colon, and the fourth in the upper part of the rectum. Sargent has collected (*Ann. of Surg.*, 1904, vol. xxxix, p. 733) 18 cases of cicatricial stricture consequent on strangulation of the intestine in hernial sacs. On 11 of these operations were performed, 4 dying, a mortality of 36.3%. Three enterectomies recovered, also an enterostomy followed by anastomoses. Two enteroplasties were successful, and one of two lateral anastomoses. Three enterostomies were followed by death.

The bad prognosis experienced in the treatment of stenoses depends on the fact that premonitory symptoms of chronic obstruction have been overlooked or remained untreated, since the surgical treatment of a cicatricial stricture is in itself unattended by serious difficulty or danger.

OBSTRUCTION BY BILIARY OR INTESTINAL CALCULI

Intestinal calculi are rare; they occur twice as frequently in men as in women.

Obstruction by biliary calculi is more common, the stone passing either by the duct, or by ulceration from the duct into the duodenum, transverse colon, or, rarely, the stomach. Those that pass into the colon seldom give trouble, but several cases of sigmoid obstruction are on record, and occasionally stones may be retained near the anus for some time. Large stones entering the duodenum more often give rise to intestinal obstruction.

Indications. The occurrence of obstruction is sometimes preceded by a history of gall-stone colic, but this may be absent. The attack presents peculiar features due to the fact that the source of obstruction is of a shifting nature. Initial pain is followed by free vomiting, which may entirely evacuate the contents of the alimentary canal above the impacted calculus. This feature, together with the fact that the primary obstruction is high, renders distension of the abdomen uncommon. A remission of the primary symptoms may therefore occur, followed by a recurrence when the progress of the moving stone again ceases. The arrest of the stone may give rise to considerable enterospasm, or even be followed by a moderate degree of intussusception. The symptoms are accompanied by resistance in the lower abdomen, sometimes localized to the right iliac fossa, and the absence of distension occasionally allows the stone to be actually palpated.

Operation. A right paramedian subumbilical incision with outward displacement of the rectus is most suitable. Search for the stone is commenced by examination of the lower ileum, the most common point of arrest. If the termination of the ileum be collapsed, the bowel is rapidly searched in an upward direction. In this particular, however, it should be borne in mind that the stone is readily felt, and the introduction of the hand into the abdomen usually allows of its localization at once, which may save considerable unnecessary manipulation of the bowel.

Certain other possibilities are to be borne in mind with regard to the point of arrest. This may be determined by the presence of local adhesions of the external surface of the bowel, or by the existence of a stenosis. Thus, in a case of tuberculous disease Mayo Robson found a gall-stone above a stenosed portion of the bowel. Again, the stone may be impacted on the proximal side of a hernia, or indeed within the confines of the hernial sac itself.

When the stone has been localized it should be passed backwards from the point at which it has been arrested, to avoid incising the bowel at a damaged spot, and the coil of gut containing it is drawn well out of the abdomen.

A long retaining clamp is applied to the base of the coil, or a small clamp is applied on either side of the stone, and the peritoneal cavity and the wound in the abdominal wall are protected by the insertion of gauze plugs. A longitudinal incision is made in the wall of the bowel at the antemesenteric aspect of sufficient extent to allow the stone to be expressed. The wound in the bowel is closed by two rows of sutures, an inner through and through, and an outer of continuous Lembert's or a series of mattress stitches. If the incision be of moderate length it is best united in the transverse axis of the bowel. The exposed coil is now thoroughly cleansed, the retaining clamp and the gauze plugs are removed, and it is returned into the abdomen.

In some cases it may prove easy to pass the stone upwards into the colon, and if this is the case, and the bowel-wall is in good condition, it is the best plan to adopt.

When the stone has been removed it may exhibit one or more facets, suggesting the existence of a second calculus. Under these circumstances the surgeon should satisfy himself that a second stone is not concerned in the production of obstructive symptoms, but a too exhaustive search in the region of the gall-bladder is undesirable, since by it adhesions between the gall-bladder and the bowel may be disturbed, leading to leakage and consequent peritonitis.

The occurrence of a period of latency in the symptoms is responsible for a certain proportion of these cases coming under the notice of the surgeon at a late date; hence, the intestine in the neighbourhood of the stone may have become gangrenous. An enterectomy is then indicated, or if the condition of the patient forbids this, an enterostomy must be established. This eventuality, in the case of the small intestine, is naturally to be avoided if possible.

Results. The results of operations for the removal of gall-stones are steadily improving, and the mortality of 40% will no doubt be materially reduced as operations are more generally undertaken at an early date.

FÆCAL IMPACTION

The simple retention of fæces may sometimes give rise to complete intestinal obstruction, but it is rare that the condition calls for surgical measures, apart from the cases in which the impaction is due to the obstruction of a narrowed portion of the bowel by a mass of hardened fæces.

The condition is most frequently met with in patients afflicted with general enteroptosis, the subjects of severe chronic constipation, the old, or the feeble-minded.

When the obstruction is complete, is accompanied by vomiting, and has proved resistant to every other means, an abdominal exploration may become necessary. Two methods of treatment then exist. The obstruction may be found to depend on the impaction of separate hardened masses, especially in the sigmoid flexure, which by manipulation may be passed downwards in the colon. If this method fails, a temporary colostomy must be established.

CHAPTER XVI

GENERAL LINES OF TREATMENT OF DIFFUSE
PERITONEAL INFECTION

DIFFUSE peritoneal infection may rarely be of hæmatogenous origin; occasionally it results from the entry of organisms by the Fallopian tube; in other instances the infection results from the migration of organisms through an intestinal wall, the vitality of which is lowered by acute distension usually accompanied by an increase of toxicity of the contents of the bowel; but as affecting surgical treatment its genesis is more common in connexion with a gross perforation of some portion of the gastro-intestinal canal than from any other cause. Certain definite lines should guide the technical treatment of the condition, with minor variations depending upon the stage to which the process has attained, the nature and situation of the occasioning primary lesion, and the variety of the organism concerned.

Indications. It may be broadly laid down that cases of acute diffuse peritoneal infection accompanied by effusion demand prompt surgical intervention, the objects of the aid afforded being the relief of the mechanical tension which favours absorption, and the provision of a free channel of exit for the infective material from the peritoneal cavity.

Need for some discrimination in the application of this indication is obvious, and very great difficulty may arise in arriving at a correct decision if more than thirty-six hours have been allowed to elapse after the occurrence of the initial infection. Exceptions to the rule may be made: (1) When the incidence is accompanied by so severe a degree of shock as to render the increase likely to follow an operation prohibitive of success, especially when the infection is in the region of the gall-bladder or in the lower abdomen. (2) When the condition has been allowed to remain untreated beyond a period of forty-eight hours, and any signs indicating localization are developing.

Operation. For some details as to the preliminary preparation of the patient for these operations, reference may be made to p. 807. The site of the primary incision will in some cases be determined by a previous diagnosis of the seat of the occasioning lesion; if doubt exists as to the nature and situation of the latter, the paramedian subumbilical incision should be chosen for the exploration.

The locality of the primary lesion should, if possible, be first determined. If it be practicable to deal with this in such a manner as to prevent any further supply of infective material, as by the suture of a wound or perforation, or sometimes by the removal of an inflamed organ, as a suppurating Fallopian tube or an infected ovarian cyst, this step should form an integral part of the operation. It is rare for a case of diffuse peritoneal infection to terminate favourably when the surgeon remains in ignorance of the initial origin of the condition; still, the state of the patient may preclude any more extensive procedure than the mere evacuation of the peritoneal effusion and the establishment of drainage, and this defective operation is preferable to the maintenance of a purely expectant attitude, since a recovery occasionally follows.

Methods of dealing with the effusion. The mere act of opening the peritoneal cavity allows the escape of a considerable amount of fluid in some cases, which may be supplemented by the introduction of a syphon tube if desired. Further steps are guided by definite rules, the essential spirit of which is the occasionment of as little disturbance of, and damage to, the peritoneum as possible. In the removal of effusion, all possible delicacy of manipulation is to be observed; the fluid should be literally *absorbed* by the introduction of soft dry sterile gauze strips into cavities made by gentle displacement of the intestine. No *scrubbing* is allowable, since this both favours immediate absorption and increase in toxæmia, and the formation of ulterior adhesions. Care should be at the same time exercised to avoid favouring absorption by the exposed tissues of the wound in the abdominal wall, which should be protected as far as possible by holding forward the margins of the peritoneum and the application of a gauze covering during the intraperitoneal manipulations.

When the infection is quite recent, the fluid consists mainly of reactionary peritoneal effusion, which should be absorbed by sterile swabs with as little disturbance of the contents of the abdomen as possible. If it be due to a perforation of the stomach or duodenum, escaped contents of the viscera require to be removed, and this process may need somewhat widespread examination of the hepato-renal pouch and the under surface of the diaphragm. In such cases reactionary peritoneal effusion has usually gravitated into the pelvis, either over the great omentum, or along the course of the ascending colon, according to the position of the primary lesion. If this be the case it is usually perfectly safe, when the perforation is not of more than twenty-four hours' standing, to neglect the intervening portion of the abdominal cavity and simply remove the fluid which has collected in the pelvis from a second hypogastric incision.

When the infection is of longer standing the difficulties may be greatly increased by the addition of peritoneal adhesions, and the fact that a part of the effusion will be much more highly infective than the remainder. When this is the case, it is preferable, if possible, to first absorb the peripheral less highly infective portion of the effusion and then protect the general peritoneal cavity with plugs before dealing with the area immediately surrounding the primary lesion, which may be to a certain extent localized. The surrounding effusion will otherwise serve as a medium for the wide diffusion of the more highly infective matter. This is especially liable to be the case in infections from the appendix or Fallopian tubes.

As a general rule the less existing adhesions are interfered with the better, since their disturbance favours local absorption and wider diffusion of the infection. Their separation can serve no useful purpose in preventing the formation of permanent adhesions, but rather favours the development of more resistant ones. None the less if it is found that adhesions include localized collections of pus, as may be the case when the condition is only attacked at a late stage, liberation of the confined pus is a matter of necessity if the operation is to be of permanent benefit.

Certain infections are less liable to be accompanied by the formation of adhesions than others; thus they are generally absent in the presence of streptococcus, usual in the presence of bacillus coli communis, common in gonococcal peritonitis, and variable when pneumococcus is the organism. In the last-named infection the condition may vary from a general bathing of the whole abdominal contents in pus without a single adhesion, to the presence of such sharply localized collections of pus in the lower abdomen that the sensation of a localized cyst may be experienced on examination.

Washing with saline solution, or other fluids, should be restricted to portions of intestine which may happen to be without the confines of the abdominal cavity; occasionally it is well to wash out a localized area of the cavity which has been serving as the seat of an operation, the remaining portion being protected with gauze plugs. Under all circumstances general flushing of the peritoneal cavity is to be avoided, as likely to enlarge the area of infection, and to favour the absorption of both bacteria and toxins. The importance of this rule, especially when portions of the cavity are affected from which diffusion is not as a rule free, such as the right hypochondriac region, the right iliac fossa, or the pelvis, is very great. Evisceration for the purpose of cleansing the intestines and the peritoneal cavity is still more strongly to be deprecated, since to the objections already raised to the process of flushing must be added great increase of shock, increase of distension of the exposed coils, and a definite lowering of their vitality.

Peritoneal Drainage. In early peritoneal infections, such as those met with in perforations of less than twenty-four hours' standing, drainage may be dispensed with, provided the initial lesion has been satisfactorily dealt with. Under these circumstances the peritoneum is perfectly capable of dealing with the degree of infection which has already taken place. When actual suppuration has developed drainage is desirable.

The question then arises whether drainage from a single opening or the introduction of several tubes after multiple incisions of the abdominal wall is indicated. Generally speaking, a single drainage aperture at a dependent spot is to be preferred if adhesions are not present.

It is to be remembered that the efficient action of a peritoneal drain is seldom continued beyond a period of twenty-four hours; again, that if adhesions are not already present, the immediate effusion tends to gravitate towards the pelvis if the patient be placed in a suitable position. The passage of any but strictly local effusion by a drainage tube ceases at a period corresponding to that at which gravitation of the general effusion also ceases to continue. Hence the action of a drainage tube, except as a purely local matter, is of short duration and utility.

Any advantage to be gained by the use of multiple incisions is therefore highly doubtful, and they should only be employed when large irregular localized collections are met with. Thus, while the advantage of separate drainage of the two iliac fossæ in appendical infections crossing by the pelvic route, or where the effusion is more or less localized in both loins, cannot be denied, yet, in general infections unaccompanied by the presence of adhesions, a single tube inserted deeply into the pelvis is much to be preferred to multiple incisions with a series of tubes emerging from the flanks and loins.

The most effective drainage is obtained by the use of large-sized rubber tubes, but when it is desired to maintain a free opening for more than twenty-four hours, it is well to supplement the tube by the passage of a gauze plug by its side; or, where two tubes are inserted in different directions from the same opening, by the introduction of a gauze plug between them so as to preserve a temporary potential space. The plugs are of use as acting by capillarity, and still more by maintaining a sufficiently free separation of the margins of the abdominal wound, which tend to rapidly contract around a simple tube. It is to be constantly borne in mind that the presence of a drain involves the formation of surrounding adhesions, hence the large gauze tampons formerly used freely are to be avoided.   The employment of such large plugs, inserted for instance in the pelvic cavity, may lead to the formation of adhesions between as much as a fourth of the whole extent of the small intestine with all its attendant risks and inconveniences.

Enterotomy and enterostomy.   In some cases of peritoneal infection accompanying acute obstruction of the intestines, and in perforative infections of some standing, great distension of the bowel combined with paresis of the wall may be present.   In such cases evacuation of the contents of the bowel may be desirable, either for convenience in manipulation in dealing with the site of the initial lesion or for the replacement of escaped bowel.   For these a temporary enterotomy suffices.   In others a marked degree of paresis of the intestinal wall, together with a highly toxic condition of the intestinal contents, may render it desirable to establish a temporary enterostomy.   For this purpose a Paul's tube may be tied in, or, if it be considered that a mere vent will suffice, the method of Witzel may be employed (see p. 689).

After-treatment.   The patient should be placed in the 'almost sitting position' of Fowler.   To maintain this attitude, which resembles that obtained by the use of the double inclined plane, a pillow is placed beneath the knees and fastened by webbing attached to its two ends to the posts at the head of the bed, and support is afforded to the feet. The position eases the respiration, and favours gravitation of the peritoneal effusion into the less absorbent area afforded by the pelvic peritoneum.   Passage downward of the fluid is also helped by the general peristaltic movements of the small intestine.

Vomiting.   That due to the anæsthetic may be treated by copious draughts of warm water, to which is added a drachm of bicarbonate of sodium.   By this method the after-effects of chloroform absorption are combated, and the stomach is washed out automatically.   Irritability of the stomach may be quieted by the administration of cocaine in quarter to half-grain doses, or by the administration of a couple of drops of tincture of iodine in a wine-glassful of water.   In more severe cases, especially if there be distension, gastric lavage may be resorted to with much benefit.

Feeding.   Should vomiting persist, feeding by the mouth is useless; in any case, nothing but sips of warm water only are to be allowed during the first twelve hours.   Later it is best to commence with albumen water, whey, or milk and soda-water.   To these may be added some of the various patent foods, and meat extracts after the first twenty-four hours.   Thirst in the early stages is best met by infusion of normal saline solution *per rectum.*

Rectal infusion.   Infusions of normal saline may be given at intervals, or the continuous method of Murphy may be employed. If the interrupted method be chosen, a pint of fluid may be given with a funnel and tube every four hours.

When practicable the continuous method is to be preferred. A convenient apparatus is shown in Fig. 409. Murphy objects to a regulating clip on the syphon tube; he says it prevents reflux to the cistern if expulsive efforts are made by the patient, and that escape takes place by the anus and the patient's bed is wetted. The delivery tube is fixed by strapping to the patient's thigh.

The fluid should be kept at a temperature of 100° F., and the flow so regulated as to allow the supply of about one and a half pints in two hours. The flask needs to be elevated only a few inches above the level of the patient's buttocks. By this method some eighteen pints may be introduced in the twenty-four hours, but watch must be kept on the patient's pulse to see that it does not become too full, and care must also be taken that pulmonary œdema is not produced.

The infusion relieves thirst, combats shock, quiets the patient, and by favouring free renal excretion aids in the elimination of toxins and organisms from the general circulation.

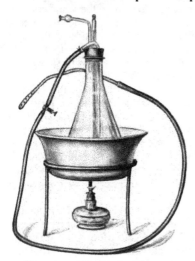

FIG. 409. FLASK PROVIDED WITH THERMOMETER, BLOW TUBE TO START THE SYPHON ACTION, AND DELIVERY TUBE TO RECTUM. It is placed in an iron basin containing water, beneath which a spirit lamp is arranged.

While normal salt was originally used, surgeons for the most part now use ordinary tap water heated to body temperature. Where there is much depletion and acidosis is threatened, 5% glucose solution or sodium bicarbonate may be added to reduce the acidity. In urgent cases where enteroclysis is not available or where fluid in addition to this seems inadvisable even as a primary measure in severe cases of dehydration from vomiting or other causes, Kanavel has advised the administration of normal salt or alkaline solution by continuous hypodermoclysis. This is advocated since the administration of normal salt at stated intervals calling for the reinsertion of the hypodermoclysis needles distresses the patient and entails much work on the part of the surgeon. He states that the following technique has been satisfactory.

The ordinary hypodermoclysis set is used with the exception that the needles are much finer than are those commonly attached and provision made so that the solution can be shut off from either needle. The needle chosen is four inches in length, No. 20. The assistants are impressed with the fact that no pain must be given the patient either during the insertion of the needles or the administration of the solution.· To obviate this the skin is blistered with a few drops of novocaine (½ per cent solution) using the finest hypodermic needle, then a few drops of the same solution is forced along the course we expect the needle to follow in the deeper tissue. The point of a fine, sharp hypodermoclysis needle is then placed against the skin and gently rotated with firm pressure. This carries the needle in absolutely without pain. After being in place, the head is wrapped in gauze so that the flange does not touch the skin and cause pressure and the needle is fixed in position with adhesive plaster. The solution is kept warm by frequently refilling the can or using a sterile hot water bottle in the can. The solution is allowed to drop in slowly, never distending the tissue to the point of pain. Whenever the patient says there is a sense of fullness, the rubber tube on that side is shut off.

In this manner continuous normal salt solution has been given for three or four days with no discomfiture or ill consequences to the patient. It has been used in children without the slightest complaint on their part. Its use has become a routine in all cases of persistent vomiting and toxæmia as peritonitis, ileus, pernicious vomiting of pregnancy, toxic nephritis, septicæmia, etc. In debilitated patients the needles have been inserted and hypodermoclysis begun at the beginning of an operation and the patient has been returned to bed with the needles in place and the administration continued indefinitely. It is used supplementary to rectal administration of tap water and in those cases where, owing to the nature of the operation, e.g. intestinal resection, this could not be used. By this method a seven-year-old child suffering from paralytic ileus was given 40,000 c.c. over a period of three days. In another case much dehydrated from persistent vomiting 13,000 c.c. were given in forty-four hours (Kanavel, Surg. Gyne. Obst., Oct., 1916, p. 483).

In cases where the heart is growing weak there has been at times a tendency to water-logging of the tissue. Therefore such cases are watched carefully so that, on the one hand, this will not occur and, on the other, we shall not overload the circulation and strain the heart.

To combat acute dilatation of the stomach and persistent vomiting of any type continual stomach lavage combined with the above has proved of great benefit. He describes his technique as follows:

For surgical purposes a stomach tube modified from the Einhorn and Rehfuss types has been devised. This modification is necessary since we wish a tube that can be inserted in the stomach and left in position days if necessary; moreover, the tube should be one that can be introduced without the active co-operation of the patient, since it should be available even though the patient be nauseated and vomiting continually or be still anæsthetized (see Fig. 410).

The tube and its carrier are constructed as follows: The bulb is of the same size as the Rehfuss bulb except that the lumen of exit is larger and it is so constructed that it is impossible for the wire carrier to slip out. The rubber tubing is of the same size as the Rehfuss tube but only

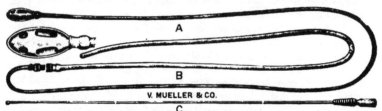

FIG. 410. STOMACH LAVAGE TUBE, BULB, AND WIRE CARRIER. (*Kanavel.*)

30 inches long, being attached to a second heavier tube 25 inches long by a screw lock. A carrier of piano wire is made to fit the first tube so that it can be introduced without difficulty. The second tube is attached after the removal of the carrier and the contents of the stomach aspirated or siphoned off.

If the patient will swallow the tube, the lumen of exit of the bulb being larger than the Rehfuss tube, the stomach contents can be aspirated with greater freedom and the mucus interferes less. This latter is of considerable importance in post-operative lavage when the mucus is generally considerable and interferes even with this tube at times. It will be seen that the bulb is so constructed that the point of the wire carrier cannot slip out of the bulb and injure the stomach. Owing to the shortening of the rubber tubing, there is less probability of the collapse of the tube upon suction and there is less difficulty in removing the carrier. This latter procedure is also aided by having the patient throw his head back, thus lessening the sharp angle in the tube.

The tube described has proved of signal benefit in the vomiting of peritonitis or persistent vomiting from any cause as well as being of great aid in the routine examination of stomach contents for diagnosis. In the former instance the tube is either introduced by the surgeon, or is swallowed by the patient. It is then attached to the chin by a piece of adhesive plaster and may be left in for days. In the regurgitation incident to peritonitis, the stomach contents are aspirated every half-hour to an hour and at regular intervals the stomach is washed out by injecting soda solution, or other liquid, through the tube and aspirating it. Between the washings the end of the rubber tube attached is placed in a basin with the end covered by fluid so that a continuous siphonage takes place. The retention of the tube is without discomfort, while the absence of stomach distention and vomiting gives the greatest relief to those distressed patients.

Fluid may be left in the stomach or medication given if desired.

Sleep. Insomnia is mainly due to toxæmia, and the use of saline infusion, and sometimes of sera or vaccines, may be of help. Morphia, as hindering free excretion and favouring the occurrence of intestinal distension, is to be avoided. The introduction of fifteen grains of aspirin into the rectal infusion is often useful, and if hypnotics are used, either veronal or sulphonal is perhaps the least objectionable.

Distension. Intestinal distension in late cases is often beyond the limits of treatment. When not due to complete atony, gastric lavage and the alternation of an occasional enema containing from half to one ounce of turpentine may help. Again, the passage of a rectal tube often allows the escape of flatus in considerable quantity. Hypodermic injections of eserin salycilate, gr. 1/100, often favour intestinal peristalsis, as do also small repeated doses of calomel, $\frac{1}{2}$ or 1 grain, which at the same time help intestinal asepsis. In bad cases large doses (up to one ounce) of sulphate of magnesia are useful.

Sera and vaccines. The acute nature of the disease restricts the early employment of sera to stock preparations. Polyvalent sera of bacillus coli communis, streptococcus pyogenes, or pneumococcus may be useful. The first injection should be made before the patient leaves the operation table. The routine inoculation of a culture tube in all cases renders it practicable to prepare a special vaccine which may be substituted for the serum later if desired.

Dressings should be frequent if discharge is free, and the surface of the abdomen should be carefully cleansed on each occasion. Drainage tubes must be retained as long as any discharge persists; they should be shortened rather than diminished in calibre prior to removal, when they have been retained for more than a couple of days. A small gauze plug may be substituted when the tube is finally removed.

Results. Those obtained by the surgical treatment of diffuse peritoneal infection due to perforations have been already referred to under the special sections devoted to that subject (pp. 669, 673, 678, 682, 803). A general numerical computation from statistical records can hardly serve any practical purpose, since authors differ so widely in their views as to what is to be designated ' diffuse ' infection.

The prognosis in any given case depends upon the nature of the infection, upon its duration, upon the extent of peritoneal surface involved, and upon the locality infected. Thus streptococcic and bacillus pyocyanic infections prove almost uniformly fatal, the rare staphylococcic are somewhat less serious, while infections by bacillus coli communis and the gonococcus are comparatively favourable. Pneumococcus infections may be rapidly fatal, or in other cases tend to localize themselves securely and lead to moderate sized abscesses. A large proportion of all peritoneal infections are of a mixed character. The treatment of acute infections of more than thirty-six hours' duration is unpromising, and when more than one-third of the peritoneal cavity is involved the prognosis is very unfavourable. Infections of the central area of the abdomen occupied by the small intestine are especially dangerous on account of the rapidity with which diffusion is effected by the peristaltic movements of the bowel, while in such comparatively quiet situations as the right hypochondrium and the right iliac fossa diffusion takes place more slowly, and localization develops more readily. Systemic absorption is much more rapid and abundant from the upper abdomen than from the pelvis.

CPSIA information can be obtained
at www.ICGtesting.com
Printed in the USA
BVHW08*1159170918
527708BV00009B/216/P